THOS. FLINT, Jr., M.D.

Formerly Senior Consultant, Emergency Department, and
Director, Division of Industrial Relations,
Permanente Medical Group and Kaiser Foundation Hospitals,
Oakland, Richmond and Vallejo, California

HARVEY D. CAIN, M.D.

Chief of Industrial Medicine and Rehabilitation,
Permanente Medical Group and Kaiser Foundation Hospital,
Sacramento, California

EMERGENCY TREATMENT AND MANAGEMENT

Fifth Edition

W. B. SAUNDERS COMPANY
Philadelphia • London • Toronto

W. B. Saunders Company: West Washington Square
Philadelphia, PA 19105

1 St. Anne's Road
Eastbourne, East Sussex BN21 3UN, England

1 Goldthorne Avenue
Toronto, Ontario M8Z 5T9, Canada

Library of Congress Cataloging in Publication Data

Flint, Thomas, 1903–

Emergency treatment and management.

Includes index.
1. Medical emergencies.   2. Medicine — Practice.
    I. Cain, Harvey D., 1930–   joint author.
    II. Title.
    [DNLM: 1. Emergencies.   WB100 F625e]

RC87.F62 1975   616'.025   74–9433

ISBN 0–7216–3728–0

Listed here is the latest translated edition of this book together with the language of the translation and the publisher:

Greek *(3rd Edition)* — Asklepios, Athens, Greece

Spanish *(3rd Edition)* — Editorial Jims, Barcelona, Spain

Italian *(4th Edition)* — Piccin Editore, Padova, Italy

Emergency Treatment and Management   ISBN   0-7216-3728-0

Last digit is the print number: 9   8   7   6   5   4

PREFACE
TO THE FIFTH EDITION

The field of emergency care, as previously predicted, is not only growing but its structure and the accreditation requirements are becoming formalized. The American College of Emergency Physicians should soon become a recognized medical specialty board of the American Medical Association. Increasingly, emergency departments are adding to their full-time staffs physicians who have had special training in the field. The same is true for registered nurses and paramedical personnel, technicians, firemen, policemen, and ambulance drivers.

Communities, recognizing the need for prompt and effective on-the-scene initiated treatment, are cooperating to coordinate the efforts of well-trained paramedical personnel in fully equipped units with hospital radio-transmitted assistance. The sparsely equipped hearse-ambulance is becoming an anachronism.

Another type of major community effort, indicative of recognition and concern for rapid communication in all types of emergencies, is the rapidly spreading use of the 911 Emergency Telephone System. Once a caller has placed a 911 call, the specially trained public safety operator will usually transfer the call to the proper agency or refer the caller to the number of that agency. Within the next 10 years this system, or some modification of it, will probably be in effect throughout the civilized world.

In the first edition of this book (1954), "Emergency Care" was defined as the examination, treatment and disposition of a person who has developed or sustained an unforeseen medical condition which is believed to call for prompt action—a definition which still is adequate. Continuing as a complex medical and legal problem is the delineation of the point at which the emergency care of a person who appears to have sustained brain death but who has cardiac activity should cease and the person be pronounced legally dead. California and several other states have passed legislation in this area. The California law reads, "A person shall be pronounced dead if it is determined by the physician that the person has suffered a total and irreversible cessation of brain function." There must be a confirmation by an independent consultant and neither of the physicians who makes a determination of brain death should participate in organ removal or organ transplantation. Electroencephalograms can be used to help make a determination of death.

As in each of the other editions we again stress that the clinical interpretations and therapy recommended do not necessarily represent the only proper method, but do represent an approach which in many instances will decrease disability and suffering and preserve life. The authors have assiduously endeavored to present safe therapeutic adult medication doses; however, pharmaceutical dosage recommendations change and the reader is advised to follow the recommendations of current pharmaceutical texts or of the manufacturers.

Illness caused by medicines, particularly by combinations of medications, is increasingly being recognized as a major health problem. These adverse reactions may involve diverse organ systems, although the skin, gastrointestinal tract, and hematopoietic systems are among the more commonly affected areas. A significant number of emergency department visits and hospital admissions stem from drug reactions. Many patients self-prescribe with across-the-counter medications in addition to taking their physician-prescribed medications. Other patients will obtain prescriptions from two or more physicians.

Relief of pain, relaxation of skeletal or smooth muscle spasm (spasm causing problems of ischemia, venous congestion, impairment of microcirculation, edema, and more pain), and relief of apprehension—all with variable degrees of effect on diverse organ function—are frequent emergency problems. Unfortunately, the precise physiologic mechanisms of pain and the exact actions of the autonomic nervous system are among the largest and oldest bastions of medical ignorance. Medication approach to therapy of these problems is sometimes not effective, for several reasons: (1) unavailability, (2) contraindications to use, and (3) therapeutic failure. Under these circumstances, various forms of reflex therapy may be used as an adjunctive measure for relief. Embryologically, the entire central, peripheral, and autonomic nervous systems are derived from ectoderm, and critical functional relationships with the skin persist throughout life. Skin stimulation and the spinal reflex suggest the existence of a dermatomyosplanchnic response, which may result in relief of pain and muscle spasm.

Modifications have been made to further simplify and expedite cross references to similar or related conditions.

We wish to express again our appreciation to Bernard Horn, M.D., Permanente Medical Group at the Kaiser Foundation Hospital, Vallejo, California, and to Alfredo Burlando, M.D., and Alan Frankel, M.D., Permanente Medical Group, Kaiser Foundation Hospital, Sacramento, California, for constructive criticism and suggestions concerning the text. We are indebted to Joyce Sparks for her meticulous typing of the manuscript, and to our wives for their efforts and tolerance.

Vallejo, California   Thos. Flint, Jr., M.D.
Sacramento, California   Harvey D. Cain, M.D.

PREFACE
TO THE FIRST EDITION

Many excellent texts are available covering first aid procedures and surgical and medical care in acute conditions. The following pages, however, have a much more limited objective – the presentation of the treatment and management of the patient by the Emergency Physician from first examination until disposition for definitive treatment can be arranged. To borrow a phrase from current labor relations, I have endeavored to outline *in a rapidly available form* "portal-to-portal" care in emergency situations.

The term "Emergency Physician" has been used throughout this book to designate the physician in charge of the patient in the emergency room, department, or private office. In large hospitals this physician may be on a full-time basis; in smaller units he may have numerous other duties, or be on part-time emergency call. Too often he is an intern, resident, or general practitioner of very limited experience in the management and treatment of acute conditions. To all these physicians whose contribution to the welfare of the patient is often overshadowed by a spectacular surgical procedure or a brilliant medical diagnosis, I am dedicating this book, with the hope that the information herein contained may be of some assistance to them in fulfilling their very great, and often unrecognized, responsibilities.

"Emergency Care" is used in this book in the sense of the examination, treatment, and disposition of a person who has developed or sustained an unforeseen condition which is believed to call for prompt action. Examination may disclose no urgent or pressing need for treatment, and reassurance of the patient or his family may be all that is necessary. On the other hand, prompt and proper handling of the case may result in saving a life, preventing a long illness, or preserving maximum function.

In the first section are grouped some important generally applicable miscellaneous medical procedures. Administrative medicolegal and clerical principles and procedures which I have found to be of value in the operation of an efficient emergency service are covered in the third section. Since, by the nature of the cases which he is called upon to handle, the physician treating emergencies is especially vulnerable to legal action, the medicolegal aspects have been outlined in considerable detail. The underlying legal principles used as the basis for the medicolegal points involved are widely accepted, although minor variations may occur in some localities.

In order to facilitate rapid reference all conditions covered in the second section are listed alphabetically, and cross references are indicated. Although in some instances the most important diagnostic points have been given, I have made no attempt to cover this aspect fully. The methods of treatment suggested are *not necessarily the only proper therapeutic methods,* but they are based upon several years of experience in the handling of a large volume of emergency cases as well as upon accepted methods of emergency care. The drugs mentioned are those available in any well equipped emergency room or office. The dosages given are for adults unless otherwise specified and should, of course, be modified for infants, children, or elderly persons. Whenever the use of Plazmoid is recommended, dextran, PVP (polyvinylpyrrolidone), serum albumin, or any of the other accepted plasma volume expanders can be substituted. If facilities for typing and cross matching are available the use of whole blood transfusions is even more desirable.

No attempt has been made to specify or suggest therapeutic measures after immediate emergency care with the exception of supportive therapy during ambulance transportation and occasional instructions to be carried out at home before receiving hospital or office treatment.

It will be noted that repetition and duplication occur rather frequently, particularly in the section covering *Poisoning, Acute* [Topic 49]. I believe that *for the purpose of quick reference* this repetition will be found to be of value.

The political and social unrest so prevalent throughout the world suggest the possibility that many physicians not familiar with emergency measures may be called upon to treat large numbers of serious civilian casualties. This possibility - remote though it may be—in my opinion justifies the presentation of this summary at this time.

I should like to express my thanks to Dr. E. M. MacKay for his encouragement, constructive criticism and guidance in the preparation of this book. I am also grateful to Dr. Glenn Lubeck for his suggestions on *Cardiac Emergencies* and to Dr. Arthur Michels for the section on *Shock*. The interpretation and clarification of the medicolegal problems by Mr. James French and Mr. C. H. Brandon have been invaluable. Finally, I wish to thank Miss Bernice Turkovich for her very great assistance in the preparation of the manuscript.

THOS. FLINT, JR.

NOTICE

Every effort has been made to prevent errata in dosage recommendations and to keep the dosages found in this text in agreement with official standards at the time of publication.

However, dosage recommendations do sometimes change; we therefore urge you to check the manufacturer's brochure, particularly before using any drug which you have used only infrequently or have not used for some time.

THOS. FLINT, JR.
HARVEY D. CAIN

CONTENTS

GENERAL MEDICAL PRINCIPLES AND PROCEDURES

CONTENTS

EMERGENCY TREATMENT OF SPECIFIC CONDITIONS

CONTENTS

CONTENTS

GENERAL MEDICAL PRINCIPLES AND PROCEDURES

1. ACHIEVEMENTS IN URGENT THERAPY

During the last few years, improvements in training guidelines and facilities for physicians have resulted in establishment of many residencies and postgraduate continuing medical education training courses in critical care medicine. Computer-assisted instruction is in the process of development.

Reduction of the time interval between injury or the onset of acute illness and institution of adequate emergency care has been accomplished by:

1. Training of ambulance attendants, physicians' assistants, licensed vocational nurses, registered nurses, allied medical personnel, firemen, and law enforcement officers in rapid and proper on-the-spot therapy.

2. Improvement in, and more frequent utilization of, two-way radio voice communication between ambulances, snow patrols, highway patrol units, helicopter rescue units, etc., with an emergency care center.

Improvements in Mechanical Equipment Related to Emergency Care

1. Better ambulances — wider, higher, better equipped (two-way radio) for on-the-spot and in-transit care.

2. Establishment of a universal telephone number for emergencies — phone number 911 now serves 250 communities in the United States — about 10% of the population. Phone numbers 03 in Russia and 999 in Great Britian serve the same purpose.

3. Equipment for near-instant temperature readings.

4. Simplification of equipment for extracorporeal dialysis.

5. Development of improved mechanical equipment for external cardiac compression.

6. Development of practical child-resistant containers for drugs, with limitation of the number of tablets per prescription.

Technical Improvements

1. Refinements in methods of determining central venous pressure (CVP).

2. Development of laboratory equipment for rapid and accurate blood gas determinations.

3. Development of simple kits for rapid identification of toxic substances.

4. Improvements in the equipment for, and technique of micro-surgery, especially for the repair of partially or completely severed nerves and blood vessels.

5. Use of naloxone hydrochloride (Narcan) to neutralize the respiratory and cardiac depressant effects of opiates and certain synthetic narcotics.

6. Development of human nervous tissue vaccine (N.T.V.) to replace duck embryo vaccine (DEV) in the treatment of rabies, with subsequent reduction of the required total number of injections from between 14 and 21 to 2 or 3.

7. Refinement and development of techniques for successful replantation of partially or completely severed limbs, especially feet and fingers. Replantation centers, with appropriate equipment and specially trained personnel, have been established in many localities.

2.   ADDICTION

Two common and unrecognized examples of addiction in everyday life are the use of caffeine-containing drinks and the use of tobacco products. Both fulfill the requirements for true addiction (increased tolerance and withdrawal symptoms), but social condemnation of habitual use of either has never become widespread, although it does occur in certain religious, sociologic and professional groups. The possible results of rigid government control (tried unsuccessfully and eventually repealed for alcohol and now in effect in varying degrees in different localities for narcotics, barbiturates, marihuana and other so-called dangerous drugs) is an interesting topic for surmise. Use of mood modifiers (hallucinogens, sedatives, stimulants, tranquilizers and psychedelics) has introduced problems which currently are requiring medical and sociologic consideration (see **49 – 64.** *Amphetamines;* **49 – 358.** *Hallucinogens*).

Public attention at present is focused mainly upon three categories of addictive agents – alcohol, barbiturates and narcotics.

2 – 1. ALCOHOL

Acute dehydration and malnutrition may make hospitalization for fluid replacement (**6**) necessary. Delirium tremens (**34 – 3**) and alcoholic neuritis (**46 – 8**) as well as degenerative mental changes (**50 – 1**. *Organic Psychoses*) may require institutional care. For the toxic picture and treatment of acute alcoholism, see **49 – 315**. *Ethyl Alcohol.*

2 – 2. BARBITURATES

Chronic addition to barbiturates rarely requires emergency care unless an overdose has been taken, but hospitalization for supportive therapy may be necessary when the drug is stopped. Too rapid withdrawal may result in convulsions, irreversible mental changes and even death.

For signs, symptoms and treatment of acute poisoning, see **49 – 111**. *Barbiturates.*

2 – 3. NARCOTICS

Whenever addition to, or self-administration of, any of the substances covered by the Narcotics Act is known or suspected, certain restrictions (**2 – 5**) apply. Most of the substances covered are included in the following list:

Alpha and beta eucaine (**49 – 324**).
Alphaprodine (Nisentil) (**7 – 2**).
Apomorphine (**49 – 85**).
Cocaine and its salts, preparations, compounds and derivatives (**49 – 218**).
Codeine and its salts, preparations, compounds and derivatives (**49 – 219**).
Dihydrocodeinone (Hycodan) (**49 – 273**).
Hemp and its extracts and compounds (**49 – 441** *Marihuana*).
Heroin (**49 – 366**).
Hydromorphone (Dilaudid) (**49 – 277**).
Laudanum (tincture of opium) (**49 – 413**).
Levorphan (Levodromoran) (**49 – 472**. *Methorphinan hydrobromide*).
Lophorphora (mescal, peyote) (**49 – 460**).
Marihuana (**49 – 441**).
Meperidine (Demerol) (**7 – 2; 49 – 245**).
Methadone (Adanon, Dolophine) (**49 – 464**).
Morphine and its salts, preparations, compounds and derivatives (**49 – 495**).
Opium and its salts, preparations, compounds and derivatives (**49 – 545**).
Pantopon (pantopium hydrochloride) (**49 – 562**).
Paregoric (camphorated tincture of opium) (**49 – 545**. *Opium*).
Racemorphan (Dromoran, methylmorphinan) (**49 – 472**. *Methorphinan hydrobromide*).

2−4. ADDICTION TO OPIATE-TYPE DRUGS

SIGNS AND SYMPTOMS

1. In spite of widespread publicity to the contrary, a habitual user of opium derivatives or opiate-like synthetics who is taking regular doses of a pure preparation at accustomed intervals will rarely show any outward evidence of dependence on the drug. Mental impairment of any type almost never occurs; neither does physical or social degeneration if the addict is financially able to support the very expensive habit without interruption and if degenerative mental or physical processes were not already present when habitual use became established.

2. Scars − old, recently healed, healing and fresh − from subcutaneous, intramuscular or intravenous injections.

3. Pinpoint nonreactive pupils or small pupils which react sluggishly to light. Pupillary signs demonstrable by the usual tests may be completely absent in persons accustomed to large doses. The nalorphine hydrochloride (Nalline) test (**15−3**) is of great diagnostic value in this type of case.

2−5. RESTRICTIONS ON TREATMENT OF NARCOTIC ADDICTION

In many states and countries all over the world, ambulatory treatment of narcotic addiction is unlawful. As a result, in these areas narcotic addicts can be treated only if they are under complete control − usually in government certified institutions. Therefore, only palliative symptomatic care (sedation, hydration, supportive therapy, etc.) can be given while arranging for disposition of the patient with the proper agencies. Ambulatory methadone substitution programs are available in some localities.

Whenever possible, patients should be encouraged to arrange voluntarily for treatment in a controlled environment by physicians especially trained in this very difficult therapy.

The usual exceptions to these restrictions are:

1. An acute condition which in itself is an indication for a narcotic drug.

2. If the patient has been booked and is in custody.

3. If the patient has a chronic, slowly progressing incurable or terminal condition. In this instance the patient must be registered with the proper enforcement agency. The following form is usually

required to be sent by registered mail within 5 days of first treatment:

```
MAIL TO:
                BUREAU OF NARCOTIC ENFORCEMENT

NAME OF PATIENT                                          AGE

ADDRESS
                    STREET                   CITY
QUANTITY AND KIND OF NARCOTIC

DAILY DOSAGE

DIAGNOSIS OF INJURY OR AILMENT


HAS PATIENT PREVIOUSLY USED NARCOTICS?        ADDICTED?
                                    YES OR NO        YES OR NO
PHYSICIAN'S SIGNATURE

ADDRESS
                    STREET                   CITY
DATE OF REPORT                        FED. REG. NO.
```

3.   DEATH CASES

3 – 1.   ABSENCE OF ACCEPTED CRITERIA FOR DETERMINING TIME OF DEATH

Modern methods of resuscitation (**11**) have been spectacularly successful—so much so that the point at which death ends human existence has become difficult to determine. Although respiratory and higher nervous system centers have been destroyed by prolonged anoxia, viability of what has been termed "a human heart-lung preparation" may be continued for lengthy periods by various means, including major organ transplants. It seems probable that at some time in the future some type of civil action—for instance, an important will contest—will result in establishment of generally accepted basic medicolegal criteria for "life," "existence" and "death."

3−2. PRESUMPTIVE SIGNS OF DEATH

No response to painful stimuli.

No pulse or heart beat by palpation or auscultation.

No breath sounds on auscultation; no fogging of a freshly polished mirror held close to the nostrils or mouth.

Complete absence of corneal and deep tendon reflexes.

Absence of evidence of blood pressure by sphygmomanometer.

A flat base line on all electrocardiographic (ECG) leads.

Doughy resistance to passive motion suggestive of developing rigor mortis.

Dependent lividity and cyanosis.

Decreased body temperature in relation to environment.

These presumptive signs are usually considered to be adequate for determination of death when they occur following severe trauma or in the terminal stages of chronic illnesses such as malignancy with metastases or uremia in a patient with whom the attending physician is thoroughly familiar. They are *not* adequate for determination of sudden and unexpected death in catastrophic emergency conditions such as acute poisoning (**49**) or myocardial infarction (**26−12**) or if the attending physician is not familiar with the patient's underlying condition; with the events leading up to and climaxed by the apparent terminal state; or with the interval (in minutes) since onset of presumptive signs of death.

3−3. CONCLUSIVE SIGNS OF DEATH

Complete partition of parts of the body incompatible with life (examples: complete decapitation, separation of the trunk into two or more completely detached parts with no one portion containing adequate vital organs, etc.).

Generalized body putrefaction.

Fully established rigor mortis.

Flat lines without evidence of rhythm in all leads of an electro-encephalographic (EEG) tracing, not modified by loud noises. When there have been no EEG or ECG changes present for one hour, (for exception, see **29−5.** *Electrical Shock*), the attending physician is justified in certifying to the death of the patient and in terminating resuscitative measures, even if agonal cardiac ventricular activity is still demonstrable by electrocardiogram. The time at which cardiac circulatory support was discontinued should be entered on the clinical record and indicated on the death certificate (**65 – 6**) as the official time of death. The clinical record should give an accurate account of findings and therapy and, if possible, should be countersigned by another physician.

3 – 4. DEAD ON ARRIVAL (DOA) CASES

These should be registered in the usual manner (**66**), using *John Doe* or *Jane Doe* if unidentified. Any available information regarding details of the illness or accident, cause of death, etc., together with external signs of trauma and other objective findings, should be entered in detail on the emergency record.

Any physician called upon to examine a suspected DOA has the very great responsibility of determining to the best of his ability if life, is, in fact, extinct. If there is any suspicion in his mind that life might still be present, immediate and vigorous resuscitative and supportive measures (**11**) should be begun. Careful recheck examinations should be done at frequent intervals until there is ABSOLUTELY no doubt in the mind of the attending physician that life is no longer present.

CASES IN WHICH A SPARK OF LIFE IS SUSPECTED, AND WHICH RECEIVE ANY TREATMENT, SHOULD NOT BE CLASSIFIED AS "DOA."

All DOA cases must be reported at once to the coroner's office and the remains, together with any personal belongings, turned over to the coroner or his representative.

3 – 5. CORONER'S OR MEDICAL EXAMINER'S CASES

The circumstances under which a death case comes under the jurisdiction of the coroner (in some areas called the medical examiner) vary in minor details in different localities, but, in general, responsibility is transferred from the attending physician to the coroner or medical examiner for the locality or political subdivision in which the death occurs, in the instances listed below. When a coroner or medical examiner assumes responsibility, his authority is supreme and completely supersedes the usual rights of the surviving spouse or next of kin (**3 – 6**).

1. All DOAs (**3 – 4**).
2. All deaths without previous medical care.
3. All attempts at self-destruction (**13.** *Suicide*).

4. All violent deaths.

5. All cases of poisoning − known or suspected.

6. All deaths resulting directly or indirectly from an accident at any time in the past.

7. All cases with reasonable grounds for suspecting that death may have resulted from criminal acts of another person or persons.

8. When the deceased had not been seen by his attending physician for 20 or more days before death.

9. When the patient had been hospitalized less than 24 hours and a definite diagnosis has not been established.

10. All instances in which the attending physician for any reason is unable or unwilling to sign the death certificate (**65 − 6**).

The attending physician CANNOT sign the death certificate (**65 − 6**) in coroner's cases unless specifically designated to do so by the coroner or his representative. The decision regarding the need for an autopsy, and its extent, is made solely by the coroner, although he may delegate the actual performance of the postmortem examination to another person. In this case the person who authorized the autopsy, not the person who actually performed it, is completely responsible.

3 − 6. AUTOPSIES (POSTMORTEM EXAMINATIONS)

CORONER'S CASES

All requests for autopsies must be signed by a representative of the coroner's office. The signature of any other person is invalid.

NONCORONER'S CASES

1. *Request and Permit for Autopsy*

Any type of postmortem examination, with or without removal of tissue or organs, requires completion of a properly signed and witnessed autopsy permit (**69 − 3**) BEFORE THE EXAMINATION IS BEGUN. Any type of postmortem examination without such permission constitutes actionable assault. There are no universal specifications in regard to the persons who may authorize postmortem examinations but, in general, priority is usually considered to be as follows:

The surviving spouse.

Surviving children over 18 years of age.

Surviving parents of the deceased.

Surviving adult siblings of the deceased.
Other surviving adult kin in order of closest blood relationship.
Although the signature of only one of several persons of the same degree of blood relationship is required by law, it is always desirable and advisable to obtain as many as practical.

2. *Limitations*

Any limitations or restrictions on the extent and scope of the postmortem examination, or unusual special instructions, must be specified on the Autopsy Permit form (**69 – 3**) and must be scrupulously observed by the autopsy surgeon or pathologist. Any examination or removal of tissues or organs in excess of, or in addition to, those specifically authorized is prima facie evidence of law violation even if, in the opinion of the autopsy surgeon, such additional examination is absolutely necessary to determine the cause of death. Example: "No brain examination."

3 – 7. DISPOSAL OF REMAINS

If the decedent leaves written instructions in a will or other document (**69 – 33.** *Uniform Donor Card*), his remains should be disposed of in accordance with his instructions even if other provisions of the will are subject to dispute. If the decedent leaves no will or written instructions, the decision regarding disposition rests with survivors, following the same priority as outlined under **3 – 6.** *Autopsies.*

Stillbirths – for definition, see **65 – 4.**

When the parents do not wish custody of a dead fetus, a permit for disposal (**69 – 10.** *Disposal of Dead Fetus*) should be properly signed and witnessed.

3 – 8. RELIGIOUS RITES

Considerable variation exists among religious groups regarding procedural rites before, at and after death. Accepted procedures, in some of which the attending physician may of necessity be forced to participate, are outlined on pages 11 and 12.

	ROMAN CATHOLIC	JEWISH	PROTESTANT
Physician's responsibility	Call a priest to administer the required sacraments of Penance, Holy Communion and Anointing of the Sick (Extreme Unction). Arrange complete privacy for confession.	Call a rabbi – preferably of the branch (Conservative, Orthodox, Reformed) to which the patient belongs.	Call a minister – preferably of the patient's own denomination. In certain instances, Holy Communion, Penance and Extreme Unction may be required. Arrange for privacy.

PREMATURE OR OTHER INFANTS IN CRITICAL CONDITION: STILLBIRTHS, ABORTIONS

	ROMAN CATHOLIC	JEWISH	PROTESTANT
	Excluding Anglo-Catholic, Eastern Orthodox and Polish National Catholic.	The Conservative, Orthodox and Reform branches specify minor differences in certain rites.	Presbyterian, Episcopalian, Lutheran, Moravian, etc.
GENERAL INSTRUCTIONS Notify the closest representative of the patient's church group, but if death is imminent, do not await his arrival.	Call a priest (addressed as *Father*).	Call a rabbi (addressed as *Rabbi*).	Call a minister (addressed generally as *Mister* or *Doctor*, never as *Reverend*; Lutheran, *Pastor*; high church Episcopal, *Father*).
BAPTISM OR CIRCUMCISION "I baptize you in the name of the Father and of the	Required for infants in danger of death and for	No Jewish males are circumcised on the 8th day	Required for all viable infants and stillbirths

PREMATURE OR OTHER INFANTS IN CRITICAL CONDITION: STILLBIRTHS, ABORTIONS

	ROMAN CATHOLIC	JEWISH	PROTESTANT
Son and of the Holy Spirit, Amen."	all products of conception, no matter how early. Water must flow on the skin. If born with membranes intact, immerse in water and break membranes. If in utero, hypodermic injection of sterile water through membranes.	after birth – no religious rites of any type for females.	(65–4), not for early products of conception. (Exceptions – Baptists and Disciples of Christ not baptized.) Water must touch skin –excess poured off – cloths, cotton, etc., used to wipe skin or head must be burned at once.
Name necessary?	No. Give full details to priest on his arrival.	No.	Yes. If no given name, specify *Baby Boy Doe.* Give full details to minister on his arrival.

DEATH CASES

	ROMAN CATHOLIC	JEWISH	PROTESTANT
Last rites	Call a priest. If last rites have not been given before death, the Sacrament of Anointing of the Sick (Extreme Unction) can be administered conditionally for several hours afterward, provided the body has not been shrouded or covered.	No last rites. Notify a rabbi or a responsible member of the Jewish community so that arrangements for disposition of remains, burial, etc., can be made.	No last rites after death.
Permission for autopsy?	No objection on religious grounds.	Because of religious objections, permission will have to be obtained through a rabbi.	No moral or religious objection to autopsy.

4. DRUG DOSAGE IN CHILDREN

Except in those instances in which a specific dose per age, dose per weight or dose per skin surface ratio is given in the text or in the brochure of the manufacturers, the following dosage tables are satisfactory for emergency use.

BY AGE

AGE	COMPARISON WITH ADULT DOSE	AGE	COMPARISON WITH ADULT DOSE
1 month	1/20	3 years	1/5
3 months	1/15	4 years	1/4
6 months	1/10	5–6 years	1/3
9 months	1/9	7–8 years	1/2
1 year	1/7	9–12 years	5/8
2 years	1/6	13–15 years	3/4

BY WEIGHT (Clark's Rule)

$$\text{Child's dose} = \frac{\text{weight in lb.}}{150} \times \text{adult dose}$$

BY SKIN SURFACE FOR AGE, WEIGHT AND HEIGHT

AGE	WEIGHT kg.	WEIGHT lb.	HEIGHT cm.	HEIGHT in.	SURFACE AREA (sq. m.)	APPROXIMATE PERCENTAGE OF ADULT DOSE*
Birth	3.4	7.4	50	20	0.21	11
3 months	5.7	12.5	60	23.5	0.29	16
6 months	7.4	16	66	26	0.36	21
1 year	10.0	22	75	29.4	0.45	26
2 years	12.4	27	87	34	0.54	31
3 years	14.5	31	96	38	0.60	35
4 years	16.5	36	103	40.5	0.68	39
5 years	19.0	41	110	43.5	0.73	42
6 years	21.5	47	116	46	0.82	47
7 years	24.1	53	123	48.5	0.90	53
8 years	26.8	59	129	51	0.97	57
9 years	29.4	65	134	53	1.05	61
10 years	32.3	71	139	55	1.12	65
11 years	35.5	78	144	57	1.20	69
12 years	39.0	86	151	59.5	1.28	74

*Based on average adult skin surface of 1.73 sq. m.

Infants are especially susceptible to the action of narcotics; therefore, from the age of 6 months to 2 years doses should be reduced below these schedules by at least one half.

DO NOT GIVE *ANY* NARCOTICS OF *ANY* KIND UNDER *ANY* CIRCUMSTANCES TO *ANY* INFANT UNDER SIX MONTHS OF AGE.

5. EMERGENCY MEDICAL BAG CONTENTS

The contents of an emergency bag will, of course, vary considerably according to the owner's type of practice and individual preferences, and with the proximity of a well-equipped emergency room or hospital. Some physicians may wish to add to or delete items from the lists suggested. However, a bag containing the basic items specified below will allow a physician called upon to handle emergency cases to give efficient and satisfactory care for almost all urgent conditions (**17**). A strongly constructed bag—18 inches long, 8 to 10 inches wide and 10 to 12 inches deep—with closable compartments, in the top, will accommodate the suggested basic equipment with a total overall weight of between 25 and 30 pounds.

The basic emergency bag suggested in the following pages contains diagnostic equipment (**5–1**), medications (**5–2**) and therapeutic supplies (**5–3**) listed alphabetically, not in order of importance. Each article should be packaged separately, labeled clearly for rapid identification and kept in a specific place in the bag. Medications (especially solutions) preferably should be in separate individual doses and not in stock bottles. Parenteral medications should be carried in single-dose sterile vials. Plastic nonbreakable bottles should be used for all liquids.

REPLACEMENT OF EACH ITEM as soon as possible after use IS IMPERATIVE! A list of items used on each call facilitates replacement as soon as the physician returns to his office.

5-1. DIAGNOSTIC EQUIPMENT

ITEM	QUANTITY	DESCRIPTION AND USE
1.	1 set	Batteries and bulb (spare) to fit diagnostic equipment. A battery-containing universal handle to fit flashlight, laryngoscope and otoscope saves space and weight. A nickel-cadmium battery unit, rechargeable in 5 minutes, obviates need for carrying spare batteries.
2.	1	Clinitest packet containing dropper, test tube and Clinitest and Acetest tablets.
3.	4	Finger cots, assorted sizes, for digital examination, finger dressings and use as *flutter valves* (**28-5**)
4.	1	Flashlight, small (1. *above*).
5.	2	Fluorescein ophthalmic solution (1%); single application packages or strips.
6.	2 pairs	Gloves, sterile, disposable, plastic or rubber.
7.	1	Laryngoscope with 3 blades (infant, medium, large) to fit universal handle (1. *above*).
8.	1	Neurologic reflex hammer with pinwheel, soft hair tuft and tuning fork incorporated.
9.	1	Ophthalmoscope-otoscope to fit universal handle (1. *above*).
10.	1	Phenylephrine hydrochloride (Neo-Synephrine), 10% solution, 5 ml. dropper vial (for funduscopic examination).
11.	2	Pontocaine, ½% solution, single application container for eye examinations.
12.	2	Rectal lubricant (K-Y Jelly), single application packages.
13.	1	Sphygmomanometer, aneroid, with self-adherent cuff.
14.	1	Spinal puncture needle with stylet (22 gauge).
15.	1	Stethoscope, folding type with flexible tubes.
16.	2	Thermometers (oral and rectal) in break-resistant cases.
17.	1	Thoracentesis needle, 4 inch, 18 gauge short bevel, with stylet.
18.	4	Tongue blades, individually packaged.

5-2. MEDICATIONS

ITEM	QUANTITY	NAME	HOW GIVEN	DESCRIPTION AND AMOUNT
19.	2	Aminophylline	I.V.	Ampules, 0.5 gm.
20.	3	Amobarbital (Amytal) sodium	I.M.	Ampules, 250 mg.
			I.V.	
21.	2	Ampicillin sodium (Polycillin N)	I.M.	Vial, 500 mg.
			I.V.	
22.	12	Ampicillin Trihydrate (Polycillin)	Oral	Capsules, 250 mg.
23.	4	Atropine sulfate	Oral	H.T., 0.4 mg.
			I.M.	
			I.V.	
24.	2	Caffeine sodiobenzoate	I.M.	Ampules, 0.5 gm.
			I.V.	
25.	2	Calcium gluconate (10%)	I.V.	Ampule, 10 ml.
26.	6	Codeine sulfate	Oral	H.T., 30 mg.
			I.M.	
27.	4	Deslanoside (Cedilanid-D)	I.M.	Ampules, 4 ml. (0.2 mg./ml.)
			I.V.	
28.	1	Dextrose in water (50%)	I.V.	Ampule, 50 ml.
29.	10	Digoxin (Lanoxin)	Oral	Tablets, 0.25 mg.
30.	1	Digoxin (Lanoxin), Pediatric Elixir	Oral	Bottle, 60 ml. (0.05 mg./ml.)
31.	1	Diphenylhydantoin	I.M.	Ampule, 250 mg.
			I.V.	
32.	2	Diphenylhydramine (Benadryl)	I.V.	Ampules, 1 ml. (50 mg./ml.)
33.	4	Epinephrine hydrochloride	I.M.	Ampules, 1 ml. of 1:1000 solution
			I.V.	

34.	4	Furosemide (Lasix)	I.V.	Ampules, 2 ml. (20 mg.)
35.	2	Heparin sodium	I.M.	Ampules, 1 ml. (1000 U.S.P. units)
			I.V.	
36.	1	Ipecac, syrup	Oral	Bottle, 30 ml.
37.	2	Isoproterenol hydrochloride (Isuprel)	I.V.	Ampules, 5 ml.
38.	1	Lidocaine (Xylocaine) hydrochloride	I.M.	Vial, 20 ml. (1%)
			I.V.	
39.	2	Metaraminol bitartrate (Aramine)	I.M.	Ampules, 1 ml. (10 mg.)
			I.V.	
40.	2	Methylergonovine maleate (Methergine)	I.M.	Ampules, 1 ml. (0.2 mg./ml.)
			I.V.	
41.	2	Methylprednisolone Sodium Succinate (Solu-Medrol)	I.V.	Mix-O-Vial, 125 mg.
42.	6	Morphine sulfate	Oral	H.T., 15 mg.
			I.M.	
			I.V.	
43.	6	Nitroglycerin	Sublingual	Tablets, 0.3 mg.
44.	1	Procainamide hydrochloride (Pronestyl)	I.M.	Vial, 10 ml. (10 mg./ml.)
45.	1	Prochlorperazine (Compazine)	I.M.	Vial, 10 ml. (5 mg./ml.)
46.	10	Secobarbital (Seconal)	Oral	Capsules, 100 mg.
47.	2	Sodium bicarbonate	I.V.	Vials, 50 ml. (3.75 gm.)
48.	2	Tetanus immune globulin, human	I.M.	Vials, 1 ml. (250 units)
49.	1	Tincture of benzoin	Local	Bottle, 30 ml.
50.	1	Tincture of merthiolate	Local	Bottle, 30 ml.
51.	2	Water (sterile)	Local	Ampules, 10 ml.
			I.M.	
			I.V.	

5 – 3.   THERAPEUTIC SUPPLIES

ITEM	QUANTITY	DESCRIPTION
52.	1 roll	Adhesive tape – 3″.
53.	1	Alcohol 70%, 60 ml. in plastic bottle with screw top.
54.	6	Alcohol-saturated gauze pads, small, individually packaged.
55.	6	Applicators, cotton-tipped, sterile, individually packaged.
56.	1	Bandage scissors (medium size).
57.	1 box	Bandages, sterile, assorted sizes (Band-Aids).
58.	2	Catheters, plastic No. 12 and No. 16 Foley, 5 ml. reservoir, sterile.
59.	2	Eye patches.
60.	1	File for opening ampules and vials.
61.	4	Gauze roller bandages, sterile, 1″ and 2″.
62.	8	Gauze pads, sterile, 2″ × 2″, individually packaged.
63.	4	Gauze pads, sterile, 4″ × 4″, individually packaged.
64.	9	Hypodermic needles, sterile, individually packaged and labeled. 2 #26 gauge, $7/8$″ long 2 #24 gauge, $1\frac{1}{2}$″ long 3 #22 gauge, 2″ long 1 #18 gauge, 3″ long 1 #14 gauge, 3″ long, for emergency airway puncture
65.	6	Hypodermic syringes, sterile, individually packaged and labeled. 1 syringe, 1 ml. (tuberculin) 1 syringe, 2 ml. 1 syringe, 5 ml. 1 syringe, 50 ml.
66.	3	Laryngeal intubation tubes (assorted sizes).
67.	1 dozen	Matches, friction type, in waterproof container.
68.	1	Pocket knife, large pointed blade.
69.	1 dozen	Safety pins, assorted sizes, in plastic box.
70.	1 roll	Scotch tape, $3/4$″ width.
71.	1	Suction cup (small), for removal of contact lenses.

5—4.   ADDITIONAL EQUIPMENT (Optional — can be carried in the car trunk)

Electrocardiograph, portable, with electrolyte jelly.

Intravenous Starter Set

ITEM	QUANTITY	DESCRIPTION
1.	1	Dextran, 500 ml.
2.	1	Dextrose, 5% in water, 500 ml. flask or 125 ml. starter bottle.
3.	1	Sodium lactate, 1/6 molar solution, 500 ml.
4.	2	Needles, short bevel, 20 gauge, 2″ long.
5.	2	Disposable tubing sets.

Lavage and Catheterization Setup

ITEM	QUANTITY	DESCRIPTION
1.	2	Adaptors (plastic or metal, *not* glass) to fit funnel, catheters, gastric lavage tubes and rubbing tubing.
2.	2	Adaptors (plastic or metal), Y-tube.
3.	4	Catheters (sterile), individually packaged, 3 male (small, medium, and large), one female (plastic, nonbreakable); with adaptors to fit plastic funnel, syringe and tubing.
4.	1	Funnel (plastic) with adaptors to fit lavage tubes, catheters and tubing.
5.	2	Gastric lavage tubes (Ewald type), small and medium.
6.	1	Syringe, large, with tubing and adaptor.

Obstetric — Gynecologic

ITEM	QUANTITY	DESCRIPTION
1.	1	Clamp (Kocher), large, sterile.
2.	1	Forceps, thumb, sterile.
3.	2 ampules	Silver nitrate solution (1%), individual dose package.
4.	2	Umbilical cord ties (sterile).
5.	1	Vaginal speculum, medium size.
6.	1	Episiotomy set (spring retractor, scissors, needle holder, sutures)

Orthopedic

ITEM	QUANTITY	DESCRIPTION
1.	1	Aluminum, sheet, malleable, 6″ × 8″ for small splints.
2.	1	Mechanic's pliers with side-cutting jaws.
3.	1	Metal shears, heavy enough to cut sheet aluminum.
4.	6 rolls	Plaster of paris 2 2″ rolls 2 3″ rolls 2 4″ rolls
5.	2 rolls	Sheet wadding 3″.
6.	1	Sling, muslin (Red Cross type).
7.	1 roll	Stockinette, bias-cut, 3″.

5 – 4. ADDITIONAL EQUIPMENT

Oxygen tank, small, portable, with face mask, rebreathing bag, tubing and adaptors.

Poison kit. Some physicians will wish to carry a separate kit for treatment of acute poisoning. This should contain the following items. Those marked with an asterisk are duplicated in the basic bag.

Acetic acid, 5%
Activated charcoal
Ammonia water, 0.2%
Amyl nitrite pearls
Amytal sodium (parenteral)*
Apomorphine (parenteral)
Atropine sulfate (parenteral)
Caffeine and sodiobenzoate (parenteral)
Calcium gluconate, 10% (parenteral)*
Dimercaprol (BAL)
Edathamil calcium disodium (EDTA)
Ipecac, syrup of*
Magnesium hydroxide (milk of Magnesia)
Metaraminol bitartrate (Aramine)*
Methylene blue, 1% aqueous (parenteral)
Methylprednisolone sodium succinate (parenteral)
Nalorphine or levallorphan
Paraldehyde
Phenylephrine hydrochloride (parenteral)
Potassium chloride (Tablets and parenteral)
Potassium permanganate
Procainamide (parenteral)*
Sodium bicarbonate (parenteral)
Sodium formaldehyde sulfoxylate
Sodium thiosulfate, 25% (parenteral)
Starch
Vitamin K_1 oxide (AquaMephyton)
Water (distilled, sterile)*

Specimen Collection Setup

ITEM	QUANTITY	DESCRIPTION
1.	2	Bottles, plastic, sterile, large mouth, screw top, 60 ml. for specimens of urine, vomitus, stool, etc.
2.	2	Culture tubes, 5 ml., plastic, screw top.
3.	1 box	Labels, gummed, small.
4.	4	Microscope slides, sterile, in container.
5.	2	Vials, sterile, 10 ml., screw top, for blood samples.

Surgical Setup

ITEM	QUANTITY	DESCRIPTION
1.	4	Clamps (hemostats), sterile, individually packaged. 2 small (mosquito or Kelly) 2 large (Carmalt or Kocher)
2.	1	Eye scalpel, bistoury point, sterile.
3.	1	Eye spud, small, sterile.
4.	3	Forceps (sterile), individually packaged and labeled. 1 thumb forceps, plain tip 1 thumb forceps, rat-tooth tip

Surgical Setup

ITEM	QUANTITY	DESCRIPTION
5.	4	Needles, surgical, cutting edge, half curved, assorted sizes, sterile, in individual envelopes.
6.	1	Probe, flexible wire, ball tip.
7.	1	Razor, safety, with package of blades.
8.	1	Scalpel handle (Bard Parker No. 3) with 3 individually packaged sterile blades, assorted shapes, to fit handle.
9.	1	Scissors, Mayo type (1 sharp, 1 rounded point).
10.	1	Ring cutter in case.
11.	6	Sutures with affixed needles in individual sterile tubes or envelopes: 2 3–0 Dermalon 2 5–0 Dermalon 1 2–0 Plain catgut 1 4–0 Plain catgut

Miscellaneous

Emergency textbook.
Prescription pad.
Road and street map.
Restraint straps (4), 1″ webbing, airplane-type quick release buckles.
Rubber tubing (2 rolls), ¼″ to ⅜″ bore, 18 to 36 inches long for use as tourniquets, etc.

5 — 5. PRECAUTIONS

The basic emergency bag, as well as optional kits, should be kept out of public view as much as possible, preferably locked in the luggage compartment. If carried on the seat or floor of the car, they should be covered. All equipment will be safer if the car does not carry M.D. identification.

When a physician receives an emergency night call, a spotlight, either transportable or mounted on the car, and a good map of any unfamiliar localities are invaluable.

If calls for emergency treatment are received from persons who are not known to the physician, or if the circumstances of the call are unusual and the patient cannot be brought to the emergency department, it may be prudent for the physician to request a police escort, particularly if the area to be visited has a high crime rate.

6. FLUID REPLACEMENT IN EMERGENCIES

Proper replacement of fluid and electrolytes is an often over-looked and neglected aspect of the care of emergency cases that in certain situations may be lifesaving. The following principles of replacement therapy may require modification because of limited facilities for laboratory determination, but in many instances clinical examination will allow institution of therapy which can be continued during transfer to a hospital where accurate confirmatory laboratory tests can be obtained. In all instances, an *accurate* record of intake, both parenteral and oral, and of output must be sent with the patient.

Calculations for repair of electrolyte imbalance are usually expressed in milliequivalents per liter (abbreviated mEq./L.).

$$\text{mEq./L.} = \frac{\text{mg./100 ml.} \times 10}{\text{atomic weight}} \times \text{valence}$$

BASIC ELEMENTS IN ELECTROLYTE BALANCE

ELEMENT	CHEMICAL SYMBOL	ATOMIC WEIGHT	VALENCE	RANGE OF CONCENTRATION IN EXTRACELLULAR FLUID (mEq./L.)
Sodium	Na	23	1	135–148
Potassium	K	39	1	4.4–5.6
Carbon dioxide combining power	CO_2	...	1	25.0–30.0
Chloride	Cl	35	1	99–108
Calcium	Ca	40	2	4.5–5.5

6−1. BASIC CONSIDERATIONS IN MANAGEMENT AND TREATMENT

1. **Estimation of magnitude of prior loss** of water, sodium and other electrolytes and of degrees of acid-base imbalance.
    a. Duration and rate of losses or lack of intake.
    b. Weight loss.
    c. Urinary specific gravity.
    d. Skin turgor.

e. Presence of loss into *third compartment* (e.g., pleural cavity and peritoneal cavity).

f. Specific determinations of urine and blood electrolytes, pH and blood volume as needed. Electrocardiograms can be of assistance in emergency evaluation of calcium and potassium levels. (See also **43—1.** *Acidosis;* **43—5.** *Alkalosis;* Table 3 under **53.** *Identification of Degree or Severity of Shock.*)

2. **Estimation of type of prior fluid loss** for deficits in water, electrolytes, plasma and whole blood.

a. History of type of losses and type of intake.

b. Evaluation of route of current losses (upper and lower gastrointestinal tract, urinary tract, respiratory tract, skin).

c. Determination of loss directly through laboratory examination of output (gastrointestinal tract, urine, sweat).

3. **Estimation or determination of rate of current abnormal losses** by magnitude and type and estimation of loss for the next 24 hours.

4. **Estimation of anticipated normal loss of water and electrolytes** for the next 24 hours.

5. **Determination of the type and rate of correction** based on the considerations above, plus the patient's age, severity of condition and cardiovascular and renal status. Specific orders should be written covering the first 24 hours of replacement therapy, giving type of fluids (**6—4**), amount of fluids, and route and rate of administration.

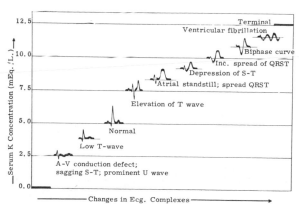

Correlation of the serum potassium concentration and the electrocardiogram (providing there is no parallel change in Na and Ca). (From Krupp, Sweet, Jawetz, and Armstrong, Physician's Handbook, 15th ed., 1968. Lange Medical Publications, Los Altos, Calif.)

6 – 2. BASIC REQUIREMENTS (FLUIDS AND ELECTROLYTES) PER DAY

Number all bottles of fluids consecutively. The following summary is useful.

Estimated losses

	WATER (ml.)	SODIUM (mEq.)	POTASSIUM (mEq.)	CHLORIDE (mEq.)	BLOOD (ml.)
Prior loss					
Current abnormal loss					
Normal loss in 24 hours					
Total loss at end of next 24 hours					
Replacement to be ordered for next 24 hours					

6 – 2. BASIC REQUIREMENTS (FLUIDS AND ELECTROLYTES) PER DAY

The amount of fluids and electrolytes required every 24 hours depends upon the patient's age, weight and skin surface (usually indicated in square meters). Approximate relationships between the weight in kilograms and the skin area (S.A.) in square meters (sq. m.) are as follows:

WEIGHT (kg.)	S.A. (sq. m.)	WEIGHT (kg.)	S.A. (sq. m.)	WEIGHT (kg.)	S.A. (sq. m.)	WEIGHT (kg.)	S.A. (sq. m.)
1.0	0.10	11.0	0.52	21.0	0.85	31.0	1.13
1.5	0.12	12.0	0.55	22.0	0.87	32.0	1.15
2.0	0.15	13.0	0.58	23.0	0.90	33.0	1.18
2.5	0.18	14.0	0.61	24.0	0.93	34.0	1.20
3.0	0.20	15.0	0.64	25.0	0.95	35.0	1.25
4.0	0.25	16.0	0.71	26.0	1.00	36.0	1.25
5.0	0.29	17.0	0.74	27.0	1.03	37.0	1.27
6.0	0.33	18.0	0.76	28.0	1.06	38.0	1.30
7.0	0.38	19.0	0.79	29.0	1.08	39.0	1.32
8.0	0.42	20.0	0.82	30.0	1.11	40.0	1.34
9.0	0.45						
10.0	0.49	S.A. of average (70 kg.) adult = 1.73 sq. m.					

Water (H₂O) requirements per day

Average physical condition	1500 ml./sq. m.
Moderately dehydrated	2400 ml./sq. m.
Severe dehydrated	3000 ml./sq. m.
Hyperventilating	500 ml./sq. m.
Hyperpyrexic	1500 ml./sq. m. + 4.5% for each Centigrade degree above normal (2.5% for each degree Fahrenheit)

Potassium ion requirements per day: 40 mEq./sq. m.

Sodium chloride (NaCl) requirements per day by age

	NaCl	
AGE	gm.	mEq.
Newborn	0.25	4
1-3 months	0.35	6
3-6 months	0.5	8
6-12 months	0.75	12
1-2 years	1.0	17
2-4 years	2.0	34
4-7 years	3.0	51
7-12 years	4.0	68
12-18 years	5.0	85
18 years up	6.0-7.0	100-120

6-3. OUTPUT

Physiologic output of fluids and electrolytes must be given full consideration in estimating replacement therapy. Pathologic processes (excessive perspiration, hyperpyrexia, rapid respiration, vomiting, diarrhea, bleeding) must also be considered. In edematous patients, no loss of electrolytes is considered to occur through the skin.

6-4. REPLACEMENT SOLUTIONS

TYPES AND APPROXIMATE AVERAGE AMOUNTS OF OUTPUT

TYPE	Na	K	Cl	HCO_3	AVERAGE OUTPUT PER DAY IN ML. (70 kg. adult)
		mEq./L.			
Bile	140	10	100	30	500
Bowel	120	10	105	25	3000
Gastric	35	12	125	...	2500
Pancreatic	140	10	75	75	700
Saliva	10	25	10	10	1000
Urine	40	30	70	...	1500
Sensible and insensible (skin and lungs)					
At rest	0	0	0		1000
Moderate activity	25	0	25		1500
Extreme activity	50	0	50		2000+

6-4. REPLACEMENT SOLUTIONS (mEq. to volume indicated)

	VOLUME OR AMOUNT	Na	K	Cl	LACTATE
Ammonium chloride (0.9% solution)	Per liter	...	...	167	...
Butler's solution	Per liter	57	25	50	25
Darrow's solution	Per liter	117	35	99	53
Normal saline	Per liter	154	...	154	...
Plasma	Per 250 ml.	35	1.2	25	...
Ringer's lactate	Per liter	131	4	110	28
Sodium bicarbonate (3.75 gm.)	Per 50 ml.	44.6	...	...	...
Sodium lactate (1/6 molar solution)	Per liter	166	...	...	166
Potassium penicillin	Per million units	...	1.7	...	...
Sodium penicillin	Per million units	1.6	...	...	...

6-5. FLUID REQUIREMENTS OF A BURNED ADULT IN THE FIRST 24 HOURS (Modified from standard procedure in Brooke Army Hospital)

DEXTROSE IN WATER (fixed amount)   2000 ml.

ELECTROLYTE SOLUTIONS

Formula: Body weight in kilograms × % of body surface burned
(**25 − 1; 48 − 14**) × 1.5 ml.

Example: 70 kg. adult with 40% S.A. burn

$$70 \times 40 \times 1.5 = 4200 \text{ ml.}$$

COLLOID SOLUTIONS (Blood, plasma, plasma volume expanders)

Formula: Body weight in kilograms × % of body surface burned
× 0.5 ml.

Example: $70 \times 40 \times 0.5 = \underline{1400 \text{ ml.}}$

Total fluids in example 5600 ml. (electrolytes and colloids)

One half of the total (2800 ml.) should be given in the first 8 hours; then one quarter of the total (1400 ml.) in the next two 8 hour periods, modified by clinical judgment.

6 − 6. ORAL SOLUTION FOR MASS CASUALTY USE

Oral intake of one to two glasses of a solution containing 1 level teaspoonful of table salt and ½ teaspoonful of baking soda dissolved in a quart of water may be lifesaving in persons who show evidence of water, saline and base depletion.

7. NARCOTICS (OPIUM DERIVATIVES AND SYNTHETICS) IN EMERGENCY CASES

For use and toxicity of other substances listed under the Narcotic Act (**2 − 3**), see **49.** *Poisons.*

7 − 1. EMERGENCY USE

Opium derivatives as well as synthetic narcotics are of great value in emergency treatment provided indiscriminate use is avoided and the following principles are kept in mind.

Definite indications for use are present:
1. Control of severe pain and acute apprehension.
2. Specific effects are desired [apomorphine to induce vomiting; naloxone hydrochloride (Narcan) to counteract overdoses of opiates and synthetic narcotics; morphine to control apprehension as well as pain].

No contraindications are present.
The most important contraindications are:
1. Head injuries (**41**). Important changes in vital signs may be masked by even small doses of narcotics.
2. Respiratory depression from any cause.
3. Chest injuries (**28**).
4. Undiagnosed abdominal pain (**19**).
5. Addiction, with or without withdrawal symptoms (**2 – 4**), unless other conditions requiring use of narcotics are present.
6. Abnormal or allergic reactions to previous doses (**21**).
7. Infancy or early childhood (**4**).
8. Pregnancy at or near term – respiratory depression may be dangerous to the child.
9. Myxedema (**33 – 5**).
10. Concomitant administration of other drugs which accentuate or potentiate the action of narcotics.

Minimal effective dosage based on the age or weight (**4**) and physical condition of the patient is used.

Proper means of administration is chosen. Oral administration is contraindicated if vomiting is present or may occur; subcutaneous or intramuscular injections may be totally ineffective if the patient is in circulatory collapse, producing an overwhelming accumulative toxic effect when the circulation improves.

The appropriate drug is used. Consideration must be given to possible side effects as well as to intensity and duration of action. Morphine sulfate is by far the most useful narcotic for general emergency use not only because of its general availability and low cost but also because of its ability to control severe pain and at the same time allay apprehension. If marked contraction of smooth muscle and decreased respiratory rate will be detrimental, meperidine hydrochloride (Demerol) may be substituted. Demerol, however, has little effect on severe pain and does not control acute apprehension; therefore, it should not as a rule be used in emergencies such as fractures and myocardial infarction. Codeine sulfate (**7 – 2**) is satisfactory for control of pain of moderate intensity and is, for practical purposes, nonaddictive.

7-2. ANALGESIC NARCOTICS (OPIATES AND SYNTHETICS) OF USE IN EMERGENCY THERAPY

NARCOTIC DRUG	AVERAGE ADULT DOSE	DURATION OF ACTION (Hours)	METHOD OF ADMINISTRATION	INDICATIONS FOR USE	CONTRAINDICATIONS TO USE	ANALGESIC EFFECT (Rise in Pain Threshold)	MINIMAL LETHAL DOSE FOR ADULTS (Approximate)*
Alphaprodine hydrochloride (Nisentil)	40 mg.	1-2	S.C.	Dental emergencies; minor surgery; obstetric analgesia	Same as morphine	++	60 to 120 mg.
Camphorated opium tincture (paregoric)	4 ml.	2-3	Oral	Pediatrics – in children over 2 years of age*	Same as morphine	+	60 ml.
Codeine sulfate	60 mg.	2-3	Oral S.C. I.M.	Control of moderate pain; headache; neuralgia; ryalgia; persistent cough	Allergic reactions in some persons, but usually well tolerated	++	0.8 gm.
Dihydrocodeinone bitartrate (Hycodan)	10 mg.	1-2	Oral	Cough depressant; does not paralyze ciliary action	None except individual hypersensitivity	+	0.3 gm.
Hydromorphone hydrochloride (Dilaudid)	2 mg.	3-4	Oral S.C. I.M. I.V.	Control of severe pain or acute apprehension; relaxation of reflex spasm	Same as morphine; slightly more toxic	+++	0.1 gm.
Meperidine hydrochloride (Demerol)	50 mg.	1-2	Oral I.M. I.V.	Moderate pain; obstetric analgesia; preoperative preparation; whenever smooth muscle contraction will be harmful	Severe pain or acute apprehension; head or chest injuries; shock	++	1 gm.
Morphine	15 mg.	4-5	Oral S.C. I.M. I.V.	Control of any type of severe pain (except psychogenic); control of acute apprehension and anxiety; shock; preoperative preparation	Head or chest injuries; respiratory depression; unstable mental make-up; when contraction of smooth muscle is detrimental	+++	0.2 gm.

*In infants (children under 2 years of age) the minimal lethal dose varies from approximately 1/100 of the adult dose in the first 2 weeks of life to 1/20 of the adult dose at the age of 2. The values given in this table do not include the occasional cases of atopic or allergic hypersensitivity.

Hydromorphone hydrochloride (Dilaudid) (**7 – 2**) is of use in some emergency situations in place of morphine not only because of its ability to control apprehension and severe pain but also because its name is not as well known. In certain circumstances it may be desirable to keep from the patient (or the family) the fact that administration of a powerful narcotic has been necessary. Its actions, side effects and addictive tendencies are similar to those of morphine (**49 – 495**), although its toxicity is slightly greater.

8. PRESCRIPTION RESTRICTIONS

8 – 1. AMOUNTS

Only small amounts of medications of any kind should be prescribed for patients seen solely on an emergency basis – enough to obtain the desired effect until the patient can report elsewhere for definitive care.

8 – 2. CONTROLLED DRUGS OR DEVICES

In many areas strict resistrictions are in effect in regard to prescription not only of narcotics (**8 – 4**) but also of a large number of drugs of various actions specified as unsafe for self-medication and classified as controlled substances. Certain instruments used in administration of drugs are also included. These classifications usually include the following:

1. Any hypnotic drug – defined as "any compounds, mixtures or preparations that may be used for producing hypnotic effect."
2. Aminopyrine and its compounds or mixtures.
3. Amphetamines (except preparations for use in the nose).
4. Cinchopen and neocinchopen.
5. Diethylstilbestrol.
6. Ergot, cotton root or their contained or derived active compounds.
7. Oils of croton, rue, savin or tansy.
8. Phenylhydantoin derivatives.
9. Sulfanilamide or substituted sulfanilamides (except topical preparations containing not more than 5% strength).
10. Thyroid and its contained or derived active compounds.

11. Any drug whose packaging bears the legend: "Caution: federal law prohibits dispensing without prescription."

12. Hypodermic syringes and needles.

QUICK REFERENCE CHART ON PRESCRIBING CONTROLLED SUBSTANCES (BASED ON FEDERAL AND CALIFORNIA REGULATIONS)*

SCHEDULE I — Not applicable to prescription of drugs for emergency care.

SCHEDULE II

- Prescription cannot be phoned in.
- Prescription must be completely handwritten in ink by the prescriber.
- Preprinted precription forms not allowed.
- Need patient's address and prescriber's Bureau of Narcotics and Dangerous drugs (BNDD) number and telephone number on prescription.
- No refills allowed.
- Must be filled within 7 days.
- Federal order form required to obtain drugs for office use.

A. Narcotics — State Triplicate Prescription Blank Required	B. Non-narcotics — regular Prescription Blank Acceptable	
Cocaine	Amphetamine	Dramamine D
Codeine	Ambar	Eskatrol
Demerol	Amodex	Methamphetamine
Dilaudid	Amytal	Nembutal
Dionin	Appetrol	Obedrin
Donnagesic Extentabs No. 2	Bamadex	Obetrol
Leritine	Benzedrine	Parest
Morphine	Biphetamine	Preludin
Paregoric	Bontril	Quaalude
Percobarb	Desbutal	Ritalin
Percodan	Desoxyn	Seconal
Percodan Demi	Dexamyl	Tuinal
	Dexedrine	

SCHEDULE III

- May be prescribed orally or in writing.
- Written prescription must be completely handwritten in ink by the prescriber.

*The controlled drugs listed are for example only; the lists are not complete.

8−2. CONTROLLED DRUGS OR DEVICES

- Preprinted prescription forms not allowed.
- Need patient's address, prescriber's BNND number and phone number on prescription.
- Oral prescription (new and refill authorization) must be personally phoned to pharmacist by the prescriber (no other person).
- Limit of 5 refllls over a 6 month time period.

A. Narcotics
Ascodeen
APC with Codeine
Citra Forte Syrup
Donnagesic Extentabs No. 1
Empirin & Codeine (Nos. 1, 2, 3, 4)
Fiorinal & Codeine (Nos. 1, 2, 3)
Hycodan
Hycomine
Paregoric mixtures
Percogesic C
Phenaphen & Codeine (Nos. 2, 3, 4)
Tussend Syrup
Tussionex Suspension
Tylenol & Codeine (Nos. 1, 2, 3, 4)

B. Non-narcotics
Butisol
Carbrital
Doriden
Fiorinal
Noludar

SCHEDULES IV AND V

- New prescription or refill authorization may be phoned in by prescriber or authorized employee (written evidence of authorization must be on file with pharmacy or provided within a reasonable time).
- Need patient's address and prescriber's BNND number and telephone number on prescription.
- Limit of 5 refills over a 6 month time period.

A. Schedule IV
Barbital
Chardonna
Chloral Hydrate
Deprol
Equagesic
Equanil
Mebaral
Meprobamate
Meprospan
Milpath
Miltown
Noctec
Phenobarbital
Placidyl
Valmid

B. Schedule V
Actifed C
Donnagel PG
Elixir Terpin Hydrate & Codeine
Lomotil
Parepectolin
Phenergan Expectorant & Codeine
Robitussin AC

NONCONTROLLED DRUGS

- New prescription or refill authorization may be phoned in by prescriber or authorized employee (written evidence of authorization must be on file with pharmacy or provided within a reasonable time.
- Need patient's address.
- Need prescriber's state license number on prescriptions.
- Refill limit discretionary with prescriber.

Examples

    Antibiotics
    Antihistamines
    Diuretics
    Oral Contraceptives

INFORMATION REQUIRED ON ALL PRESCRIPTIONS IN CALIFORNIA, REGARDLESS OF THE DRUG'S CLASSIFICATION

1. Name and address of patient.
2. Name, strength and quantity of drug or device prescribed.
3. Directions for use.
4. Date of issue.
5. Signature of prescriber.
6. License classification of prescriber (M.D., D.D.S., etc.).
7. Name, address, and telephone number of prescriber (either rubber stamped, typed, printed by hand or typeset).

8-3. NARCOTICS

Although regulations regarding prescription of narcotics vary in different countries, it is usually required that the prescription be completely in the physician's handwriting and his office address, telephone number and narcotic registration number be given. Only the minimal amount necessary to obtain the desired effect should be used in adjusting the dose to the age in children (**4**) and in elderly or debilitated persons. Such prescriptions, as a rule, cannot be refilled. Some states require the use of triplicate forms.

For restrictions on prescription of narcotics for treatment of addiction, see **2-5**.

8-4. SOMNIFACIENTS

Antihistaminics, hypnotics, muscle relaxants, narcotics, sedatives and tranquilizers are among the commonly used drugs which may cause drowsiness and slowing of reflexes. Therefore, persons for whom any of these drugs have been prescribed should be cautioned against operating any type of motor driven vehicle during the duration of the effect of the drug. The same warning should be given to persons exposed to changes in barometric pressure (**23**).

9. RAPE

The legal definition of rape is "the carnal knowledge, to a lesser or greater degree, of a female, not the wife of the assailant, without her consent and by compulsion, either through fear, force or fraud, singly or in combination." As long as the penis enters any portion of the female genitalia the assailant need not have an orgasm, or even an erection. Many states have established "the age of consent" (usually 16 to 18 years) below which sexual intercourse, even with the girl's consent, constitutes statutory rape.

Examination for possible rape should never be done, even when requested by law enforcement officers, without a properly witnessed written consent (**69 – 14**) of the patient or, if she is a minor, of a parent (both parents, if possible) or legal guardian.

Examination and treatment should cover the following:
1. Care of physical injuries.
2. Prevention or treatment of psychological damage.
3. Prevention or treatment of venereal disease or pregnancy.
4. Medicolegal documentation.

Questioning and examination should always be done in the presence of a third person (preferably a nurse, certainly a woman) and should cover the points listed below. Negative as well as positive findings should be noted in detail in the Emergency Department record.

Date and time of the alleged act.

The patient's statement regarding the circumstances of the alleged act and of previous sexual relations.

Physical examination as soon as possible after the alleged act. In a small child general anesthesia may be necessary.

The report on this examination should include notations regarding the condition of the clothing, development of the genitalis, external signs of injury (abrasions, lacerations, contusions, edema, bleeding, etc.), presence or absence of excessive secretion (type ?), abrasions or lacerations of the vaginal canal and condition of the hymen. Evidence of injuries to parts of the body other than the genital area should be noted and recorded.

Collection of specimens of secretion using a pipet, from the labia, introitus and cervix. These specimens of secretion should be examined IMMEDIATELY as wet preparations and the presence or absence of motile or nonmotile sperm noted. If no sperm are found (many men have had vasectomies) tests for seminal fluid (**15−7**) should be made on intravaginal specimens and on dried secretions on the vulva or upper thighs. Smears from the same areas should be made, carefully labeled for possible later identification and sent to a qualified laboratory for staining and confirmatory examination for spermatozoa and for gonococci.

Material for cultures should also be obtained. All smears should be preserved as permanent records for at least 2 years.

In some localities, examination for rape requires that a blood sample (10 ml.), marked carefully for identification, be sent to a laboratory for serology tests. Arrangements should be made to have these tests repeated in about 6 weeks.

Evidence of rape (attempted or accomplished) must be reported at once to the proper law enforcement authorities. For permit for examination and release of information, see **69−14**. Even if there is no evidence of penetration or seminal emission, findings indicative of trauma to the external genitalia are often considered to be presumptive evidence of criminal assault.

10. REPORTABLE DISEASES

Public health regulations regarding certain diseases require that special forms be completed and signed by the physician who established the diagnosis. The list of reportable diseases usually includes the following:

Amebiasis (**37−20**)
Anthrax (**30−1**)
Botulism (**49−141**)
Brucellosis (undulant fever) (**30−35**)
Chancroid (**60−2**)
Chickenpox (varicella) (**30−3**)
Cholera
Coccidioidomycosis
Conjunctivitis, acute infections of the newborn (gonorrheal ophthalmia, ophthalmia neonatorum, and babies' sore eyes in the first 21 days of life)
Dengue (**62−4**)
Diarrhea of the newborn (**48−21**)
Diphtheria (**30−4**)
Dysentery, bacillary (see **30−5**. *Shigella infections*)
Encephalitis, acute (**62−5**)

10. REPORTABLE DISEASES

Epilepsy (**29 – 7**)
Food poisoning (**49 – 339**)
Gonococcus infection (**60 – 3**)
Granuloma inguinale (**60 – 4**)
Hepatitis, infectious (**62 – 8**)
Hepatitis, serum (**62 – 8**)
Leprosy (Hansen's disease) (**30 – 12**)
Leptospirosis, including Weil's disease
Lymphogranuloma venereum (lympho-
   granuloma inguinale) (**60 – 4**)
Malaria (**30 – 14**)
Measles (rubeola) (**30 – 15**)
Meningitis, meningococcal or meningo-
   coccemia (**30 – 16; 48 – 41**)
Mumps (**30 – 17**)
Paratyphoid fever, A, B and C (see **30 –
   33; 49 – 339.** *Food Poisoning)*
Pertussis (whooping cough) (**30 – 38**)
Plague (**30 – 20**)
Pneumonia, primary infectious (**52 – 14**)
Poliomyelitis, acute anterior (**30 – 21;
   46 – 9; 48 – 49**)
Psittacosis (**30 – 22**)

Q fever
Rabies, human or animal (**62 – 17**)
Relapsing fever
Rheumatic fever, acute
Rocky Mountain spotted fever (**24 – 22**)
Salmonella infections (exclusive of typh-
   oid fever) (**30 – 33; 49 – 339.** *Food
   Poisoning*)
Scarlet fever (**30 – 27**)
Shigella infections (**30 – 5**)
Smallpox (variola) (**30 – 30**)
Streptococcal infections (including scar-
   let fever and streptococcal sore throat)
   (**30 – 9**)
Syphilis (**60 – 5**)
Tetanus (**30 – 31**)
Trachoma (**30 – 32**)
Trichinosis (**37 – 20**)
Tuberculosis
Tularemia
Typhoid fever, cases and carriers (**30 – 33**)
Typhus fever (**30 – 34**)
Yellow Fever (**30 – 39**)

Official cards (see below) for reporting these cases should be completed as soon as the diagnosis is made and mailed to the local health officer. Botulism, cholera, dengue, relapsing fever, plague, smallpox, typhus (louse-borne epidemic type) and yellow fever must be reported immediately to the director of the state department of public health by telephone or telegraph.

Morbidity Report Form

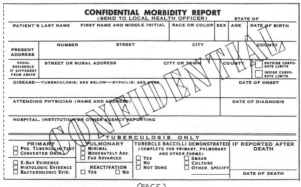

(FACE)

```
                    SYPHILIS  Diagnostic Information-
          INFECTIOUS                      NON-INFECTIOUS
    □ PRIMARY                         □ LATE LATENT
    □ SECONDARY                       □ NEUROSYPHILIS, ASYMPTOMATIC
    □ EARLY LATENT                    □ NEUROSYPHILIS, CLINICAL
    EPIDEMIOLOGIC NOTE:  TO MINIMIZE SPREAD,  □ CARDIOVASCULAR
    PROMPT  CONTROL  MEASURES  ARE  ESSENTIAL. □ OTHER LATE
    PLEASE PHONE REPORTS FOR INFECTIOUS CASES. □ CONGENITAL        SPECIFY
    REMARKS




    _____



    REQUEST    NUMBER              NAME AND ADDRESS
    MORBIDITY
    BOOKS
                                        DEPARTMENT OF PUBLIC HEALTH
```

(REVERSE SIDE)

11. RESUSCITATION

See also **22.** Asphyxiation; **22−3.** Drowning; **26−7.** Cardiac Arrest; **48−53.** Smoke Inhalation in Children.

Absent pulses, absent respirations and lifeless appearance are the obvious initial signs of collapse of cardiopulmonary function. When these conditions are present, resuscitative measures in order to be effective must be begun immediately and carried out vigorously according to a comprehensive preconceived and practiced plan. However, not every person with presumptive evidence of death (**3−2**) should be subjected to such efforts.

Vigorous cardiopulmonary resuscitation measures should be begun if:

1. Presumptive evidences of death (**3−2**) occur suddenly and unexpectedly.

2. The state and duration of biologic death of the central nervous system would not preclude return to functional life. With rare exceptions, extensive biologic death occurs if cardiopulmonary function is absent for 4–6 minutes.

3. The primary disease process is treatable to a point of restoration of functional life.

Effective cardiopulmonary resuscitation consists of 2 major parts—(a) insurance of adequate blood oxygenation and gas exchange to prevent irreversible tissue damage and (b) adequate blood perfusion of vital organs, dependent upon a functional heart rate, rhythm and stroke volume. The body's reserve capacity for survival following cessation of either or both of these functions is consumed rapidly; therefore, resuscitation measures must be started immediately.

11–1. ARTIFICIAL VENTILATION

EXPIRED AIR METHODS

Mouth-to-mouth

1. Remove obstructing substances (blood, food, mucus, dentures) from the mouth with fingers or handkerchief.

2. Place one hand under the nape of the neck and hyperextend it as far as it will go (unless there is evidence of severe neck injury). This will bring the tongue and lower jaw forward and open the airway (Fig. 1).

3. Place the opposite hand on the patient's forehead, pressing down, compressing the nostrils with the fingers. Take a deep breath; then breathe directly between the patient's lips. The lips

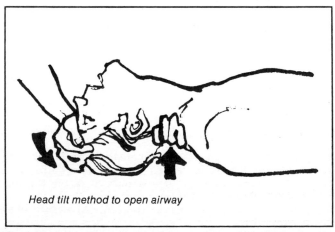

Head tilt method to open airway

Figure 1. Mouth-to-mouth artificial ventilation. Reprinted with permission of the American Heart Association, Inc.

must form an airtight seal. Watch the chest for adequate expansion (Fig. 2).

4. Allow the patient to exhale.

5. Repeat every 4 to 5 seconds for an adult, slightly faster for a child. Regular rhythm is not as important as adequate ventilation volume per minute.

6. In a small child, cover the mouth and nose with lips and blow into them very gently.

Mouth-to-nose

Same as mouth-to-mouth (above) except that the mouth is held closed with the fingers of one hand and air is blown into the nostrils.

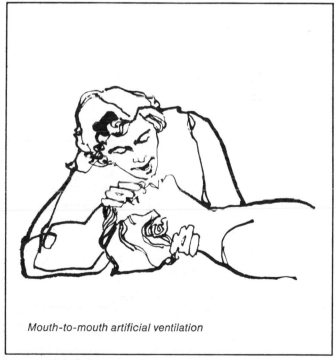

Mouth-to-mouth artificial ventilation

Figure 2. Mouth-to-mouth artificial ventilation. Reprinted with permission of the American Heart Association, Inc.

11−1. ARTIFICIAL VENTILATION

Mouth-to-airway
Proceed as for mouth-to-mouth; make seal of patient's lips around tube as tight as possible. (Not preferred because of air leakage at mouth around tube.)

Mouth-to-mask
Success depends upon holding the mask firmly in place and keeping the airway patent.

Advantages of Expired Air Methods
These expired air methods have the following advantages over manual push-pull techniques (Schaefer, Sylvester, Holger-Nielsen, etc.):

1. Better pulmonary ventilation—enough to sustain life.

2. The rescuer's hands are free to extend the head and pinch off the nostrils.

3. Special positioning is not necessary; therefore, expired air respiration can be performed in cramped or unusual circumstances —for instance, while bringing a drowning victim to shore, or treating a patient in the upright position (i.e., electrical linemen).

4. The presence of an obstruction can be recognized. If it is impossible to force air in, an obstruction in the upper respiratory tract is present.

5. Can be used in the presence of fractures of the upper extremities or thorax.

MANUAL METHODS

All of the well-known manual methods (Schaefer, Sylvester, Holger-Nielsen) are inefficient and unsatisfactory and do not supply enough ventilation to sustain life. The only exception is in infants in whom the Richard prone-tilting visceral shift "teeter board" method is of value.

TECHNIQUE

1. Place the infant face down on the operator's supinated forearm flexed to 90 degrees at the elbow.

2. Insert the middle finger in the mouth to insure a clear airway by holding the tongue down and the jaw forward. The remaining digits should be pressed against the infant's face for stability.

3. Hold the infant on the forearm with the opposite hand.

4. Alternately extend to 180 degrees and flex the arm to 90 degrees at the elbow. The weight of the infant's abdominal organs will result in enough tidal air flow to insure aeration of the lungs and prevent irreversible central nervous system changes from hypoxia.

MECHANICAL METHODS

1. Face mask and rebreathing bag (air or oxygen) (Fig. 3).

2. Oxygen under intermittent positive pressure by face mask or endotracheal catheter and rebreathing bag (Fig. 3).

3. Intermittent pressure ventilatory apparatus (Bennett, Bird, Ohio 560, Emerson, etc.). These types of equipment can be used

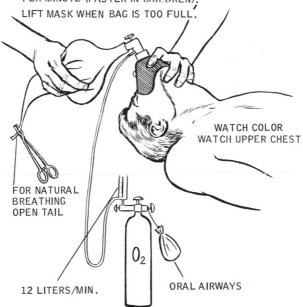

BAG-MASK-OXYGEN RESPIRATION

REMOVE EXCESSIVE MUCUS.
PLACE MASK SNUGLY OVER MOUTH AND NOSE.
SUPPORT ANGLES OF JAW - TILT HEAD BACK.
SQUEEZE BAG INTERMITTENTLY 10 TO 12 TIMES
PER MINUTE (FASTER IN CHILDREN).
LIFT MASK WHEN BAG IS TOO FULL.

WATCH COLOR
WATCH UPPER CHEST

FOR NATURAL
BREATHING
OPEN TAIL

O₂

12 LITERS/MIN.

ORAL AIRWAYS

Figure 3. Bag-mask-oxygen respiration. (Adapted from Safar, P., and McMahon, M. C.: *Resuscitation of the Unconscious Victim—A Manual for Rescue Breathing.* 2nd ed. Springfield, Illinois: Charles C Thomas, 1961.)

when external cardiac compression is being administered; however, it is easier to coordinate resuscitation with an Ambu or similar type of bag.

4. Coordinated intermittent positive pressure apparatus and external cardiac compression apparatus now available offer the best method for sustaining combined mechanical ventilation and cardiac resuscitation.

11−2. CARDIAC COMPRESSION (See also 26−7. Cardiac Arrest)

CLOSED CHEST (EXTERNAL) CARDIAC COMPRESSION

1. Start with three rapid effective artificial ventilations (11−1), demonstrated by inspiratory filling of the upper chest. The patient should be supine on a hard surface. If the patient must remain in bed, a bed board should be slid under him. For the resuscitating individual to perform with adequate technique and effective pressure, he must kneel at the patient's side.

2. Check the size of the pupils; even under powerful miotic drugs such as morphine the pupils dilate with inadequate oxygenation of the brain.

3. Check the pulse. (Palpation of the carotid or femoral arteries is most convenient.)

4. Strike the left upper chest forcibly with the closed fist. This precordial thump takes little time and on rare occasions has resulted in resumption of a normal heart beat, especially in victims of electric shock (29−5).

5. Call for help as loudly and as frequently as can reasonably be expected to bring assistance while instituting the following:

6. Start cardiac compression by placing the heel of one palm over the distal (inferior) portion of the body of the sternum, avoiding the xiphoid process. Cover this hand crosswise with the heel of the other hand and exert forcible downward pressure. Keep the fingers and elbows straight; let the shoulders and body weight do the work. Pressure (usually amounting to 60 to 120 pounds for an average sized adult) should be applied with a forceful thrust, followed by a quick release. In children and infants, pressure should be made with less force by placing the hands near the center of the sternum and using the fingers only.*

---

*Prior practice with a manikin such as ResusciAnn (available through local chapters of the American Heart Association) will give the operator a greater appreciation of proper technique and desired pressures.

7. Repeat chest compression at a rate not less than 60 times per minute. Repeat the series of 2 expired air ventilations and 15 closed chest massages 4 times per minute.

8. Check the skin color, pulse and pupillary size. If deterioration (cyanosis and dilating pupils) is occurring, review the technique of resuscitation carefully. When the first assistant (Resuscitator #2) arrives, he makes sure that more help is on the way and assists Resuscitator #1 in heart-lung resuscitation. When Resuscitator #3 arrives, he relieves Resuscitator #1, who then administers intravenous sodium bicarbonate and starts an intravenous portal, preferably with a catheter device, and an infusion of 5% dextrose in water.

9. Use defibrillator as soon as available. For technique see page 44.

10. Inject sodium bicarbonate solution (3.75 gm. in 50 ml. of solution) intravenously and repeat immediately or in 5 minutes and then every 10 minutes to combat rapidly developing metabolic acidosis. Use 25 ml. doses in children and 10 to 15 ml. doses in infants.

11. Inject 2 to 10 ml. of 1:10,000 epinephrine hydrochloride (Adrenalin) intravenously and repeat every 5 to 10 minutes as necessary.

12. Recheck the pulse and pupils. Determine heart action clinically and confirm by cardiac monitor electrocardiographic tracing.

External manual cardiac compression and efficient ventilation may result in restoration of an adequate heartbeat without further measures. If this does not occur, continuation of adequate ventilatory assistance and external manual cardiac compression by the previously outlined techniques will allow time for arrival of additional assistance, special apparatus, instruments and consultation.

If the heart is in standstill (by electrocardiographic determination)

1. Continue external cardiac compression, ventilation and general measures as previously outlined. Inject 5 ml. of 1:10,000 epinephrine hydrochloride (Adrenalin) intravenously every 5 to 10 minutes. Larger doses may be given if necessary. If a well running intravenous catheter has been placed and adequate cardiac compression has been instituted, the intravenous route has the advantage over intracardiac injection of not interfering with external cardiac compression.

2. Inject sodium bicarbonate (3.75 gm. in 50 ml. of solution) intravenously; repeat immediately or in 5 minutes and then every 10 minutes as long as electrical standstill persists.

3. Reinforce a feeble heart beat with synchronized manual com-

pression every 3rd or 4th beat as required. External or intracardiac pacing may be of value.

If the heart is fibrillating (as suspected clinically or determined by electrocardiographic monitoring)

1. Inject epinephrine hydrochloride (Adrenalin) intravenously as outlined previously. Larger doses are indicated if the quality of fibrillation potentials is weak.

2. Continue external cardiac compression, ventilation by expired air or mechanical methods and intravenous sodium bicarbonate injections as outlined previously until the defibrillator is ready and between attempts at defibrillation.

3. Adjust the defibrillator controls for external defibrillation, using the setting recommended by the manufacturer. For alternating current (A.C.), this is usually 440 to 880 volts (220 volts for children) for 0.25 seconds, repeated as often as necessary; for direct current (D.C.), which is preferred, use 100 to 400 watt-seconds (joules). Begin with 400 watt-seconds for an average adult. If the patient has been on digitalis therapy, a lower initial voltage or watt-seconds is recommended.

4. Apply electrolyte jelly (*not* K-Y jelly) to the paddle electrodes and to the patient's chest (Fig. 4). Press the electrodes firmly in place, one over the apex of the heart and the other over the right

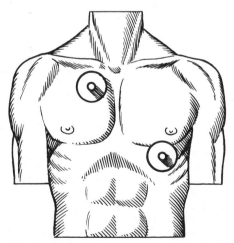

Figure 4. Position of paddle electrodes for countershock.

parasternal 2nd interspace. Too much electrolyte jelly may cause the current to jump from paddle to paddle, with resultant burns. Stand clear of the patient and the bed. Make sure that any assistants do likewise.

5. Press the switch for defibrillation charge and evaluate results; repeat 2 or 3 times within 15 to 20 seconds. Increase the voltage or watt-seconds if less than maximum was used initially.

6. Check results by palpation of the carotid or femoral pulse or by monitor. Between shocks, resume cardiac compression, artificial ventilation and intravenous sodium bicarbonate as indicated.

7. Give 50 to 100 mg. (5 to 10 ml. of 1% solution) of lidocaine (Xylocaine) intravenously; follow in 3 minutes by a 400 watt-second direct current shock. Procainamide (Pronestyl) (100 mg., intravenously) or quinidine gluconate (100 mg., intravenously) may be used instead of lidocaine.

8. Add 200 mg. metaraminol bitartrate (Aramine) or 8 ml. levarterenol bitartrate (Levophed) to 500 ml. of 5% dextrose in water and give intravenously by rapid drip. Check if it is time to repeat intravenous sodium bicarbonate (10 minute schedule).

9. Repeat 400 watt-second shock.

10. Inject 2 to 5 ml. of 1:10,000 solution of epinephrine hydrochloride (Adrenalin) intravenously every 5 to 10 minutes.

11. Repeat 400 watt-second shock.

12. Inject 5 ml. of 10% calcium chloride solution intravenously or directly into the heart.

13. Repeat 400 watt-second shock.

14. Check if it is time to repeat intravenous epinephrine hydrochloride and sodium bicarbonate (10 minute schedule).

The steps outlined above should be continued for 1 hour or longer, depending on developments. A fibrillating heart is a strong heart, with a much better chance of recovery than an asystolic heart. Ventricular fibrillation is a more common cause of cardiac arrest than cardiac standstill.

Successful resuscitation after cardiac arrest requires a combination of the following factors:

Prompt institution of corrective measures.

Adequate pulmonary ventilation.

Adequate coronary artery flow and adequate perfusion of vital organs with oxygenated blood.

Adequate correction of acidosis and electrolyte imbalance.

Adequate defibrillating current for an effective time with good skin contact of the electrodes with the chest.

Restoration of a functional cardiac rate, rhythm and stroke volume, with assistance of an artificial pacemaker if necessary. When functional rhythm, rate and stroke volume have been established, supportive cardiac compression and artificial ventilation as needed should be continued for at least 5 minutes more. At the end of this period, the following measures to facilitate recovery can be begun:

Determination and treatment of the cause of cardiac arrest (**26−7**); further treatment of shock (**53−7**).

Intravenous supportive or replacement therapy (**6.** *Fluid Replacement in Emergencies;* **14−13.** *Transfusions*) based on frequent arterial pH, blood gas and electrolyte determinations.

Vasopressor drugs if indicated for hypotension.

Continuous electrocardiographic monitoring.

Cardiac pacemaker (external or intracardiac via intravenous route) on operative or standby basis is indicated with 2nd and 3rd degree atrioventricular (A-V) blocks and some sinus rhythms with intraventricular block.

Resuscitative measures should cease if after 1 hour the pupils are widely dilated and the electrocardiograph reveals either no activity or progressive decrease in amplitude and widening of the QRS ventricular fibrillation pattern.

OPEN CHEST (DIRECT) CARDIAC COMPRESSION

Since the cardiac output obtained by external cardiac compression is, for practical purposes, as good as that obtained by direct open chest compression, there are few indications for the open chest procedure. However, among these are:

1. If the patient is in the operating room under anesthesia when the arrest occurs and the surgeon in charge and his surgical team are familiar with the technique of open cardiac massage.

2. If the chest has already been opened for some operative procedure.

3. Presence of chest wall fractures or restricting deformities.

11−3. HEART-LUNG RESUSCITATION BY A SINGLE INDIVIDUAL (Fig. 5)

1. Expired air ventilation (**11−1**), 3 times immediately.

2. Closed chest cardiac compression (**11−2**), 15 times (rate of 80 times per minute).

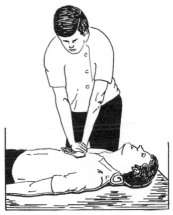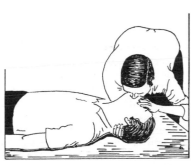

Figure 5. Heart-lung resuscitation by one individual.

3. Expired air ventilation (**11 – 1**), 2 times (rate of 8 times per minute).

4. Alternate steps 2 and 3 above at the same ratio, 4 times per minute, shifting from the same kneeling position until assistance is available or until spontaneous and stable circulation and ventilation has been reestablished. This procedure is rapidly fatiguing for a single resuscitator.

HEART-LUNG RESUSCITATION BY TWO INDIVIDUALS (Fig. 6)

1. Expired air ventilation (**11 – 1**), rapidly 3 times immediately by Resuscitator #1.

2. Closed chest cardiac compression (**11 – 2**), continuously at a rate of 1 per second by Resuscitator #2.

3. Expired air ventilation by Resuscitator #1, once between every fifth cardiac compression maneuver.

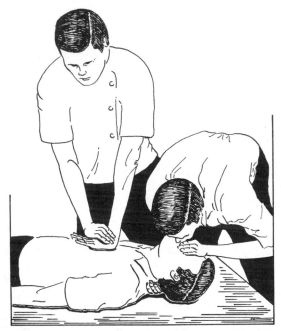

Figure 6. Heart-lung resuscitation by two individuals.

12. SERUM SENSITIVITY AND DESENSITIZATION

Although hypersensitivity of the skin to animal serum does not necessarily parallel systemic hypersensitivity, intradermal (intracutaneous) skin tests should always be done before injections of antisera of any type are given. The injection must be made into, and not through, the skin and must not draw blood. A syringe containing 1 ml. of 1:1000 epinephrine hydrochloride (Adrenalin) should be available for immediate use; deaths have occurred from anaphylactic reactions (**21—1**) to diluted antitoxin used for skin tests. Ophthalmic tests for sensitivity to antisera should never be used — severe reactions may result in permanent eye damage. Scratch tests are of no value.

If an indurated wheal (with or without pseudopods) is present 20 minutes after intradermal (intracutaneous) injection of 0.1 ml. of 1:10 dilution, the test should be considered as positive and the need for passive protection by antitoxin should be reevaluated very carefully. If indicated, the following desensitization procedure should be carried out as a considered risk:

Inject	0.01 ml. of antitoxin subcutaneously
20 minutes later	0.02 ml. of antitoxin subcutaneously
20 minutes later	0.04 ml. of antitoxin subcutaneously
20 minutes later	0.10 ml. of antitoxin subcutaneously
20 minutes later	0.25 ml. of antitoxin subcutaneously
20 minutes later	0.58 ml. of antitoxin subcutaneously
Total	1.00 ml.

Twenty minutes later 1 ml. of antitoxin may be injected subcutaneously or intramuscularly, accompanied by 0.5 to 1 ml. of a 1:1000 solution of epinephrine hydrochloride (Adrenalin) subcutaneously.

Following this desensitization procedure, large amounts of antisera can be given with relative safety provided no local erythema, urticaria, asthmatic breathing, nausea, vomiting or chills have occurred. If such reactions do develop at any time during the procedure outlined above, the last dose should be repeated after a 20 minute wait; two reactions make further attempts at administration of the particular antiserum (usually equine or bovine) inadvisable. Similar skin testing with available antisera derived from other animals (i.e., bovine instead of equine, etc.) may be practical. As an alternative, bicillin and tetracycline therapy have been reported as effective. Human tetanus immune globulin (TIG) should always be used in place of tetanus antitoxin (**16.** *Tetanus Immunization*).

Oral administration of an antihistaminic (preferably in sustained action form) at the time the antitoxin is given and daily for 10 days thereafter may prevent, or decrease the severity of, serum sickness (**21–4**).

13. SUICIDE

All cases of attempted or successful suicide are reportable to the closest law enforcement agency. Any physician called upon to examine or treat this type of case should protect the hospital emergency department and himself by reporting any cases in which, in his opinion, self-destruction may have been attempted through asphyxiation, drowning, falls, poisoning, shooting, lacerations or other means. ANY PERSON KNOWN TO HAVE ATTEMPTED SUICIDE, OR SUSPECTED OF THE ATTEMPT, SHOULD BE KEPT UNDER CLOSE OBSERVATION WITH A PHYSICALLY ABLE ATTENDANT IN THE ROOM AT ALL TIMES WHILE HE IS UNDER EMERGENCY MEDICAL CARE.

If toxic substances in any form are known or suspected as the means of attempted suicide, ALL BODY CAVITIES ACCESSIBLE TO THE PATIENT (especially the rectum and vagina) SHOULD BE EXAMINED AS SOON AS POSSIBLE AND EMPTIED IF INDICATED. A specimen of any suspect material obtained from each site (including the stomach and bladder)—as well as a blood specimen—should be collected and placed in a labeled container for possible later toxicologic examination and identification. Blood alcohol level should be determined routinely.

For suicidal tendencies, see **50—2.** *Psychogenic Psychoses.*

14. SURGICAL AND EMERGENCY PROCEDURES AND TECHNIQUES

14—1. ARTIFICIAL RESPIRATION

For expired air, manual and mechanical methods, see **11—1.**

14—2. CARDIAC COMPRESSION

For closed chest (external) and open chest (internal) cardiac compression, see **11—2.**

14—3. CATHERIZATION (Bladder)

Insertion of any type of tube into the bladder invites infection; therefore, a clean catch or second glass specimen should usually be used for routine diagnostic purposes. If acute retention (**38—19**) or need for determination of kidney function (**53—5**. *Determination of Severity of Shock*) requires catheterization, careful sterile technique should be used.

MALE

1. Cleanse the penis thoroughly with soap and water and place on a sterile towel.
2. Put on sterile gloves.
3. Insert a sterile catheter by using gentle, steady pressure and holding the dorsum of the penis upward toward the abdominal wall to straighten the urethral curve.
4. If obstruction is encountered so that the bladder cannot be entered on two or three gentle attempts, or if there is bleeding, a sedative should be given and the patient referred for urologic care. If bladder distention is acute and urologic care is not immediately available, the bladder can be decompressed by inserting a 3 inch No. 18 needle with stylet suprapubically in the midline, using sterile technique. This is a relatively simple and safe procedure which can be repeated as often as necessary.

FEMALE

In female patients, catheterization can be done easily, preferably by a nurse, using a sterile nonbreakable catheter.

14—4. GASTRIC LAVAGE

When emetics are ineffective or contraindicated, washing the stomach may be necessary. Since the object of lavage is rapid, complete emptying of the stomach, as large a tube as possible should be used. Even small children will tolerate passage through the mouth of relatively large tubes. Attempted lavage through an intranasal tube is utterly unsatisfactory. A CHILD MUST BE MUMMIFIED BY BEING WRAPPED TIGHTLY IN A SHEET AND PLACED ON HIS BACK WITH THE HEAD TURNED TO ONE SIDE AND THE HIPS SLIGHTLY ELEVATED. The lavage tube should be smooth and well lubricated with a water-soluble preparation. A large syringe or funnel or an irrigating can suspended above the patient's head and equipped with a two way stopcock is satisfactory for introduction of the solution. Repeated washings with small amounts of solution should be done until the return solution is clear. Overfilling of the stomach should be avoided because of the danger of regurgitation and aspiration. The tube should be pinched off, or gentle suction retained, during removal to prevent aspiration. In cases of suspected or known poisoning, a specimen of vomitus or stomach washings should be collected, marked for identification and saved for possible later analysis.

14—5. INTRAGLOSSAL INJECTIONS

In unconscious patients whose veins are collapsed or impossible to locate without a cutdown, a small amount (up to 2 ml.) of a vasopressor drug injected into the tongue is rapidly absorbed without residual ill effects. Enough effect can usually be obtained to allow location of a peripheral vein for conventional venous infusion.

TECHNIQUE
1. Grasp the tongue by the tip and pull it upward toward the nose.
2. Using a short bevel, 20 or 22 gauge needle, inject the solution into the muscles on the underside of the base of the tongue, avoiding the large veins on each side of the midline.
3. Only rapidly absorbable, nonirritating medications should be used except as a lifesaving measure.

14—6. NASAL PACKING

ANTERIOR

Several methods are satisfactory. Topical anesthesia often is required.
1. Pack tightly with petrolatum gauze.
2. Pack firmly with a gauze strip moistened with 1:1000 epinephrine hydrochloride (Adrenalin).
3. Fill a rubber finger cot or glove finger loosely with gauze and insert into the nostril; then moisten the gauze. The resultant swelling of the gauze will cause uniform and even pressure. Medicated gauze (especially iodoform gauze) should not be used for nasal packing.

POSTERIOR (NASOPHARYNGEAL)

Gauze Packing

1. Give a preliminary injection of morphine sulfate to older children and adults to allay apprehension. A pentobarbital sodium (Nembutal) suppository should be substituted in children under 10 years of age. Topical anesthesia may be indicated in hypersensitive persons.

2. Pass a small, soft rubber catheter through a nostril and into the pharynx.

3. Grasp the slotted end of the catheter with forceps and bring it out through the mouth.

4. Attach to the slotted end of the catheter the ends of a 12 inch length of No. 30 or No. 40 cotton suture to the middle of which is fastened a piece of soft, nonmedicated selvage-edged gauze attached to another 12 inch length of cotton suture.

5. Pull the gauze gently but firmly into the posterior nares by withdrawing the catheter through the nose.

6. Unfasten the catheter and tie the cotton ligatures extruding from the nostril and mouth loosely together over a piece of gauze placed on the upper lip below the nostrils, avoiding pressure on the columella. Tape the mouth string to the side of the cheek.

7. Hospitalize for observation. Evaluate for coagulation disorders.

Insertion of a Foley catheter with filling of the tip reservoir with saline and application of gentle traction.

14—7.   PERICARDIAL SAC ASPIRATION (See also 26—15. Pericardial Effusion)

The only equipment needed for this procedure, which may be lifesaving if cardiac tamponade (**26—22**) is present, is a 3 inch or 4 inch 18 gauge short-beveled hypodermic needle and a medium Luer syringe. (For electrocardiographic monitoring for position of the needle tip, see **26—15.** Pericardial Effusion)

SITES OF ASPIRATION (In order of desirability)

1. Slightly to the left of the xiphoid process of the sternum with the needle directed superiorly and posteriorly.

2. Through the left fourth interspace ½ inch to the left of the sternocostal junction.

3. Through the posterior chest slightly to the right of the inferior angle of the left scapula. This method transverses the lung and should not be used if there is any possibility of pericardial sac empyema.

TECHNIQUE

1. Cleanse the selected area thoroughly with soap and water and pHisoHex and paint with Ioprep.

2. Insert a short-beveled 3 inch long 18 gauge needle attached to a 10 or 20 ml. syringe through the chest wall into the pericardial sac and aspirate gently. Either fresh or defibrinated blood may be obtained. Relief from tamponade may be obtained from removal of as little as 5 ml. The procedure may be repeated as often as necessary for relief, but immediate thoracotomy is indicated if aspiration gives no relief, if no blood is obtained or if signs and symptoms of tamponade recur in spite of repeated aspirations.

14-8. PERITONEAL ASPIRATION

With a small (No. 22) abdominal paracentesis trocar with obturator or a large bore spinal puncture or thoracotomy needle with stylet, abdominal aspiration can be performed safely and easily. The urinary bladder should be empty. This is a valuable diagnostic procedure, especially in abdominal contusions (**55-1**). Fresh blood is usually an indication for immediate exploratory laparotomy. For the technique of insertion of a trocar, see **14-9**.

14-9. PERITONEAL DIALYSIS

This very simple procedure is of great value in the treatment of certain types of poisoning (**49-3**. *General Principles of Treatment of Poisoning*) and in systemic diseases such as hepatic coma (**29-10**).

TECHNIQUE (See Fig. 7)

1. Prepare a site on the abdomen by shaving and by presurgical skin preparation. The patient should be supine and in bed. The site of choice is in the midline 4 cm. below the umbilicus. Any scarred areas should be avoided because of the probability of adjacent intra-abdominal adhesions. The urinary bladder should be empty.

2. After anesthetizing the area, insert a No. 22 paracentesis trocar through a stab wound. In the absence of ascites, 500 ml. of

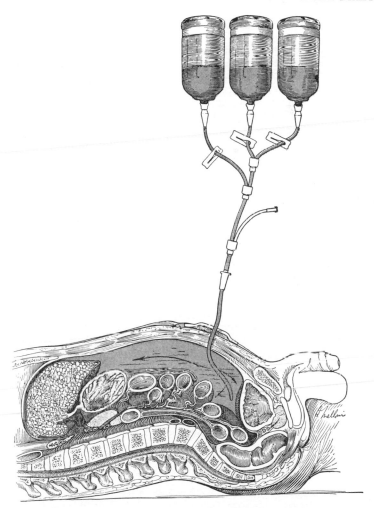

Figure 7. The position of the peritoneal dialysis tube in the pelvis and the method of attachment of three intravenous bottles are demonstrated. Dialysis fluid shown in gray. (Modified from Palmer, E.: Amer. Family Physician, Vol. 4, No. 3, 1963.)

air should be injected preliminarily; if there is ascites, this is not necessary.

3. Push the trocar with the obturator in place through the peritoneum; remove the obturator and substitute a previously prepared dialysis tube—a 12 inch section of plastic intravenous tubing with elliptical holes cut at frequent intervals in the distal 4 inches is satisfactory. Gently work the dialysis tube into the pelvis.

4. Remove the trocar and suture the skin around the dialysis tube.

5. Connect the dialysis tube to a piece of tubing at least 36 inches long. The tubing, in turn, should be connected through a three way stopcock or double Y connectors to three flasks containing the following solutions (if commercial dialysate solutions are not available):

Normal saline, 1000 ml.

Dextrose, 5% in water, 1000 ml.

Sodium bicarbonate (100 ml. of 10% solution) in 1000 ml. of 5% dextrose in saline.

(Potassium, 5 mEq./liter, is added or deleted according to the clinical problem.)

6. With the solution bottles elevated on an intravenous stand, adjust the flow so that $1\frac{1}{4}$ to $1\frac{1}{2}$ hours are required for all to empty into the abdomen. (Two liters of commercial dialysate solution may be substituted for the solutions specified above and used according to the manufacturer's directions.)

7. When about 20 ml. remain in each bottle, remove them from the intravenous stand and place them on the floor and allow the fluid from the abdomen to run out by gravity.

8. Collect specimens of fluid for analysis as required.

9. Substitute new solution bottles and elevate to the intravenous stand.

10. Repeat the procedure above as needed, governed by the patient's clinical condition and analysis of the returned dialysis fluid.

11. Keep an accurate input-output record.

14—10. REDUCTION OF DISLOCATIONS

ACROMIOCLAVICULAR DISLOCATIONS See **44—8.**

ANKLE DISLOCATIONS See **44—9.**

CARPAL DISLOCATIONS See **40—6; 44—16; 44—19.**

CERVICAL SPINE DISLOCATIONS See **44—58; 46—8; 46—11.**

ELBOW DISLOCATIONS See **44 – 12; 44 – 21.**

EPIPHYSEAL DISLOCATIONS See **44 – 30.**

FINGER DISLOCATIONS See **44 – 20.**

HIP DISLOCATIONS

Hip dislocations are difficult to reduce and usually require hospitalization for general anesthesia. Open operation may be necessary.

JAW DISLOCATIONS See **44 – 26.**

LUNATE DISLOCATIONS See **44 – 16.**

NASAL BONE AND CARTILAGE DISLOCATIONS See **45 – 4.**

PATELLAR DISLOCATIONS See **44 – 18.**

PERILUNAR DISLOCATIONS See **44 – 19.**

PHALANGEAL DISLOCATIONS See **44 – 20.**

RADIAL HEAD SUBLUXATIONS See **44 – 21.**

SHOULDER DISLOCATIONS

All persons with known or suspected shoulder dislocation should be checked carefully before and after reduction for evidence of nerve and/or blood vessel pressure and for fractures around the glenoid.

Arm-weight Traction Method (Stimson)

1. After preliminary administration of morphine sulfate, place the patient face down on a narrow examination table with the arm on the injured side hanging down.

2. Make prolonged firm gentle traction on the wrist with gentle external rotation. If after 15 to 20 minutes reduction has not been accomplished, other methods should be tried, with hospitalization for reduction under general anesthesia if the heel-in-axilla and Kocher's methods are unsuccessful.

Heel-in-Axilla Method

With the victim and operator lying recumbent on the floor and the emergency physician's heel in the axilla as a fulcrum, reduction can be often be accomplished by prolonged traction and manipulation. If two attempts are unsuccessful, refer for hospitalization and reduction under general anesthesia.

Kocher's Method

The maneuvers described below should be done extremely gently —forcible manipulation may cause additional damage around the shoulder joint and is never justified. If gentle manipulation is not successful, the patient should be referred for reduction under general anesthesia.

1. Relaxation of the muscles around the shoulder by firm gentle traction on the elbow with lateral pressure on the humeral head.
2. Adduction of the elbow with slow forcible external rotation of the forearm.
3. Slow internal rotation of the forearm with the elbow held close to the body until the hand is on the opposite shoulder.
4. Confirmation of reduction by x-ray or fluoroscopic examination (**18**).
5. Application of a snug Velpeau bandage.

SPINAL DISLOCATIONS See **44−11.** *Cervical Spine Dislocations;* **44−58.** *Neck Injuries*

STERNOCLAVICULAR DISLOCATIONS See **44−24.**

TARSAL DISLOCATIONS See **44−25.**

TEMPOROMANDIBULAR DISLOCATIONS See **44−26.**

TOE DISLOCATIONS See **44−27.**

14−11. SPINAL PUNCTURE

Although spinal puncture usually has no use as a therapeutic measure in emergency situations, it is a valuable diagnostic adjunct in conditions in which intracranial or spinal cord disease is suspected. The principal contraindication is evidence of increased intracranial pressure thought to be due to an intracranial mass (unless preparations have been made for immediate remedial surgery). Spinal puncture is necessary in the presence of acute fulminating infections with signs of meningeal irritation so that the offending organism can be identified and prompt treatment begun (**30−16.** *Meningitis;* **48−42.** *Meningococcemia in Children;* **48−63.** *Waterhouse-Friderichsen Syndrome*).

Technique

1. Place the patient on his side with the knees drawn up to decrease the normal lumbar lordosis and spread the spinous processes.

2. Scrub the skin over the full width of the back from the lower thoracic to midsacral area with pHisoHex, paint with Ioprep and drape.

3. Inject a local anesthetic into the space between the spinous processes of the 4th and 5th lumbar vertebrae. The space between the 3rd and 4th vertebrae may be used in adults but not in infants and children.

4. Insert a short-beveled No. 22 spinal puncture needle between the spinous processes in the midline with the obturator in place, keeping the bevel of the needle in the plane of the long axis of the body to minimize dural tears (see **27—28.** *Spinal Puncture Headaches*). A definite resistance will be felt as the tip of the needle passes through the dura.

5. Remove the obturator stylet, connect the manometer and record the initial cerebrospinal fluid pressure in millimeters.

6. Collect a total of 5 to 6 ml. of cerebrospinal fluid in three sterile vials and observe for color, viscosity and translucency. Send the collected specimens at once to the laboratory for necessary tests — for example, cell count (RBCs, WBCs and differential), smears for microorganisms, cultures and sensitivity tests, chemistry [chlorides (as NaCl), glucose and total proteins] and Kolmer complement fixation test.

7. Note variation in the manometer column with respiration.

8. Test for evidence of block by the Queckenstedt maneuver if spinal subarachnoid block is suspected.

9. Record the final manometric pressure in millimeters of CSF.

10. Disconnect manometer and remove needle gently. Apply a sterile pad over the puncture site.

11. If signs and symptoms of acute meningeal irritation are present and the spinal fluid is grossly purulent, start massive systemic antibacterial therapy and symptomatic and supportive care at once without waiting for laboratory results (**30—16.** *Meningitis;* **48—42.** *Meningococcemia in Children;* **48—63.** *Waterhouse-Friderichsen Syndrome*). Do a gram stain at once as a guide to therapy.

12. Keep the patient prone for one hour to minimize gravity seepage of cerebrospinal fluid. If postpuncture cephalgia develops (incidence, 10–20%), treat as outlined under **27—28.** *Spinal Puncture Headaches.*

CEREBROSPINAL FLUID – NORMAL VALUES

Amount (adults)	100–140 cc.
Appearance	Clear, colorless
Pressure (on side, relaxed)*	
Newborn	30–80 mm. of CSF
Children	50–100 mm. of CSF
Adults	70–200 mm. of CSF
Specific gravity	1.003–1.009
pH	7.35–7.40
Total cell count	
Infants	0–20 per cu. mm. (no PMNs)
Adults	0–10 per cu. mm. (no PMNs)
Proteins, total	20–45 mg. %
Glucose	50–75 mg. %
Chlorides (as NaCl)	120–130 mEq./L.

*Apprehension, excitement, straining, crying or excessive flexion of the neck or trunk may give above normal readings which should not be interpreted as indicating organic disease.

14 – 12. TRACHEOSTOMY

INDICATIONS

1. Emergency bypass or removal of airway obstruction not attainable by other methods.

2. Need for prolonged ventilatory assistance (many times an endotracheal tube will suffice for 12 to 36 hours).

Tracheostomy May Be Necessary In:

Angioedema (**21 – 2.** *Allergic Reactions;* **48 – 4.** *Angioedema in Children*).

Burns (usually of the flash type with flame inhalation) (**25 – 18.** *Mucous Membrane Burns*).

Cerebral vascular accidents with respiratory muscle involvement (**59 – 2.** *Intracranial Bleeding*).

Debilitated and severely ill persons with impaired respiratory function (**29 – 6.** *Emphysema*).

Foreign bodies lodged above the second tracheal ring (**36 – 4; 48 – 29; 48 – 44**).

Laryngeal paralysis, bilateral (**30 – 4.** *Diphtheria*).

Poliomyelitis, bulbar type (**30 – 21; 46 – 9**).

Poisoning resulting in coma [**29 – 13; 49** (see names of poisons)].

Respiratory obstruction from any cause (**52.** *Respiratory Tract Conditions*).

Surgical procedures (repair of jaw injuries, neck dissections, etc.).
Tetanus (**30−31**).
Transverse myelitis, cervical, usually traumatic, high enough to
affect respiratory muscles (**46−9**).
Trauma
    Chest injuries (**28**).
    Facial injuries.
    Fractures and dislocations of the cervical spine with spinal cord
    injury (**46−11**).
    Head injuries (**41; 48−32.** *Head Injuries in Children*).
    Soft tissue injuries of the throat and neck with resultant
    edema (**44−58.** *Neck Injuries;* **55−38.** *Tracheobronchial Injuries*).

METHODS

Cricothyroid Membrane Puncture

This procedure may be a lifesaving measure and can be done with
any sharp instrument, such as sharp-pointed scissors, knife blade
or nail file. It must be supplanted by a regular tracheostomy within
2 days.

1. Locate the space between the two most prominent cartilages
with the neck slightly hyperextended.

2. Make a 1 inch transverse incision in the soft space between
the cartilages. This incision should go through the skin only (Figs.
8 and 9).

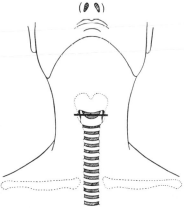

Figure 8. Drawing of cricothyroid membrane. Solid line shows incision. (Nicholas, T. H.,
and Rumer, G. F.: J.A.M.A., Vol. 179:1933, 1960.)

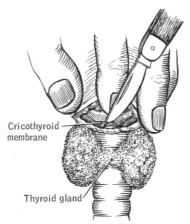

Cricothyroid membrane

Thyroid gland

Figure 9. Cricothyroid membrane puncture. To establish an emergency airway, a 1-inch transverse skin incision is made over the cricothyroid membrane. The larynx is stabilized between the thumb and middle finger on the left hand. A sharp instrument is then passed along the nail of the index finger, which is pressed firmly into the membrane. (Modified from Nicholas, T. H., and Rumer, G. F.: Mod. Med., April 17, 1961.)

3. Stabilize the larynx between the left thumb and middle finger; press the index fingernail firmly into the exposed cricothyroid ligament.

4. Using the index fingernail as a guide and holding the instrument blade transversely, work the blade through the ligament and into the trachea (Fig. 9). Avoid excess pressure with damage to the posterior wall.

5. Spread by turning the blade through 90 degrees.

6. If necessary, substitute a key or pen barrel for the blade. DO NOT USE SMALL OBJECTS WHICH MIGHT BE ASPIRATED.

Low Tracheostomy (Method of choice)

1. Place the patient on his back with the neck slightly hyperextended by a support under the shoulders.

2. Under local anesthesia, make a longitudinal incision through the skin and subcutaneous tissue from below the cricoid to just above the sternal notch.

3. Separate the muscles by blunt dissection.

4. Locate the inferior border of cricoid with the finger trans-

versely. Avoid the inferior thyroid veins. If necessary, clamp, suture and retract the thyroid isthmus after cutting between clamps, exposing the 1st through 5th tracheal rings.

5. Incise the 3rd and 4th tracheal rings vertically and pick up the edges with hooks.

6. Insert the cannula followed by the inner tube. Complete hemostasis is important. If ventilatory assistance is required, use an inflatable cuffed tube.

7. Suture the upper angles of the wound loosely to allow escape of air.

8. Fasten the tapes snugly around the neck.

9. Arrange for tracheostomy care. Specific instructions regarding suction, aspiration of the bronchi and cleansing of the tube should be given (Figs. 10 and 11).

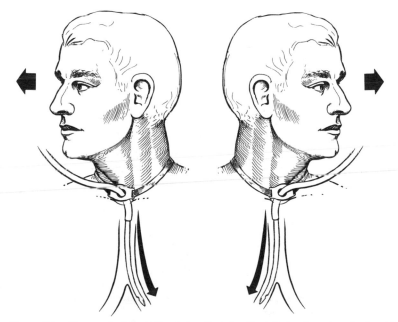

Figure 10. Placement of aspirating tube. To enter the left stem bronchus, the head is turned sharply to the right and the chin elevated. Reverse the procedure to enter the right stem bronchus. (From Samson, P. C.: Hosp. Med., Vol. 1, No. 4, 1964.)

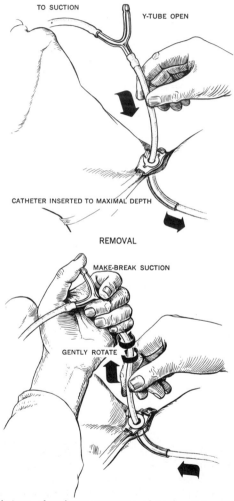

INSERTION

TO SUCTION

Y-TUBE OPEN

CATHETER INSERTED TO MAXIMAL DEPTH

REMOVAL

MAKE-BREAK SUCTION

GENTLY ROTATE

Figure 11. Technique of catheter aspiration of tracheostomy. (From Samson, P. C.: Hosp. Med., Vol. 1, No. 4, 1964.)

10. Check the position of the tracheostomy tube by fluoroscopy or x-ray when the patient's condition will permit.

14—13. TRANSFUSIONS

Transfusions of whole blood are the most efficient means of maintaining and increasing blood volume and oxygen-carrying ability, replacing toxic circulating blood and enhancing blood coagulation. In emergency situations, the urgency of the need for blood modifies the details of administration.

If immediate transfusion of blood is required

1. Collect 20 ml. of blood from the patient and send to the laboratory for possible future typing and cross-matching.

2. Give type O Rh negative (*universal donor*) bank (storage) blood by intravenous catheter, using a cutdown if necessary. The blood should be warmed to room temperature before infusion.

3. Use as many sites of injection as are necessary for the amount of blood required. Multiple sites are more effective and safer than attempted rapid injection at one site.

4. Use type O Rh negative blood for further emergency transfusions. After two weeks without transfusions, the patient should be typed and properly cross-matched blood given if necessary.

If transfusion can safely be delayed until the patient's blood can be typed and cross-matched (usually about 2 hours)

1. Before any plasma volume expander is given, collect 20 ml. of venous blood and send to the laboratory for immediate typing and cross-matching.

2. Give plasma volume expanders (Dextran, polyvinylpyrolidone) intravenously as required for circulatory support.

3. Substitute properly cross-matched blood for plasma volume expanders as soon as possible.

4. Use packed RBCs if severe anemia without hypovolemia is a primary problem.

Hazards of Blood Transfusions

Acidosis. The pH of bank (storage) blood varies from 6.4 to 7.2. This can be controlled by intravenous injection of 10 ml. of sodium bicarbonate solution (3.75 gm. in 50 ml. of solution).

Air Embolism. Sixty to 80 ml. of air is required to stop the heart — smaller amounts are usually well tolerated. Intra-arterial transfusions — the usual cause of massive air embolism — have an extremely limited place in the treatment of emergencies.

Allergic Reactions. See **21.**

Bacterial and Viral Contamination.

Citric Intoxication (see also **49—215.** *Citric Acid*). This occurs most frequently in exchange transfusions in erythroblastotic infants and can be prevented by intravenous administration of 10% calcium gluconate.

Hemolytic Reactions. Hemolytic reactions are usually dangerous only if more than 250 ml. of incompatible blood have been given. In all instances, the first 100 ml. of blood should be given under close observation. If there is evidence of hemolysis, the transfusion should be stopped at once and 100 ml. of 20% mannitol in water given intravenously followed by intravenous sodium bicarbonate solution and prednisone. Development of acute apprehension and/or low back—especially sacral—pain calls for immediate cessation of the transfusion.

Hypothermia. These reactions can be avoided by warming the blood to room temperature before and during administration.

Overtransfusions. Serial central venous pressure determinations may be of assistance in avoiding this rare problem.

Pyrogenic Reactions. Pyrogenic reactions are due to nonbacterial pyrogens and are characterized by a rapid temperature rise to 40°C. (104°F.). Full recovery in a short time is to be expected.

Runaway Catheters. See **36—9.** *Foreign Bodies in the Venous System.*

15. TESTS APPLICABLE TO EMERGENCY CASES

No attempt has been made in this section to list or describe the numerous clinical and laboratory tests which constitute an essential and invaluable part of efficient diagnosis, treatment and management of emergency cases. The tests outlined below, however, are peculiarly valuable in emergency situations, even though in some instances their interpretations may be suggestive and not conclusive.

15—1. ALCOHOL INTOXICATION TESTS

Measurements of the alcohol content of the breath, blood and urine can be made without difficulty and are of approximately equal accuracy. The admissibility of the results of chemical tests for alcohol as evidence in courts is becoming more widespread year by year. The results of breath analysis tests at the present time are not accepted as legal evidence in some localitities but may be of great value to law enforcement officers. Tests for alcohol content of the breath are often made by law enforcement officers without any signed authorization. Drawing of blood for determination of the alcohol level requires a signed and witnessed authorization (**69—4**). In many localities, refusal to submit to a breath, blood or urine alcohol test results in automatic revocation of the license to operate a motor vehicle.

BREATH ANALYSIS

Various modifications of 4 main types of breath analyzers are in common use. These types are the Breathalyzer (Borkenstein), the Drunkometer (Harger), the Intoximeter (Forrester) and the Alcometer (Greenberg). All 4 types depend upon the analysis of expired alveolar air collected in a plastic or rubber balloon. Breath forced into the balloon is generally considered to contain $5/8$ alveolar air and $3/8$ corridor air (from the nares, mouth and nasopharynx). Since the alveolar air-blood ratio for alcohol is known (about 1:2100) and the alveolar air contains about 5.5% carbon dioxide, by weighing the amount of carbon dioxide and determining the amount of alcohol in a given specimen, the blood alcohol concentration can be determined very accurately.

BLOOD ANALYSIS

All tests for alcohol in the blood depend upon a complex chemical analysis of blood obtained from a vein by a technique which avoids possible contamination with alcohol from outside sources.

Method of Obtaining Blood Specimen

1. On request of a patient, his legal guardian or a law enforcement officer, blood may be drawn by a physician for blood alcohol determination, provided the permission of the patient or his legal guardian is obtained in writing without misrepresentation or coercion. For a satisfactory permit form, see **69—4**. Before the permis-

sion is signed, the patient or his guardian should be informed in simple nontechnical language of the purpose of the test. It is the physician's responsibility to determine that the patient is sufficiently in possession of his faculties at the time of signature to understand the reason for, purpose of and possible consequences of the test. Tacit permission for withdrawal of blood for the test is assumed if the patient, after having been given the information above, makes no active attempt to prevent completion of the procedure.

2. No alcohol, or substance containing alcohol, can be used in cleansing the skin.

3. Syringes, needles and vials used in collecting the blood specimen must have been sterilized by a nonalcohol technique.

4. Special containers, marked for identification, must be used. These should be labeled carefully for identification and initialed by at least 2 witnesses before being sent to the laboratory for analysis.

5. The exact time that the specimen is taken should be indicated on the container.

CLINICAL EXAMINATION FOR ALCOHOLIC INTOXICATION

History and Habits

1. Occupation (deep-sea or sports diver, caisson worker, exposure to narcotic or inebriating gases at work, etc.).

2. Injuries or diseases which might modify interpretation of results of tests.

3. Medications, especially narcotics, hypnotics, sedatives, mood modifiers, muscle relaxants and antihistaminics.

4. Consumption of alcoholic beverages:
   Daily or periodic drinker.
   Average daily amount.
   Time, kind and amount of last drink.
   Companions or witnesses—name of bar, etc.

5. Treatment in past for acute or chronic alcoholism, delirium tremens, addiction to any substances or neuropsychiatric complaints.

Physical Examination

A fair and accurate conclusion regarding alcohol intoxication requires comparison of the original examination findings with the results of previous examination or of reexamination several hours later, preferably by the same physician. The following points should be covered:

1. Odor of alcoholic beverages on the breath. In spite of the claims of the manufacturers of various proprietary compounds, this odor cannot be masked or dissipated by any known method.

2. Red ("bloodshot") or watery eyes.

3. Impairment of speech (indistinctness, slurring).

4. Unbuttoned or disarrayed clothing.

5. Evidence of vomiting, bowel or bladder incontinence or seminal emission.

6. Mental alertness and attitude (euphoria, sullenness, belligerence, depressions, etc.).

7. Evidence of recent trauma — especially head injuries (**41**).

8. Muscular coordination

Gait — broad base, straddling, unsteady.

Balance — ability to walk a straight line and to execute rapid turns.

Joint sense — finger to nose or ear, foot to opposite knee, etc.

Specialized motions — picking up pins or coins, comparison of handwriting with previous or subsequent samples.

9. Evidence of unrelated injuries or of local or systemic conditions which could be mistaken for alcoholic intoxication.

INTERPRETATION OF RESULTS OF BLOOD ALCOHOL TESTS

PER CENT ALCOHOL IN BLOOD (by weight)	MILLIGRAMS OF ALCOHOL PER MILLILITER OF BLOOD	CLINICAL EFFECT (Average)	SLOWING OF REACTION TIME (Average)	LEGAL INTERPRETATION: UNDER INFLUENCE OF ALCOHOL?
0.01 to 0.05	10 mg./100 ml 50 mg./100 ml.	None	Possibly slight	No
0.06 to 0.10	60 mg./100 ml. 100 mg./100 ml.	Decreased coordination and visual fields, blurred vision, impaired control and restraint, euphoria, slurred speech, impairment of special senses	2 ×	Possibly
0.11 to 0.30	110 mg./100 ml. 300 mg./100 ml.	Staggering, mental confusion, stupor	4 ×	Definitely
0.31 to 0.45	310 mg./100 ml. 450 mg./100 ml.	Respiratory and circulatory impairment, subnormal temperature, coma, sometimes death	Total loss	Completely
0.46 up	460 mg./100 ml.	Complete respiratory and circulatory paralysis, death	Total loss	Irreversibly, often terminally

Modifying Factors

The amount of alcohol necessary to produce the different stages of alcoholism outlined above may be modified by:

1. Individual sensitivity (constitutional tolerance, age, sex).
2. Acquired tolerance (habituation).
3. Mental condition.
4. Environment and circumstances (climate, temperature, exercise, type of work).
5. Diet—recent intake of food.
6. Medications.
7. Unrelated organic pathology. Among these diseases and pathologic conditions are:

Metabolic disturbances such as diabetic hypoglycemia, acidosis, uremia, effects of increased barometric pressure, etc.

Pulmonary diseases, such as emphysema with carbon dioxide retention.

Myocardial infarction; angina pectoris.

Hypertension.

Senility.

Postsurgical and postanesthetic reactions.

Intracranial pathology.

15—2. CERVICAL SPINE INJURY TEST

Determination of the possibility of cervical spine injury in the presence of other injuries which may mask discomfort in the neck is often very important, since presence of cervical injuries makes modifications in handling and transportation essential. The patient must be conscious for this test to be of value. X-rays of the cervical spine (anteroposterior, lateral and obliques) should be taken at the earliest possible opportunity, using a portable machine if necessary.

1. Gently move the head so that the neck is comparatively straight (do NOT do this in the presence of obvious deformity or malalignment or of evidence of cord injury).
2. Place one hand on the top of the head and tap it lightly with the other, with the force in the long axis of the spine.

If cervical pathology is present, the patient will show subjective signs of discomfort by protest, objection or facial grimace.

15 — 3. NARCOTIC ADDICTION TEST

For clinical signs of addiction, see **2 — 4.**

For signs and symptoms of acute intoxication from overdosage, see **49 — 366.** *Heroin;* **49 — 495.** *Morphine.*

NALORPHINE HYDROCHLORIDE (Nalline) TEST

1. Have the patient (or his legal guardian if he is a minor or mentally incompetent) give written permission for the test in the presence of 2 witnesses. The permission form must include a statement that the purpose of the test has been explained to, and is understood by, the signer and that no coercion has been used in obtaining the signed permission.

2. Measure the size of the patient's pupils, using a piece of cardboard pierced or marked in 0.5 mm. gradations from 0.5 mm. to 3 mm.

3. Inject 3 mg. of nalorphine hydrochloride (Nalline) subcutaneously, having means at hand for combating sudden severe withdrawal symptoms (step 6 below).

4. Wait 30 minutes.

5. Remeasure the size of the pupils with exactly the same amount of life present as in step 2 above.

6. Treat withdrawal symptoms if necessary by subcutaneous or intravenous injection of an effective amount of morphine sulfate.

7. Interpret the results of the test as follows:

PUPILLARY SIZE	USING ADDICTIVE NARCOTICS?
Decreased	No
No change	Occasionally (or normally has small pupils)
Increased	Yes (addict)

The injections suggested in steps 3 and 6 must be performed by a licensed physician.

15 — 4. OPIUM DERIVATIVE TEST

For therapeutic or medicolegal reasons rapid identification of drugs found on an emergency patient may be important. Opium and its narcotic derivatives (heroin, hydromorphone and morphine) may be identified as follows:

15−5. PELVIC-FEMORAL INTEGRITY TEST

1. Place a drop of concentrated nitric acid on a glass slide or in an evaporating dish.
2. Scrape a few particles from the suspect tablet into the acid.
The formation of a cherry-red color indicates the probable presence of a derivative of opium. Synthetic nonopiate narcotics show no characteristic color change. The results of this test should always be confirmed by a qualified laboratory.

15−5. PELVIC-FEMORAL INTEGRITY TEST

Determination of the possibility of bone injury to the femur and pelvis is of extreme importance, especially in elderly or debilitated persons with impaired stability.
1. With the patient supine, press a stethoscope firmly against the exact center of the symphysis pubis.
2. With the legs straight and the quadriceps completely relaxed, tap firmly against the anterior surface of each patella and listen for a difference in sound intensity between the injured and uninjured sides. Suggestive (not conclusive) findings are as follows:

Equal intensity on both sides−no bony injury.

Lack of transmittal on one side−fracture, probably displaced, of the femur or pubic rami.

Decreased intensity on one side−suggestive of fracture with impaction.

Emergency handling can be based on the results above, with diagnostic x-rays as soon as possible.

15−6. SALICYLATE INGESTION TEST

Because of the delay in the development of signs and symptoms such as hypernea after ingestion of salicylates, and because of the too frequent uncertainty on the part of parents as to what their child may have swallowed, the following simple, rapid test is of value for emergency use:
1. Heat a specimen of urine gently to rule out presence of acetone bodies.
2. To 5 ml. of urine add 1 ml. of 10% ferric chloride solution.
3. Shake gently and observe the color. Development of a purple color indicates presence of acetylsalicylic acid (aspirin), methyl, phenyl or sodium salicylate or phenol derivatives.
Presence of a purple color will indicate the ingestion of as little

as one 0.3 gm. aspirin tablet between 30 minutes and 12 hours before examination. The test is not quantitative.

15–7. SEMINAL FLUID TEST

This test is essential for complete examination for rape (**9**) and is based on the presence of acid phosphatase in seminal fluid. The test should be done on intravaginal specimens and on dried secretions on the vulva and upper thighs.

TECHNIQUE

1. To a solution of the suspect material add 2 drops of a solution of sodium alpha naphthol phosphate.

2. Add 1 or 2 drops of naphthanil diazoblue B.

A characteristic purple color indicates the presence of acid phosphatase and is considered as legal evidence of rape (**9**).

15–8. VENTILATION TEST (Snider)

As an index of expiratory volume and flow rate, the following match test is of value in estimating changes in respiratory physiology in potentially progressive conditions.

1. Have the patient remove dentures if present.

2. Hold a lighted half-burned book-type match 6 inches from his mouth.

3. Instruct the patient to blow out the match. (Several positions should be used to compensate for facial weaknesses, etc.).

4. Inability to blow out the flame indicates a forced expiratory volume of less than 1000 ml. and a flow rate of less than 120 liters per minute.

16. TETANUS IMMUNIZATION

See also **12.** *Serum Sensitivity and Desensitization;* **30–31.** *Tetanus;* **48–59.** *Tetanus in Children.*

Because the mortality from established tetanus (**30–31**) is greater than 50%, protective injections should be given without hesitation following soft tissue injuries after as efficient a wound toilet as possible has been done (**55–20**. *Lacerations, Debridement*). Failure to recognize the need for active or passive immunization against tetanus and to institute proper protective and therapeutic measures at once may be actionable (**68–1**). The majority of cases of active tetanus (**30–31**) follow minute or unrecognized breaks in the skin and occur in children and elderly persons.

16–1. CONDITIONS REQUIRING IMMUNOLOGIC PROTECTION AGAINST TETANUS (Tetanus-prone Wounds)

All penetrating wounds (**55–26**) and all puncture wounds, even if minute (**55–28**).

All animal, bat, snake or spider bites (**24**).

All open (compound) fractures (**44–3**).

All wounds that are deep, crushing or grossly contaminated with dirt, dust or soil, especially if possible contamination with animal excreta is present.

All friction and pavement burns (**25–21**).

All cold injuries with local necrosis (**57–1**).

All gunshot wounds (**55–26**).

All penetrating injuries involving the central nervous system.

All wounds (including minute abrasions and lacerations) in which firearms or explosives of any type (dynamite, fireworks, gunpowder, cap pistol ammunition) may have been factors.

All wounds with necrosis due to vascular insufficiency.

All wounds in which adequate debridement (**55–20**. *Lacerations, Debridement*) has not been possible because it would involve sacrifice of essential structures (nerves, major blood vessels, tendons, joint cartilages, etc.), or in which complete obliteration of dead spaces has not been accomplished.

All home or other nonhospital deliveries in which the umbilical cord has been severed under unsterile conditions.

All wounds for which treatment has been neglected, inadequate or delayed beyond 24 hours.

16–2. INDICATIONS FOR USE OF HUMAN TETANUS-IMMUNE GLOBULIN (TIG) (Passive Protection)

Human tetanus-immune globulin (TIG) has supplanted the equine antitoxin for passive immunologic protection against tetanus. It should be given intramuscularly if:

16−3. INDICATIONS FOR USE OF TETANUS TOXOID

a. There is no history of previous adequate active immunization (series of toxoid injections), or if the history is indefinite or uncertain. A history given by the patient of "tetanus shots" may mean only a skin test and an injection of antitoxin given for temporary passive protection following an injury. In these instances active immunization with tetanus toxoid also should be begun, giving the toxoid in a different extremity from the TIG, with specific instructions to the patient regarding completion of the series.

b. Adequate active immunization (2 or 3 toxoid injections followed by a booster in 8 to 12 months) is incomplete or was completed more than 10 years previously with no interval boosters.

c. *Immediate* protection is required following massive contamination. Since passive protection from TIG lasts for a limited time only (not over 21 days), further injections may be necessary if a grossly infected tetanus-prone type wound is present. In addition, large doses of penicillin [benzathine penicillin G (Bicillin), 1,200,000 units intramuscularly for 5 days] or oxytetracycline (Terramycin), 1 gm. orally for 7 to 10 days, may be indicated.

Human tetanus-immune globulin (TIG) should always be given intramuscularly. The dosages recommended below can be doubled with safety in the presence of massive or neglected wounds.

Dosage by age:

0–5 years	75 units
5–10 years	125 units
10 years and over	250 units

Dosage by weight is 4 units per kilogram of body weight. No intradermal, ophthalmic or other tests for sensitivity are required before injection of TIG. Anaphylactic and allergic reactions are rare, but if they do occur they should be treated as outlined under **21.** *Allergic Reactions.*

d. There is active tetanus (**30−31**) present or suspected.

16−3. INDICATIONS FOR USE OF TETANUS TOXOID
(Active Protection)

An injection of 0.5 ml. of tetanus toxoid should be given intramuscularly if:

a. The patient has never been actively immunized by a series of 2 or 3 injections of tetanus toxoid or has not received a booster of toxoid 8 to 12 months after the initial series. TIG (**16−2**) should also be given for temporary protection in this instance. The patient should be encouraged to complete the active immunizing series.

b. Active immunization by injections of toxoid (including a booster 8 to 12 months after the initial series) has been completed more than 10 years previously.

c. A booster injection has not been given within 10 years. If injections of TIG and toxoid are given at the same visit, different extremities should be used, i.e., arm and opposite thigh. Tetanus toxoid is of no value in treatment of established tetanus (**30 – 31**).

17. URGENCY EVALUATION (TRIAGE)

Rapid classification of emergency cases by the urgency with which treatment is required (triage) is one of the most important functions and responsibilities of a physician called upon to treat such cases (**71**). Accurate urgency evaluation, often complicated by the presence of multiple serious conditions in the same individual and almost always in an unstable excited environment, calls not only for extensive basic knowledge of surgery, medicine, toxicology, psychology (especially crowd psychology) and psychiatry, but also for the ability to translate this knowledge into immediate effective action under stressful circumstances. In mass casualty situations, the physician in charge of triage should be the best trained and most experienced available.

In contrast to many of the conditions encountered on a busy emergency service, immediate recognition and prompt, effective and correct management of the conditions listed below may be lifesaving.

Cessation or acute embarrassment of respiration (**11. *Resuscitation***).

Massive bleeding from major vessels (**42. *Hemorrhage;* 59 – 1. *Vascular Disorders*).

Cardiac arrest (**26 – 7**).

Severe heatstroke with rapidly rising temperature (**57 – 4. *Heat Hyperpyrexia***).

Profound shock from any cause (**53**).

Drowning (**22 – 3**).

Rapidly acting poisons (**49**).

Anaphylactic reactions (**21—1**).

Acute epidural hemorrhage (**41—19; 48—26.** *Extradural Hemorrhage in Children*).

Acute overwhelming bacteremia and toxemia (**30—16.** *Meningitis;* **48—41.** *Meningitis in children;* **48—12.** *Meningococcemia in Children;* **48—63.** *Waterhouse-Friderichsen Syndrome in Children*).

Acute adenocortical insufficiency (**33—1**).

Severe head injuries with rapid deterioration of vital signs (**41**).

Penetrating wounds of the pleura (**28—9**) or pericardium (**26—22**).

Rupture of a viscus (**28—1; 28—3; 28—6.** *Chest Injuries;* **55—1.** *Abdominal Injuries*).

Acute maniacal states (**50.** *Psychiatric Emergencies*).

Only through experience and confidence in his own knowledge and judgment will the emergency physician develop the ability to distinguish between an individual dying from an uncontrollable irreparable condition and a less spectacularly injured or sick person for whom immediate and proper therapy may be life or function saving.

18. X-RAYS

18—1. INDICATIONS

A surprisingly large percentage of injury cases requiring emergency care are potentially medicolegal problems, especially if industrial coverage (**75**) or liability or subrogation factors (**67**) are involved. Malpractice actions (**68**) are all too frequently based on the first treatment received by the patient. Therefore, to protect the patient, the attending physician and the hospital, x-rays should be taken whenever bony injuries, or other conditions demonstrable roentgenologically, are suspected, provided that moving and positioning the patient will not be harmful. If the presence of a neck injury is suspected, a cross-table lateral using portable x-ray equipment should be taken and examined before any movement of the neck is allowed. Normal ("negative") x-rays may have as much medicolegal value as those showing traumatic or other pathology. If a splint or cast has been applied, x-rays should be taken before the patient is allowed to leave the immediate control of the emergency physician.

18 — 2. INTERPRETATION

The attending physician's interpretation of the recently developed films must often be used as a basis for emergency therapy and disposition. The presence or absence of pathology can be determined from wet films with reasonable accuracy and a working diagnosis established. This original interpretation of the x-rays should be confirmed or modified by a qualified roentgenologist as soon as possible, and a report of the final interpretation of the films incorporated in the patient's record.

18 — 3. TRANSFERRAL OF X-RAYS

X-rays essential to definitive care should be sent with the patient whenever transfer to any hospital is arranged. If referral to another physician's office is made, the films should be held awaiting his request except in those instances when adequate treatment requires their immediate presence (fractures, dislocations, head injuries, etc.). If x-ray films for any reason leave the direct control of the physician by whom they are ordered, a receipt should be signed by the person to whom they are consigned for transportation. Return of the x-rays as soon as possible should be required, with careful follow-up in a reasonable time.

18 — 4. OWNERSHIP OF X-RAYS

No matter who pays for them, x-ray films are the property of the physician who orders them and not of the patient, the hospital or laboratory where they are taken, other medical attendants, attorneys, insurance companies or other interested persons. Since the films (NOT the reports based on them) must be produced when designated by due process of law (**73.** *Subpoenas*), they must be safeguarded in the same manner as the clinical record (**66.** *Emergency Case Records*).

18 — 5. FLUOROSCOPIC EXAMINATION

If a fluoroscope is available, it will be found to be of assistance in some instances in the determination of cardiac and gastrointestinal tract disease and in the reduction of fractures and dislocations. An x-ray technician should if possible be present whenever the fluoroscope is used, but, *to protect himself and the patient,* any physician using the equipment should personally, carefully and invariably observe the following safety factors:

Always wear a protective apron and, if possible and practical lead-impregnated gloves.

Never use more than 5 milliamperes (5 ma.).

Never use more than 80 kilovolts (80 kv.).

Always limit each exposure time to not more than 3 seconds.

Never use more than 10 exposures.

18—6. PROTECTION OF GONADS

Although the danger from gonadal radiation has been greatly overemphasized in the lay press, shielding of the lower abdomen and external genitalia is a simple procedure and should be done whenever practical, especially in children, in males in the reproductive age and in women during the 1st trimester of pregnancy.

18—7. X-RAY BURNS (See also 25—32.)

Unless there has been a gross miscalculation of dosage, or a defect in the operation or calibration of the equipment, radiation burns are usually the result of x-ray therapy. In this instance, the temporary uncomfortable erythema and subsequent atrophic changes represent a calculated risk of which the patient had been, or should have been, informed. For treatment, see **25—32.** See also **63—4.** *Ionizing Radiation Effects, Gamma Rays.*

EMERGENCY TREATMENT OF SPECIFIC CONDITIONS

19. ABDOMINAL PAIN

Distinguishing an acute surgical abdomen from less serious or less fulminating conditions may require blood counts and other more sophisticated laboratory procedures not available in an emergency situation. However, in a high percentage of cases a tentative diagnosis can be made from the history and physical examination; certainly, from the history and clinical picture the attending physician should be able to determine whether or not immediate hospitalization is indicated. Unless a definite diagnosis of a nondangerous condition has been established, any person with persistent or recurrent severe abdominal pain should be hospitalized as soon as possible for thorough examination, diagnosis and treatment.

Some of the numerous conditions in which acute abdominal pain may be the main symptom are included in the following incomplete list:

Accumulation of gas (in infants)
Alcoholic hepatitis (sclerosing hyaline necrosis of the liver)
Aneurysm (**59–3**)
Appendicitis (**37–7**)
Arthritis (**44–1**) and fractures of the dorsolumbar spine (**44–2**)
Bowel obstruction (**37–2**)
Caisson disease (**23–3**)
Cholecystitis (**37–8**)
Cirrhosis of the liver
Coronary disease and infarction (**26–12**)
Cystitis (**38–10; 48–31.** *Genitourinary Tract Emergencies in Children*)
Decompression sickness (**23–3**)
Diabetes (hyperglycemia) (**29–3**)
Diverticulitis (**37–10**)
Dysentery (**37–9; 48–21.** *Diarrhea in Children*)
Ectopic pregnancy, ruptured (**47–2**)
Enteritis, acute bacterial or regional (**37–2**)
Epilepsy, abdominal (**31.** *Convulsive Seizures;* **50–11.** *Episodic Unconsciousness — Differential Diagnosis*)
Esophageal perforation (**37–3**)
Fecal impaction (**37–2.** *Obstruction, Mechanical*)
Foreign bodies (**36–5**)
Gallbladder disease (**37–8**)
Gastroenteritis (**37–11.** *Esophagitis and Gastritis;* **48–30.** *Gastrointestinal Tract Emergencies in Children*)
Gonococcal perihepatitis
Hepatitis, acute (**62–8**) or traumatic (**55–21**)
Hernia — diaphragmatic (**48–35**), femoral (**48–35**), inguinal (**37–5** and **48–35**), and umbilical (**48–35**)
Herniation of an intervertebral disk
Herpes zoster (**27–15** and **46–8**)

Hypoglycemia (**29 – 3**. *Coma,* **43 – 16**. *Metabolic Disorders;* **48 – 37**. *Hypoglycemia in Children*)
Ileus (**48 – 38**. *Intestinal Obstruction in Children*)
Infarcts of abdominal viscera
Infections, acute systemic
Intestinal obstruction (**37 – 2**)
Intestinal parasites (**37 – 20**)
Intraperitoneal perforation (**37 – 3**)
Intussusception (**48 – 38**. *Intestinal Obstruction in Children*)
Kidney stones (**38 – 20**)
Leptospirosis
Liver disease (**29 – 10**. *Hepatic Coma;* **55 – 21**. *Liver Injuries*)
Lupus erythematosus (systemic)
Mediastinitis (**37 – 3**. *Esophageal Perforation*)
Mesenteric thrombosis and embolism; lymphangitis (in children)
Migraine (**27 – 21** and **48 – 43**. *Migraine in Children*)
Mittelschmerz (**39 – 8**)
Myocardial infarction (**26 – 12**)
Nephritis (**38 – 14**)
Neuritis, intercostal
Obstruction of the gastrointestinal tract (**37 – 2**)
Orchitis, traumatic (**38 – 3**)
Ovarian cyst with torsion of the pedicle (**39 – 13**)
Pancreatitis, acute (**37 – 19**) or traumatic (**55 – 25**)
Parathyroid crises (**33 – 3**)
Peptic ulcer with or without perforation (**37 – 3**)
Pericardial trauma (**26 – 22**. *Cardiac Trauma – traumatic hemoperitoneum with tamponade;* **48 – 15**. *Cardiac Emergencies in Children*)
Peritonitis, acute (primary, from trauma or infections, periodic, eosinophilic)
Pleurodynia (**62 – 15**)
Pneumonia (**52 – 14, 48 – 45**. *Pneumonia in children;* **62 – 11**. *Interstitial Pneumonia*)
Poisoning, acute. See **49**. *Poisoning,* under entries listed below unless other references are given.

Antimony (**49 – 81**)
Arsenic trioxide (**49 – 90**)
Aspidium (**49 – 100**)
Barium (**49 – 112**)
Bichloride of mercury (**49 – 128**)
Botulism (**49 – 141**)
Cadmium (**49 – 156**)
Carbon tetrachloride (**49 – 173**)
Chromates (**49 – 207**)
Colchicine (**49 – 220**)
Copper salts (**49 – 223**)
Croton oil (**49 – 232**)
Cyanides (**49 – 235**)
Diethylstilbestrol (**49 – 271**)
Ergot (**49 – 306**)
Fluorides (**49 – 336**)
Formaldehyde (**49 – 340**)
Gasoline (**49 – 349**)
Kerosene (**49 – 408**)

Lead (**49 – 420**. *Lead Salts*)
Methyl alcohol (**49 – 475**)
Morphine (**49 – 495**)
Mushrooms (**49 – 502**)
Organic phosphate pesticides (**49 – 546**)
Phenolphthalein (**49 – 591**)
Physostigmine (**49 – 603**)
Solanine (**49 – 712**)
Spider venom (**24 – 20**. *Spider Bites;* **49 – 716; 61**. *Venoms*)
Squill (**49 – 718**)
Staphylococcal food poisoning (**49 – 339**)
Sulfapyridine (**49 – 731**. *Sulfonamides*)
Thallium (**49 – 768**)
Tung nuts (**49 – 814**)
Turpentine (**49 – 815**)
Veratrum viride (**49 – 825**)
Viosterol (**49 – 827**)

Porphyria (**43 – 22**)
Premature separation of the placenta (**47 – 4**)
Pyelonephritis (**38 – 14.** *Nephritis*)
Pyloric stenosis (**48 – 38.** *Intestinal Obstruction*)
Rectus abdominis muscle hemorrhage
Renal colic (**38 – 20**)
Round ligament spasm during pregnancy
Rupture of a viscus
Salpingitis (**39 – 9.** *Pelvic Inflammatory Disease*)
Subdiaphragmatic abscess (**20 – 29**)
Tabes dorsalis (**60 – 5**)
Tetany (**43 – 25**)
Thrombosis or thrombophlebitis, portal or hepatic vein
Torsion of testicle (**38 – 7**)
Trauma, direct – especially to the liver (**55 – 21**) and spleen (**55 – 31**)
Tubal pregnancy (**47 – 2**)
Tubo-ovarian abscess (**39 – 9**)
Tumors, space consuming or malignant
Uremia (**29 – 15**)
Ureteral stone (**38 – 20**)
Vascular purpura (Henoch's purpura)
Volvulus (**48 – 38.** *Intestinal Obstruction*)
Withdrawal symptoms, narcotics (**2 – 4.** *Addiction;* **49 – 366.** *Heroin;* **49 – 495.** *Morphine*)

If after a careful history and physical examination and utilization of available laboratory tests the emergency physician is unable to determine the cause of persistent or recurrent abdominal distress, the patient should be hospitalized. Because of the possibility that they will mask signs and symptoms, no opiates or synthetic narcotics of any kind should be given for control of pain or relief of apprehension until a definite diagnosis has been established; even then, barbiturates or phenothiazines in small doses are preferable.

A detailed summary of all laboratory tests, observations and findings, especially changes in condition, and of all treatment should be sent with any patient with abdominal pain who is being transferred to a hospital or referred to a private physician's office. To protect the patient and himself, the emergency physician should be sure that the patient understands the need for further medical care (**64 – 2**).

20. ABSCESSES

GENERAL CONSIDERATIONS

Early abscesses without localization or fluctuation should be treated expectantly by local application of heat. Many will be absorbed under this regimen; others will localize in a short time.

Small superficial abscesses may be incised and drained under ethyl chloride spray or procaine or lidocaine (Xylocaine) block anesthesia.

Large deep abscesses should be treated conservatively by application of heat until localization occurs, then referred for hospitalization and wide drainage, usually under a general anesthetic.

ABSCESSES REQUIRING SPECIAL MANAGEMENT

20 – 1. ALVEOLAR ABSCESSES

Alveolar abscesses arise from infection at a tooth root and are often exquisitely painful (**58.** *Toothache*).

TREATMENT

Early Cases

1. Codeine sulfate and acetylsalicylic acid (aspirin) for pain.
2. Penicillin intramuscularly or tetracyclines by mouth.
3. Reference to a dentist for drilling (not extraction).

Late Cases with fluctuation at the gingival margin (*gum boils*)

1. Drainage through a small incision parallel to the border of the gum. No anesthetic is required and relief is immediate.
2. Reference for dental care.

20 – 2. ANORECTAL ABSCESSES

Anorectal abscesses may be superficial or deep, but all require incision and drainage under general or low spinal anesthesia.

Control of pain while hospitalization is being arranged is the only emergency treatment required.

20 – 3. APICAL ABSCESSES   See **20 – 1.** *Alveolar Abscesses*

20 – 4. BARTHOLIN ABSCESSES   See **39 – 3.**

20 – 5. BOILS

TREATMENT

1. Application of local heat until localization and fluctuation develop or spontaneous resolution takes place.
2. Incision and drainage under ethyl chloride spray anesthesia, with insertion of a rubber dam drain and application of an absorbent dressing after obtaining material for cultures.

3. Ringing of the draining sinus with petrolatum gauze to minimize mechanical spreading.

4. Reference for further medical care.

20−6. BRAIN ABSCESSES

Brain abscesses may follow head injuries (especially fractures), otitis media and mastoiditis. Suspicion of the presence of a brain abscess is an indication for immediate hospitalization.

20−7. BREAST ABSCESSES

Breast abscesses may give severe pain, with general malaise and elevated temperature.

TREATMENT

1. Start local heat at once.

2. Have the patient wear an oversize brassiere for support.

3. Refer for surgical drainage and cultures, with antibiotic therapy if indicated.

20−8. CARBUNCLES

Carbuncles are multilocular abscesses with multiple individual compartments.

TREATMENT

1. If possible, avoid incision and drainage by:

Control of pain by acetylsalicylic acid (aspirin), or small doses of narcotics.

Application of local heat.

Limitation of activity.

Search for and treatment of underlying metabolic abnormalities such as diabetes mellitus and Cushing's syndrome.

2. Refer for hospitalization if surgical drainage becomes necessary.

20−9. COLD ABSCESSES

Cold abscesses are usually due to attenuated organisms following antibiotic therapy or to tuberculosis and are rarely encountered as an emergency unless sudden spontaneous drainage occurs. Fluctuation may be present, but the usual signs of inflammation (redness, local heat, tenderness) are absent.

No emergency treatment is needed, but the importance of adequate medical care should be stressed to the patient.

20—10. COLLAR-BUTTON ABSCESSES

Collar-button abscesses are infections in the webs between the fingers which cause acute palmar tenderness and swelling but which point on the dorsal surface of the hand.

TREATMENT

Early
1. Immobilization with a splint and sling.
2. Frequent hot soaks.
3. Control of pain by elevation, anodynes and, if necessary, small doses of narcotics.

Advanced
1. Incision and drainage through two incisions, a curved incision along the edge of the volar swelling and a small incision over the dorsal web. This procedure should be done under nerve block or general anesthetic, preferably in a hospital. Cultures and sensitivity tests should be obtained.
2. Insertion of a rubber dam drain.
3. Application of a hand splint and sling.
4. Administration of appropriate antibiotics.
5. Careful and frequent follow-up care.

20—11. DENTAL ABSCESSES See 20—1. *Alveolar Abscesses;* 58. *Toothache*

20—12. EPIDURAL ABSCESSES

Epidural abscesses are characterized by low back pain, progressive flaccid weakness of the legs and urinary retention, and represent an acute emergency. Immediate hospitalization for drainage is mandatory.

20—13. FELONS (Whitlows)

Felons or whitlows require immediate drainage through an extensive fish-mouth or through-and-through incision of the fingertip. Care must be taken to open every infected compartment. Digital nerve block at some distance above the infected area is usually adequate for anesthesia.

20−14. GAS ABSCESSES

If crepitus, foul odor and tenderness with severe systemic signs and symptoms develop in a previously comfortable wound 2 to 4 days after injury, immediate hospitalization for exploration and removal of necrotic tissue is required.

Penicillin in massive doses (up to 12 million or more units a day) is indicated, with large doses of tetracyclines. Treatment with gas gangrene antitoxin is of no value.

20−15. ISCHIOANAL ABSCESSES

These abscesses develop suddenly, with extreme pain, fever and chills, a feeling of fullness in the rectum and urinary retention.

TREATMENT

Superficial ischioanal abscesses:

1. Preliminary sedation with sodium phenobarbital (Luminal), pentazocine (Talwin) or a small dose of morphine sulfate.

2. Intracutaneous infiltration of a local anesthetic over the point of localization between the anus and the ischial tuberosity.

3. Incision and drainage with insertion of a drain.

4. Reference for follow-up care. Late fistulectomy is often necessary.

Deep or extensive abscess with severe toxic symptoms and signs:

1. Control of pain by pentazocine (Talwin), codeine or morphine sulfate intramuscularly.

2. Hospitalization for drainage under general anesthesia. Cultures should be obtained and antibiotics given as indicated by sensitivity tests.

20−16. MIDDLE EAR ABSCESSES See 32−13. *Otitis Media*

20−17. NASAL SEPTUM ABSCESSES

Nasal septum abscesses may follow trauma or operative procedures.

TREATMENT

1. Start antibiotic therapy at once.

2. Refer to an otolaryngologist for incision and drainage.

20—18. PALMAR SPACE ABSCESSES See **20—10.** *Collar-button Abscesses;* **40—2.** *Cellulitis of the Hand.*

20—19. PARONYCHIA

Throbbing pain accompanied by redness and swelling adjacent to the border of a finger or toenail can be relieved only by incision and drainage.

20—20. PERIANAL ABSCESSES See **20—15.** *Ischioanal Abscesses*

20—21. PERINEAL ABSCESSES

Perineal abscesses require emergency care only if pressure causes partial or complete urinary retention. All cases should be referred to a urologist for care.

20—22. PERITONSILLAR ABSCESSES (Quinsy)

Signs and symptoms consist of severe agonizing pain on one side of the throat, acute dysphagia, high temperature, extreme general malaise and bulging in the supratonsillar fossa.

TREATMENT

If the abscess is fluctuant and can be accurately localized:

1. Infiltration of the mucous membrane only with 1% procaine or lidocaine (Xylocaine).

2. Incision with a sharp knife with adhesive tape wrapped around the blade 3/8 inch from the point as a guard against too deep penetration.

3. Irrigation with warm saline.

4. Administration of antibiotics after cultures and tests for sensitivity.

5. Reference to an otolaryngologist for follow-up care.

If the abscess is deep and no area of fluctuation can be determined:

1. Control of pain by adequate doses of morphine sulfate.

2. Reference to an otolaryngologist for further care.

Do not attempt to *explore* the throat. Deaths have occurred from uncontrollable hemorrhage from the ascending pharyngeal, external carotid and internal carotid arteries and from the internal jugular vein.

20 – 23. PERIURETHRAL ABSCESSES

Periurethral abscesses arise from acute urethritis or from infection of the glands in the area and usually point near the base of the shaft of the penis.

TREATMENT
1. Incision and drainage under local anesthesia.
2. Antibiotic therapy based on sensitivity tests.
3. Reference to a urologist for further care.

20 – 24. PILONIDAL ABSCESSES

TREATMENT
1. Control of pain by anodynes or narcotics as required.
2. Hospitalization for incision and drainage under spinal or general anesthesia.

20 – 25. PSOAS ABSCESS See 20 – 9. *Cold Abscesses*

20 – 26. RETROPERITONEAL ABSCESSES

Retroperitoneal [anterior, posterior (perinephric) and retrofascial] abscesses require immediate hospitalization for surgical drainage.

20 – 27. STITCH ABSCESSES

Stitch abscesses may be superficial or deep and can be drained easily by removal of the offending stitch (cutting it close to the uninfected side). Spreading of the incision may be necessary.

20 – 28. SUBURETHRAL ABSCESSES

These abscesses should not be opened externally if this can be avoided. Reference to a urologist is indicated as soon as the diagnosis has been made.

20–29.   SUBDIAPHRAGMATIC ABSCESSES

Hospitalization for treatment is required.

20–30.   TENDON SHEATH ABSCESSES (Tenosynovitis) See 40–2. *Cellulitis of the Hand.*

20–31.   TUBO-OVARIAN ABSCESSES See 39–9. *Pelvic Inflammatory Disease*

20–32.   WHITLOWS See 20–13. *Felons*

21.   ALLERGIC REACTIONS

A bracelet or necklace giving information regarding special medical problems such as heart trouble or allergic reactions to drugs or other substances may be lifesaving. Additional emergency information can be obtained by telephone on a 24 hour basis from the central agency.*

Four types of acute allergic reactions require immediate, sometimes lifesaving, emergency measures. These are anaphylactic shock, acute angioedema, asthma with acute bronchospasm and serum shock.

21–1.   ANAPHYLACTIC SHOCK

Anaphylactic shock usually develops within a few seconds or minutes of exposure to the allergen but may be delayed for a few hours. Its onset may be overwhelming, and death may occur from rapid respiratory and circulatory collapse before any treatment can be given.

TREATMENT

1. Immediate injection of epinephrine hydrochloride (Adrenalin) at the first evidence of anaphylaxis. No time should be spent look-

---

*Medic Alert, P.O. Box 1009, Turlock, California 95380, telephone number (209) 634-4917.

ing for an available vein—instead, 1 to 2 ml of 1:10,000 Adrenalin should be injected into the center of the vascular plexus at the base of the tongue (**14 — 5.** *Intraglossal Injections*) repeated every 20 minutes until the evidence of vascular collapse or cardiorespiratory failure lessens. Additional injections of 1:10,000 Adrenalin should then be given intravenously as needed.

2. If the anaphylactic reaction results from an injection or an insect sting (see **56 — 1.** *Bee Stings;* **61.** *Venoms*), a tourniquet should be applied and 0.25 ml. of 1:1000 Adrenalin injected into and around the site of entry of the antigen. The tourniquet should be loosened, but not completely released, for 2 to 3 minutes every 20 minutes. Application of ice may slow absorption.

3. Insurance of a clear airway by removal of false teeth, suction, positioning and support of the angles of the jaw.

4. Administration of expired air respiration (**11 — 1**) followed by oxygen under positive pressure by face mask or endotracheal catheter and rebreathing bag. An emergency cricothyreotomy (**14 — 12**) may be necessary.

5. Removal or neutralization of the allergen if known or suspected.

6. Intramuscular or intravenous injection of ephedrine sulfate (0.25 to 0.5 ml.) followed by levarterenol bitartrate (Levophed) or metaraminol bitartrate (Aramine) intravenously (**53 — 7**) if hypotension is extreme.

7. Intravenous injection of 200 mg. of hydrocortisone sodium succinate (Solu-Cortef) or of 50 mg. of prednisolone sodium hemisuccinate (Meticortelone). Repeat as necessary.

8. Intramuscular or intravenous injection of antihistaminic drugs.

9. Hospitalization after the above measures. The patient should be kept under close observation for at least 24 hours.

21 — 2. ANGIOEDEMA (See also **48 — 4.** *Angioedema in Children*)

In addition to the measures outlined under **21 — 1.** *Anaphylactic Shock,* it may be necessary to perform a conventional tracheostomy (**14 — 12**) to replace the previously performed cricothyreotomy.

21 — 3. ASTHMA WITH ACUTE BRONCHOSPASM See **48 — 6.** *Asthma in Children;* **52 — 1.** *Asthma*

21 − 4.   SERUM REACTIONS (See also **48 − 50.** *Serum Reactions in Children*)

SERUM DISEASE

ONSET.   Seven to 12 days after injection of antiserum. Horse serum is the most common offender.

The clinical picture of serum disease consists of severe headache accompanied by a high temperature, diffuse erythema, urticarial wheals, severe itching, marked edema, nausea, vomiting, abdominal cramping, generalized adenopathy and severe joint and muscle pain.

TREATMENT

Mild Cases

1. Control of itching by sodium bicarbonate paste or calamine lotion, with 1% phenol. (Do not compress.)

2. Tripelennamine hydrochloride (Pyribenzamine), 50 to 100 mg. orally every 4 hours.

Severe Cases

1. Epinephrine hydrochloride (Adrenalin), 0.5 to 1.0 ml. of 1:1000 solution intramuscularly, or, in extremely severe cases, intravenously, repeated as necessary.

2. Procaine (0.5% solution) injected slowly intravenously. The usual dose is 4 mg. per kilogram of body weight administered over a 20 to 30 minute period. The development of any of the symptoms of an atopic or toxic blood level procaine reaction (**49 − 72.** *Anesthetics, Local*) calls for immediate discontinuance of the injection.

PROGNOSIS.   There is usually complete recovery, although uncomfortable and sometimes disabling symptoms may persist for 10 to 14 days.

SERUM SHOCK

ONSET.   Immediately following injection. As in anaphylactic shock (**21 − 1**) death may occur in a few minutes from respiratory and circulatory collapse. For immediate treatment, see **21 − 1.**

PROPHYLACTIC TREATMENT

1. Prevention is the only sure effective treatment. Intracutaneous (intradermal) tests for sensitivity (**12**) should always be done before antiserum of any type is given, although the absence of dermal hypersensitivity does not always indicate that there will be no general hypersensitivity reaction. If the intracutaneous test is positive, the method for desensitization as outlined under **12.** *Serum Sensitivity*

and Desensitization should be used if administration of antitoxin is essential and no other animal or human antiserum is available. Preliminary oral intake of a sustained release capsule of an antihistaminic may prevent or decrease the severity of the hypersensitivity reaction.

Any person who has had a severe systemic reaction to an insect sting should carry, and be familiar with the use of, an emergency kit (**56 – 1.** *Bee Stings*). Hyposensitization to insect allergens is highly effective.

2. Hospitalization for observation and treatment if the patient survives the initial shock. This applies even if complete recovery apparently has taken place.

PROGNOSIS. Full-fledged serum shock may be overwhelming and rapidly fatal, but if the patient survives for 5 minutes or more, there is a good chance of complete recovery.

21 – 5. LESS SERIOUS ALLERGIC REACTIONS

Less serious allergic reactions are common and may cause varying degrees of edema, urticaria and pruritus.

TREATMENT

1. Remove from contact with or stop intake of the offending agent if known or suspected.

2. Inject epinephrine hydrochloride (Adrenalin), 0.5 to 1 ml. of 1:1000 solution intramuscularly. For home administration a 1:100 solution used with a nebulizer may be prescribed, with specific instructions regarding its use.

3. Prescribe tripelennamine hydrochloride (Pyribenzamine), 50 mg. by mouth 3 times a day for swelling and wheals and trimeprazine tartrate (Temaril), 2.5 mg. 4 times a day for severe itching, unless the offending drug is an antihistaminic (**49 – 80**).

4. Apply calamine lotion with 1% phenol to the itching areas.

5. Refer severe or stubborn cases to an internist or allergist for follow-up care.

22.   ASPHYXIATION

See also **11.** *Resuscitation;* **29.** *Coma.*

22 — 1.   ASPHYXIA

Asphyxia or suffocation is caused by lack of oxygen and accumulation of carbon dioxide in the blood and is characterized by the signs and symptoms of air hunger (acute anxiety, increasing lividity, cyanosis), coma and death.

CAUSES

1. Mechanical obstruction of the respiratory passages by edema (**21 — 2.** *Angioedema;* **55 — 38.** *Tracheobronchial Injuries*) and foreign body (**36 — 4.** *Foreign Bodies in the Larynx, Trachea or Bronchi;* **48 — 29.** *Foreign Bodies in Children;* **48 — 44.** *Obstruction of the Respiratory Tract in Children).*

2. Acute depression or paralysis of the respiratory center by drugs such as morphine (**49 — 495**).

3. Filling of the alveolar air spaces with fluid (**22 — 3.** *Drowning;* **28.** *Chest Injuries;* **51.** *Pulmonary Edema*), fumes (**49.** *Poisoning*) or products of infection (**52 — 14.** *Pneumonia*).

4. Disturbances in the oxygen-carrying ability of the red blood cells (**49 — 172.** *Carbon Monoxide*).

5. Paralysis of the muscles concerned with respiration by disease (**46 — 9.** *Paralysis*), drugs which act on the motor end plates (**49 — 234.** *Curare*), cervical trauma (**44 — 3.** *Vertebral Fractures;* **44 — 58.** *Neck Injuries*) or intracranial pathology (**41.** *Head Injuries;* **59 — 2.** *Cerebrovascular Accidents*).

TREATMENT

1. Removal from exposure.

2. Insurance of an adequate airway by digital removal of secretions, postural drainage, suction, support of the angles of the jaw, intubation or emergency cricothyreotomy or tracheostomy (**14 — 12**).

3. Removal of foreign bodies blocking the airway (**36 — 4**).

4. External cardiac compression (**11 — 2**) if indicated.

5. Immediate expired air respiration (**11 — 1**). Other methods of nonmechanical manual artificial respiration are less efficient and do not result in enough oxygenation to preserve life, but should be made use of if for any reason mouth-to-mouth, mouth-to-nose or mouth-to-adjunct techniques (**11 — 1**) cannot be used. Of the manual

methods, the Holger-Nielsen chest pressure armlift method is the most effective for adults; the Rickard prone-tilting visceral shift (**11 – 1**) is sometimes useful for infants.

6. Mechanical artificial respiration as soon as equipment is available. Air or oxygen under intermittent positive pressure should be administered by face mask and rebreathing bag, by endotracheal catheter and rebreathing bag or by mechanical respirators of various types.

7. Avoidance of dependence on analeptics. Drugs such as α-lobeline, caffeine sodiobenzoate and pentylenetetrazol (Metrazol) are of no value until cardiorespiratory function has been reestablished.

22 – 2. ASPHYXIA NEONATORUM See **48 – 5**.

22 – 3. DROWNING

Mouth-to-mouth respiration (**11 – 1**) while bringing a drowning person to shore may be lifesaving. As soon as the victim has been removed from the water, the following routine should be followed.

1. Insure a patent airway by digital removal of false teeth and secretions from the mouth and throat. Postural drainage ("rolling over a barrel") is of limited value.

2. Support the angles of the jaw with the neck in moderate hyperextension.

3. Start expired air respiration (**11 – 1**) and closed chest cardiac compression (**11 – 2**). For technique by a single rescuer see **11 – 3**.

4. As soon as help is available arrange for transportation to a hospital even if apparent improvement has taken place. Immersion in fresh water for lengthy periods often results in delayed ventricular fibrillation (**26 – 23**) or massive hemolysis from osmosis. Transfusions of whole blood may be necessary. Lower nephron nephrosis is a serious complication. The possibility of a preliminary heart attack, an acute neck injury or an overwhelming allergic reaction (**21**) to some type of marine life (**61.** *Venoms*) should be considered in all "drowning" persons.

As soon as the patient reaches a hospital, sodium bicarbonate should be given intravenously to combat metabolic acidosis. The dose is 3.75 gm. in 50 ml. of solution for adults, repeated in 5 minutes and as necessary; give children 25 ml. and infants 10 to 15 ml.

Frequent blood gas monitoring should be done, and the patient should be kept under close observation until the results are within normal limits.

Recurrence of coma after initial apparent improvement indicates a poor prognosis.

22 — 4.   ELECTROCUTION See **11.** *Resuscitation;* **25 — 11.** *Electrical Burns;* **29 — 5.** *Electric Shock*

Remember that the usual criteria for death (**3 — 3**) sometimes do not apply in electrical shock (**29 — 5**).

22 — 5.   SMOKE INHALATION (See also **48 — 53.** *Smoke Inhalation in Children*)

Although inhalation of smoke by persons trapped in burning buildings and by firemen causes acute symptoms (cyanosis, cough, bronchospasm), fatalities are usually the result of acute carbon monoxide poisoning or of thermal damage to the respiratory tract. For treatment, see **49 — 172.** *Carbon Monoxide;* **25 — 18.** *Mucous Membrane Burns (Burns of the Respiratory Tract).* Hyperbaric oxygen therapy often is indicated in severe cases.

23.   BAROTRAUMA

Changes in atmospheric pressure — both decreases and increases — can cause numerous conditions which may require emergency care.

23 — 1.   ALTITUDE SICKNESS (See also **23 — 6.** *Mountain Sickness*)

Although individual ceilings vary, above 8000 feet many persons develop signs and symptoms of hypoxemia of varying degrees, ranging from increased pulse and respiration and euphoria to gradually decreasing mental and physical efficiency with eventual loss of consciousness. Posthypoxemic symptoms such as headache, nausea, vomiting, tinnitus and deafness are common but usually clear spontaneously in 2 or 3 days.

TREATMENT
1. Return to an accustomed atmospheric pressure.
2. Oxygen inhalations under positive pressure by face mask and rebreathing bag.
3. Dimenhydrinate (Dramamine), 50 to 100 mg. by mouth.
4. Circulatory stimulation by caffeine sodiobenzoate, 0.5 gm. intramuscularly.
5. Reference for care by an otolaryngologist if ear symptoms persist.

23 — 2. BENDS See **23 — 3.** *Caisson Disease*

23 — 3. CAISSON DISEASE (*Bends,* Compressed Air Sickness, Decompression Sickness)

Caisson disease may occur in divers who breathe air or oxygen through any type of mechanical equipment (**23 — 5**) and in persons who work in air locks under increased atmospheric pressure. If decompression is not gradual, bubbles of nitrogen are released into the blood and produce a variety of signs and symptoms. The most common of these are severe throbbing pain which shifts its location frequently and involves especially muscles, joints and bones. Abdominal pain may be acute enough to be confused with an acute surgical abdomen. Vertigo (**46 — 13**) is often severe enough to cause staggering which may be mistaken for drunkenness. Intense pruritus and mottling and erythema of the skin may be present. Among frequent nervous system symptoms are numbness and tingling of the extremities, bizarre paresthesias, bladder and bowel incontinence, hemiplegia, paraplegia, quadriplegia, strabismus, nystagmus, diplopia and paresis. Acute dyspnea may occur several hours after apparently successful recompression and decompression and be followed by collapse and unconsciousness.

TREATMENT
Recompression and gradual decompression is the only treatment of any value. While this is being arranged the following supportive measures may be necessary:
1. Continuous artificial respiration by any feasible method (**11 — 1**) — mouth-to-mouth and mechanical are the most satisfactory.
2. Inhalation of pure oxygen or oxygen-helium mixtures.
3. Injection of caffeine sodiobenzoate, 0.5 gm. intramuscularly.

23 – 4. COMPRESSED AIR SICKNESS See **23 – 3.** *Caisson Disease*

23 – 5. DIVING HAZARDS

The problems, limitations and hazards of deep water diving with air hose, suit and metal helmet have long been recognized. Commercial divers are required to be in good physical condition and are trained and instructed in accordance with stringent safety regulations. In contrast, the recent development, commercial exploitation and wide use of various types of self-contained underwater breathing apparatus (commonly abbreviated to SCUBA) by inexperienced, untrained, unsupervised and unlicensed persons diving for sport have resulted in the need for recognition and treatment of various physical, metabolic and mental disturbances resulting from exposure to an unfamiliar and potentially dangerous environment.

Skin divers (who can remain under water only as long as they can hold their breath) are subject only to the usual well-known hazards of diving and swimming. *Snorkel* divers are exposed to these hazards plus the additional danger of thoracic squeeze if an overly long (more than 18 inch) breathing tube is used.

GENERAL PRINCIPLES OF MANAGEMENT AND CARE

1. Artificial respiration – expired air respiratory assistance (**11 – 1**) – to dyspneic, cyanotic, unconscious or "drowned" divers, continued not only during rescue and en route to the pressure chamber but also in the chamber during recompression, may be lifesaving.

2. Knowledge of the location of, the shortest route to, and the indications for use of the closest pressure chamber equipped for recompression and gradual decompression.

3. Recompression and slow supervised decompression of any seriously ill, stuporous or comatose diver who has been 30 feet or more under water using any type of air- or gas-filled diving apparatus, no matter how long an interval has elapsed since the dive. Recompression and gradual controlled decompression in a pressure chamber is harmless not only to the diver, but also to an attendant, and under certain circumstances may prevent serious, permanent, even terminal, aftereffects. *When in doubt, recompress!*

4. The conditions listed in the following table are related directly or indirectly to underwater pressure or subsurface environment and may require emergency management.

CONDITION	SKIN DIVERS (Breath-holding)	SNORKEL DIVERS (Tube-to-Surface)	SCUBA DIVERS	HELMET-SUIT-AIR HOSE DIVERS	CAUSE	SIGNS AND SYMPTOMS	RECOMPRESSION IN PRESSURE CHAMBER?	ARTIFICIAL RESPIRATION?	OTHER TREATMENT AND COMMENTS
Air embolism	No	No	Yes	Yes	Holding breath during ascent	Any picture—indistinguishable from decompression sickness	Yes	Yes	Sedatives and anodynes for pain. Permanent sequelae may require symptomatic therapy
Anoxia	No	No	Closed circuit only	Air supply cut off	Failure of breathing apparatus	Unconsciousness without warning	Yes	Yes	Failure of oxygen supply is often associated with air embolism and/or decompression sickness caused by too rapid rescue
Bends	No	No	Yes	Yes	Decompression sickness	Pain in legs and/or abdomen	Yes	No	Sedatives and narcotics for pain. See 23–3. *Caisson Disease.*
Carbon dioxide poisoning	No	No	Yes, closed circuit	No	CO_2 absorbent inadequate	Rapid breathing, unconsciousness	Yes	Yes	Prevention—avoidance of deep breathing exercises before starting dive
Carbon monoxide poisoning	No	No	Yes, open circuit	No	Impure air in cylinder	Sudden loss of consciousness	Yes	Yes	See 49–172
Chokes	No	No	Yes	Yes	Decompression sickness	Dyspnea, cough, chest pain	Yes	Yes	Must be adequately recompressed immediately. See 23–3. *Caisson Disease.*
Cold	Yes	Yes	Yes	Yes	Low water temperature	Slowing of functions, shivering	Often	Often	Shivering makes holding mouthpiece impossible, or slowed mental and physical responses may lead to other complications.

CONDITION	SKIN DIVERS (Breath-holding)	SNORKEL DIVERS (Tube-to-Surface)	SCUBA DIVERS	HELMET-SUIT-AIR HOSE DIVERS	CAUSE	SIGNS AND SYMPTOMS	RECOMPRESSION IN PRESSURE CHAMBER?	ARTIFICIAL RESPIRATION?	OTHER TREATMENT AND COMMENTS
Conjunctival hemorrhage	No	No	Yes	No	Tight goggles — excessive depth	Bleeding may be retrobulbar	No	No	Symptomatic treatment only. Recovery complete
Decompression sickness	No	No	Yes	Yes	Rapid ascent from deep dives	May give any picture. Onset may be delayed for many hours	Yes	Often	Sedatives and anodynes for pain. See 23-3. *Caisson Disease.*
Drowning	Yes	Yes	Yes	Yes	Hypoxia, water in lungs	Unconsciousness, absent vital signs (see 3-2)	Often	Yes	Any "drowned" diver using any type of gas-containing breathing apparatus requires recompression at once
Ear drum rupture	Yes	No	Yes	Yes	Barotrauma, previous disease	Pain, hearing loss	No	No	Shrinking of eustachian tubes. Nothing into ear. Antibiotics may be necessary
Emphysema (subcutaneous, mediastinal)	No	No	Yes	Yes	Air embolism	Crepitus of soft tissues, dyspnea	Yes	Often	Subcutaneous emphysema usually clears; mediastinal often recurs after decompression
Epistaxis	Yes	Yes	Yes	Yes	Barotrauma, previous disease	May vary from slight oozing to severe hemorrhage	No	No	Symptomatic treatment only
External ear squeeze	No	No	Yes	Yes	Nonequalizing air-containing apparatus	Redness, bleb formation, bleeding	No	No	Symptomatic only — recovery complete in short time

CONDITION	SKIN DIVERS (Breath-holding)	SNORKEL DIVERS (Tube-to-Surface)	SCUBA DIVERS	HELMET-SUIT-AIR HOSE DIVERS	CAUSE	SIGNS AND SYMPTOMS	RECOMPRESSION IN PRESSURE CHAMBER?	ARTIFICIAL RESPIRATION?	OTHER TREATMENT AND COMMENTS
Hemoptysis	Yes	Yes, if tube too long	Yes	Yes	Usually air embolism; occasionally too long snorkel or barotrauma	Bloody froth indicative of lung sinus, or middle ear damage from attempts to equalize pressure on descent	Yes	Often	In snorkel or skin divers, supportive therapy only; in SCUBA or helmet-suit–air hose divers immediate recompression and slow decompression may be lifesaving
Neurologic disturbances	No	No	Yes	Yes	Air embolism or decompression sickness	All types. Onset may be deferred many hours or occur after apparent recovery from other conditions	Yes	May be necessary	Neurologic abnormalities in a diver who has descended more than 30 feet using any type of breathing apparatus requires recompression and slow decompression at once
Otitis externa	Yes	Yes	Yes	Yes	Water in external canal	See *External ear squeeze* (above)	No	No	If irritation or maceration of canal is present, drying after each dive is indicated. (Also see **32–12**.)
Otitis media	Yes	Yes	Yes	Yes	Frequent wetting, chilling	Pain, tinnitus	No	No	See **32–13**
Oxygen poisoning	No	No	Yes	Yes	Excessive depth, inadequate lung ventilation	Vertigo, nausea, muscle twitching, followed by convulsions	Yes, usually	Yes, usually	Usually complete recovery if rescued before drowning, air embolism, or decompression sickness occurs

CONDITION	SKIN DIVERS (Breath-holding)	SNORKEL DIVERS (Tube-to-Surface)	SCUBA DIVERS	HELMET-SUIT-AIR HOSE DIVERS	CAUSE	SIGNS AND SYMPTOMS	RECOMPRESSION IN PRESSURE CHAMBER?	ARTIFICIAL RESPIRATION?	OTHER TREATMENT AND COMMENTS
Paralysis	No	No	Yes	Yes	Air embolism	Any part of body may be involved. Onset may be deferred many hours	Yes	May be necessary	Permanent paralysis may remain in spite of recompression and controlled decompression
Pneumothorax	No	No	Yes	Yes	Usually air embolism and/or decompression sickness, but may occur independently	Dyspnea, cyanosis, chest pain	Usually	Occasionally	After reexpansion in pressure chamber symptoms may recur when pressure is lowered
Respiratory arrest	Yes	Yes	Yes	Yes	Air embolism, decompression sickness, CO or CO_2 intoxication	Not breathing	Often	Yes	Immediate oxygenation by mouth-to-mouth, or mechanical artificial respiration continued during transportation to, or institution of, other therapy

23 – 6. MOUNTAIN SICKNESS

Acute mountain sickness, characterized by sleeplessness, lethargy, poor appetite, nausea and vomiting, is common among nonaccustomed persons above 17,000 feet. The condition is self-limiting and clears slowly under symptomatic treatment or on descent to a lower altitude. Frequent complications are pulmonary edema (**51**) and thrombophlebitis (**59 – 11**).

23 – 7. RESTRICTIONS ON AIR TRAVEL

Although modern commercial aircraft are equipped with pressurized cabins which limit the effects of barotrauma to those caused by ascent to and descent from a maximum of 8000 feet, persons with certain physical ailments may develop uncomfortable, possibly serious, symptoms if they travel by air. Among these conditions are:

1. Valvular heart disease or other severe or decompensated cardiac conditions, extreme hypertension, angina pectoris and coronary disease which could be seriously aggravated by altitude sickness (**23 – 1**), air sickness (**43 – 4**) or motion sickness (**43 – 18**).

2. Conditions in which the normal expansion of body gases (1.75 at 8000 feet, compared to 1.0 at sea level) might be detrimental. Among these are glaucoma, acute or chronic sinusitis, nasopharyngitis and otitis; large unsupported hernias; intestinal obstruction; acute appendicitis, peptic ulcers or postoperative conditions (eye surgery, pneumonectomy, intestinal anastomosis, etc.) in which increased gas volume might cause acute complications.

3. Fractured jaw. Unless some method of quick release in case of vomiting has been substituted for the usual wiring, persons with broken jaws should not travel by air.

4. Conditions in which slight hypoxia (90% arterial oxygen saturation at 8000 feet, compared to 96% at sea level) might be detrimental; among these are shock, status asthmaticus and severe pulmonary emphysema with limited respiratory reserve. It should be remembered that the oxygen masks available above each seat commercial aircraft have a flow rate of only 1.5 liters per minute or less than the flow rate (5 to 10 liters per minute) necessary for ment of acute hypoxemic states.

Conditions associated with profound anemia. This includes the ce of S and C hemoglobins in some Negroes; sickling and sis may occur.

6. Psychoses.
7. Communicable diseases.
8. Pregnancy beyond the 32nd week.

24. BITES

See also **56.** *Stings;* **61.** *Venoms.*

24—1. ANT BITES (See also **24—10; 56—2**)

The bites of many common varieties of ants can cause transient discomfort and occasional allergic reactions (**21**). The venom of the fire ant (**56—5**) is injected not by its jaws but by an abdominal stinger, causing severe localized reactions and systemic effects which may be dangerous.

24—2. BARRACUDA BITES

These voracious fish have tremendously long jaws armed with large, sharp serrated teeth which can inflict serious lacerations requiring extensive debridement and repair. Pound for pound they are much more dangerous than any variety of shark.

24—3. BAT BITES

Certain varieties of carnivorous and insectivorous bats may be rabid (**62—17**). In addition, they may carry other infectious viruses in their salivary glands. Orchitis, oophoritis and aseptic meningitis have been reported following bat bites.

24—4. BLACK WIDOW SPIDER BITES

The female of this species of spider (*Latrodectus mactans*)— easily identifiable by an hourglass-shaped, bright orange coloration of the abdomen—is responsible for many of the severe toxic effects following spider bites. The bite of the drab male is harmless.

In spite of wide publicity to the contrary, black widow spider bites are rarely fatal in adults unless an exceptionally vascular part of the body is bitten. However, in infants the mortality rate is high; it decreases progressively with age. The toxic picture (developing from 1 to 2 hours after the bite) is characterized by severe headache, cramping of the extremities, nausea, vomiting and intense local and abdominal pain which may be severe enough to be mistaken for an acute surgical abdomen. Severe shock (**53**) may be present.

TREATMENT

1. Treat shock at once (**53—7**).

2. Relieve apprehension and pain with rapid-acting barbiturates or opiates. Sodium pentobarbital, 0.2 to 0.3 gm. intramuscularly, should be given first; if no relief, 10 to 15 mg. of morphine sulfate should be given slowly intravenously.

3. Give 500 to 1000 ml. of 5% dextrose in saline intravenously. Force fluids by mouth.

4. Control the characteristic acute myalgia by intravenous injection of 10 ml. of 10% calcium gluconate solution. Magnesium sulfate, 10 ml. of a 25% solution, given slowly intravenously, also may be of value for this purpose.

5. Transfer to a hospital as soon as shock and acute pain have been controlled.

6. Antiserum may be necessary in severe cases but should not be given as a part of emergency therapy unless a long delay before hospitalization is anticipated. If antiserum is to be given, inject 0.02 ml. intracutaneously to test for sensitivity. If no wheal or indurated area is present after 20 minutes, give 2.5 ml. intramuscularly. If the intradermal test is positive, administration should be postponed until the patient has been hospitalized and desensitization procedures (**12**) have been carried out.

24—5. BROWN SPIDER BITES

Volume for volume the venom of a brown spider (*Loxosceles reclusa,* false hackled band spinner) is much more toxic than that of a rattlesnake, and of about the same potency as that of the female black widow spider (**24—4**). The venom contains levarterenol and a powerful hemolysin. The brown recluse spider is easily identified by a violin-shaped mark on its head.

Mild reactions to brown spider bites are characterized by slight discomfort (less than a bee sting) at the time of the bite, gradually increasing over a period of 8 hours to agonizing pain. Bleb formation surrounded by an area of intense ischemia develops, followed in 24 to 48 hours by formation of a tough black eschar surrounded by purplish induration. On removal there is a deep irregular, necrotic-based ulcer which heals very slowly with extreme scarring and usually with surrounding permanent pigmentation.

TREATMENT

1. Antihistaminics.

2. Anodynes for pain. Narcotics may be necessary, since the pain may be agonizing.

3. Calcium gluconate, 10 ml. of a 10% solution intravenously, for arthralgia.

4. Local infiltration of phentolamine (Regitine) to limit necrosis.

Severe reactions are indicated by a generalized morbilliform eruption, fever up to 40°C. (104°F), recurrent fainting spells, severe arthralgia, shock and hemoglobinuria.

TREATMENT

1. Treatment of shock (**53 — 7**).

2. Control of arthralgia with intravenous calcium gluconate, 10 ml. of a 10% solution.

3. Hospitalize for symptomatic and supportive therapy (**49 — 4**). Antivenin has been used with excellent results against certain South American varieties, but no antivenin for the North American variety is as yet commercially available.

PROGNOSIS. Prognosis for recovery is good unless a massive dose of venom has been received. Repeated bites apparently cause immunity. Disfigurement by scars and pigmentation is common.

24 — 6. CAMEL BITES

Because of the tremendous leverage resulting from the unusual shape of the jaws and the peculiar dentition (long incisors in the upper jaw which imbricate with the canines) of these vicious animals, camel bites usually result in fractures and dislocations in addition to extensive crushing, tearing and avulsion of soft tissues. Extensive reconstructive surgery is often required.

24 — 7. CAT BITES

Cat bites and scratches, even if minute, may cause a benign low-grade infection (cat scratch fever). For local treatment, see **24 — 9**. *Dog Bites.*

24 – 8. CHIGGER BITES

The small larvae of thrombiculid mites (chiggers) – which often are parasitic to birds and reptiles – may cause uncomfortable but rarely serious local irritation, especially in children. Infestation usually occurs from playing in damp, swampy areas of scrub vegetation and is characterized by papules and vesicles at the site of the bite, especially around the genitalia, sometimes causing difficulty in voiding. Itching, redness and swelling, lasting 3 to 5 days, may occur with secondary cellulitis and lymphadenitis, or occasionally bacteremia, from scratching.

TREATMENT
1. Scrubbing with soap and water.
2. Trimming fingernails.
3. Application of a lotion containing 1% gamma benzene hexachloride.
4. Antipruritic ointments and lotions.
5. Antibiotics for secondary infection.

24 – 9. DOG BITES

Dog bites vary in extent from slight contusions, superficial abrasions and fang puncture wounds to deep tearing lacerations if the animal or the victim attempts to pull away.

TREATMENT
1. Contusions usually require no treatment provided the skin is not broken. See **62 – 17**. *Virus Infections – Rabies.*
2. Abrasions and puncture wounds require thorough local treatment (**55 – 2; 55 – 28**) followed, if indicated, by specific measures against tetanus (**16**) and rabies (**62 – 17**).
3. Lacerations require thorough debridement, irrigation and closure (**55 – 20**), protection against tetanus (**16**) and consideration of the need for protection against rabies (**62 – 17**). Whenever possible, the dog should be kept under observation by the appropriate animal control agency. If the animal has been killed, the body should be turned over to the local health authorities for disposition. Under no circumstances should the body be destroyed.

24 – 10. FLEA BITES

Flea bites may cause severe local reactions with surrounding edema, wheals, cellulitis and intense itching.

TREATMENT
1. Cold compresses.
2. Application of sodium bicarbonate paste or calamine lotion.
3. Tripelennamine hydrochloride (Pyribenzamine), 30 to 50 mg. by mouth.
4. Referral to a dermatologist for possible desensitization in extreme cases.

24—11. GILA MONSTER BITES

Gila monster bites cause severe local reactions but are rarely dangerous except in infants and small children.
TREATMENT
1. Immediate use of ice packs.
2. Application of a tourniquet proximal to the bite if on an extremity, with slow release over a period of 1 hour.
3. Thorough cleansing, with debridement and primary closure under local anesthetic if necessary.
4. Protection against tetanus (**16**).
5. Administration of prophylactic antibiotics.

24—12. HORSE BITES

Severe horse bites are rare because of the shape of the front teeth. If the skin is broken, treatment is the same as that outlined for dog bites (**24—9**), except that rabies prophylaxis is not necessary.

24—13. HUMAN BITES

Human bites often result in severe infections. Treatment consists of thorough debridement, irrigation and repair (**55—20**) followed by antibiotics—preferably after culture and sensitivity tests. Inoculation against rabies and protection against tetanus is not necessary.

24—14. INSECT BITES

Although severe systemic diseases may be transmitted by insect bites [i.e., malaria (**30—14**), yellow fever (**30—39**), typhus (**30—34**), etc.], local reactions are usually mild. Systemic allergic reactions, however, may be extremely severe and require immediate and extensive care (**21.** *Allergic Reactions;* **61.** *Venoms*).

24 — 15. LLAMA BITES

Llama bites have the same peculiarities and characteristics as camel bites (**24 — 6**).

24 — 16. MOSQUITO BITES

Therapy is the same as that given for flea bites (**24 — 10**). See also **30 — 14.** *Malaria;* **30 — 39.** *Yellow Fever.*

24 — 17. RAT BITES

Infants living in squalid surroundings may be injured severely by rat bites. The treatment is similar to that outlined under dog bites (**24 — 9**). Severe systemic conditions such as bubonic plague (**30 — 20**) may be transmitted by rat fleas.

24 — 18. SANDFLY BITES. See **62 — 18.** *Sandfly Fever*

24 — 19. SNAKE BITES

"Bites" of poisonous snakes are not caused by closing of the jaws, but by strikes or thrusts with the mouth open, with introduction of the venom through needle-like hollow fangs.

All of the 4 species of poisonous snakes inhabiting North America (rattlesnake, copperhead or highland moccasin, water moccasin or cottonmouth, and coral or harlequin snake) are pit vipers and can be identified by elliptical pupils, pits posterior to the nostrils, fangs and a single row of subcaudal plates on the ventral surface (Fig. 12). By far the most common is the rattlesnake, which may vary in length (from 6 inches to over 7 feet) and in color and markings with its environment. The fer-de-lance group — the tropical rattler, the cantril and the bushmaster — is common in tropical Central and South America. Many varieties of cobras and kraits occur in southeastern Asia and India. Several varieties of sea snakes are extremely toxic. One variety [the yellow-bellied seasnake *(Pelamus platurus)*] is found on the Pacific coast of Mexico and is ten times as toxic as cobras or kraits (**61.** *Venoms*).

Snake venoms contain hemotoxic and neurotoxic substances in varying proportions and amounts, depending on the species (**61.** *Venoms*). Antitoxins are available for some, but not all, varieties in the areas in which they occur.

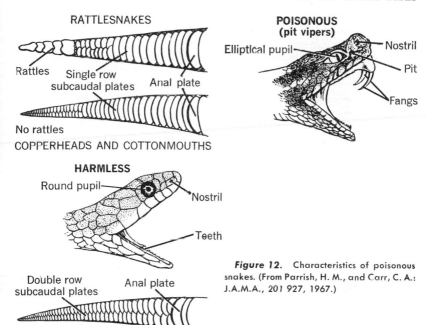

RATTLESNAKES

Rattles
Single row subcaudal plates
Anal plate

No rattles

COPPERHEADS AND COTTONMOUTHS

POISONOUS (pit vipers)

Elliptical pupil
Nostril
Pit
Fangs

HARMLESS

Round pupil
Nostril
Teeth

Double row subcaudal plates
Anal plate

Figure 12. Characteristics of poisonous snakes. (From Parrish, H. M., and Carr, C. A.: J.A.M.A., 201 927, 1967.)

Signs and symptoms of snakebite consist of typical fang marks—2 distinct punctures. A row of small superficial wounds from the lower teeth may be present. Local pain, ecchymosis, edema and local hemorrhage may be present with some varieties, absent with others. Progressive respiratory and circulatory depression and neurologic signs and symptoms, depending upon the toxic properties of the venom (**61**), develop within a short time.

TREATMENT

1. Apply a tourniquet about 2 inches proximal to the bite or swelling if on an extremity, tight enough to occlude the lymphatics and venous return but not tight enough to shut off the arterial blood supply. The tourniquet should not be removed until the patient can receive definitive care, but can be loosened slightly every 20 to

30 minutes for a few minutes and advanced as necessary to keep it 2 inches proximal to the swelling extending from the bite.

2. Keep the patient as calm and quiet as possible. Excessive activity may result in more rapid spread of the venom. If possible, kill the snake for identification.

3. Give morphine sulfate cautiously through subcutaneous, intramuscular or intravenous routes for severe pain and apprehension. The smallest possible effective doses should be used because of the danger of increasing respiratory depression. If necessary, the depressant effect of the narcotic can be neutralized by intravenous naloxone hydrochloride (Narcan).

4. Incise the bite (including the fang marks) linearly, down to the fat and extending slightly beyond each fang mark. Do not make any cruciate incisions. Massage the bite area digitally to express venom. Suction should be applied by suction cup or other means. Mouth suction can be used without danger, but may result in secondary infection of the incised area. Suction of some type should be continued for at least 1 hour.

5. Support the circulation. Large amounts of black coffee by mouth, or caffeine sodiobenzoate (0.5 gm. intramuscularly or intravenously), usually is effective. If circulatory depression is acute, support by administration of vasoconstrictor drugs may be necessary. See *Vasopressor and Cardiotonic Medications,* under **53−7.** *Treatment of Shock.*

6. Inject anti-snakebite serum after testing for sensitivity to horse serum (**12**) in adequate amounts as soon as possible, even if the victim is moribund. The usual North and South American Antiserum (antivenin) is polyvalent for every variety of rattlesnake, copperhead, moccasin, fer-de-lance group, cantril and bushmaster. It is not effective against coral snakes, cobras, kraits and poisonous seasnakes. An antiserum against coral snake venom has recently become available in the United States. In other parts of the world, special types of antisera effective against indigenous poisonous snakes are prepared and available, usually through local public health authorities. After testing for sensitivity to horse serum (**12**), 5 ml. of antivenin (or appropriate antiserum) should be injected subcutaneously and intramuscularly around the bite to prevent sloughing and necrosis. The remainder of the ampule should then be injected intramuscularly at some distance from the bite. This initial injection of antiserum represents only a small fraction of the total amount required for adequate treatment. Four or 5 ampules may be required to adequately neutralize the venom of large or

tropical species. Children usually require 2 to 3 times the adult dose. If coma, paralysis or other evidences of massive envenomization are present, intravenous injections of antivenin may be necessary. If the intravenous route is used, 0.25 ml. of a 1:100 dilution of antivenin should be given; if after 10 minutes no reaction has occurred, 3.0 ml. should be given, followed in 10 minutes by the full dose intravenously.

7. Inject human tetanus-immune globulin (TIG). Tetanus toxoid may be indicated if the patient has ever been actively immunized (**16**).

8. Give broad spectrum antibiotics in large doses.

9. Transfer all patients to a hospital as soon as possible for further antivenin, necessary supportive therapy and close observation for at least 4 days. Dangerous relapses may occur after apparent marked improvement as long as 3 days after the bite. Less serious complications may require medical care for 2 weeks or more.

10. DO NOT cauterize the punctured area with acids, potassium permanganate crystals, iodine or hot metallic objects. Alcohol-containing drinks are of no therapeutic value, although they may result in a beneficial temporary decrease in anxiety and activity. Corticosteroids, antihistaminics and cryotherapy are of no value in the emergency treatment of snake bite.

24—20. SPIDER BITES

Except for the 3 varieties listed below, spider bites result in mild local reactions only and require no specific therapy.

Black widow spider. The female is characterized by an hourglass-shaped, bright orange marking on the belly (**24—4**). The male is smaller, dun-colored and harmless.

Brown spider. Characterized by a violin-shaped darker brown or black coloration on the back (**24—5**).

Tarantulas. Characterized by large size and hairiness of legs and body (**24—21**).

24—21. TARANTULA BITES

Tarantula bites cause no systemic reactions, but locally the reaction may be severe, especially in children. Thorough cleansing followed by debridement of the wound under procaine or lidocaine (Xylocaine) infiltration anesthesia, often is necessary.

Human tetanus-immune globulin (TIG) or toxoid (**16**) should be given routinely.

24 − 22. TICK BITES

Tick bites are characterized by burying of the head of the tick. The following procedures may be necessary to release the head from the tissues: gentle rotation of the body; application of kerosene, turpentine or gasoline; careful approximation of the glowing end of a cigarette close to the body of the tick or excision of the buried head under local anesthesia.

Rocky Mountain spotted fever, transmitted by both the wood tick and the dog tick, is endemic in the United States and represents an often overlooked cause of severe local and general symptoms.

TREATMENT

1. Frequent inspection for and removal of ticks, especially from the scalp.

2. Hospitalization for agglutination tests and definitive therapy, if the clinical picture is suggestive of Rocky Mountain spotted fever. If a delay in hospitalization is anticipated, large doses of broad spectrum antibiotics are indicated.

TICK PARALYSIS

Bites of certain varieties of wood ticks (*Dermacentor andersoni*) and dog ticks (*Dermacentor variabilis*) may cause severe, even fatal, paralysis. Some type of powerful neurotoxin absorbed from the head of the gravid female tick apparently is the toxic agent. Tick paralysis is often ascending and progressive and can be distinguished from the paralysis of anterior poliomyelitis and Guillain-Barré syndrome only by the absence of fever and spinal fluid changes.

TREATMENT

1. Surgical removal of the buried head. Except in moribund patients, this will result in progressive improvement starting 2 to 3 days after excision with ultimate complete recovery.

2. Energetic supportive therapy until improvement begins.

24 − 23. WILD ANIMAL BITES

Wild animal bites are notorious for causing severe infections: they require energetic treatment. Bites on the face are especially dangerous. Lacerations and deep puncture wounds may require debridement, irrigation and secondary closure (**55—20**). All cases should be given human tetanus-immune globulin (TIG) or toxoid (**16**) and broad spectrum antibiotics. Follow-up care in 24 hours should be arranged. *Cauterization with fuming nitric acid—*as suggested in some first aid texts—*should never be done.* For details of prophylactic treatment following bites of nonrabid and rabid animals, see **62—17.** *Virus Infections—Rabies.*

24—24. BITES OF UNIDENTIFIED ETIOLOGY

Bites of unidentified etiology should be treated symptomatically as follows:

1. Application of a tourniquet, if on an extremity, with release for 1½ minutes every half hour.
2. Chilling of the site of the bite by ice packs.
3. Control of severe pain by appropriate anodynes.
4. Debridement, irrigation, antitetanus prophylaxis and antibiotics, as outlined under **24—23.** *Wild Animal Bites.*
5. Intravenous injection of 10 ml. of 10% calcium gluconate for acute myalgia. If relief is obtained, this injection can be repeated as needed; if not, the tourniquet and ice packs with symptomatic measures should be continued until the patient can be hospitalized for observation.

For prophylactic treatment against rabies, see **62—17.**

25. BURNS

See also **48—14.** *Burns In Children.*

25—1. PRINCIPLES OF EVALUATION

Emergency therapy, disposition and prognosis in all types of burns are based on five basic factors which must be considered at the first evaluation of the patient.

PER CENT OF BODY SURFACE AFFECTED

The body surface of an average-sized (70 kg. of 154 lb.) adult is about 1.73 square meters or 18½ square feet. Disposition, treatment and prognosis depend upon estimation of the amount of body surface involved.

PRINCIPLES OF EVALUATION

The *Rule of Nines* is accurate enough for emergency use. For variations in infancy and childhood, see **48 — 14.**

PART OF BODY	% OF BODY SURFACE
Head, face and neck	9
Right arm, forearm and hand	9
Left arm, forearm and hand	9
Thorax — front	9
Thorax — back	9
Abdomen — lower ribs to inguinal creases	9
Back — lower ribs to subgluteal creases	9
Right thigh, leg and foot — front	9
Right thigh, leg and foot — back	9
Left thigh, leg and foot — front	9
Left thigh, leg and foot — back	9
Genitalia	1
	100%

DEPTH See Fig. 13.

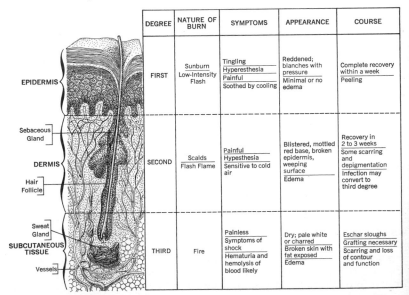

	DEGREE	NATURE OF BURN	SYMPTOMS	APPEARANCE	COURSE
EPIDERMIS	FIRST	Sunburn Low-Intensity Flash	Tingling / Hyperesthesia / Painful / Soothed by cooling	Reddened; blanches with pressure / Minimal or no edema	Complete recovery within a week / Peeling
Sebaceous Gland / DERMIS / Hair Follicle	SECOND	Scalds Flash Flame	Painful / Hyperesthesia / Sensitive to cold air	Blistered, mottled red base, broken epidermis, weeping surface / Edema	Recovery in 2 to 3 weeks / Some scarring and depigmentation / Infection may convert to third degree
Sweat Gland / SUBCUTANEOUS TISSUE / Vessels	THIRD	Fire	Painless / Symptoms of shock / Hematuria and hemolysis of blood likely	Dry; pale white or charred / Broken skin with fat exposed / Edema	Eschar sloughs / Grafting necessary / Scarring and loss of contour and function

Figure 13. Diagnosis of burn depth. (From Sako, Y.: Hosp. Med., Vol. 1, No. 2, 1964.)

1. Superficial (first degree). Erythema, dry, painful.
2. Partial Skin Thickness (second degree). Bleb formation, bases reddened; moist, painful.
3. Deep (third degree). Involvement of the full thickness of the skin and the subcutaneous and deeper tissues with discoloration, charring and loss of substance. Usually not painful.

LOCATION

Shock (**53**) is much more common if the head, face, hands, genitalia and feet are damaged. Severe pain may be present if highly specialized areas (such as the face or hands) or freely movable areas (such as flexion creases or joints) are involved.

Time elapsed since the burn.   The danger of shock and infection varies directly with the interval between injury and treatment.

Age and general physical condition.   Children under 5, elderly persons and all individuals whose resistance is below normal for any reason are especially susceptible to the systemic effects of burns.

25 — 2.   PRINCIPLES OF TREATMENT

Localized: involving less than 35% of body surface in adults (for children, see **48 — 14**)

TREATMENT
1. Wash thoroughly with nonmedicated white soap and water.
2. Apply a petrolatum gauze dressing; in very mild cases, apply a soothing lotion.
3. Prescribe sedatives for restlessness and acetylsalicylic acid (aspirin) for pain.
4. Arrange for follow-up care.

Extensive: involving more than 35% of body surface in adults, less in children (**48 — 14**)

TREATMENT
1. Wash thoroughly with a mild detergent that does not contain hexachlorophene, followed by soap and water.
2. Apply petrolatum gauze dressings, or wrap in sterile towels or sheets. If the patient is hospitalized, substitute sulfamylon cream for the petrolatum gauze dressings. Sulfamylon cream (10% para-aminomethylbenzene sulfonamide acetate in a water soluble base) is applied directly to the cleansed burn area with the sterile gloved hand and should be washed off and reapplied twice a day. The appli-

cation may be painful enough to require small doses of narcotics. Because of this discomfort and because no protective bandage is applied, sulfamylon cream is not suitable for ambulatory care.

3. Control apprehension, restlessness and pain, using narcotics if necessary. In infants and children under 4 years old, a pentobarbital sodium (Nembutal) suppository should be substituted for narcotics.

4. Hospitalize if the location or extent of the burn makes ambulatory or home care impractical.

Partial Skin Thickness (second degree) **or Deep** (third degree) **Burns**
TREATMENT

1. Control apprehension, restlessness and pain by subcutaneous, intramuscular or intravenous barbiturates and/or narcotics, as indicated.

2. Combat shock (**53 – 7**).

3. Gently remove all clothing from the involved areas.

4. Using aseptic technique, cleanse the burned areas thoroughly with a mild detergent followed by soap and water and irrigate with sterile saline solution. Gross contamination and loose devitalized tissue should be removed, but no attempt at thorough debridement should be made.

5. Apply a sterile dressing of one of the following types:

Petrolatum gauze held in place by bias-cut stockinette or loosely wrapped elastic bandage.

A cellulose pad faced with fine mesh gauze held in place by bandage or adhesive.

Pads of gauze, sterile towels or sheets saturated with sterile saline if immediate hospitalization has been arranged. These dressings should be replaced by sulfamylon cream as soon as possible.

6. Apply splints if necessary to prevent motion of the burned areas.

7. Administer tetanus-immune globulin (TIG) or toxoid (**16**).

8. Hospitalize as soon as possible if:

More than 35% of body surface is involved. (For children, see **48 – 14**.)

The patient has been or remains in severe shock (**53**).

The head, eyes, face, respiratory tract, hands, feet or genitalia are extensively involved.

The areas involved, or other factors, preclude ambulatory or home care.

BURNS REQUIRING SPECIAL MANAGEMENT

25 — 3.   ACID BURNS

TREATMENT

1. Wash thoroughly in running water for a lengthy time as soon as possible after contact with acid.

2. Control restlessness and pain by administration of barbiturates and narcotics as needed. Combat shock if present (**53**).

3. Manage as indicated under *Principles of Treatment* (**25 — 2**). See also **25 — 13**. *Eye Burns;* **35 — 31**. *Conjunctival Injuries;* **35 — 32**. *Corneal Injuries;* **49 — 26**. *Acids.* For treatment of hydrofluoric acid burns, see **49 — 378**.

25 — 4.   ALKALI BURNS

TREATMENT

1. Wash thoroughly for a lengthy time with running water.

2. Control restlessness and pain by administration of barbiturates and narcotics as needed. Treat shock if necessary (**53 — 7**).

3. Manage as outlined under *Principles of Treatment* (**25 — 2**). See also **25 — 13**. *Eye Burns;* **35 — 31**. *Conjunctival Injuries;* **35 — 32**. *Corneal Injuries;* **49 — 39**. *Alkalies,* **49 — 432**. *Lye.*

25 — 5.   ASPHALT OR TAR BURNS

TREATMENT

1. Control apprehension and pain by barbiturates and narcotics as indicated. Combat shock if necessary (**53 — 7**).

2. Wash thoroughly with soap and warm water.

3. Remove adherent congealed asphalt or tar if the area involved is relatively small and the site permits by:

Soaking with solvents such as skin cleanser, ether, mineral oil or Scriptoil. Certain substances can be removed most easily by freezing with ice or an ethyl chloride spray.

Peeling off with forceps.

4. Wash thoroughly with soap and warm water, followed by irrigation with sterile saline.

5. Apply a petrolatum gauze dressing and hold in place by a bias-cut stockinette or a loosely applied elastic bandage.

6. Splint if necessary.

7. Give tetanus-immune globulin (TIG) or toxoid if indicated (**16**).

8. Hospitalize if the congealed asphalt or tar covers a large portion of the body or involves an area which will not permit removal without anesthetic. Hot asphalt and tar burns are usually much deeper than first examination would seem to indicate.

25−6. ATOMIC ENERGY BURNS See 63−4.

25−7. CAUSTIC BURNS See 25−4. *Alkali Burns*

25−8. CEMENT OR CONCRETE BURNS See 25−4. *Alkali Burns*

25−9. CHEMICAL BURNS See 25−3. *Acid Burns;* 25−4. *Alkali Burns;* the specific chemical involved; 49. *Poisons*

25−10. EAR BURNS

Of the soft tissues. Treat as outlined under *Principles of Treatment* (**25−2**), except that open treatment without bandaging is often practical.

Of the canals—usually from hot slag or metal. No treatment is required except removal of the foreign body (**36−1**). The patient should be warned against putting medications or plugs of any type into the ear canal.

Of the ear drums. If slight, removal of the foreign body (**36−1**) is all that is required. If the foreign body is burned in or has perforated through the drum:

1. Control pain.
2. Apply a pad over the ear.
3. Refer at once for specialist care.

25−11. ELECTRICAL BURNS (See also 29−5. *Electric Shock*)

Passage of an electrical current through living tissues often does far more damage than is apparent on superficial examination. Immediate death from ventricular fibrillation (**26−23**) may occur. Respiratory failure requiring artificial respiration (**11−1**) is common. Low voltage currents are more dangerous than high tension, and alternating current is more lethal than direct current.

Treatment

1. If the patient is in coma or in circulatory or respiratory collapse, defer all local treatment until the measures outlined under **29 – 5.** *Electric Shock* have been carried out and the patient's condition has stabilized.

2. Identify the points of entrance and exit of the current (the latter often is overlooked). By estimating the path of the current some idea of the organs which may have been damaged can be obtained.

3. Debride both the entrance and exit wounds thoroughly under local anesthesia, removing all charred or devitalized structures. Close with loose, interrupted, nonabsorbable sutures and apply sterile dressings. Relaxing incisions and skin grafting may be necessary.

4. Hospitalize for observation for at least 48 hours if the patient has been unconscious, if cardiac irregularities have been noted or if the burned areas are deep, extensive or involve important structures.

25 – 12. ESOPHAGEAL BURNS (See also **25 – 18.** *Mucous Membrane Burns;* **49 – 26.** *Acids;* **49 – 39.** *Alkalies;* **49 – 432.** *Lye).*

Strictures requiring dilatation may occur.

25 – 13. EYE BURNS (See also **35 – 31.** *Conjunctival Injuries;* **35 – 32.** *Corneal Injuries)*

ACID, ALKALI OR CAUSTIC BURNS

1. Irrigate for at least 15 minutes with tap water, sterile water or normal salt solution. Never attempt to use neutralizing solutions in the eyes.

2. Instill 2 drops of 0.5% tetracaine (Pontocaine) solution to control pain.

3. Apply an eye patch.

4. Refer at once to an ophthalmologist.

HOT ASPHALT, TAR, SLAG OR METAL BURNS

1. Instill 2 drops of 0.5% tetracaine (Pontocaine) solution.

2. Remove any loose or superficially embedded foreign bodies (**35 – 31; 35 – 32**). If deep or firmly adherent, do not attempt removal.

DO NOT attempt to use the solvents previously recommended for asphalt and tar (**25 – 5**).

3. Apply an eye patch.

4. Refer at once to an ophthalmologist.

25 – 14. FLASH BURNS

Nuclear fission bomb flash burns are characterized by involvement of the side of the body toward the point of explosion and by bizarre patterns of several depths resulting from the varying absorbabilities of different clothing fabrics. The treatment is the same as outlined under **25 – 2**. *Principles of Treatment – Burns;* **63 – 4** and **63 – 6**. *Wartime Emergencies.*

Welder's flash burns (Photophthalmia). See **35 – 31**. *Conjunctival Injuries.*

25 – 15. FRICTION BURNS

Friction burns usually involve the palmar surface of the hands ("rope burns") or those portions of the body not protected by heavy clothing [*Pavement Burns* (**25 – 21**)]. Friction burns may range in severity from slight superficial abrasions to shredding and avulsion of charred and blackened tissues. For treatment, see **25 – 2**. *Principles of Treatment – Burns;* **40**. *Hand Injuries;* **55 – 2**. *Abrasions.*

25 – 16. GASOLINE (Distillate, Fuel Oil, Kerosene) BURNS

TREATMENT

1. Remove all contaminated clothing at once.

2. Wash the affected areas thoroughly with mild, nonmedicated soap and water.

3. Apply a bland ointment to areas of erythema. Second degree burns are not common, but if present they should be dressed with petrolatum gauze.

4. Watch carefully for evidence of upper respiratory tract irritation caused by aspiration or inhalation of fumes or flames; if present, antibiotics followed by hospitalization is indicated.

25 – 17. MAGNESIUM BURNS (See also 49 – 434)

TREATMENT

1. Paint the burned area with copper sulfate solution, watching closely for evidence of copper toxicity (**49 – 223**).

2. Irrigate with large amounts of saline solution.

3. Remove superficially embedded particles of metal by sharp dissection, using local anesthesia or regional nerve blocks if necessary.

4. Apply a petrolatum gauze dressing, or, if the patient is hospitalized, apply sulfamylon cream with the sterile gloved hand twice a day.

5. Give broad spectrum antibiotics.

6. Watch carefully for development of crepitation, ulceration or sloughing.

25 – 18. MUCOUS MEMBRANE BURNS

Mucous membrane burns are usually mild, but in some instances they may result in extreme edema and severe pain. Three sites are common: mouth, throat and respiratory tract.

In the mouth and throat [except for acid burns (**25 – 3**) and alkali burns (**25 – 4**)], burns are usually caused by swallowing extremely hot foods or drinks. As a rule, these burns are more uncomfortable than serious. Symptomatic treatment is all that is required.

In the respiratory tract, burns are caused by the inhalation of flame or hot gases. Symptoms of acute carbon monoxide poisoning (**49 – 172**) may be present.

TREATMENT

1. Administration of sedatives. In severe cases, small doses of narcotics for control of reflex spasm may be necessary.

2. Insurance of an adequate airway by removal of secretions by postural drainage and suction. If marked edema, dyspnea or cyanosis is present, emergency cricothyreotomy or tracheostomy (**14 – 12**) may be necessary.

3. Prescription of a soothing cough mixture.

4. Immediate hospitalization if evidence of lung damage is present. Terminal pulmonary edema (**51**) may occur, usually as a delayed development.

In the vagina, the use of strong caustic medications as douches or as attempts to induce abortions (see **49 – 618.** *Potassium Permanganate*) may cause mucous membrane injury ranging from slight edema to necrosis and perforation.

TREATMENT

1. Mild cases require only sedation and copious, frequent, nonirritating douches.

2. Moderate cases require adequate frequent careful cleansing to prevent secondary infection.

3. Severe cases with extreme edema and ulceration or perforation must be hospitalized at once. Surgical debridement and repair under general anesthetic may be necessary.

25 – 19. MUSTARD GAS BURNS See 49 – 833. *War Gases.* (Vesicants); 63 – 11. *Poison Gases*

25 – 20. NAPALM BURNS

Spraying of burning gasoline or distillate mixed with a contact adhesive is now a common offensive weapon in war and results in severe burns with the characteristics of hot asphalt burns (25 – 5) and upper respiratory tract burns (25 – 18. *Mucous Membrane Burns, Respiratory Tract*).

25 – 21. PAVEMENT BURNS

Persons thrown from moving vehicles often slide along abrasive surfaces with considerable momentum. Friction and abrasion, with grinding into the skin, subcutaneous tissues and underlying structures of multiple small foreign bodies, can result in injuries peculiarly susceptible to infection, tattooing and permanent scarring.

TREATMENT. See 25 – 15. *Friction Burns;* 55 – 2. *Abrasions.*

25 – 22. PHOSPHORUS BURNS (See also 49 – 602. *Phosphorus*)

The use of rockets and flares in modern warfare has resulted in a large number of serious second and third degree burns from phosphorus, which has the physical property of igniting spontaneously, even in the tissues, on exposure to air. Systemically, absorption of phosphorus may result in liver and kidney damage and depression of the blood forming organs.

TREATMENT

1. As soon as possible after injury, flood with large quantities of water or 2% sodium bicarbonate solution.

2. Coat with 5% copper sulfate solution applied directly to the phosphorus particles.

3. Debride all necrotic or loose tissue at once, removing all particles of phosphorus by forceps or sharp dissection. The severity of systemic reactions is directly proportionate to the amount of phosphorus left in the tissues.

4. Irrigate the wound thoroughly with normal saline solution to remove excess copper, which in itself may give serious toxic effects (**49 — 223**).

5. Apply sodium perborate solution or sulfamylon cream directly to the burned areas.

6. Transfer for prompt and adequate follow-up medical care for systemic effects — ecchymoses, gastrointestinal bleeding, jaundice, hypoglycemia, hematuria and blood changes.

25 — 23. RADIATION BURNS See **25 — 32.** *X-ray Burns;* **63 — 4.** *Wartime Emergencies, Nuclear Bombs*

25 — 24. RESPIRATORY TRACT BURNS See **22 — 5.** *Smoke Inhalation;* **25 — 18.** *Mucous Membrane Burns*

25 — 25. ROPE BURNS See **25 — 15.** *Friction Burns*

25 — 26. SCALP BURNS

Mild cases require only application of a soothing lotion. In severe cases, after clipping the hair and shaving the area around the burn, treat as outlined under **25 — 2.** *Burns, Principles of Treatment.*

25 — 27. SLAG BURNS

In the ear. See **25 — 10.**
In the eye. See **25 — 13; 35 — 31.** *Conjunctival Injuries;* **35 — 32.** *Corneal Injuries.*

25 — 28. SUNBURN

Mild cases require only sedatives or anodynes and local application of a soothing lotion.

Severe cases with bleb formation should be treated as outlined under **25 — 2.** *Burns, Principles of Treatment.* Hospitalization may be required if over 40% of the skin surface (less in children —

see **48−14**) is affected. Death can occur from extensive severe sunburn with involvement of a large percentage of the body surface. For systemic effects, see **57−8**. *Sunstroke.*

25−29. TEAR GAS BURNS See **49−832**. *War Gases*

25−30. TITANIUM TETRACHLORIDE BURNS See **49−787**

Do not use water for original treatment.

25−31. VAGINAL BURNS See **25−18**. *Mucous Membrane Burns;* **49−618**. *Potassium Permanganate*

25−32. WAR GAS BURNS See **49−832**

Tear gas burns respond well to early use of topical steroids.

25−33. X-RAY BURNS

Roentgen therapy in large doses (**18−7**) may result in an uncomfortable erythema. Industrial use of x-ray equipment (determination of defects in metals, etc.) is resulting in an increasing number of x-ray burns.

TREATMENT
1. Sedation by barbiturates, preferably by mouth.
2. Control of pain by acetylsalicylic acid (aspirin), 0.6 gm., with 0.03 gm. of codeine sulfate by mouth every 4 hours.
3. Limitation of painful motion by splinting.
4. Application of petrolatum gauze dressings.
(See also **63−4**. *Gamma Rays from Nuclear Bombs*)

26.   CARDIAC EMERGENCIES

See also **11**. *Resuscitation;* **48−15**. *Cardiac Emergencies in Children;* **53**. *Shock;* **59**, *Vascular Disorders.*

Definitive therapy of acute cardiac disease varies with the etiologic background of the illness or injury and usually requires more than brief treatment under emergency conditions. There is, however, a distinct group of cardiac emergencies in which prompt and rational action on the part of the attending physician may be the deciding factor in the patient's chance for survival. When life-threatening heart conditions, resulting from either mechanical or electrical failure, are present, or circumstances conducive to their development occur, the patient must be given immediate emergency supportive therapy, continued during careful and safe transportation to a well staffed and adequately equipped intensive or coronary care unit.

Direct current cardioversion is being more commonly used not only for ventricular fibrillation (**26 – 23**) but also for serious or life-threatening arrhythmias refractory to conventional forms of treatment and not induced by digitalis toxicity (**26 – 9**) or electrolyte imbalance.

26 – 1. ANEURYSM, VENTRICULAR

Occurring to some degree in 10 to 20% of myocardial infarctions, ventricular aneurysms may rupture and cause sudden death, although in some instances ventricular septal ruptures may be amenable to corrective surgery.

In the early postmyocardial infarction period, exacerbation of chest pain, increase or appearance of congestive heart failure (**26 – 8**) or shock (**53**), development of a coarse systolic murmur or progressive change in electrocardiographic vector should alert to the possibility of ventricular aneurysm, ventricular septal rupture or rupture of the chordae tendineae. Echocardiography aids in providing rapid, safe and non-invasive diagnosis. Referral for surgical evaluation and possible emergency intervention (ablation of the adynamic area, closure of septal rupture, placement of a prosthetic valve or prosthetic chordae replacement) is indicated in such situations.

26 – 2. ANGINA PECTORIS

Angina pectoris is characterized by rapid onset of substernal or precordial pain, usually squeezing or burning in character, which is often associated with increased cardiac work.

This acute discomfort usually clears in not more than 15 minutes with no treatment except rest. More rapid relief can be obtained by sublingual absorption of glyceryl trinitrate (nitroglycerin), 0.3 to 0.6 mg. repeated every 5 minutes. If 3 doses do not cause marked relief of symptoms, the patient should be evaluated for possible myocardial infarction (**26 – 12**). Smaller doses of nitroglycerin may be indicated if hypotension or severe throbbing headaches develop.

Note: Glyceryl trinitrate (nitroglycerin) tablets gradually deteriorate and lose their effect on exposure to air and should be replaced approximately twice a year.

26 – 3. ATRIAL FIBRILLATION (See Fig. 14, G)

If it occurs with a rapid ventricular rate, atrial fibrillation may cause acute pulmonary edema (**51**) from ventricular failure. Treatment under these circumstances consists of rapid intravenous digitalization with single or (preferably) divided doses of 0.8 to 1.6 mg. of deslanoside (Cedilanid-D) or, if conditions permit, with divided doses of 1.5 mg. of digoxin.

If the condition is life-threatening and remains refractory to digitalis therapy (and was not induced by digitalis), cardioversion with initially reduced current (50 watt-seconds) may be tried.

26 – 4. ATRIAL FLUTTER (See Fig. 14, F)

This condition usually demonstrates a rapid regular atrial rate of about 300 per minute and may have a variable A-V block, usually 2:1. It may occur during the course of treatment of atrial fibrillation with quinidine. The acuteness of the problem varies with the cause, degree of block and ventricular rate. As with atrial fibrillation (to which atrial flutter may revert during treatment), basic treatment consists of rapid intravenous digitalization with deslanoside (Cedilanid-D). Quinidine, sometimes recommended, should not be used unless the patient is fully digitalized. Electrical cardioversion should be considered.

26 – 5. ATRIAL PAROXYSMAL TACHYCARDIA (Fig. 14, I) See 26 – 21. *Supraventricular Tachycardia*

26 – 6. BACTERIAL ENDOCARDITIS, ACUTE

Usually secondary to a primary streptococcal, staphylococcal or pneumococcal focus elsewhere in the body, this endocardial and valvular infection is suggested by septicemia, murmur, diffuse electrocardiographic ST-T changes, bacterial growth in blood cultures and signs of emboli.

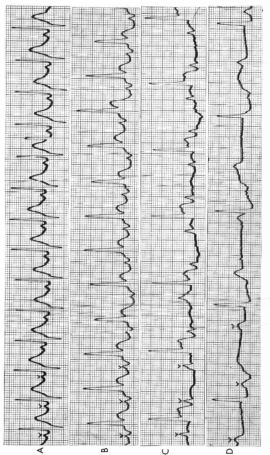

Figure 14. Electrocardiographic tracings. *A,* Sinus tachycardia. *B,* First degree A-V block. *C,* Second degree A-V block. *D,* Third degree A-V block.

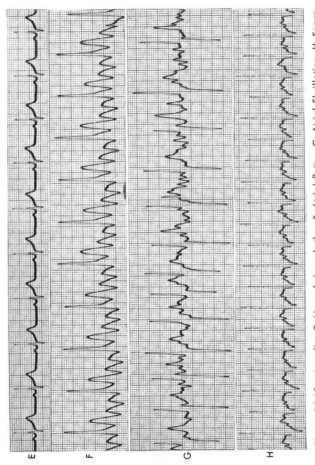

Figure 14 (Continued). *E*, Normal sinus rhythm. *F*, Atrial flutter. *G*, Atrial fibrillation. *H*, Supraventricular tachycardia, nodal.

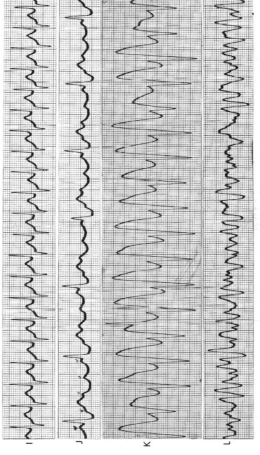

Figure 14 (Continued). I, Supraventricular tachycardia, atrial. J, Atrial tachycardia with 4:1 A-V response. K, Ventricular tachycardia. L, Ventricular fibrillation. (Tracings B, C, F, H, I and J made from instructional rhythm strip tapes available from the Physiologic Training Company, San Marino, California.)

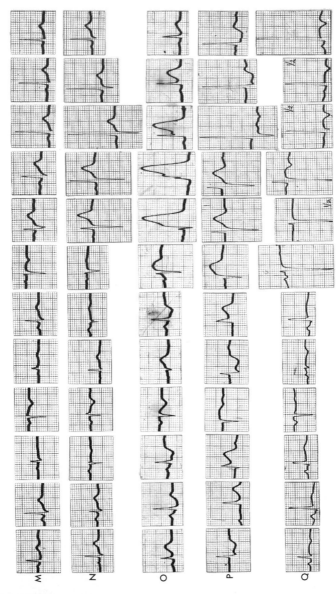

W

N

O

P

Q

Figure 14 (Continued). *M*, Normal electrocardiogram, intermediate position. *N*, Normal electrocardiogram, horizontal position. *O*, Acute anterior myocardial infarction. *P*, Acute inferior myocardial infarction (plus third degree atrioventricular block). *Q*, Pericarditis (typical limb leads; T wave of precordial leads usually upright early and invert later).

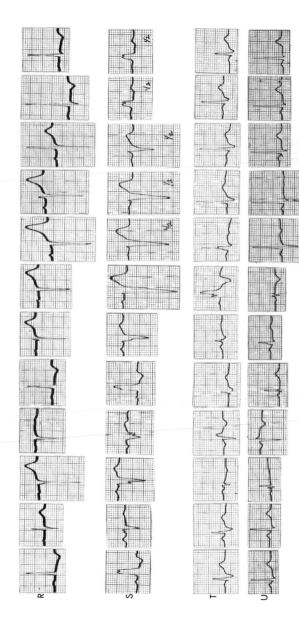

Figure 14 (Continued). *R*, Left ventricular hypertrophy (plus first degree atrioventricular block and q wave in aVF due to probable old inferior myocardial infarction). *S*, Complete left bundle branch block (r wave in V₁ and V₂ may be absent). *T*, Complete right bundle branch block. *U*, Incomplete right bundle branch block.

TREATMENT
1. Obtain six blood cultures rapidly, within 1 hour.
2. Start massive antibiotic therapy parenterally based on the probable cause of the primary infection without waiting for results of cultures and sensitivity tests. For appropriate antibiotics, **see 30 – 41.** *Antimicrobial Drugs of Choice.*

26 – 7. CARDIAC ARREST (For treatment, see 11 – 1. *Artificial Respiration;* 11 – 2. *Cardiac Compression*)

Characterized by loss of arterial pulse, pulse pressure and respiration, arrest may be due to cardiac standstill or to ventricular fibrillation (**26 – 23**) (*asystole cordis, convulsion of the heart*). It represents one of the most urgent conditions which may be encountered in the practice of medicine. Rapid recognition of the condition and prompt reestablishment of adequate oxygenation and circulation represent the only possible chance of saving the patient's life. Because severe hypoxemia for more than 3 to 5 minutes will usually result in irreparable damage to the higher centers of the brain, success depends upon carrying out an already planned course of action without delay.

CAUSES OF CARDIAC ARREST

Too rapid or unregulated administration of, or overdosage of, any anesthetic (inhalation, intravenous, spinal or local), with lack of close observation for and recognition of changes in condition.

Obstruction of the respiratory tract [mucus, vomitus, foreign bodies (**36**), trauma, angioedema (**21 – 2**), bronchospasm (**21 – 3**)].

Preexistent conditions [acute anxiety states (**34.** *Excitement States*), anemia, cardiac disease, dehydration, hyperpyrexia, pulmonary edema (**51**), shock (**53**)].

"Shotgun" preoperative medications.

Insufficient preanesthetic administration of atropine sulfate.

Mechanical errors (faulty gauges, mislabeled tanks, poor valves, etc.).

Position of the patient. The sitting position (sometimes used for throat operations) and the deep Trendelenburg are the most dangerous positions. Rapid shifting on the operating table may precipitate cardiac arrest.

Electric shock (**25 – 11.** *Electrical Burns;* **29 – 5**).

Air emboli (**59 – 4**), rare.

PRELIMINARY WARNING SIGNS OF INCIPIENT CARDIAC ARREST

1. Signs of respiratory obstruction (cyanosis, gasping respiration, tracheal tug, increased rate and shallowness of respiration).
2. Pulse irregularities and rate changes with a fall in pulse pressure. A resting pulse rate above 120 suggests shock; a rate of below 50 suggests decreased cardiac output.
3. Incipient cardiac decompensation and atrial fibrillation.
4. Electrocardiographic evidence of multifocal premature ventricular systoles.
5. Muscular twitching.
6. Dilation of the pupils; coldness and clamminess of the skin.

MEDICOLEGAL ASPECTS OF CARDIAC ARREST

1. Failure to recognize the preliminary warning signs of incipient cardiac arrest and to institute prompt and proper treatment has been held to constitute negligence (**68−1**).
2. Closed chest cardiac compression (**11−2**) is now accepted as the proper resuscitative measure, unless the chest is already open and the heart readily accessible for direct open chest manual cardiac compression or there is a fixed thoracic deformity or unstable thorax from fractures.
3. Lack of constant attendance during the recovery period from cardiac arrest has been construed as indicating negligence (**68−1**) on the part of the attending physician.

TREATMENT

For detailed therapy, see **11−1**. *Artificial Respiration;* **11−2**. *Cardiac Compression.*

26−8. CONGESTIVE HEART FAILURE (See also **51**. *Pulmonary Edema*)

This serious condition is due to pump failure of the ventricles (left, *forward failure;* right, *backward failure*) and is characterized by gradual increase in intra- and extravascular fluid volume, increased venous pressure, delayed circulation time (arm to tongue; arm to lung), pulmonary rales, edema of the liver and extremities, orthopnea, paroxysmal nocturnal dyspnea, exertional dyspnea, decreased effort tolerance and tachycardia.

Causes of the cardiac failure may be complex (coronary atherosclerosis, hypertension and fibrosis, myxedema, thyrotoxicosis, constrictive pericarditis, vitamin deficiency, valvular or septal defect or combinations thereof). Hospitalization may be required for definitive studies and appropriate treatment of the primary cause.

GENERAL MEASURES IN TREATMENT

1. Rest; decrease in cardiac work demand until compensated.
2. Low sodium diet.
3. Furosemide (Lasix), 40 to 80 mg. orally in a single dose, or 20 to 40 mg. intramuscularly or intravenously.
4. Digitalization (unless interrogation indicates recent use).
Slow: by digoxin, 0.5 mg. orally, then 0.25 mg. every 8 to 12 hours until signs of adequate digitalization are present. Slow digitalization is preferable in elderly or debilitated patients.
Intermediate: by digoxin, 0.75 to 1.0 mg. orally, followed by 0.25 to 0.5 mg. every 8 hours until digitalized.
Rapid: by deslanoside (Cedilanid-D), 1.2 to 1.6 mg., or by digoxin, 1.0 to 1.5 mg. intravenously, in a single injection or (preferably) in divided doses. One eighth to one quarter of the original dose should then be given at 4 hour intervals until the patient is digitalized.
5. Oxygen under positive pressure (6 liters per minute) by nasal catheter.
6. Sedation by chloral hydrate, 0.5 to 1.0 gm. orally, repeated every 4 to 6 hours if necessary.

26 – 9. DIGITALIS TOXICITY (See also 49 – 272)

The latitude between therapeutic and toxic doses of digitalis is small. Toxicity may result from overdosage, low tolerance (as in elderly patients) or disturbances in renal digitalis excretion or electrolyte balance (low serum potassium level).

Patients taking digitalis preparations who have previously had atrial fibrillation and who convert to a regular rhythm (i.e., complete atrioventricular block with regular nodal rhythm take-over have digitalis toxicity until proved otherwise and require serial evaluation with electrocardiograms. Right carotid sinus pressure for 5 seconds may assist in determining the presence of early toxic states. The electrocardiographic signs of toxicity described below may increase during the period of carotid stimulation.

SIGNS OF DIGITALIS TOXICITY (In order of increasing severity)

1. Mild malaise, anorexia, occasional unifocal premature ventricular contractions on ECG.

2. Nausea, vomiting, diarrhea, blurred vision, cephalgia and an increase in electrocardiographic findings − first degree conduction block (see Fig. 14, *B*), wandering pacemaker, frequent unifocal premature ventricular contractions.

3. Disorientation, partial heart block (especially paroxysmal atrial tachycardia with 2:1 block and atrioventricular dissociation), complete heart block, multifocal premature ventricular contractions, atrial fibrillation (**26−3**) and ventricular fibrillation (**26−23**) or ventricular tachycardia (**26−24**).

TREATMENT

Mild overdosage

1. Withholding of digitalis preparation for several days or up to three weeks, depending on the excretion rate of the particular drug in use and the observed clinical improvement.

2. Correction of any potassium deficit.

3. Reinstitution of a lower maintenance dose.

Severe toxicity

Hospitalize at once. For details of treatment, see **49−272**.

26−10. HEART BLOCK, COMPLETE (See Fig. 14, *D*)

Third degree atrioventricular block is diagnosed electrocardiographically and suspected clinically by the presence of slow ventricular rate (approximately 30 to 40 per minute) with unappreciable increase with activity, and is often heralded by syncope (Stokes-Adams attack). Intravenous administration of isoproterenol (Isuprel), 0.02 to 0.04 mg. in a single dose or by drip infusion of 2 mg. of Isuprel in 500 mg. of 5% dextrose in water, or 10 to 15 mg. every 4 to 6 hours sublingually, institution of any necessary resuscitative measures (**11−2**) and hospitalization for insertion of a temporary or permanent cardiac pacemaker are indicated.

26−11. HYPERTENSIVE CRISES AND ENCEPHALOPATHY

Significant further increments in diastolic blood pressure, particularly in individuals with backgrounds of chronic diastolic hypertension and associated degenerative effects, may precipitate cardiac failure (**26 — 8**), coronary ischemia (**26 — 12**), severe headaches, nausea, vomiting, confusion, coma and focal cerebral neurologic signs. These clinical signs and symptoms may be due to edema, major vessel vasospasm or hemorrhage (**59.** *Vascular Disorders*). Appropriate diagnostic tests must be performed.

TREATMENT

1. Reduction of diastolic blood pressure towards normal at a rate and degree consistent with maintenance of effective arterial perfusion pressure of vital organs.

2. Antihypertensive medications. When immediate reduction in blood pressure is essential, 300 mg. of diazoxide (Hyperstat) intravenously given rapidly (in less than 30 seconds) will cause a drop in a few minutes. The dose may be repeated in 30 minutes if the initial response is inadequate. If a slower drop in blood pressure is indicated, 2.0 to 2.5 mg. of reserpine is given intramuscularly, unless there is known or suspected hypersensitivity to reserpine. If adequate reduction of diastolic blood pressure still does not occur, a 2nd dose of 2.5 to 5.0 mg. can be given in 4 to 8 hours. Ganglionic blocking agents may be added cautiously if required. A tilt bed with the head elevated increases effectiveness. Maintenance therapy is usually necessary after establishment of a satisfactory blood pressure level; the medications listed above and thiazides are of value.

Neither guanethidine nor methyldopa should be used in the presence of pheochromocytoma (**33 — 1**) or in association with monoamine oxidase inhibitors such as isocarboxazid (Marplan), nialamide (Niamid), phenelzine sulfate (Nardil) and tranylcypromine (Parnate).

3. Lumbar puncture (see **14 — 11.** *Spinal Puncture.*) This procedure not only may be of diagnostic value but also in some instances may be of assistance in control of convulsions and severe cephalgia.

4. Limitation of sodium intake.

26 — 12. MYOCARDIAL INFARCTION, ACUTE (Fig. 14, *O*)

Whenever possible, persons with suspected or proved myocardial infarction should be started on treatment while arrangements for hospitalization are being made.

1. Have the patient remain quietly in a position of comfort.

2. If the patient is not in shock (**53**), mix morphine sulfate, 10 to

15 mg. in 10 ml. of distilled water, and inject 1 ml. portions slowly intravenously until acute pain and apprehension lessen or respirations slow.

3. Keep the intravenous portal open by slow infusion of 5% dextrose in water.

4. Start oxygen under positive pressure (6 liters per minute) by intranasal catheter or face mask.

5. If acute pulmonary edema develops, treat as outlined under **51**.

6. If evidence of shock (**53**) is present, give 5 to 10 mg. of metaraminol bitartrate (Aramine) intramuscularly and start an intravenous infusion of 5% dextrose in water.

7. Transfer the patient to the hospital by ambulance, not by private auto, continuing supportive and resuscitative therapy (supervised by a trained attendant) en route. Smooth and safe transportation, not excessive speed, should be emphasized.

8. On arrival at the hospital move the patient directly to the coronary care or intensive care unit. Start electrocardiographic monitoring immediately.

9. If symptoms of shock (**53 – 4**) progress, start a second infusion containing levarterenol bitartrate (Levophed), 4 mg. in 500 to 1000 ml. of 5% dextrose in water, given via a well placed intravenous catheter. This infusion should be given slowly for its inotropic effect rather than for its peripheral vasoconstrictive effect, and titrated to give an adequate carotid pulse and a urinary output of about 1 ml. per minute. Frequent blood pressure determinations are indicated and central venous pressure monitoring can be of assistance, especially in elderly persons. If intravenous infusion of smaller amounts of a plasma volume expander (e.g., 250 ml. of low molecular weight dextran) appears to be indicated, watch carefully for early signs of pulmonary edema (**51**).

10. For treatment of serious premature ventricular beats (6 or more per minute, 2 or more in a row or any premature ventricular beats occurring in the T waves), give 50 to 100 mg. (5 to 10 ml. of 1% solution) of intravenous lidocaine (Xylocaine), repeated in 5 minutes if necessary, followed by intravenous infusion of 1000 to 2000 mg. of lidocaine (Xylocaine) in 100 ml. of 5% dextrose in water every 12 to 24 hours.

11. Treat cardiac arrest (**26 – 7**) as indicated under *Resuscitation* (**11 – 1**. *Artificial Respiration;* **11 – 2**. *Cardiac Compression*).

26 – 13. NODAL PAROXYSMAL TACHYCARDIA (See Fig. 14, *H*)

Differentiating this condition from atrial tachycardia (**26 – 5**) by clinical and electrocardiographic examination may be difficult. Both may be grouped together for treatment under supraventricular tachycardia (**26 – 21**). Particularly dangerous are those attacks with heart rates of 250 to 300 per minute in which the low ejection volume may cause cerebral hypoxemia, syncope and cardiac failure. Treatment is directed at 2 objectives: (1) reducing the excessively rapid ventricular rate by decreasing the excitability and propagation of the atrioventricular node; and (2) preventing recurrences of the attacks.

26 – 14. PACEMAKER FAILURE

As the prevalence of implanted cardiac pacemakers increases, so does the frequency with which physicians will encounter problems associated with occasional ineffective operation. Episodic or complete malfunction may be caused by mechanical factors (wire breakage, loss of adequate contact, penetration of leads through the myocardium) or failure of the battery. An altered heart rate (more than 5 beats per minute for fixed rate pacemakers; more than 10 beats per minute for demand pacemakers) over the usual established heart rate (approximately 70 per minute) may be a sign of pending battery failure, as may be a relative decrease in voltage of ventricular complexes on the electrocardiogram. Use of an Avionics electrocardiocorder may help to determine if any malfunction of the pacemaker is occurring during episodic syncopal attacks or during periods of pulse alteration or absence. If a defective pacemaker is suspected or proved, referral for definitive care, including replacement, is indicated, with any necessary intervening supportive treatment (**11.** *Resuscitation;* **26 – 10.** *Heart Block*).

26 – 15. PERICARDIAL EFFUSION

Diagnosis and treatment of the primary cause (septic, aseptic, viral, traumatic) and treatment of pain are usually of greatest importance. Occasionally signs of cardiac tamponade may appear:
Increasing venous engorgement with inspiratory filling rather than collapse.
Increased heart rate.

Decreased pulse pressure, and heart tones.

Pulsus paradoxus.

Abnormal Valsalva response (no slowing of heart rate within 9 to 10 beats after ceasing 15 seconds of Valsalva's maneuver).

Decreasing voltage of ventricular complexes of electrocardiogram.

Characteristic abnormal echocardiogram pattern.

If signs of cardiac tamponade are appearing, a pericardiocentesis is indicated for drainage. This is most safely performed by attaching the C lead of the ECG to the hub of a Luer-Lok syringe with a 3 way stopcock in between and using a 4 inch 20 gauge needle; the tip of the needle becomes an exploring electrode and an enormous *current of injury pattern* will appear immediately on the electrocardiogram if the needle touches the epicardium. If this occurs, the needle is then withdrawn a few millimeters until the ST segment elevation disappears. The pericardial effusion is removed as adequately as possible and a specimen saved for any necessary diagnostic tests (cytology, cultures, smears). If septic pericardial effusion is present, infusion of antibacterial solution through the same needle at the time of the procedure may be advisable. Rapid recurrence of effusion with tamponade is an indication for surgical referral regarding pericardiotomy.

26 – 16. PERICARDITIS (Fig. 14, Q)

Inflammation of the pericardial sac may develop slowly or rapidly and may be due to:

Septic causes (pneumococcus, meningococcus, tuberculosis).

Viruses (particularly Coxsackie).

Fungi.

Aseptic causes (uremia, myocardial infarction, collagen diseases, postpericardiotomy).

Trauma (chest crush injuries, particularly compression from steering wheels).

TREATMENT

1. Prompt removal of pericardial fluid (**26 – 15**) if cardiac tamponade is occurring.

2. Appropriate antibiotics after cultures if from a septic cause.

3. Discontinuation of anticoagulants if being used, e.g., as in treatment of myocardial infarction.

4. Pain may be mild to severe and require aspirin, dextropropoxyphene (Darvon), codeine (32 mg., orally or by hypodermic injection every 4 to 6 hours), pentazocine lactate (Talwin), 30 mg. intramuscularly every 3 to 4 hours, or meperidine (Demerol), 50 to 100 mg. intramuscularly every 3 to 6 hours.

5. Intercostal nerve blocks with lidocaine (Xylocaine) or alcohol may be required for persistent and severe pain.

6. Prednisone, 40 to 80 mg. in divided daily doses and tapering off over a 7 to 10 day period, is an adjunct in aseptic or viral cases with severe pain.

26–17. PULMONARY EDEMA, ACUTE

For signs, symptoms and treatment, see **51**. *Pulmonary Edema.*

26–18. SINUS TACHYCARDIA (Fig. 14, *A*)

Sinus tachycardia occurring at rest infrequently is an emergency situation in and of itself, but attention must be given to diagnosis and treatment of the underlying cause [infection, anemia, hyperthyroidism (**33–5; 43–15**), shock (**53**), congestive heart failure (**26–8**), myocardial infarction (**26–12**), anxiety states (**34**. *Excitement States*)].

26–19. SHOCK See **53; 48–51**. *Shock in Children*

26–20. STOKES-ADAMS SYNDROME (See also **11**. *Resuscitation;* **26–10**. *Heart Block;* **26–23**. *Ventricular Fibrillation;* **26–24**. *Ventricular Tachycardia;* **48–15**. *Cardiac Emergencies in Children*)

Sudden intermittent unconsciousness, due usually to periods of ventricular standstill or complete atrioventricular block or occasionally to ventricular fibrillation or tachycardia, may revert spontaneously to a cardiac rhythm consistent with life, or sudden death may occur. The number of fatalities can be reduced by immediate supportive measures given in accordance with a preconceived plan (**11**. *Resuscitation;* **26–10**. *Heart Block*) pending definitive defibrillation or external or internal cardiac pacing.

26 – 21. **SUPRAVENTRICULAR TACHYCARDIA** (See also **26 – 9.** *Digitalis Toxicity;* **26 – 13.** *Nodal Paroxysmal Tachycardia*)

TREATMENT OF ACUTE ATTACKS

1. Rest in a recumbent position.

2. In milder cases (heart rate, 160 to 180 per minute), sedation by pentobarbital (Nembutal), 100 mg. intramuscularly.

3. Application of Valsalva's maneuver:

Have the patient sit up in bed with his head bent forward between his flexed knees.

Have him expel a deep breath against a closed glottis or blow into a sphygmomanometer tubing to maintain a pressure of 40 mm. of mercury for 15 to 30 seconds. With short intervening rest periods, this procedure may be repeated several times.

4. Begin carotid sinus massage by using gentle pressure. Massage the right carotid sinus area (over the middle portion of the carotid artery at the level of the hyoid) for several seconds, monitoring the heart rate. If a satisfactory decrease in rate is not obtained, the duration of massage may be increased to 10 seconds and the pressure may be increased but not enough to occlude blood flow in the carotid artery. Massage of the left carotid sinus may be tried but not simultaneously with the right carotid.

PRECAUTIONS

Have the patient lying supine, preferably with equipment for cardiopulmonary resuscitation immediately available.

Keep a syringe containing atropine sulfate, 0.4 to 0.6 mg., at hand for immediate intravenous injection if excessive vagal stimulation occurs.

Do not massage both sides of the neck at the same time.

5. Increase peripheral arterial pressure through reflex vagal stimulation by intravenous injection of 5 to 10 mg. of methoxamine hydrochloride (Vasoxyl) diluted in 10 ml. of solvent, monitoring response. This approach is preferably limited to young people.

6. Digitalize by deslanoside (Cedilanid-D), 0.8 to 1.6 mg. in a single dose or divided doses, intravenously; or by digoxin orally, initial dose, 1 mg., followed by 0.25 mg. every 4 hours until digitalized. The type of digitalis preparation and route of administration used will depend upon the rapidity of effect required.

7. If the patient has been on digitalis therapy prior to the acute episode of tachycardia (or if the history regarding prior use of

digitalis is indefinite), propranolol hydrochloride (Inderal) can be given intravenously or orally (**26-9**).

8. Direct current countershock should be considered in infrequent cases refractory to the more common methods outlined above, particularly if cardiac decompensation is occurring because of the rapid heart rate and if digitalis toxicity (**26-9**) is not present.

PREVENTION OF RECURRENCES

1. Provision for adequate physical and emotional rest.

2. Limitation of use of tobacco and alcohol.

3. Maintenance digitalization. Quinine, procainamide hydrochloride (Pronestyl) or propranolol hydrochloride (Inderal) may be used instead of digitalis if repetitive attacks still occur.

26-22. CARDIAC TRAUMA

Penetrating or severe concussive chest injuries may cause injury to the myocardium or endocardium and bleeding within the pericardium with cardiac tamponade (**14-7**. *Pericardial Sac Aspiration;* **26-15**. *Pericardial Effusion*). Contusions of the heart are treated similarly to myocardial infarction (**26-12**), except anticoagulants should not be used. If a person with chest or sternal injuries (**28**) or a penetrating injury to the neck or abdomen is in unexplained or therapy-resistant shock, an electrocardiogram revealing myocardial damage may clarify the picture. Treat shock (**53**) according to the predominant cause—hemorrhage, cardiac (myocardial) contusion or mechanical constriction (cardiac tamponade); smaller penetrating chest injuries (not more than 1 cm.) are candidates for treatment of pericardial sac hemorrhage by aspiration alone. If the external injury is larger, if shock is refractive to treatment or if tamponade recurs following aspiration, immediate surgical consultation regarding thoracotomy is warranted.

26-23. VENTRICULAR FIBRILLATION (Fig. 14, *L*) For treatment, see **11**. *Resuscitation*

This extremely serious arrhythmia, incompatible with life if not rapidly corrected, may occur:

As a result of electric shock (**25-11**. *Electrical Burns;* **29-5**).

Following excessive doses of catecholamines.

With excessive dosage of digitalis (**26-9; 49-272**), potassium ions and quinidine (**49-641**).

During cyclopropane anesthesia (**49—70.** *Anesthetics, Inhalation*).

With acute myocardial infarction (**26—12**).

The lack of effective cardiac output causes signs and symptoms of cardiac arrest (**26—7**).

PROPHYLAXIS AGAINST VENTRICULAR FIBRILLATION

1. Cautious use of therapeutic agents which are conducive to development of ventricular fibrillation.

2. If frequent premature ventricular contractions or short runs of ventricular tachycardia are seen by electrocardiograph or cardiac monitor, inject lidocaine (Xylocaine), 25 to 100 mg. (2.5 to 10 ml. of 1% solution), intravenously. Then place on maintenance doses of lidocaine, 0.5 to 2.0 mg. per ml. of 5% dextrose in water by slow intravenous infusion until monitoring shows clearing of the abnormal fluctuations.

AGONAL ARRHYTHMIAS

Ventricular fibrillation followed by cardiac standstill is the common agonal arrhythmia seen terminally in persons with serious chronic diseases. Management of ventricular fibrillation under these circumstances when death is anticipated should be approached with discernment.

26—24. VENTRICULAR TACHYCARDIA (Fig. 14, *K*)

Since ventricular tachycardia can result in ineffective cardiac output, signs of cardiac arrest (**26—7**) may appear, although not as readily as with ventricular fibrillation (**26—23**). Although life may be maintained for long periods of time in the presence of this condition, treatment should commence as soon as it is recognized. Ventricular tachycardia may occur from various causes—myocardial infarction (**26—12**), valvular heart disease and toxic effects of certain drugs, including digitalis (**26—9; 49—272**), procainamide (**49—624**) and quinidine (**49—641**).

TREATMENT

Treatment is aimed at restoration of normal sinus rhythm and rate; it varies with the severity and exciting cause.

1. If digitalis toxicity (**26—9**) is a likely cause and adequate perfusion levels and urinary output are being maintained:

Stop digitalis intake.

Give an intravenous infusion of 40 to 80 mEq. of potassium in 500 ml. of 5% dextrose in water at a rate of 100 to 200 ml. per hour, controlled by cardiac monitoring. Urine output should be adequate (45 ml. per hour), and there should be no hyperkalemia when starting therapy.

Give 0.5 to 1 mg. of propranolol hydrochloride (Inderal) slowly intravenously at 10 minute or more intervals (total not to exceed 3 mg.) until electrocardiographic monitoring shows reversion to a sinus mechanism or the rhythm present before onset of ventricular tachycardia.

Do not attempt electrical conversion.

2. If pressor amine-resistant shock is present and the patient is not overdigitalized, direct current cardioversion may be a rapid and lifesaving method of restoring a normal sinus rhythm.

3. If there is no evidence of development or presence of complete atrioventricular block, give procainamide hydrochloride (Pronestyl), 1000 mg. in 100 ml. of 5% dextrose in water intravenously. The rate should not exceed 10 ml. (100 mg.) per minute; the rate of infusion and amount should be controlled by evaluation of the patient's condition and electrocardiographic monitoring.

4. In the presence of complete atrioventricular block, quinidine and procainamide hydrochloride (Pronestyl) are absolutely contraindicated. Isoproterenol (Isuprel) by intravenous drip may be of benefit.

PROPHYLAXIS AGAINST VENTRICULAR TACHYCARDIA

1. Cautious use of drugs conducive to ventricular tachycardia.

2. Intravenous infusion of lidocaine (Xylocaine), 500 to 1000 mg. in 500 ml. of 5% dextrose in water, if premature ventricular contractions are observed while monitoring a patient with acute myocardial infarction (26 − 12).

27. CEPHALGIA

Many types of headache may be severe enough to cause the sufferer to seek emergency medical care. Although the etiology in many instances is obscure and requires more thorough study for determination than is practical in an emergency setting, there are certain types which can be recognized and given at least temporary relief on an emergency basis.

27–1. ALCOHOLIC EXCESS ("Hangover") HEADACHES (See also 49–315. *Ethyl Alcohol*)

Inhalations of oxygen, administration of fluids and acetylsalicylic acid (aspirin) may help. Barbiturates and all types of opiates and synthetic narcotics should be avoided.

27–2. ALTITUDE SICKNESS See 23–1; 23–6. *Mountain Sickness*

27–3. ARTHRITIS OF THE CERVICAL SPINE

Arthritis of the cervical spine (with or without aggravation by trauma) may cause severe headaches, usually localized to the distribution of the greater or lesser occipital or the posterior auricular nerves on one or both sides. Occasionally the pain may be frontal or postorbital.

TREATMENT
Treatment consists of salicylates, muscle relaxants and sedation. Application of a Thomas collar or cervical traction may be necessary. (See also 44–1. *Arthritis.*)

27–4. ASTHENIA DUE TO ADDISON'S DISEASE See 33–1. *Adrenal Emergencies*

27–5. BRAIN TUMORS

Brain tumors may cause frontal or generalized headaches, aggravated by changes in position.

TREATMENT
Acetylsalicylic acid (aspirin), with or without codeine sulfate, may give temporary relief. If a brain tumor is suspected, referral to a neurologist for thorough investigation and definitive treatment is mandatory.

27–6. CAFFEINE-WITHDRAWAL HEADACHES

In habitual coffee drinkers, abstinence may cause severe, often completely disabling, headaches.

27 – 7.   CONCUSSION HEADACHES

Treatment
Coffee by mouth, caffeine sodiobenzoate, 0.5 gm. intramuscularly, amphetamine sulfate, 5 mg orally, or oxygen inhalations will give immediate relief.

27 – 7.   CONCUSSION HEADACHES

Concussion headaches follow direct trauma to the head, but the severity of the headache has little, if any, relationship to the intensity of the trauma. In mild cases rest, reassurance and acetylsalicylic acid (aspirin) are all that is necessary. Severe cases require treatment as outlined under **41 – 1.** *Head Injuries.*

27 – 8.   CONSTIPATION

The remedy is obvious.

27 – 9.   ECLAMPSIA See 47 – 7

27 – 10.   EPILEPSY See **29 – 7.** *Coma;* **31.** *Convulsive Seizures*

27 – 11.   EYE STRAIN

Treatment
Treatment consists basically of avoiding excessive use of the eyes, especially at close or fine work. Dark glasses may be of assistance if photophobia is present. Acetylsalicylic acid (aspirin) will often give temporary relief. The patient should be instructed to see an ophthalmologist as soon as possible.

27 – 12.   FEBRILE HEADACHES

Febrile headaches may be caused by any condition which results in a high fever. Administration of acetylsalicylic acid (aspirin), cold packs or iced saline enemas may be used to bring the fever down, while serious conditions such as meningitis (**30 – 16**), poliomyelitis (**30 – 21**) and pneumonia (**52 – 14**) are being ruled out by careful examination.

27 – 13.   FOOD ALLERGY HEADACHES

Food allergy headaches may occur following the ingestion of almost any kind of food by susceptible individuals. The most common offenders, especially in children, seem to be cabbage, chocolate, garlic, green peppers and peanuts. Antihistaminics give rapid relief.

27—14. HEMORRHAGE FROM A PEPTIC ULCER

Hemorrhage from a peptic ulcer may be accompanied by a very severe headache which disappears with supportive therapy or cessation of bleeding.

27—15. HERPES

Herpes of the posterior auricular or greater or lesser occipital nerves may cause severe localized headache with or without severe burning. The diagnosis can usually be made from the distribution of the lesions and by the type of pain.

TREATMENT

1. Protection of the herpetic lesions from infection by petrolatum gauze or butacaine (Butyn) and nitromersol (Metaphen) ointment dressings. If the lesions are on the scalp above the hair line, chlortetracycline (Aureomycin) ointment, rubbed in gently, is effective.

2. Control of pain:

If moderate, by acetylsalicylic acid (aspirin) and barbiturates.

If severe, by:

Codeine sulfate, 0.03 to 0.06 gm., orally or intramuscularly.

Meperidine hydrochloride (Demerol), 50 to 100 mg. intramuscularly.

Pentazocine lactate (Talwin), 15 to 30 mg. intramuscularly or intravenously.

If exquisite, by:

Morphine sulfate, 10 to 15 mg. intramuscularly, or, in extreme cases, intravenously.

Methadone (Amidon, Dolophine), 10 mg. orally. The analgesic effect of this drug given by mouth lasts from 8 to 12 hours.

Hospitalization in severe or stubborn cases or if the eyes are involved (**35—14**).

27—16. HISTAMINE HEADACHES

Histamine headaches (cluster headache, Horton's cephalgia) are severe, throbbing and often associated with unilateral redness and lacrimation of the eye. They may be precipitated or aggravated by alcohol ingestion. Measures such as jugular pressure which raise the spinal fluid pressure and decrease the blood supply will temporarily relieve the cephalgia, as may analgesics. Severe cases require hospitalization.

27 − 17. HUNGER HEADACHES

Hunger headaches are usually hypoglycemic and are relieved by food, especially proteins. There may be enough time lag to require acetylsalicylic acid (aspirin).

27 − 18. HYPERTENSIVE HEADACHES

Hypertensive headaches are usually present in the morning and wear off by noon. Acetylsalicylic acid (aspirin) will give temporary relief. Sleeping with the head elevated may prevent attacks. Appropriate treatment of the hypertension is indicated.

27 − 19. HYPOTENSIVE HEADACHES

Hypotensive headaches are caused by any of the many conditions which produce a drop in blood pressure and often are accompanied by vasodepressor syncope (**59 − 5**).

27 − 20. MENINGEAL IRRITATION

Severe and persistent headaches associated with fever and stiff neck require immediate spinal puncture to determine the etiology (**30 − 16.** *Meningitis;* **48 − 42.** *Meningococcemia in Children;* **48 − 63.** *Waterhouse-Friderichsen Syndrome;* **62 − 1.** *Arboviral Infections*).

27 − 21. MIGRAINE HEADACHES

In adults. Relief from the acute discomfort of migraine-type head pain can sometimes be obtained through a combination of the following measures:

1. Absolute rest in a darkened room.
2. Oxygen inhalations.
3. Ergotamine tartrate (Gynergen), 2 to 3 mg. by mouth or 0.5

mg. subcutaneously, followed by 1 mg. every 2 hours by mouth. *The total oral dose should not exceed 10 mg.* A slower effect can be obtained by 2 tablets of Cafergot (ergotamine tartrate, 1 mg. with caffeine sodiobenzoate, 100 mg.) orally, repeated in 2 hours only *once,* or by rectal suppository.

Ergot in therapeutic doses has many undesirable side effects (**49 — 306**), including myalgia, fatigue, nausea, vomiting, tingling and numbness of the hands and feet, and even myocardial infarction. Atropine sulfate, 0.4 mg. subcutaneously, will neutralize some of these side effects; calcium gluconate, 10 ml. of a 10% solution intravenously, will decrease muscle pain. Numbness or tingling of the extremities, a cold feeling or cyanosis calls for immediate discontinuance of ergot in any form.

4. Pentazocine lactate (Talwin), 15 to 30 mg. intramuscularly.

5. Nicotinic acid, 50 to 75 mg. orally.

6. Amphetamine (Benzedrine) sulfate, 10 to 15 mg. orally.

7. Dimenhydrinate (Dramamine), 50 to 100 mg. intramuscularly. The same dose by slow intravenous injection will give almost immediate relief. For intravenous use each milliliter (50 mg.) of dimenhydrinate must be diluted with 10 ml. of normal salt solution.

8. Isometheptene (Octin), 50 mg. subcutaneously. If a rise in blood pressure occurs, Octin therapy must be stopped at once; if there is no rise in ½ hour, 260 mg. by mouth, may be given.

9. Hospitalization in severe or intractable cases.

PROPHYLAXIS. Although it is of no value in treatment, methysergide maleate (Sansert), 2 mg. by mouth 3 times a day may prevent the development of migraine. Possible serious side effects require careful follow-up care.

In children. See **48 — 43.** *Migraine in Children.*

27 — 22. MYOFIBROSITIS (FIBROMYOSITIS, MYOFASCITIS)

Myofibrositis of the upper portion of the neck from trauma (**27 — 3**), postural strain (television headache) or infection (especially viral) may cause severe unilateral or bilateral headache, usually occipital but sometimes localized to the distribution of the posterior auricular or greater or lesser occipital nerves on one or both sides. Treatment of the underlying cause is necessary for permanent relief. Symptomatic relief can be given by the measures outlined for whiplash injuries (**44 — 58**).

27 – 23. ORTHOSTATIC HEADACHES See **27 – 19.** *Hypotensive Headaches*

27 – 24. POLIOMYELITIC HEADACHES See **27 – 20.** *Meningeal Irritation Headaches*

27 – 25. PSYCHOGENIC HEADACHES

Psychogenic headaches are characterized by complaints of a tight band around the head or a pulling sensation over the vertex and usually are caused by anxiety, depression or tension – singly or in varying combinations (see also **27 – 33**).

27 – 26. RELAXATION HEADACHES

Relaxation (Sunday morning) headaches are probably due to peripheral vasodilation. They can usually be relieved by small doses of acetylsalicylic acid (aspirin) or by mental or physical activity.

27 – 27. SINUS HEADACHES

Sinus headaches often can be relieved temporarily by shrinking the nasal mucous membranes, postural drainage or ultrasonic therapy. If these measures do not give relief, the patient should be referred to an otolaryngologist.

27 – 28. SPINAL PUNCTURE HEADACHES

Spinal puncture headaches occur in 10 to 20% of cases whether or not local anesthetics or the preventive measures outlined below are used.

CYCLE OF DEVELOPMENT

1. The cerebrospinal fluid pressure is decreased by puncture.
2. The difference between the spinal fluid pressure and intracranial venous pressure is increased.
3. Dilation of the intracranial venous structures results in increased volume of the brain with resultant stimulation of the intracranial pain centers.

PREVENTIVE MEASURES

1. Use of a small needle with the bevel parallel to the long axis of the body to minimize dural tears.
2. Avoidance of any motion of the spine while the needle is in place.
3. Limitation of amount of fluid removed to not more than 6 ml.
4. Maintenance of the prone position for 1 hour after completion of the procedure.
5. Intravenous administration of 5% dextrose in water (unless contraindicated by some systemic condition). Caffeine sodiobenzoate, Pituitrin, erogotamine and nicotinic acid have been used empirically but probably are of no value.

SYMPTOMATIC TREATMENT

1. Acetylsalicylic acid (aspirin) in mild cases; codeine sulfate in small doses if the discomfort is acute. The drugs listed under tension headaches (**27–33**) may be of benefit.
2. Application of a tight abdominal binder, especially following puncture for obstetric spinal anesthesia.
3. Hospitalization if the headache persists or is unaffected by postural changes.

PROGNOSIS. Complete recovery is the rule although in some cases 7 to 10 days may be required for complete relief. The patient may or may not develop symptoms if spinal puncture is repeated at a later date.

27–29. SPONTANEOUS RUPTURE OF AN INTRACRANIAL ARTERY

Spontaneous rupture of an intracranial artery (**59–2**) is characterized by sudden onset of severe occipital pain if extensive subarachnoid hemorrhage has taken place. Progressive involvement of the vital centers, which may be fatal, often occurs.

27–30. STARCH OR SUGAR HEADACHES

Ingestion of excessive amounts of sweet or starchy foods may cause severe headaches, which persist until the dietary imbalance is corrected. No emergency treatment except advice is necessary, unless rebound hypoglycemia is present.

27 – 31. SUNLIGHT HEADACHES

Sunlight headaches are caused by peripheral vasodilation from unaccustomed exposure to bright sunlight. They often precede heat cramps (**57 – 2**), heat stroke (**57 – 4**) and sunstroke (**57 – 8**).

27 – 32. SYPHILIS (Cerebral) See **60 – 5**.

27 – 33. TENSION HEADACHES

Tension headaches is an overworked catchall for many cases of mixed etiology. Although extreme mental stress and strain may cause severe headaches in certain individuals, a thorough history and examination will usually disclose a specific causative factor. Administration of some of the following drugs may give relief while the basic cause is being determined.

1. Acetylsalicylic acid (aspirin), 0.6 gm. by mouth every 4 hours.
2. Pentazocine lactate (Talwin), 15 to 30 mg. intramuscularly.
3. Meprobamate (Miltown, Equinil), 400 mg. orally 3 times a day.
4. Valoctin [a combination of isometheptene (Octin), 0.06 gm., and monobromoisovalerylurea (Bromural), 250 mg.] 1 tablet by mouth, repeated in 4 hours.
5. Reserpine, 0.25 to 0.8 mg. orally.
6. Chlorpromazine hydrochloride (Thorazine), 10 to 25 mg. orally 3 times a day. (See also **27 – 21**. *Migraine;* **48 – 43**. *Migraine in Children.*)

27 – 34. TOOTHACHES OR EARACHES

Toothaches (**58**) or earaches secondary to middle ear infection (**32 – 13**) may cause severe generalized headaches.

27 – 35. TOXIC HEADACHES

Ingestion, inhalation or absorption through the mucous membranes or the intact skin of many substances may cause severe headaches, usually frontal in location, but sometimes orbital, occipital or diffuse. Among the more common substances whose toxic pictures are characterized by headache are:

Alcohol – amyl (**49 – 67**), ethyl (**49 – 315**) and isopropyl (**49 – 403**).

Ammonia fumes (**49 — 59**).

Benzene — inhalation or ingestion (**49 — 119**).

Chlorine (**49 — 191**).

Epinephrine hydrochloride (Adrenalin) — from overzealous use of a nebulizer or from hypodermic administration. See **49 — 302**.

Hydrochloric acid vapors. See *Acids* **49 — 26**.

Iodine — inhalation of the fumes (**49 — 393**).

Kerosene fumes (**49 — 408**).

Lead and its salts — from inhalation of the fumes or dust, or ingestion. Chronic lead poisoning (plumbism) is often characterized by severe headaches (**49 — 420**).

Metal fumes (**49 — 461**).

Methyl acetate fumes (**49 — 474**).

Naphthalene fumes (**49 — 510**).

Nicotine (**49 — 523**).

Nitrates (**49 — 528**).

Ozone — in certain hypersensitive persons, inhalation of even minute concentrations of this gas will cause very severe frontal headaches (**49 — 558**).

Phosphorus pentachloride fumes (**49 — 602**).

Pyrethrum dust or powder (**49 — 631**).

Tobacco — inhalation of dust or ingestion. See *Nicotine* (**49 — 523**).

Zinc oxide — inhalation of dust. See *Metal Fumes* (**49 — 461**).

27 — 36. TRAUMATIC HEADACHES See **27 — 7**. *Concussion headaches*

27 — 37. TRIGEMINAL NEURALGIA (Tic Douloureux) See **46 — 8**

27 — 38. UREMIA

Uremia (**29 — 15**) may be accompanied by a very distressing type of headache which will persist until the causative condition is remedied. Sedatives and anodynes are of very little value in treatment.

27 — 39. VASOPRESSOR HEADACHES

Vasopressor headaches may be caused by administration of phenylephrine hydrochloride (Neo-Synephrine), epinephrine hydrochloride (Adrenalin) (**49 – 302**) and other rapidly acting vasopressor drugs. Unless excessively large doses have been given or individual hypersensitivity is present, the effect is transient only and requires no emergency treatment.

28. CHEST INJURIES

28–1. NONPERFORATING INJURIES TO THE CHEST

Acute restlessness and apprehension in a patient who gives a history of severe rib cage compression are often the only indications of intraalveolar or mediastinal bleeding. Even in the absence of external evidence of trauma, supportive therapy should be begun at once.

Respiratory depressants, especially opiates and synthetic narcotics, should never be administered to a patient with any type of chest injury until the nature and extent of the injury have been definitely determined.

28–2. FRACTURES

A patient with simple fractures of ribs or sternum usually requires no treatment except limitation of activity and control of pain. Local application of cold will often decrease immediate discomfort; after 24 hours heat may give relief. Blocking of the intercostal nerves proximal to the fractures with a local anesthetic may be necessary for relief if overriding, depression or displacement is present. Binding or strapping the chest may be dangerous, because it limits to some extent the aeration of the lungs and increases the possibility of the development of a traumatic pneumonitis. This is especially true in elderly persons. Marked sternal depression requires immediate hospitalization.

Multiple rib fractures in a patient with the loss of ability of the thorax to expand on inspiration may result in "paradoxical respiration," often associated with severe shock (**53**). Insertion of towel clips into the rib fragments, with overhead suspended weights attached to the clips for countertraction, may be lifesaving. Immediate hospitalization is always required if paradoxical respiration is present.

28—3. CONTUSIONS—CRUSHING AND COMPRESSION INJURIES

Especially in children, sudden forcible compression of the chest may cause serious intrathoracic damage without external evidence of injury. Slowly progressive bleeding due to alveolar rupture may result from the "accordion action" of the resilient rib cage. Plasma volume expanders should be started intravenously if a young patient with a history of possible thoracic compression is acutely and persistently apprehensive and restless. This should be done even if signs and symptoms of hemorrhagic shock (**53**) are absent and there are no other indications of intrathoracic injury. Hospitalization for careful and frequent observation for changes in vital signs and hematocrit levels is indicated for at least 24 hours after injury.

28—4. TRAUMATIC PNEUMOTHORAX

Traumatic pneumothorax should be ruled out by careful clinical and x-ray examination. Its presence requires hospitalization after careful observation for and treatment of latent or delayed shock (**53**).

28—5. TENSION PNEUMOTHORAX

Tension pneumothorax, caused by leakage of air from the lung into the pleural cavity with an intact chest wall, is a very serious condition which requires hospitalization as soon as possible for water-seal drainage. Before transportation of the patient, a large bore (No. 16 or No. 18) hypodermic needle with a rubber glove finger or finger cot with a small hole in the tip fastened to the needle base should be inserted into the pleural cavity between the 2nd and 3rd ribs in the midclavicular line to act as a flutter valve.

28—6. RUPTURE OF THE DIAPHRAGM

Rupture of the diaphragm may be caused by direct nonpenetrating trauma over the lower ribs on either side, or less commonly, by penetrating wounds. Dyspnea and cyanosis may be acute. Shock, usually the result of mediastinal shift, may require treatment (**53—7**) before and during transportation to a hospital equipped for open chest surgery. Small defects in the diaphragm are very difficult to detect and are potentially more dangerous than large rents because of the increased chances of obstruction and strangulation.

28 — 7. THORACIC SQUEEZE

Thoracic squeeze occurs in underwater swimmers using a snorkel tube. See **23 — 5**.

28 — 8. COSTOCHONDRAL SEPARATION

The treatment is the same as outlined in **28 — 2**. *Fractures.*

28 — 9. LACERATIONS THROUGH THE PLEURA (Stab and knife wounds, etc.)

TREATMENT

1. Cover the surface laceration with petrolatum gauze and a pressure bandage.
2. Treat shock (**53 — 7**).
3. If dyspnea or cyanosis is marked, give air or oxygen under positive pressure by face mask or intranasal catheter and rebreathing bag, after cleansing the airway by suction.
4. Use gentle restraint as needed. Opiates or synthetic narcotics are contraindicated because of their respiratory depressant effects.
5. As soon as possible transfer by ambulance for hospitalization, continuing respiratory assistance and restraint in the ambulance if necessary.

28 — 10. OPEN (COMPOUND) FRACTURES OF RIBS

Treatment is the same as outlined for pleural lacerations (**28 — 9**) — use towel-clip countertraction if paradoxical respiration (**28 — 2**. *Multiple Rib Fractures*) is present.

28 — 11. BULLET WOUNDS

TREATMENT

1. Cover the wound of entry (and of exit if present) with sterile petrolatum gauze; apply a firm pressure bandage.
2. Give oxygen inhalations after determining that the airway is clear.
3. Treat shock (**53 — 7**), and give tetanus prophylaxis (**16**) as necessary.
4. Apply gentle manual restraint as needed.

5. When the patient's condition has stabilized, transfer by ambulance, continuing oxygen and intravenous therapy if needed, to a hospital equipped for major chest surgery.

6. *Do not*

Probe for a foreign body (bullet, shot, etc.).

Give excessive amounts of intravenous fluids – pulmonary edema may result (**51**).

Administer morphine sulfate, synthetic narcotics or other respiratory depressants.

28 – 12. TRAUMATIC HEMOPERICARDIUM See **14 – 7.** *Pericardial Sac Aspiration;* **26 – 22; 48 – 15.** *Cardiac Emergencies in Children (Pericardial Tamponade)*

29. COMA

Common causes of coma (reduced awareness from which a patient cannot be aroused by usual stimuli, in contrast to sleep) are as follows:

I. *Intracranial pathology*
   1. Head injury
   2. Cerebrovascular accidents
   3. Convulsive disorders
   4. Infection
   5. Intracranial tumors – usually space-consuming
   6. Psychopathology
II. *Systemic conditions*
   1. Asphyxia (suffocation)
   2. Toxic substances (poisons, drugs, etc.)
   3. Cardiac pathology
   4. Temperature variation injuries – cold or heat
   5. Metabolic abnormalities

For clinical approach to management and treatment of coma of undetermined origin, see **29 – 17.**

29 – 1. ACUTE INFECTIOUS DISEASES

Especially in children, acute infectious diseases may cause deep coma. Treatment depends upon the causative condition (see **30.**

Contagious and Communicable Diseases; **48.** Pediatric Emergencies; **62.** Viral Infections).

29 — 2. CARDIAC DECOMPENSATION See **26.** Cardiac Emergencies; **48 — 15.** Cardiac Emergencies in Children

29 — 3. DIABETES MELLITUS

Two conditions directly related to diabetes may require emergency care, hyperglycemia (diabetic coma) and hyperinsulinism (insulin shock). Each may be fatal if not recognized promptly and treated adequately; however, each usually responds spectacularly to proper therapy.

Laboratory determinations of blood sugar levels and carbon dioxide combining power are sometimes essential for differential diagnosis, but, unfortunately, they are not always available immediately in emergency situations. Therefore, the attending physician may be forced to base his diagnosis on any history which he may be able to obtain from members of the family, friends or persons who observed the onset of the condition and on careful clinical examination and observation (**29 — 17**). If there is any doubt concerning the differential diagnosis, a small amount of dextrose given intravenously is a valuable diagnostic test. If the coma is hyperglycemic, no harm will result; on the other hand, additional insulin may be fatal to a person already in insulin shock.

TREATMENT OF DIABETIC COMA (HYPERGLYCEMIA)

When the patient is first seen, not in a hospital:

1. Draw 20 ml. of blood for serum sugar, serum acetone, potassium, BUN, HCO_3, pH and for typing and crossmatching when facilities are available. This blood specimen must be sent with the patient to the hospital.

2. Start intravenous infusion of 500 ml. of 1/6 molar sodium lactate solution. Give sodium bicarbonate intravenously if severely acidotic (**43 — 1**).

3. Give 100 units of regular insulin intravenously at once through the infusion tubing if Kussmaul's respiration and a 4 plus acetone and sugar in the urine are present.

4. Treat shock (**53 — 7**). Keep the patient warm but not hot; room temperature is satisfactory.

5. Transport the patient immediately to an adequately equipped hospital.

DIFFERENTIAL DIAGNOSIS

	HYPERGLYCEMIA WITH KETOSIS (Diabetic Coma)	HYPERINSULINISM (Insulin Shock or Reaction)
History	Known diabetes; increasing thirst, air hunger, sleepiness; nausea and vomiting	Rapid onset following insulin; may not have eaten usual meal before or after dose; may have taken too much insulin
Diet	Too much food	Not enough food
Nausea and vomiting	Often present	Seldom present
Fever	May be present	Seldom present
Thirst	Intense	Absent
Facies	Looks toxic	Looks pale and weak
Vision	Dim	Diplopia
Eyeballs	Soft	Normal
Mouth	Dry; ketotic fruity odor	Drooling
Skin	Dry and flushed	Moist and pale
Blood pressure	Low	Normal or low
Respiration	Rapid and deep	Normal
Abdominal pain	Common; may simulate an acute surgical abdomen	Absent
Tremor	Absent	Frequent
Mental state	Gradual development of coma	Sudden onset of delirium, deep coma and bizarre neurologic picture
Convulsions	None	Late
Infection	May bring on symptoms	No effect
Insulin	May have omitted usual dose	Always has taken dose, sometimes too much
Urine	Sugar and diacetic acid present	Sugar may be present and diacetic acid absent in 1st specimen; in 2nd specimen, both absent
Blood sugar (normal, 80–120 mg.%)	Above normal (also serum acetone present)	Below normal
CO_2 combining power (normal, 21-30 mEq./L.)	10 mEq./L. or less	Normal
Response to treatment	Slow	Rapid (may be delayed if protamine zinc or NPH insulin overdosage)

When the patient reaches the hospital:

1. Complete the blood tests specified above.

2. Obtain a hematocrit, white blood count and differential.

3. Obtain a urine specimen without catheterization if possible; otherwise, insertion of an indwelling catheter (**14–3**) is mandatory.

4. Start hourly urine volume, sugar and acetone determinations.

5. Obtain an electrocardiogram.

6. If febrile, culture and start antibiotic therapy based on gram stain results and sensitivity determinations.

7. Wash the stomach; continue suction through a nasogastric tube until the patient becomes responsive and cooperative.

8. Start an intravenous infusion of 750 ml. of 1/6 molar sodium lactate plus 250 ml. of normal saline. When the urine output is adequate and the ECG does not show evidence of an increased potassium level (**6–1**) add 40 to 80 mEq. of potassium chloride, depending on the need. Do not add dextrose until the blood sugar level is under 250 mg. %. Adjust the rate of infusion according to the degree of dehydration. Five to 7 liters of fluid plus electrolytes (**6.** *Fluid Replacement in Emergencies*) may be required in the first 24 hours. If indicated, give 500 ml. of whole blood or plasma concomitantly with the 1/6 molar lactate-normal saline infusion.

9. Inject 200 units of regular insulin intravenously every 2 hours until the blood sugar level is less than 300 mg. %, then decrease the regular insulin to 40 units or less subcutaneously. Continue close observation and recording of vital signs every hour until stabilized.

TREATMENT OF INSULIN SHOCK OR REACTION

1. Give 30 ml. of 50% dextrose in water intravenously.

2. Inject 0.5 to 1.0 mg. of glucagon hydrochloride (Glucagon) intramuscularly or intravenously.

3. When the patient is conscious enough to swallow, give orange juice or sweet soft drinks by mouth. Dextrose solution can also be given through the nasogastric tube.

4. Watch carefully for relapses which may occur in the presence of long-acting hypoglycemic agents if therapy is not continued.

29–4. ECLAMPSIA See **47–7.** *Eclampsia;* **47–8.** *Pre-eclamptic Toxemia*

29 — 5.   ELECTRICAL SHOCK (See also 25 — 11. *Electrical Burns*)

Severe cases are usually caused by contact with low voltage circuits and are characterized by ventricular fibrillation (26 — 23) and respiratory paralysis. Once the former is established, resuscitative measures are rarely successful; however, striking the chest forcibly with the fist, closed chest cardiac compression (11 — 2) and expired air respiration (11 — 1) should be tried, with external defibrillation (11 — 2) when and if equipment is available. When in doubt, defibrillate!

If there is perceptible heart action:

1. Start expired air respiration (11 — 1) and continue until mechanical methods such as close-fitting face mask or intranasal catheter and rebreathing bag can be substituted. Closed chest (external) cardiac compression (11 — 2) may be required as an adjunct to weak or irregular heart action. Resuscitation should be continued for at least 4 hours before declaring the patient dead. The attending physician should remember that the presumptive signs of death (3 — 2) often do not apply following an electrical shock and that normal breathing and heart action have been reestablished as long as 8 hours after contact with the current.

2. Keep the patient comfortably warm, but not hot, during resuscitative measures.

3. Do not give stimulant (analeptic) drugs; they are of no value until the breathing center has recovered and spontaneous respiration has been established. Narcotics (natural and synthetic) are contraindicated because of their respiratory depressant effects.

29 — 6.   EMPHYSEMA

Comatose patients with pulmonary emphysema are frequently and mistakenly considered as being beyond aid. However, recognition of the condition and immediate institution of the following measures may result in restoring persons with emphysema to useful activity:

1. Cleansing of the airway by suction to remove mucous plugs from the large bronchi.

2. Intermittent positive pressure breathing (IPPB) by use of a volume or other mechanical respirator. Depression of the respiratory center by intravenous morphine sulfate may be necessary to allow the apparatus to function efficiently. Moisture should be supplied by a saline spray.

3. Tracheostomy (**14 – 12**), with insertion of a large cuffed tube.

4. Restoration of normal fluid-electrolyte balance (**6.** *Fluid Replacement in Emergencies*).

5. Administration of broad spectrum antibiotics.

6. Obtaining of arterial pH, Pco_2 and CO_2 determinations.

29 – 7. EPILEPSY (See also **31.** *Convulsive Seizures*)

Prevention of injury is all that can be done in emergencies of this type. Cerebral stimulants to shorten the unconscious periods are definitely contraindicated; they may result in severe prolonged headaches and extreme exhaustion. Complete recovery is the rule and hospitalization is rarely necessary. The need for carefully supervised long-term therapy should be stressed.

First Aid For An Epileptic Seizure

1. Keep calm. The person is usually not suffering or in danger.

2. Help him to a safe place but **DO NOT** restrain his movements. Loosen tight clothing.

3. After the jerking of the seizure has subsided, and if he is still unconscious, turn the victim on his side with his face turned downward.

4. DO NOT put anything between his teeth.

5. DO NOT attempt to give him anything to drink.

6. Stand by until the person has recovered consciousness and from the confusion which sometimes follows a seizure.

7. Let him rest if he feels tired, then encourage him to go about his regular activities.

8. If the patient is a child notify parents or other persons responsible for him.

29 – 8. EPISODIC OR RECURRENT UNCONSCIOUSNESS See **50 – 11** (*Differential Diagnosis Chart*)

29 – 9. EXCESSIVE HEAT See **57 – 3.** *Heat Exhaustion;* **57 – 4.** *Heat Hyperpyrexia;* **57 – 6.** *Iatrogenic Heat Stroke;* **57 – 8.** *Sunstroke*

29 – 10. HEPATIC COMA

TREATMENT

1. Treatment of shock (**53 – 7**) and hemorrhage (**42**).

2. Reduction of body protein breakdown by intravenous infusion of 800 calories of dextrose in hypertonic solution per day.

3. Reduction of intestinal ammonia caused by bacterial decomposition. Give 1.0 gm. of neomycin orally every 6 hours.

4. Sedation with chloral hydrate or paraldehyde as needed.

5. Balancing of fluid input and output, with avoidance of saline, if hepatorenal symptoms are present. Protein intake should be sharply limited.

6. Administration of vitamin K (Phytonadione) intramuscularly.

7. Cautious treatment of anemia.

29 – 11. INTRACRANIAL PATHOLOGY See 41. *Head Injuries;* 48 – 32. *Head Injuries In Children;* 59 – 2. *Vascular Disorders*

29 – 12. MYXEDEMA See 33 – 5. *Thyroid Emergencies*

29 – 13. POISONS

The poisons listed in this section are those which are characterized by rapid action, with coma usually the main or presenting symptom in severe cases.

Alcohol. See 49 – 315. *Ethyl Alcohol.*

Barbiturates. See 49 – 111.

Carbon monoxide. See 49 – 172.

Chloral hydrate. See 49 – 184.

Morphine and related opiates. See 7. *Narcotics;* 49 – 366. *Heroin;* 49 – 495. *Morphine.*

29 – 14. SHOCK (53) FOLLOWING TRAUMA, SEVERE BURNS (25; 48 – 14. *Burns in Children*), HEMORRHAGE (42) or POISONING (49)

29 – 15. UREMIA

If uremic convulsions or coma have developed, symptomatic and supportive treatment is all that can be done. Sedatives, hypnotics and narcotics may be given in the smallest possible effective doses while hospitalization for definitive care is being arranged.

29–16.   RARE CAUSES OF COMA

Rare causes of coma are brain tumors, encephalitis (**48–24.** *Encephalitis in Children;* **62–1; 62–5**), malaria (**30–14**), syphilis of the central nervous system (**60–5**) and tuberculosis (acute miliary, meningeal form).

These conditions require only supportive and symptomatic care before and during transfer for hospitalization.

29–17.   COMA OF UNDETERMINED ETIOLOGY

Probably the emergency condition which requires the most careful immediate thought for correct diagnosis, treatment and management is deep coma of undetermined origin. A preset schedule, such as that outlined below, is essential for management of cases of this type.

Check vital signs (heart rate, respiratory rate and type, blood pressure, rectal temperature).

Clear and maintain an adequate airway.

Maintain adequate ventilation and circulation (**11.** *Resuscitation*).

If no one is available to give any accurate information, delegate some person (preferably with professional experience) to trace, if possible and as soon as possible, the patient's background. This should include:

1. Location where patient was found and the circumstances.
2. State of consciousness when found.
3. Presence of medications or instructions for their use.
4. History of prior episodes of coma.
5. Condition and complaints before development of coma. Observe the patient closely—first fully clothed, then completely undressed—covering the following points:

1. Clothing—mud, blood, semen, grease, grass, corrosive agents or other stains; alcohol or other odors; holes or tears; burns.
2. Identification data—"dog tags" around neck or wrist.
3. Skin (including scalp)—puncture wounds, ticks, thermal or electric burns, contusions, ecchymoses, pallor, sweating, cyanosis of lips or fingernails, swelling, effusions, lacerations of the genitalia, evidence of pregnancy.
4. Musculoskeletal misalignment.
5. Breath—alcohol, acetone, uremia, carbon tetrachloride, gasoline, the "musty" odor of hepatic failure.

6. Respiratory pattern—rate, rhythm, paradoxical respiration, use of accessory muscles.

7. The patient as a whole—make-up, tattooing, type of clothing, body hygiene, expression.

Draw a specimen of blood for hematocrit, white blood count and differential, typing and cross-matching and blood chemistry [sugar, blood urea nitrogen (BUN), CO_2, pH and serum acetone].

Save 5 ml. of blood serum.

Start an intravenous infusion of 5% dextrose in water or saline, preferably with a radiopaque plastic intravenous catheter.

Perform a complete physical examination and a neurologic examination covering the sensorium, cranial nerves, cerebellar and meningeal signs, motor and sensory responses and reflexes [superficial (corneal, abdominal, cremasteric and rectal sphincter), deep tendon reflexes (biceps, triceps, patellar, Achilles) and pathologic reflexes (Babinski)]. *Remove any contact lenses* (**35—39**).

Catheterize (**14—3**); leave a Foley catheter in place and note volume output in 15 minutes; save for 24 hour specimen. Refer a specimen of urine for routine urinalysis (specific gravity, pH, color, proteins, sugar, acetone and microscopic examination).

Lavage the stomach; save a specimen of vomitus or aspirate for later laboratory analysis.

Check the mouth, rectum and vagina as depositories for toxic substances.

Perform a lumbar subarachnoid puncture (**14—11.** *Spinal Puncture*), unless contraindicated. Examine cerebrospinal fluid at once for pressure, color, turbidity, protein and sugar content and cells (including Gram stain).

Save a specimen of cerebrospinal fluid for culture if indicated.

Take x-ray films as indicated below, but only if necessary positioning will not be harmful to the patient.

   a. Skull series. One lateral should be taken on a large enough film to show any gross misalignment of the cervical spine.

   b. Chest films if signs of thoracic or pulmonary pathology have been noted.

   c. Areas of suspected injury as based on physical examination.

Take an electrocardiogram for evaluation of cardiac status and for information regarding electrolytic balance.

Continue observation and investigation until a definite reason for coma has been determined. More than one factor may be contributory!

Institute specific therapy as indicated while continuing diligent supportive therapy.

29−18. PROLONGED POSTOPERATIVE COMA

Modern anesthetic techniques usually result in rapid postoperative recovery of consciousness; however, because emergency procedures sometimes do not allow complete preoperative investigation of intercurrent diseases, drug idiosyncrasies or other complicating factors, postoperative coma can be abnormally prolonged. In this case the following conditions must be considered:

ANESTHESIA AND MEDICAL DISEASES AND DRUGS

Certain diseases interfere with detoxification and elimination of anesthetic agents, so that usual amounts may cause prolonged postanesthetic coma. Among these are:

Addison's disease (**33−1.** *Adrenal Insufficiency*).
Diabetes (**29−3.** *Diabetes mellitus*).
Liver disease (**29−10.** *Hepatic Coma*).
Muscular dystrophies.
Myxedema (**33−5.** *Hypothyroid Emergencies*).
Porphyria (**43−22.**).
Renal disease (**38**).

Certain drugs potentiate and prolong the action of anesthetic agents. Particularly in elderly persons, a history of daily administration of some of these drugs may not be obtainable prior to emergency surgery.

Corticosteroids (**49−226.** *Corticotropin;* **49−227.** *Cortisone*)

Monamine oxide inhibitors [Iproniazid (Marsalid), (**49−397**), isoboxazid (Marplan), nialamide (Niamid), phenoxypropazine (Drazine), tranylcypromine (Parnate)].

Phenothiazines (**49−592**)

Sedatives (**49−111.** *Barbiturates;* **49−144.** *Bromides.*)

ANESTHETIC OVERDOSAGE

See **49−70.** *Anesthetics, Inhalation;* **49−71.** *Anesthetics, Intravenous*

CARBON DIOXIDE RETENTION

A high oxygen content in the anesthetic mixture may mask serious underventilation, which becomes apparent when postoperative breathing of air is resumed. Carbon dioxide retention is characterized by flushing, excessive perspiration, elevated pulse and hypertension. The respiration is "jerky," with a tracheal tug.

TREATMENT

1. Cautious hyperventilation, avoiding too rapid elimination of carbon dioxide which may in itself cause hypotension, cardiac arrhythmias and ventricular fibrillation (**26 – 23**).

2. Control of bronchospasm (**52 – 1**).

3. Control of respiratory acidosis by intravenous injection of 50 ml. of 8.4% sodium bicarbonate solution (1 mEq./ml.), repeated if improvement does not take place.

4. Monitor with serial arterial pH, Pco_2 and CO_2 content determinations.

CEREBRAL HYPOXIA

Delayed recovery of consciousness after anesthesia, or delayed relapse into coma after a period of semiconsciousness, may be due to hypoxic brain damage with edema. If improvement does not occur in a short time, 50 ml. of 50% glucose should be given slowly intravenously and repeated if necessary in 30 minutes.

CEREBROVASCULAR DISORDERS

Cerebral thrombosis or emboli (**59 – 4**) identifiable by focal signs, occur occasionally and result in prolonged postanesthetic coma. Cerebral hemorrhage (**59 – 2**) is very rare, except as a concomitant condition with other traumatic or degenerative conditions.

FAT EMBOLISM

This condition can practically never be diagnosed in an emergency situation but may occur following severe crush injuries to the soft tissues, long bone fractures, burns, and decompression sickness. Orthopedic procedures and inadvertent intravenous contrast media injections are iatrogenic causes. Most of the fat globules are deposited in the lungs, but involvement of the brain, kidneys and liver does occur. The urine frequently shows free fat. Treatment is symptomatic and supportive. Prophylactically, 50 ml. of 50% glucose every 8 hours intravenously has been reported as decreasing the incidence of fat emboli in multisystem injured patients.

HYPOTHERMIA (See also **57−5**).

Especially in infants, elderly persons and myxedematous patients, a decrease in body temperature may result in prolonged post-anesthetic coma. Treatment consists of rewarming as soon as possible.

METABOLIC ACIDOSIS

See **43−1.** *Acidosis;* **48−2.** *Acidosis in Children*

SHOCK

See **53; 48−51.** *Shock in Children*

30. CONTAGIOUS AND COMMUNICABLE DISEASES

30−1. ANTHRAX (Malignant Pustule, Wool Sorters' Disease)

Usually anthrax occurs in industry (**75.** *Industrial Cases*) in persons who handle, cure or process animal hides. The incubation period is 1 to 7 days. No quarantine is required, but the patient should be isolated until any drainage from superficial lesions clears.

TREATMENT

Symptomatic, plus large doses of penicillin; penicillin-sensitive patients should be given erythromycin or a tetracycline.

30−2. CHANCROID See **60−2**

30−3. CHICKENPOX (Varicella) See **30−40.** *Common Exanthems*

TREATMENT
1. Isolation for 10 days.
2. Sedation as required, with close observation regarding development of interstitial pneumonia (**48−45.** *Pneumonia in Children*).
3. Dressings to prevent scratching.
4. Trimeprazine tartrate (Temaril), 2.5 mg., by mouth every 4 to 6 hours for relief of itching.

30−4. DIPHTHERIA

Affects chiefly children between 1 and 10 years, mostly 2 to 5 years. Incubation period is 2 to 5 days. Average mortality is 5%. Spread by direct and indirect contact; carriers common.

TREATMENT

1. Immediate administration of adequate doses of diphtheria antitoxin is imperative if the clinical findings are suggestive of diphtheria. This applies even if smears are negative or inconclusive. Infants should be given 5000 units of diphtheria antitoxin; older children, 8000 to 20,000 units. Before administration, 0.1 ml. of undiluted serum should be injected intramuscularly. If no wheal appears in 20 minutes, the whole dose can be given. If a wheal does develop, 0.05 ml. of a 1:1000 solution should be injected intradermally, followed by desensitization (**12**) if necessary.

2. Serious cases require hospitalization. Mild cases may be treated at home with quarantine until 2 consecutive nose and throat cultures taken at 24 hour intervals show no diphtheria bacilli.

3. Emergency intubation or tracheostomy (**14−12**) may be indicated. Marked respiratory difficulty from edema must be relieved *before transfer of the patient.* Although in extreme emergencies a tracheostomy may be performed by simply passing a knife-blade in the midline between the cricoid and thyroid cartilages (**14−12**), this method may cause laryngeal damage. A more satisfactory method which avoids important structures and allows introduction of the tube under visual control is at the level of the 3rd and 4th tracheal rings. For technique see **14−12.**

30−5. DYSENTERY (Bacillary)

This disease, which affects persons in all age groups, is spread by indirect contact. Incubation period is 1 to 9 days (usually less than 4 days). Isolation is indicated until stool cultures no longer show the bacilli responsible. Fluid and electrolyte replacement (**6**) is essential. Tetracyclines and furazolidone (Furoxone) are important therapeutic agents.

30−6. GERMAN MEASLES (Rubella) See **30−40.** *Common Exanthems*

30−7. GONOCCAL INFECTIONS See **60−3.**

30−8. GRANULOMA INGUINALE See **60−4.** *Lymphopathia Venereum*

30−9. HEMOLYTIC STREPTOCOCCAL INFECTIONS

These organisms may cause septic sore throat, scarlet fever (**30−40.** *Common Exanthems*) and various other serious conditions. Incubation period is 1 to 5 days; it is spread by both direct and indirect contact. Since communicability lasts from first symptoms until complete recovery, patients should be isolated until afebrile and all discharges have cleared. Recovery from a condition caused by one type of hemolytic streptococcus does not result in immunity to other types.

TREATMENT
1. Bed rest under isolation precautions and symptomatic care.
2. Penicillin or erythromycin in large doses continued for at least 1 week after the acute picture has cleared.

30−10. HEPATITIS See 62−8.

30−11. INFLUENZA (See also 62−10)

The various types of influenza are viral diseases which are usually characterized by high fever, coryza, myalgia and tracheobronchitis, but delirium, convulsions and coma may simulate meningitis, especially in children (**48−41**). The incubation period is 1 to 5 days.

TREATMENT
Symptomatic treatment only is indicated. Extremely severe cases should be hospitalized to prevent complications, but the usual case does very well on home care. No quarantine is required.

30−12. LEPROSY

The incubation period is very long; the method of transmittal is not fully known. Quarantine in specially designated hospitals is required.

30−13. LYMPHOPATHIA VENEREUM See 60−4.

30−14. MALARIA

Quarantine or isolation is not required. Incubation period: 14 days.

TREATMENT

Quinine, 1 gm., 3 times a day for 3 days, then 0.65 gm. for 8 days, is the usual treatment for acute malaria caused by P. *falciformis;* however, the possibility of a quinine-resistant organism or of the development of hemolysis *(blackwater fever)* must always be considered. Chloroquine phosphate (Aralen) or pyrimethamine (Daraprim) may be required. P. vivax malaria, more common in the United States, usually responds satisfactorily to chloroquine therapy.

30 – 15. MEASLES (Rubeola) See **30 – 40.** *Common Exanthems*

TREATMENT

1. Complete isolation for 2 weeks.
2. Rest in a darkened room or protection of the eyes by dark glasses.
3. Steam inhalations; ear drops.
4. Early recognition and treatment of complications such as otitis media, bronchopneumonia and encephalitis.
5. Prophylactic injection of gamma globulin for contacts under 2 years old, pregnant women and elderly or debilitated persons.

30 – 16. MENINGITIS (See also **48 – 41.** *Meningococcemia in Children;* **48 – 63.** *Waterhouse-Friderichsen Syndrome in Children; 62 – 1. Arboviral Infections*)

The incubation period of epidemic (meningococcal) meningitis is 2 to 10 days; the quarantine period is 21 days or longer.

Evidence indicative of meningococcal septicemia (**48 – 42.** *Meningococcemia in Children*) requires immediate administration of large doses of antibiotics and readily absorbable sulfonamides, preferably intravenously. (See **30 – 41.** *Antimicrobial Drugs of Choice.*)

30 – 17. MUMPS

The incubation period is 12 to 26 days, usually 16 to 18 days.

TREATMENT

1. Bed rest in isolation until the fever and glandular swelling subside.
2. Ice packs to swollen areas.

3. Careful mouth hygiene.

4. Early recognition and treatment of complications (orchitis, pancreatitis, meningoencephalitis). Early administration of corticosteroids (prednisone) orally, 60 mg. at once and then 20 mg. 3 times a day, may relieve symptoms and possibly prevent sterility from pressure necrosis of the testicles. Gradual tapering off of the steroid should accompany decrease of edema.

30 — 18. PARATYPHOID FEVER See **30 — 33.** *Typhoid Fever*

30 — 19. PERTUSSIS See **30 — 38.** *Whooping Cough*

30 — 20. PLAGUE

The incubation period for both the bubonic and pneumonic forms is 3 to 7 days. Quarantine until complete recovery is mandatory. Streptomycin in large doses intramuscularly and a sulfonamide orally are the drugs of choice for treatment (**30 — 41**).

30 — 21. POLIOMYELITIS (Infantile Paralysis) (See also **46 — 9; 48 — 49.** *Respiratory Paralysis in Children*)

Three causative viral strains have been identified. Spread is by both direct and indirect contact. Incubation period is from 3 to 35 days (usually 7 to 14 days).

TREATMENT

1. Immediate hospitalization for spinal puncture (**14 — 11**) to establish the diagnosis if the history and clinical examination suggest the possibility of poliomyelitis. (See also **24 — 22.** *Tick Paralysis.*) The puncture may be done by the emergency physician if equipment and laboratory facilities are available.

2. Isolation for 1 week from the onset of 1st symptoms or while febrile.

3. Control of pain by sedatives and anodynes. Narcotics are contraindicated if there is any respiratory weakness.

4. Artificial respiration by mechanical or other methods (**11 — 1**) if respiratory difficulty is present. Emergency tracheostomy (**14 — 12**) may be necessary.

5. Orthopedic support of paralyzed parts to prevent contractures and other deformities.

30—22.   PSITTACOSIS (Ornithosis, Parrot Fever)

A history of contact with parrots, parakeets, lovebirds, laboratory birds or animals infected with the disease is essential for a provisional diagnosis of psittacosis. The disease has also been reported in pheasants and barnyard fowl. The causative organism is an obligate intracellular parasite. *Chlamydia psittaci.*

Incubation period is 5 to 21 days.

SIGNS AND SYMPTOMS.   Acute onset with chills, general malaise and fever to 40.6°C. (105°F.). The pulse remains relatively slow. The patient usually complains of a splitting headache and of photophobia. There is usually nausea and vomiting, herpetic skin lesions and acute sore throat. Pulmonary involvement with persistent cough and signs of patchy consolidation may develop in a few hours. Severe cases may show pinkish oval papular lesions on the trunk and may develop diplopia, hallucinations and stupor.

TREATMENT

1. Control of headaches by oral administration of codeine sulfate, 0.06 gm., and acetylsalicylic acid (aspirin), 0.6 gm., every 4 hours.

2. Morphine sulfate or meperidine hydrochloride (Demerol) may be given in small doses subcutaneously for very severe pain, but if possible their use should be avoided. Pentazocine lactate, 15 to 30 mg., intramuscularly or intravenously is effective.

3. Tetracycline hydrochloride (Achromycin) or chloramphenicol (Chloromycetin), 250 mg., orally every 4 hours (**30—41**).

4. Transfer as soon as possible to a hospital equipped to handle acute infectious diseases.

30—23.   RABIES See 62—17.

30—24.   RUBELLA (German Measles) See **30—40.** *Common Exanthems*

TREATMENT

1. Keep the patient indoors until acute symptoms subside.

2. Symptomatic care. Complications are rare; however, an uncomfortable polyarthritis with fibrositis, paresthesias, myalgia and muscle weakness lasting as long as 2 weeks may occur. Thrombocytopenic purpura is a rare complication.

30—25.   RUBEOLA See **30—15.** *Measles;* **30—40.** *Common Exanthems*

30—26. SALMONELLA INFECTIONS See **30—33**. *Typhoid Fever;* **49—339**. *Food Poisoning*

30—27. SCARLET FEVER See **30—9**. *Hemolytic Streptococcal Infections;* **30—40**. *Common Exanthems*

TREATMENT
1. Simple cases may be cared for at home.
2. Toxic or septic cases require immediate hospitalization. Delirium and convulsions are complications which may require emergency treatment.

30—28. SEPTIC SORE THROAT See **30—9**. *Hemolytic Streptococcal Infections;* **30—41**. *Antimicrobial Drugs of Choice*

30—29. SHIGELLA INFECTIONS See **30—5**. *Dysentery (Bacillary)*

30—30. SMALLPOX See **30—40**. *Common Exanthems*

TREATMENT
1. Immediate isolation as soon as the diagnosis has been established, with sterilization of the examination room and its contents after the patient has been transferred. Whenever possible, isolation should be in a suitable single dwelling or isolation unit and not in a general hospital.
2. Immediate vaccination of all persons who have come in contact with the case.

30—31. TETANUS (Lockjaw) (See also **16**. *Tetanus Immunization*)

The incubation period of tetanus is from a few hours in infants to 3 weeks or longer in older children and adults. Although about 50% of cases follow puncture wounds and lacerations, cases have been reported following injections, abortions, animal kicks, gum and tooth infections and animal bites. The diagnosis of tetanus is based on clinical findings. Early signs are abdominal and paravertebral muscle spasm, trismus, risus sardonicus and difficulty in swallowing. Stimulation of the posterior pharynx with a tongue blade produces characteristic masseter spasm.
TREATMENT
1. Protection from unnecessary stimuli in a private, quiet but not excessively darkened, room.

2. Efficient and painstaking nursing care, with minimal handling.

3. Lessening of spasm and reflex irritability by administration of muscle relaxants [diazepam (Valium), 10 to 20 mg. intramuscularly or intravenously every 2 to 4 hours] and sedatives [sodium amobarbital (Amytal Sodium) intramuscularly or intravenously or chloral hydrate rectally]. A combination of a muscle relaxant and a sedative is more effective and less toxic than either one separately. Narcotics should be avoided because of their respiratory depressant effect.

4. Human tetanus-immune globulin (TIG), 5000 units, intramuscularly in divided doses given at several sites, including adjacent to the wound, may be of value. Tetanus toxoid (**16**) is ineffective in treatment of established tetanus.

5. Wide surgical excision of the site of infection with removal of all potentially traumatized or infected tissues. The operative site should be left open and irrigated or compressed daily with hydrogen peroxide.

6. Penicillin, 30 million units the first day, followed by 10 million units per day for as long as necessary. If penicillin allergy is present, tetracycline intravenously should be substituted; initial dose of 500 mg., followed by 250 mg. every 4 hours.

7. Tracheostomy (**14—12**) if airway obstruction from acute laryngospasm is present or if the patient is developing difficulty in clearing secretions from the pharynx. A sterile tracheostomy set should be available at bedside at all times. For treatment of acute bronchospasm, see **52—1.**

8. Daily monitoring of serum and urine electrolytes, with replacement (**6**) as indicated. Adequate potassium replacement may require 80 to 150 mEq. per day. Continuous ECG monitoring is a valuable adjunct to therapy.

9. Careful supportive therapy to prevent complications which in themselves may act as irritating stimuli to the underlying condition. Among these are urinary retention, fecal impaction, gastrointestinal tract bleeding, thrombophlebitis and secondary infections.

30—32. TRACHOMA

This very infectious conjunctivitis is due to an obligate intracellular parasite, *Chlamydia trachomatis,* spread by personal contact. It may cause severe scarring and blindness.

30-33. TYPHOID FEVER

TREATMENT
1. Instruction regarding disposition of infected handkerchiefs, towels, etc.
2. Oral and topical tetracycline (**30-41**).
3. Sulfadiazine, 0.5 to 1 gm. by mouth 3 times a day (**30-41**).
4. Chloramphenicol (Chloromycetin) ophthalmic drops.
5. Reference to an ophthalmologist.

30-33. TYPHOID FEVER

Incubation period is 10 to 15 days.
TREATMENT
As soon as the diagnosis is established or suspected, the patient should be hospitalized for confirmatory diagnosis, chloramphenicol (Chloromycetin) therapy and careful supportive treatment. Severe epistaxis may require packing (**14-6**) before transfer. Quarantine is required until 2 consecutive negative stool cultures have been obtained.

30-34. TYPHUS FEVER

This rickettsial disease is transmitted from man to man by the human body louse with man as the reservoir of infection or, in certain instances, by chiggers or other mites carried by rodents and other wild animals. The usual incubation period is 12 days, but the disease may occur years after the patient has left a known typhus area. Contacts must be quarantined for 14 days. Treatment consists of control of hyperpyrexia and pain, prevention of complications and administration of large doses of tetracyclines or chloramphenicol (Chloromycetin), preferably intravenously. Penicillin is ineffective in treatment and sulfonamides are contraindicated. Although convalescence may be slow, permanent ill effects rarely occur.

30-35. UNDULANT FEVER

Incubation period is 5 to 21 days, occasionally longer. Quarantine is not required.

30-36. VARICELLA See **30-3**. *Chickenpox;* **30-40**. *Common Exanthems*

30 – 37.   VARIOLA See **30 – 30.** *Smallpox;* **30 – 40.** *Common Exanthems*

30 – 38.   WHOOPING COUGH (Pertussis)

Caused by a gram-negative bacillus, *Bordetella pertussis,* whooping cough usually lasts for about 6 weeks. Its incubation period is usually 7 to 10 days, but it may be as long as 21 days. Spread is by direct and indirect contact. It is communicable from about 7 days after exposure (when symptoms appear to be those of a common cold) until 3 weeks after onset of the typical spasmodic cough. Exclusion from schools, theaters and other public places is usually required but no strict quarantine.

TREATMENT

1. Cautious sedation for control of the paroxysmal cough by oral codeine sulfate in small doses, chloral hydrate by mouth or retention enema, paraldehyde orally or intramuscularly or pentobarbital sodium (Nembutal) by rectal suppository.

2. Insurance of a patent airway with supplemental oxygen therapy if evidence of hypoxia is present.

3. Control of vomiting which often follows paroxysms of coughing. Small doses of tincture opii camphorata (Paregoric) usually are effective.

4. Frequent oral intake of small amounts of fluids.

5. Ampicillin, 100 mg. per kilogram of body weight per day, or a tetracycline, 25 mg. per kilogram of body weight per day in 4 divided doses, orally for 1 week or until the temperature has been normal for 3 days.

6. Hyperimmune pertussis gamma globulin, 2.5 ml., daily for 5 days to decrease the intensity of paroxysms.

7. Early recognition and treatment of complications such as bronchopneumonia (**48 – 45.** *Pneumonia;* **62 – 11.** *Interstitial Pneumonia*), gastric tetany, rectal prolapse following paroxysms of coughing or vomiting (**37 – 5**), meningitis (**48 – 41**) and encephalitis (**48 – 24; 62 – 5**).

30 – 39.   YELLOW FEVER

In this age of rapid transportation when intercontinental travel within the 3 to 6 day incubation period is not only possible but common, the physician must be aware of this very serious virus infection transmitted by the *Aedes aegypti* mosquito. Yellow fever is still endemic in parts of South America and Africa.

COMMON EXANTHEMS –

CONDITION	INCUBATION (Days)	PERIOD OF COMMUNICABILITY
Chickenpox (Varicella). For treatment, see **30 – 3.**	12–21	From 1 day before onset of symptoms until about 6 days after appearance of rash
Drug rash	History of use of drug	None
Exanthema subitum (Roseola infantum)	Probably 7–10	Unknown, although blood and washings from the throat may be infective during the first day of rash
German measles (Rubella). For treatment, see **30 – 24.**	14–21	From 1 day before onset of symptoms until 1 day after disappearance of rash
Infectious mononucleosis	5–15	Undetermined
Measles (Rubeola). For treatment, see **30 – 15.**	7–15	From 2 to 4 days before appearance of rash until 2 to 5 days thereafter
Scarlet fever (Scarlatina). For treatment, see **30 – 27.**	3–5	Usually from 24 hours before onset of symptoms until 2 to 3 weeks thereafter; longer if complications occur
Smallpox (Variola). For treatment, see **30 – 30.**	10–14	From 1 to 2 days before onset of symptoms until all crusts have disappeared

DIFFERENTIAL DIAGNOSIS

SYMPTOMS AND SIGNS	SITE	ERUPTION – ONSET, DURATION AND CHARACTER
Chills, moderate fever, headache, malaise	Usually 1st on trunk, later face, neck and extremities; infrequently on palms and soles	Develop day after onset of symptoms; persist for 1 to 2 weeks. Lesions discrete; progress from macules to papules to vesicles which rupture and form crusts. Appear in crops – various forms may be present simultaneously
Variable, including fever, malaise, arthralgia, nausea, photophobia, pruritus	Generalized; sometimes restricted to exposed surfaces	Varies in time of onset and duration – may be morbilliform, scarlatiniform, erythematous, acneform, vesicular, bullous, purpuric, or exfoliative
Infants affected. High fever, usually postoccipital lymphadenopathy	Chest and abdomen, with moderate involvement of face and extremities	This diffuse macular or maculopapular rash appears on the 4th day, usually at the same time the temperature drops to normal; lasts 1 to 2 days
Malaise, fever, headache, rhinitis, postauricular and postoccipital lymphadenopathy	Face, neck, spreading to trunk and limbs.	Develop 1 to 2 days after symptoms; lasts 1 to 3 days. Fine pinkish macules which become confluent
Malaise, headache, fever, sore throat, splenomegaly and generalized lymphadenopathy	Most prominent over trunk	In about 15% of cases, a morbilliform, scarlatiniform, or vesicular rash appears 5 to 14 days after symptoms; lasts 3 to 7 days
Fever, coryza, cough, conjunctivitis, photophobia, Koplik's spots, pruritus	Forehead, face, neck, and then spreading over trunk and limbs	Develops 3 to 5 days after symptoms; lasts 4 to 7 days. Maculopapular; brownish pink; irregularly confluent
Chills, fever, sore throat, vomiting, strawberry tongue, cervical lymphadenopathy, circumoral pallor	Face, neck, chest, abdomen, spreading to extremities. Entire body surface may be involved	Develops on 2nd day; lasts 4 to 10 days. Diffuse pinkish red flush of skin, with punctate "gooseflesh" feel. Positive blanching reaction
Abrupt onset with chills, fever, rapid pulse and respiration, nausea, vomiting, severe headache, backache and pains	First face, neck, upper chest, hands. Most on exposed surfaces; may involve palms, soles, pharynx	Develops on 3rd or 4th day; persists for 2 to 5 weeks. Shot-like papules changing to vesicles and umbilicated pustules which enlarge and become confluent. Usually only 1 crop of lesions

page 181

Incubation period is 3 to 6 days.

Quarantine period:
   Patient – 3 to 5 days after development of acute symptoms.
   All contacts – 6 days.

SIGNS AND SYMPTOMS

Initial Stage

1. Sudden onset of chills and fever associated with severe headache particularly in the frontal area.

2. Temperature to 40°C. (104°F.). *The pulse goes down while the fever goes up.*

3. Generalized acute myalgia.

4. Red eyes; bloated face.

5. Anorexia, nausea, occasionally vomiting.

6. Apparent remission after 2 to 3 days.

Middle Stage

1. Severe vomiting with coffee-ground appearance of the vomitus.

2. Extreme thirst; acute dehydration.

3. Gastrointestinal hemorrhage.

4. Extreme generalized jaundice.

5. Anuria or scanty urine with marked albuminuria.

Final Stage

A crisis usually occurs on the 6th or 7th day; either the patient dies or the beginning of recovery is indicated by rapid fall of body temperature and increased secretion of urine.

TREATMENT

No specific therapy is known. Immediate hospitalization is indicated since the outcome will depend to a considerable extent upon adequate nursing care. Symptomatic treatment, especially for dehydration, should be given before and during transfer for hospitalization.

30 – 40. COMMON EXANTHEMS – DIFFERENTIAL DIAGNOSIS

See table on pages 180–181.

30 – 41. ANTIMICROBIAL DRUGS OF CHOICE

Before any of the antimicrobial agents specified in the table on pages 183 to 185 are administered, the manufacturer's brochure or a pharmacology text should be consulted for method of administration, dosages, toxicity and side effects.

ANTIMICROBIAL DRUGS OF CHOICE

INFECTING ORGANISM	DRUGS OF FIRST CHOICE	ALTERNATIVE DRUGS
BACILLI		
Acid-fast		
Mycobacterium tuberculosis	isoniazid plus p-aminosalicylic acid and streptomycin	cycloserine; ethionamide; pyrazinamide; viomycin
Gram-negative		
Aerobacter aerogenes	a tetracycline	chloramphenicol; cephalothin
Bordetella pertussis (30–38)	ampicillin	a tetracycline
Donovania granulomatis (granuloma inguinale)	a tetracycline	chloramphenicol; streptomycin
Escherichia coli		
enteropathogenic sepsis	kanamycin (oral) or neomycin (oral) kanamycin (parenteral) or neomycin (parenteral)	ampicillin; a tetracycline chloramphenicol; a tetracycline; polymyxin B or colistimethate
urinary infections (38–10)	a sulfonamide	ampicillin; a tetracycline; nitrofurantoin
Fusobacterium (Vincent's infection, 54–19)	a penicillin	a tetracycline; erythromycin
Hemophilus ducreyi (chancroid, 60–2)	a tetracycline	a sulfonamide; chloramphenicol; streptomycin
Hemophilus influenzae respiratory infections (62–10)	ampicillin	a tetracycline; chloramphenicol
meningitis (30–16; 48–42)	chloramphenicol	a tetracycline; ampicillin
Pasteurella pestis (bubonic plague, 30–20)	streptomycin with or without a sulfonamide	a tetracycline; chloramphenicol
Proteus mirabilis and other Proteus	carbenicillin with gentamicin	gentamycin, colistin, polymyxin B
Pseudomonas aeruginosa	carbenicillin with gentamycin	gentamycin, colistin, polymyxin B
Salmonella (30–33. *Typhoid*; 49–339. *Food poisoning*)	chloramphenicol	ampicillin; cephalothin
Shigella (30–5)	ampicillin	kanamycin (oral) or neomycin (oral); a tetracycline; cephalothin; furazolidone
Vibrio comma (cholera)	a tetracycline	chloramphenicol; streptomycin
Gram-positive		
Bacillus anthracis (30–1 *Anthrax*)	a penicillin	erythromycin; a tetracycline

ANTIMICROBIAL DRUGS OF CHOICE—*Continued*

INFECTING ORGANISM	DRUG OF FIRST CHOICE	ALTERNATIVE DRUGS
Clostridium perfringens	a penicillin	a tetracycline; clindamycin
Clostridium tetani (**30**−**31**)	a penicillin	a tetracycline
Clostridium welchii (gas gangrene, **20**−**14**)	a penicillin	a tetracycline
Corynebacterium diphtheriae (**30**−**4**)	a penicillin	erythromycin; cephalothin
COCCI		
Gram-negative		
Gonococcus (**60**−**3**)	a penicillin	erythromycin; cephalothin; a tetracycline
Meningococcus (**30**−**16**; **48**−**42**)	a penicillin	ampicillin; cephalothin; erythromycin; a sulfonamide
Gram-positive		
Enterococcus	a penicillin with streptomycin	ampicillin; cephalothin or erythromycin erythromycin with streptomycin
Pneumococcus (**52**−**14**)	a penicillin	erythromycin; cephalothin; clindamycin
Staphylococcus aureus non-penicillinase producing	a penicillin	erythromycin; cephalothin
penicillinase producing	a penicillinase-resistant penicillin	cephalothin; lincomycin; vancomycin
Streptococcus anaerobius	a tetracycline	a penicillin
Streptococcus faecalis	a penicillin with streptomycin	Vancomycin with streptomycin or erythromycin with streptomycin (if endocarditis is present)
Streptococcus pyogenes groups A, B, C and G	a penicillin	erythromycin; cephalothin; clindamycin
Streptococcus viridans	a penicillin with streptomycin	cephalothin; clindamycin vancomycin

FUNGI

Coccidioides immitis	amphotericin B
Cryptococcus neoformans	amphotericin B

OBLIGATE INTRACELLULAR PARASITES

Chlamydia venerii [lymphogranuloma venereum (60–4)]	a tetracycline	chloramphenicol; a sulfonamide
Chlamydia psittaci [Psittacosis (30–22)]	a tetracycline	chloramphenicol
Chlamydia trachomatis [Trachoma (30–32 and 35–26)]	oral or topical tetracyclines plus an oral sulfonamide	topical chloramphenicol
Mycoplasma [atypical viral pneumonia (62–11)]	a tetracycline	chloramphenicol

RICKETTSIA [Rocky Mountain spotted fever (24–22), typhus (30–34), Q fever]

	a tetracycline	chloramphenicol

SPIROCHETES

Leptospira	a penicillin	a tetracycline
Spirillum minus (rat bite fever)	a penicillin	erythromycin; streptomycin
Treponema pallidum [syphilis (60–5)]	a penicillin	erythromycin; a tetracycline
Treponema pertenue (yaws)	a penicillin	erythromycin; a tetracycline

Smears and cultures for identification and sensitivity tests should be taken before an antimicrobial agent is given for definitive treatment, but emergency therapy based on clinical findings as a rule should not await laboratory results.

31. CONVULSIVE SEIZURES

See also **34.** *Excitement States;* **48 – 18.** *Convulsions in Children.*
Persons of any age may develop convulsive seizures either for the first time or on a recurrent basis. Subsequent episodes are frequently, though not invariably, related to prior causes.

The underlying factors responsible for convulsions vary with age.

Neonatal and infant age group
  Birth injury
  Developmental abnormalities.
  Bacterial and viral central nervous system infections (**48 – 24.** *Encephalitis;* **48 – 41.** *Meningitis in Children*).

Children and adolescents. Same as above, with addition of *Trauma* [especially head injuries (**48 – 9.** *Brain Concussion;* **48 – 32.** *Head Injuries in Children*)].
  Idiopathic causes (**29 – 7.** *Epilepsy;* **48 – 25.** *Excitement States in Children*).

Adults
  Trauma (**41.** *Head Injuries*).
  Idiopathic causes (**29 – 7.** *Epilepsy*).
  Metabolic abnormalities (**43**).
  Effects of drugs (**49**).
  Toxemias of pregnancy (**47 – 5**), including acute atrophy of the liver (**47 – 6**) and eclampsia (**47 – 7**).
  Vascular conditions (**59 – 2.** *Intracranial Bleeding*).
  Neoplasms.

TREATMENT
The vigor with which emergency treatment is applied will depend largely on the state of the patient at the time he is first seen by the physician, since frequently the acute episode will have subsided.

1. Protection from injury by gentle restraint and maintenance in a lying position at a safe level.

2. Maintenance of an unobstructed airway during the postictal state. The patient should be placed in a prone or semiprone position with the head turned to one side.

3. Institution of cooling measures by sponging, tepid tub baths and cool water enemas if the convulsions are caused by hyperpyrexia.

4. Administration of salicylates when the convulsive seizures are associated with hyperpyrexia.

5. Sodium amobarbital (Amytal), 200 to 500 mg. intravenously, at a rate not to exceed 30 mg. per minute until some decrease in intensity of the convulsive seizure occurs. Sodium phenobarbital, 200 to 300 mg. intramuscularly, will usually prevent recurrence after the seizure has stopped.

6. Inhalation anesthesia followed by hospitalization in severe cases.

7. Paraldehyde, 1 to 3 gm. intramuscularly or orally, or chloral hydrate, 0.5 to 1.0 gm. orally or by retention enema. These drugs are particularly valuable if respiratory depression must be avoided.

8. Diphenylhydantoin sodium (Dilantin), 200 mg. intramuscularly, for prophylaxis against further episodes. Dilantin has no effect on the immediate seizure.

9. Treatment of causative condition. Some of the most common causes encountered are:

Acute infections (**30 – 16.** *Meningoencephalitis;* **48 – 41.** *Meningitis in Children;* **48 – 42.** *Meningococcemia in Children;* **48 – 63.** *Waterhouse-Friderichsen Syndrome;* **62 – 1.** *Arboviral Infections*).

Delirium tremens (**34 – 3**).

Eclampsia (**47 – 7**).

Epilepsy (**29 – 7**).

Heat stroke (**57 – 4**).

Hyperventilation (**34 – 6**).

Hypoglycemia (**29 – 3.** *Diabetes Mellitus;* **33 – 2.** *Endocrine Disorders, Pancreas;* **43 – 16**).

Poisoning, acute. For treatment see under the specific causative poison (**49**).

10. Ultimate management. Any person with convulsions of undetermined origin should have a thorough investigation including:

History of medications and alcoholic intake.

Family history.

Complete physical and neurologic examination as outlined under **29 – 17.** *Coma of Undetermined Etiology.*

Lumbar puncture (**14—11.** *Spinal Puncture*), unless contraindicated by the possibility of increased intracranial pressure.

Sugar and calcium level determinations of blood specimens taken at the time of the convulsion.

Electroencephalograms.

Definitive care. This will depend upon type and cause of the convulsions and may require trial of several regimens for control.

32. EAR CONDITIONS

32—1. ABSCESSES OF MIDDLE EAR See **32—13.** *Otitis Media*

32—2. BURNS See **25—10.**

32—3. COLD INJURIES See **57—1.**

32—4. CONTUSIONS

The marked cosmetic blemishes caused by bleeding into the helix, concha and lobule ("cauliflower ears") can often be prevented by immediate aspiration or surgical drainage of the hematoma, followed by application of pressure.

32—5. DEAFNESS

TREATMENT

1. If caused by an upper respiratory infection with eustachian salpingitis, the underlying condition should be treated. Shrinking of the nasal mucous membrane by 0.25% phenylephrine hydrochloride (Neo-Synephrine) drops or spray may give marked relief. Cocaine solutions (**49—72.** *Anesthetics, Local;* **49—218**) and naphazoline hydrochloride (**49—623.** *Privine*) should not be used or prescribed because of the relatively high incidence of untoward effects.

2. If it is due to impacted cerumen, the ear can be cleansed safely, provided the condition of the drum is known. Any evidence of perforation is an absolute contraindication to irrigation or instilla-

tion of any substance into the canal. Removal of the wax can be accomplished by the following method:

a. Fill the external auditory canal with triethanolamine poly-peptide oleate (Cerumenex) drops.

b. Plug with cotton for 15 to 30 minutes.

c. Irrigate with warm water, using a soft rubber syringe.

3. If caused or aggravated by concussion (explosions, etc.) or by sudden or prolonged exposure to intense noise (jackhammers, amplified modern "music," riveting, etc.), symptomatic treatment only is indicated. The patient should be referred to an otolaryngologist for examination and care.

32 – 6. EARACHE

Acute earache can often be relieved by anodynes and treatment of underlying infection of the middle ear and upper respiratory tract with broad spectrum antibiotics. Provided otoscopic examination shows no evidence of drum perforation, antipyrine ear drops may give relief. Persistent earache requires care by an otolaryngologist.

32 – 7. EUSTACHIAN SALPINGITIS See 32 – 13. *Otitis Media*

32 – 8. FOREIGN BODIES See 36 – 1.

32 – 9. LACERATIONS See 55 – 20.

32 – 10. MASTOIDITIS

This complication of otitis media (**32 – 13**) has become rather rare since the advent of sulfonamides and antibiotics. Recently, however, an increase in cases has become apparent, probably as a result of inadequate treatment of otitis media with antibiotics. If mastoiditis is proved or suspected, immediate hospitalization is indicated.

32 – 11. MENIERE'S DISEASE See 46 – 8. *Neuritis*

32 – 12. OTITIS EXTERNA (See also 23 – 5. *Diving Hazards*)

Inflammation of the external auditory canal requires no emergency treatment and should be distinguished from middle ear involvement (**32 — 13.** *Otitis Media*). The patient should be advised to consult an otolaryngologist if the irritation of the canal persists.

32 — 13. OTITIS MEDIA

Acute inflammation of the middle ear is often encountered as an emergency in children. Formerly uncommon in adults, it is now a fairly common occurrence in sports divers (**23 — 5**).

TREATMENT

1. Ampicillin or penicillin plus sulfisoxazole in younger children (**4**); penicillin or ampicillin orally in older children and adults.

2. Hot compresses. *No medication should be given into the canal* unless there has been rupture of the drum with drainage of frank pus; in this case hydrogen peroxide ear drops may be of benefit.

3. Acetylsalicylic acid (aspirin), 0.06 to 0.3 gm., depending on age or weight (**4**), every 4 hours. Codeine sulfate orally or subcutaneously or pentazocine lactate (Talwin) intramuscularly may be necessary for control of severe pain [dosage by age, weight or skin surface (**4**)].

4. Paracentesis of the drum (Fig. 15). Whenever possible, the patient should be hospitalized if the bulging of the drum is acute and indicates the possibility of the need for this procedure. If emergency paracentesis is required, the incision should be limited to the postero-inferior segment of the drum but should be wide enough to allow free drainage. Cultures and sensitivity tests should be obtained and appropriate antibiotic therapy instituted (**30 — 41.** *Antimicrobial Drugs of Choice*).

5. Decongestants and use of a vaporizer may help relieve eustachian tube inflammation and obstruction.

6. *Complete* control of the infection is essential in all cases of otitis media. Inadequate therapy, especially with antibiotics, may result in apparent alleviation of acute symptoms; however, later development of a suppurative mastoiditis may occur.

32 — 14. OTORRHEA

Drainage of cerebrospinal fluid from the ears is prima facie evidence of basal skull fracture (**41 — 17**). Unless massive, it usually clears spontaneously.

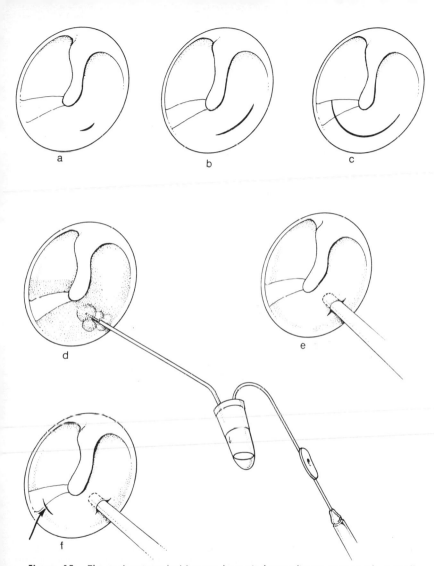

Figure 15. The myringotomy incision can be varied according to your needs: a small incision (a) is adequate for evacuating serous fluids; you might want one a little larger (b) for thicker fluids, especially in "glue ear," or for office inspection of the middle ear; and a wide incision (c) may be necessary for prolonged drainage of pus in refractory purulent otitis. Fluid can also be removed with a paracentesis needle and collected in a trap for later examination (d). A suction tip can be inserted through the incision (e) and if the fluid has become pocketed in a resistant case of otitis, a counterincision (f) may promote evacuation by letting air into the middle ear. (From Emergency Medicine, Vol. 4, No. 10, p. 149, October, 1972.)

32−15. TINNITUS

Tinnitus may be severe enough to require anodynes. All cases of severe or persistent tinnitus should be referred to an otolaryngologist.

33. ENDOCRINE EMERGENCIES

33−1. ADRENAL

Acute adrenal cortical insufficiency. This severe life-threatening situation, manifested by nausea, vomiting, shock, stupor and frequently high fever, occurs in persons with chronic adrenal insufficiency who omit their maintenance dose or whose requirements increase because of stress of some type. Primary acute cases may be associated with rampant infections and adrenal hemorrhage.

TREATMENT

1. Inject 50 to 100 mg. of hydrocortisone hemisuccinate intravenously.

2. Give 100 to 300 mg. of hydrocortisone in 1000 ml. of 5% dextrose in normal saline at a rate of 250 to 500 ml. per hour.

3. Treat shock with pressor amines (**53−7**).

4. Prescribe cortisone or hydrocortisone, 50 mg. orally, every 6 hours.

5. Treat contributing causes.

Pheochromocytoma. The urgent hypertensive complications that occur with this tumor are usually related to investigation of or surgical procedures for the tumor. A histamine test may elicit a profound hypertensive episode and may require 5 mg. of phentolamine (Regitine) intravenously, repeated at 10 to 20 minute intervals as needed. During surgical excision of the tumor, epinephrine or norepinephrine may be released; the resultant hypertension may necessitate phentolamine (Regitine) therapy. After surgical removal severe hypotension may develop, requiring phenylephrine (Neo-Synephrine) or mephentermine (Wyamine) subcutaneously, levarterenol bitartrate (Levophed), 4 ml. in 1000 ml. of 5% dextrose in water intravenously, and plasma or blood transfusions.

33 − 2. PANCREAS

Diabetic coma. See **29 − 3**. *Diabetes Mellitus;* **48 − 20**. *Diabetic Coma in Children.*

Insulin shock. See **29 − 3**. *Diabetes Mellitus;* **48 − 20**. *Diabetic Coma in Children.*

Hypoglycemia secondary to islet cell tumor manifested by coma with or without convulsions, prior increase in appetite and body weight and hypoglycemia secondary to insulin rebound in post-gastrectomy patients.

1. Treatment of acute symptoms. See insulin shock under **29 − 3**. *Diabetes Mellitus.*

2. High protein, low carbohydrate diet in frequent feedings.

3. Referral for definitive work-up and treatment.

33 − 3. PARATHYROID

Hypoparathyroidism. The neuromuscular excitability indicated clinically by carpopedal spasm, facial muscle twitching following tapping, convulsions and laryngeal stridor is due to low serum calcium concentration, usually a complication of thyroidectomy. Signs and symptoms may become evident from hours to months after the surgery.

TREATMENT

1. Collection of a blood specimen for determination of the serum calcium level prior to administration of 1 gm. of calcium gluconate intravenously (give cautiously if the patient is digitalized).

2. Sedation with barbiturates.

3. Referral to a hospital for stabilization and institution of a long-range program (dihydrotachysterol, calciferol and low phosphorus, high calcium diet).

Acute parathyroid intoxication. This uncommon emergency is characterized by hypercalcemia (**43 − 12**), profound weakness, nausea, vomiting and lethargy progressing to coma.

TREATMENT

1. Hydrocortisone, 100 mg. intravenously.

2. Normal saline solution, 1000 ml. intravenously.

3. Potassium salts intravenously to neutralize the effects on the heart of hypercalcemia.

4. Low calcium-phosphorus intake.

5. Acidification of the urine, with measures to insure a large output.

6. Use of chelating agents should be considered.

Definitive treatment consists of surgical exploration for possible removal of a parathyroid tumor.

33 — 4. PITUITARY

Emergencies related to the pituitary gland are usually related to: hypofunction of the various target organs [particularly the adrenal (**33 — 1**) and thyroid (**33 — 5; 43 — 15.** *Hyperthyroid Crises*)] following surgical or radiation ablation of the pituitary. Destruction or damage to the posterior pituitary may occur with resultant diabetes insipidus characterized by high urine volume of low specific gravity, polydipsia and dehydration.

TREATMENT

1. Vasopressin (Pitressin), 0.5 ml. (10 I.U.) subcutaneously every 4 to 6 hours, or 0.4 ml. of vasopressin (Pitressin) tannate in oil intramuscularly at longer intervals, usually 24 to 36 hours.

2. Correction of dehydration (**6.** *Fluid Replacement*).

3. In acute cases, hospitalization for evaluation and determination of Pitressin requirements.

33 — 5. THYROID

HYPERTHYROID EMERGENCIES (THYROID STORM) (See also **43 — 15.** *Hyperthyroid Crises*)

Hyperpyrexia, coma and marked tachycardia characterize this serious condition, usually precipitated by stress or by over-zealous palpation and manipulation of the gland of a hyperthyroid patient. Thorough preoperative preparation of hyperthyroid patients with antithyroid medications will usually prevent occurrence of thyroid storm.

TREATMENT

1. Reduction of fever — see **57 — 4.** *Hyperpyrexia.*

2. Placement in an oxygen tent; minimal handling.

3. Sodium iodide, 1 gm. intravenously.

4. Thiamine (Vitamin B_1), 30 to 50 mg. in 1000 ml. of 5% dextrose in normal saline intravenously.

5. Hydrocortisone-21-phosphate (Hydrocortone), 100 mg. intravenously, repeated as often as necessary with a limit of 1 gm. in 24 hours.

6. Reserpine, 2 mg. intramuscularly, repeated in not less than 4 hours, or propranolol (Inderal), 10 to 30 mg. orally every 6 hours, with monitoring of cardiac tolerance.

7. Propylthiouracil, 250 mg., or methimazole (Tapazole), 20 mg. orally every 8 hours.

8. Hospitalization for close observation and definitive therapy.

HYPOTHYROID EMERGENCIES

Myxedema coma. These patients have the classical picture of myxedema plus hypothermia and stupor or unconsciousness.

TREATMENT

1. Artificial ventilation (**11—1**) as needed for respiratory depression.

2. Liothyronine (Cytomel), 2.5 mcg., every 6 to 12 hours orally.

3. Hydrocortisone-21-phosphate (Hydrocortone), 50 mg. intramuscularly every 6 hours, followed by a maintenance dosage of dexamethasone (Decadron) orally.

4. Hypothermia is partially protective to tissues; elevation to normal body temperature must be accomplished slowly and with caution.

Myxedema compounded by narcotics. Persons with myxedema are extremely sensitive to narcotics; ordinary doses may cause shock, acute respiratory depression and coma.

TREATMENT

Treat as outlined for myxedema coma (above) plus nalorphine hydrochloride (Nalline), 5 to 10 mg. intravenously, repeated as necessary.

34. EXCITEMENT STATES

See also **48—25.** Excitement States in Children; **50—2.** Psychogenic Psychoses.

The most common causes of acute excitement states in adults are as follows:

34—1. ALCOHOLISM (See also **2—1.** Addiction; **15—1.** Alcohol Intoxication Tests; **34—3.** Delirium Tremens; **49—315.** Ethyl Alcohol)

An acute excitement state may precede the onset of coma (**29**); therefore, care should be used in administering sedation for control.

Chlorpromazine hydrochloride (Thorazine), 100 mg. intramuscularly or 100 to 150 mg. by mouth, is rapid, effective and safe, provided barbiturates or opiates have not been given previously. Paraldehyde intramuscularly is also of value. Physical restraint should be used only while sedation is taking effect. Syrup of ipecac, 8 to 12 ml. by mouth, usually will induce vomiting and in addition have a delayed sedative effect. Gastric lavage should not be attempted unless the cooperation of the patient can be obtained except when emetics do not result in satisfactory emptying of the stomach. Other causes for acute excitement (**34**) must be ruled out in all cases of apparent acute alcoholism.

34–2. CHEST INJURIES

Air hunger following nonperforating chest injuries (**28–1**), rib fractures (**28–2**), penetrating chest wounds (**28–9**. *Lacerations Through the Pleura;* **28–11**. *Bullet Wounds*) and severe crushing injuries of the thorax (**28–3**) may cause acute excitement states. Unless cardiac tamponade (**26–22**) is present, gentle manual restraint, cleansing of the airway, administration of oxygen under positive pressure by face mask and rebreathing bag, and treatment of shock (**53–7**) are generally adequate until hospitalization can be arranged.

34–3. DELIRIUM TREMENS (See also **2–1**. *Addiction;* **15–1**. *Alcohol Intoxication Tests;* **34–1**. *Alcoholism*)

This acute type of insanity may be precipitated in heavy drinkers by acute infectious diseases, trauma, (especially fractures and severe crushing injuries) and sudden withdrawal of alcoholic drinks. There is usually a prodromal period of 1 to 2 days characterized by depression, uneasiness and insomnia and followed by development of a coarse tremor and hallucinations, usually of sight.

TREATMENT

1. Paraldehyde, 10 to 15 ml. by mouth, or 5 to 10 ml. intramuscularly, is the drug of choice for sedation. It may be given with safety 3 or 4 times a day. Chloral hydrate by mouth or as a retention enema may be given as necessary for long-continued sedation.

2. Chlorpromazine hydrochloride (Thorazine), 50 to 100 mg., or prochlorperazine (Compazine), 10 to 15 mg. intramuscularly, is safe and effective.

3. Hydration with normal salt solution.

4. Restraint may be necessary but should be avoided if possible. As a rule, if restraint is required, sedation is inadequate.

5. Opiates, synthetic narcotics and alcohol should never be used.

6. Hospitalization in an institution equipped for the care of such cases.

34 — 4. HEAD INJURIES (See also 41; 48 — 9. *Brain Concussion in Children;* 48 — 26. *Epidural Hemorrhage in Children;* 48 — 32. *Head Injuries in Children*)

Injury to the head can cause hyperactivity symptoms ranging from slight restlessness to homicidal mania. Physical restraint should be kept to a minimum; however, to prevent further injury to the patient or injuries to attendants, physical control may be necessary until adequate sedation has been accomplished. Rapid-acting barbiturates, chloral hydrate, chlorpromazine hydrochloride (Thorazine), paraldehyde or prochlorperazine (Compazine) may be used with caution to quiet the patient, but opiates or synthetic narcotics should never be used unless other severe injuries make their use imperative.

34 — 5. HEART FAILURE See 26 — 8. *Congestive Heart Failure;* 48 — 15. *Cardiac Emergencies in Children*

34 — 6. HYPERVENTILATION

Rebreathing into a paper bag held over the face or inhalations of Carbogen by face mask and rebreathing bag usually will result in complete recovery in a short time. In severe cases with profound alkalosis (43 — 5), the following measures should be kept in mind:

1. Copious fluids by mouth if patient will cooperate; if not, normal salt solution intravenously.

2. Ammonium chloride, 1 gm. orally.

3. Weak hydrochloric acid, 0.6 ml. in 200 ml. of water, by mouth.

4. Calcium gluconate, 10 ml. of 10% solution intravenously.

In most cases the signs and symptoms subside rapidly and the patient can be given a sedative and sent home with a member of the family. If the history suggests mental stress as a causative factor, psychiatric evaluation should be recommended.

34 – 7. INFECTIONS

Rarely an important contributory cause in adults, acute infections are a frequent cause of excitement states in infants and children. Sedatives should be given before any attempt is made to treat the underlying acute condition. Pentobarbital sodium (Nembutal) suppositories, 0.03 to 0.06 gm., are effective in infants and children under 4 years of age. Older children tolerate other sedatives well, provided the dosage is adjusted to age or weight (**4.** *Drug Dosage in Children*).

34 – 8. MANIC-DEPRESSIVE PSYCHOSIS (See also **50 – 2.** *Psychogenic Psychoses)*

During the excitement stage physical restraint may be necessary until control by adequate doses of rapid-acting barbiturates, chloral hydrate, chlorpromazine hydrochloride (Thorazine), paraldehyde or prochlorperazine (Compazine) has been accomplished. An attendant must be with the patient *at all times* until transfer for psychiatric evaluation and care has been completed. No patient who shows evidence of an actual or impending excitement state should ever be left alone.

34 – 9. PHENOTHIAZINE EXTRAPYRAMIDAL REACTIONS (See also **49 – 592**)

Idiosyncrasy to phenothiazine drugs is relatively common, especially in children and elderly persons. Rapid subsiding of the acute excitement state usually occurs as the offending medication is metabolized.

34 – 10. THYROTOXICOSIS (Thyroid Storm) See **33 – 5.** *Hyperthyroid Emergencies*

35. EYE CONDITIONS

An estimate of the vision of each eye should be recorded in the patient's record before further examination is performed for any eye condition. Vision should be tested if possible by the Snellen or

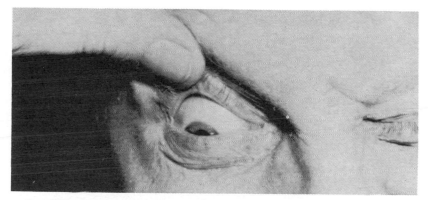

Figure 16. Stabilization of the eye for examination. To have the eye under control, press the upper lid against the bony rim of the orbit. The eye must be under constant control so that injury is not increased. (From Gordon, D. M., Hospital Medicine, Vol. 5, No. 5, p. 21, May, 1969.)

Jaeger test charts; if these charts are not available, finger perception or reading tests are satisfactory.

To prevent further damage during examination, the eye should be stabilized (Fig. 16). Indirect lighting (or the use of a slit lamp) is essential. Except in simple cases, cultures of any discharge or excessive secretion should be taken.

If fluorescein solution is used to locate and evaluate corneal defects, individual sterile ampules or diagnostic strips should be utilized instead of a stock dropper bottle. Local medication (antibiotics, etc.) should be in the form of ophthalmic drops, not ointments. If an eye patch is indicated it should be applied in such a way that it does not cause pressure on the eye (Fig. 17).

NONTRAUMATIC EYE CONDITIONS

35—1. ANGIOEDEMA (See also 21. *Allergic Reactions*)

TREATMENT

1. Apply cold or heat, whichever is more comfortable for the patient.

2. Inject epinephrine hydrochloride (Adrenalin) (1:1000 solution), 0.5 to 1 ml. subcutaneously; repeat in ½ hour if necessary.

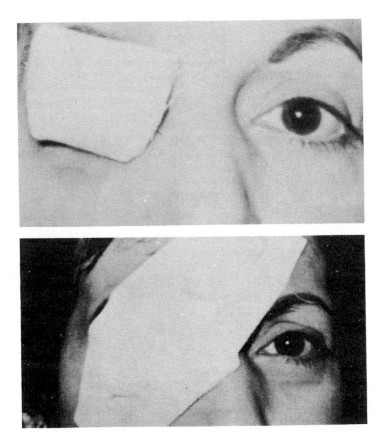

Figure 17. Application of an eyepatch. If corneal epithelium has been lost a double patch is used to immobilize the eye. (From Gordon, D. M., Hospital Medicine, Vol. 5, No. 5, p. 21, May, 1969.)

3. Prescribe tripelennamine hydrochloride (Pyribenzamine), 25 mg. by mouth, every 4 hours.

4. Refer to an ophthalmologist if the condition persists.

35–2. BLEPHARITIS

TREATMENT

1. Examine for and remove ingrowing or turned under eyelashes.

2. Cleanse the lids and remove scales from the eyelashes. Chewing gum can be removed from the lids and lashes with ordinary cooking oil or by chilling with an ice cube.

3. Prescribe antibiotic eye drops.

4. Refer to an ophthalmologist if marked irritation is present.

35–3. CHALAZION

No emergency treatment is necessary. Refer to an ophthalmologist.

35–4. CHOROIDITIS

This condition causes no pain and is not the immediate result of trauma; therefore, it is for practical purposes never encountered as an emergency.

35–5. CONJUNCTIVITIS (See also 35–41. *Differential Diagnosis Chart*)

TREATMENT

1. Irrigate thoroughly and frequently.

2. Instill sodium sulfacetamide drops (30%) every 4 to 6 hours during the day; apply an antibiotic ointment at night.

3. Prescribe iced compresses 2 to 3 times a day.

4. If condition persists for more than 48 hours, instruct the patient to consult an ophthalmologist.

35–6. CORNEAL ULCERS (For traumatic ulcers, see 35–32. *Injuries to the Cornea*)

TREATMENT

1. Determine the extent of the ulceration by staining with fluorescein, using the reagent-soaked strip method or individual sterile ampules.

2. Give emergency treatment as outlined for keratitis (**35—20**).

3. Instruct every patient with a corneal ulcer to report to an ophthalmologist within 24 to 48 hours.

35—7. DACROCYSTITIS

TREATMENT

1. Acute. Apply frequent hot compresses and give local and systemic broad spectrum antibiotics; refer to an ophthalmologist within 24 hours because of the danger of development of orbital cellulitis.

2. Chronic. No emergency treatment is necessary. Evaluation by an ophthalmologist should be recommended.

35—8. ECTROPION (Eversion of Lid)

No emergency treatment is needed. The patient should be advised to consult an ophthalmologist.

35—9. EDEMA OF THE EYELIDS

Inflammatory (from styes, dacrocystitis, sinusitis, etc.).

TREATMENT

1. Apply hot compresses.

2. Give sedation and control pain as necessary.

3. Refer for determination and treatment of the underlying cause.

Systemic (renal or cardiac). No emergency treatment is needed. The importance of complete investigation of the cause should be stressed to the patient.

Allergic. Usually due to some type of local application or medication (mascara, eye shadow, lash curlers and dyes, eye drops, ophthalmic ointments, etc.). Recovery is usually rapid after stopping use of the offending substance.

35—10. EMPHYSEMA OF THE LIDS

Crepitus from air in the soft tissues generally means a fracture of the sinus wall.

TEATMENT

1. Apply a firm pressure bandage.

2. Warn the patient against blowing his nose.
3. Hospitalize immediately for head injury care.

35 — 11. ENTROPION (Inversion of Lid)

TREATMENT
1. Hold the lid in proper position if possible by Scotch tape.
2. Refer to an ophthalmologist for definitive treatment.

35 — 12. EVERSION OF EYELIDS See 35 — 8. *Ectropion*

35 — 13. GLAUCOMA (See also 35 — 41. *Differential Diagnosis Chart*)

TREATMENT
1. Whenever examination indicates the possibility of increased intraocular tension, refer *at once* to an ophthalmologist.
2. Rapid failure of sight, violent headache and severe ophthalmic pain, sometimes associated with nausea, vomiting and general depression, should suggest the possibility of a "glaucomatous attack" and call for immediate hospitalization.

35 — 14. HERPES

Herpes simplex (see also **62 — 9**). Immediate referral to an ophthalmologist if the condition is suspected or proved. Treatment with 5-iodo-2-deoxyuride (IDU) or adenine arabinoside (Ara A) may result in complete healing without vision loss.

Herpes zoster ophthalmicus
1. Control severe pain by codeine sulfate or morphine sulfate intramuscularly.
2. Apply a protective bandage (Fig. 17).
3. Refer to an ophthalmologist for treatment at once. Steroid therapy should be directed by an ophthalmologist.

35 — 15. HORDEOLUM See 35 — 24. *Stye*

35 — 16. INVERSION OF EYELASHES See 35 — 27. *Trichiasis*

35 — 17. INVERSION OF EYELIDS See 35 — 11. *Entropion*

35 — 18. **IRIDOCYCLITIS** See **35 — 19.** *Iritis;* **35 — 41.** *Differential Diagnosis Chart*

35 — 19. **IRITIS** (Iridocyclitis, Uveitis) (See also **35 — 41.** *Differential Diagnosis Chart)*

TREATMENT
1. Apply hot compresses, not over 38°C. (100.4°F.).
2. Apply an eye patch (Fig. 17).
3. Arrange for immediate treatment by an ophthalmologist.

35 — 20. **KERATITIS**

TREATMENT
1. Examine thoroughly for and remove any foreign bodies.
2. If pain is severe, phenacaine (Holocaine), dibucaine (Nupercaine) or ethylmorphine (Dionin) ophthalmic drops may be used as necessary. Cocaine in any form should not be used.
3. Apply an eye patch (Fig. 17).
4. Impress on the patient the need for immediate care by an ophthalmologist.

35 — 21. **PANOPHTHALMITIS**

Relieve the pain by anodynes or opiates and hospitalize *at once* for care by an ophthalmologist.

35 — 22. **PTERYGIUM**

No emergency treatment is needed. Refer to an ophthalmologist.

35 — 23. **SCLERITIS**

TREATMENT
1. Apply hot compresses.
2. Arrange for immediate care by an ophthalmologist.

35 — 24. **STYE** (Hordeolum)

TREATMENT
1. Apply hot compresses.
2. Incise and drain if the condition is localized.

3. Prescribe 1% chlortetracycline (Aureomycin) or 5% sulfathiazole eye drops for home application.

35 – 25.   SYMBLEPHARON (Conjunctival Adhesions)

Refer to an ophthalmologist.

35 – 26.   TRACHOMA

This very infectious conjunctivitis is due to *Chlamydia trachomatis,* an obligate intracellular parasite (**30 – 32**), which is spread by personal contact. It may cause severe scarring and (occasionally) blindness.

TREATMENT

1. Sulfadiazine, 0.5 to 1 gm. by mouth 3 times a day.
2. Tetracycline, 250 mg. orally 3 times a day.
3. Tetracycline or chloramphenicol ophthalmic ointment for use at night.
4. Instruction regarding disposal of infected handkerchiefs, towels, etc.
5. Referral to an ophthalmologist.

35 – 27.   TRICHIASIS (Inversion of Lashes)

If only a few lashes are inverted, they may be removed with cilia forceps. If multiple lashes are involved or if severe pain, lacrimation, photophobia or ulceration is present, the case should be referred to an ophthalmologist.

35 – 28.   UVEITIS See **35 – 19.** *Iritis;* **35 – 41.** *Differential Diagnosis Chart*

TRAUMATIC EYE CONDITIONS

In all cases of suspected eye injury, vision of each eye should be tested before detailed examination, by the Jaeger or Snellen chart method or by reading tests or finger visualization, and results recorded in the patient's chart.

35 – 29.   INJURIES TO THE CHOROID

Rupture of the choroid can be caused by a severe contusion of the eyeball. The diagnosis as a rule cannot be made on emergency examination, but suspicion of its presence requires immediate reference to an ophthalmologist.

Penetrating wounds may cause suppurative iridochoroiditis with exquisite pain, requiring codeine or morphine sulfate for relief. Hospitalization and care by an ophthalmologist should be arranged as soon as possible.

35 — 30. INJURIES TO THE CILIARY BODY

Injuries of this area are in the so-called "danger zone" of the eye and not infrequently result in sympathetic ophthalmia (**35 — 38**). Immediate reference to an ophthalmologist is indicated if an injury to the ciliary body is suspected.

35 — 31. INJURIES TO THE CONJUNCTIVA

Burns (see also **25 — 13**). Thorough irrigation with tap water is the only treatment needed in mild cases. Moderately severe cases require cold or iced compresses and application of antibiotic ophthalmic drops after thorough irrigation. No attempt should be made to irrigate with a neutralizing solution. An eye patch should be applied and arrangements made for the patient to consult an ophthalmologist within 24 hours. Severe cases, especially electrical, acid or alkali burns, require immediate referral to an ophthalmologist.

Foreign bodies. Many foreign bodies are found lying on the inner surface of the upper lid and can be removed with or without 1% tetracaine hydrochloride (Pontocaine) anesthesia by turning back the lid (Fig. 18) and brushing with a cotton applicator dampened with saline. If acute conjunctivitis or corneal irritation is present, antibiotic ophthalmic drops should be prescribed and an eye patch applied (Fig. 17). If an abrasion is present, recheck examination by an ophthalmologist should be arranged within 2 days.

Injuries caused by intense light (Welder's Flash, Photophthalmia). (See also **25 — 14.** *Flash Burns*). Patients' stories are often inaccurate; therefore, a thorough search should be made for foreign bodies in the conjunctival sac, under the lids and on the cornea before a diagnosis of photophthalmia is made. If none is found and the history is indicative of a "flash," the following routine should be used:

1. Instill 2 drops of 1% tetracaine hydrochloride (Pontocaine) solution.

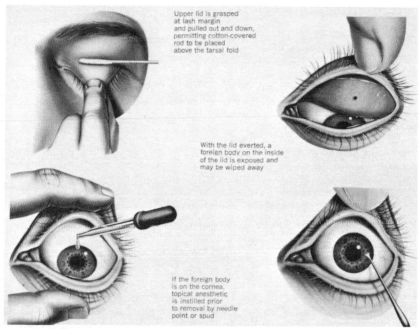

Figure 18. Eversion of eyelid for removal of a foreign body. (From Gordon, D. M., Hospital Medicine, Vol. 5, No. 5, p. 21, May, 1969.)

2. Cover with cold (preferably iced) compresses for 5 minutes.
3. Instill 2 drops of the following solution:

Phenylephrine (Neo-Synephrine) hydrochloride (1% sol.)	12.5 ml.
Tetracaine hydrochloride (Pontocaine)	0.25 ml.
Isotonic solution (buffered) q.s. ad	100.00 ml.

4. Cover with cold compresses for 5 minutes.
5. Instill 2 drops of castor oil.
6. Instruct the patient to apply cold or iced compresses and castor oil drops at home and to arrange for further medical care in 24 hours if acute discomfort persists.

Lacerations. No attempt should be made to suture cuts in the surface of the conjunctiva. A sterile eye patch should be applied (Fig. 17) and the patient referred at once to an ophthalmologist.

35—32. INJURIES TO THE CORNEA

Burns. If corneal burns are small and superficial, treatment is the same as for conjunctival burns (**35—31**); if extensive or deep, immediate care by an ophthalmologist is essential.

Contusions. Usually caused by some blunt object, contusions as a rule clear spontaneously (and slowly) without treatment. Internal bleeding and dislocation of the lens require immediate care by an ophthalmologist.

Foreign bodies

1. A history of any object striking the eye makes a thorough search for foreign bodies mandatory. Fluorescein (1 or 2%) is harmless and may be used to demonstrate breaks in the external layers of the cornea. The eye must be irrigated thoroughly after examination. A fresh solution of fluorescein should always be used, preferably from individual dose sterile ampules. Fluorescein-impregnated strips are satisfactory. Exact localization of embedded or intraocular radiopaque foreign bodies can often be obtained by special radiologic techniques.

2. Foreign bodies on or embedded superficially in the cornea may be removed under 1% tetracaine hydrochloride (Pontocaine) anesthesia, using a damp cotton applicator or an eye spud (Fig. 18). An excellent eye spud can be improvised from a short bevel 25 gauge needle, using the barrel of a small syringe as a handle. Removal of any residual rust ring requires reference to an ophthalmologist and should not be attempted as emergency treatment.

3. No attempt should be made to remove deeply embedded foreign bodies as an emergency measure. An eye patch should be applied unless the pressure of the pad might cause further penetration, and the patient should be referred at once to an ophthalmologist.

4. An electromagnet should never be used except under the direction of an ophthalmologist.

5. Defects (ulcers) of the cornea following removal of foreign bodies require application of 5% sulfathiazole or 1% chlortetracycline (Aureomycin) eye drops, protection of the eye with a patch and reference to an ophthalmologist within 48 hours. Cycloplegic eye drops should not be used unless a definite indication is present.

Wounds

Superficial. These generally heal without complications, provided they are kept clean.

TREATMENT
1. Irrigation followed by antibiotic eye drops.
2. Application of an eye patch.

Penetrating. Immediate care by an ophthalmologist is mandatory. X-ray films should be taken to rule out or localize buried radiopaque foreign bodies.

35 – 33. INJURIES TO THE EYELIDS

Ecchymosis (Black Eye). Direct trauma in the region of the eyes severe enough to cause ecchymosis may also cause severe underlying injuries. The following conditions, which require immediate care by an ophthalmologist, should be ruled out:
1. Lacerations of the cornea (**35 – 32**).
2. Fracture of the orbital wall (see **35 – 10.** *Emphysema of the Lids;* **35 – 35.** *Injuries to the Orbit*). Special x-rays, including Waters' views, usually are necessary.
3. Detachment of the retina, partial or complete (see **35 – 36.** *Injuries to the Retina*).

TREATMENT
Cold compresses for 24 hours, followed by hot compresses and gentle massage. Injection of hyaluronidase in 1% procaine hydrochloride often is very effective. If a fracture is suspected from clinical or x-ray examination, the patient should be hospitalized for observation and treatment.

Insect bites (See also **21.** *Allergic Reactions;* **24.** *Bites;* **56.** *Stings;* **61.** *Venoms.*)
Cold compresses are indicated for control of swelling, which may be extreme. Antihistaminics may be of value.

Lacerations. Because loss of tissues of the eyelids may result in ectropion (**35 – 8**) or entropion (**35 – 11**), lacerations in this area should be thoroughly irrigated but not debrided before suturing (Fig. 19). Antibiotics and tetanus-immune globulin (TIG) or toxoid (**16**) should be given if gross contamination is present.

Especially in vertical lacerations, suturing should be done with great care in order to prevent contractures (Fig. 19). If the laceration extends through the eyelid, careful examination for damage to the eyeball should be made before suturing. If a through-and-through laceration is jagged or extensive, or if there is avulsion or loss of tissue, a sterile bandage should be applied and the patient hospitalized at once for operative repair and possible skin grafting.

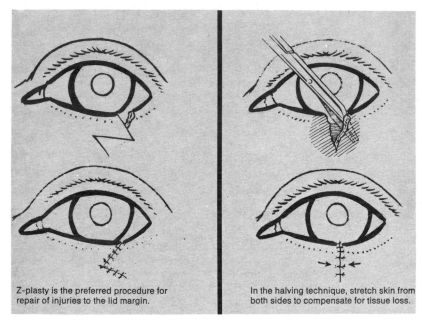

Z-plasty is the preferred procedure for repair of injuries to the lid margin.

In the halving technique, stretch skin from both sides to compensate for tissue loss.

Figure 19. Repair of eyelid lacerations. (From Emergency Medicine, Vol. 3, No. 1, p. 40, January, 1971.)

35–34. INJURIES TO THE IRIS

Nonpenetrating. Concussion with subsequent traumatic mydriasis is the most frequent cause. After instillation of 1 or 2 drops of 1% pilocarpine hydrochloride and application of an eye patch, the patient should be referred to an ophthalmologist.

Penetrating. This condition calls for application of an eye patch and immediate reference to an ophthalmologist for care.

35–35. INJURIES TO THE ORBIT

If injury to the orbit is suspected from clinical or x-ray examination, immediate hospitalization for head injury care (**41**) is indicated. Fractures of the margins or floor of the orbit (Fig. 20) require immediate surgical repair to avoid impaired vision.

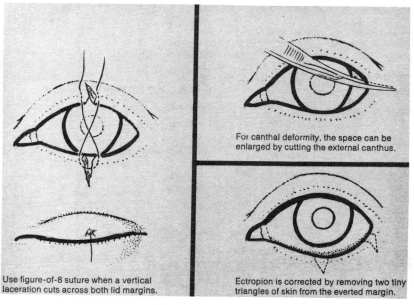

For canthal deformity, the space can be enlarged by cutting the external canthus.

Use figure-of-8 suture when a vertical laceration cuts across both lid margins.

Ectropion is corrected by removing two tiny triangles of skin from the everted margin.

Figure 19. (Continued)

35 – 36. INJURIES TO THE RETINA

Suspected or proved incomplete or complete detachment of the retina requires immediate reference to an ophthalmologist.

35 – 37. INJURIES TO THE SCLERA

If injury to the sclera is suspected, the patient should be referred to an ophthalmologist *without delay* for examination and treatment. X-ray films should be taken to rule out embedded radiopaque foreign bodies if the history is suggestive (**35 – 32**).

35 – 38. SYMPATHETIC OPHTHALMIA

This extremely serious condition practically never occurs unless there has been a penetrating injury of the opposite eye at some time

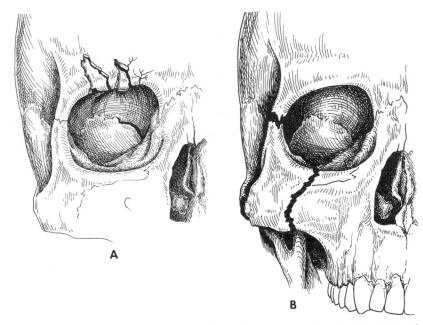

Figure 20.   A, Superior rim fracture with a moderate amount of comminution. B, Tripod fracture of the zygoma with downward displacement.

in the past. Recognition in the stage of sympathetic irritation may result in preventing total blindness. The usual signs and symptoms of this stage are marked photophobia and lacrimation, with dimness of close vision, bizarre bright and colored sensations and neuralgic pain in and around the eye.

Any person with a history of a perforating injury to an eye at any time in the past who complains of any of the signs and symptoms listed above in the uninjured eye should be referred immediately to an ophthalmologist.

35–39. REMOVAL OF CONTACT LENSES

Modern contact lenses are made of plastic and are of 2 types:
1. *"Hard."* These cover the cornea only and measure 8 to 9 mm. in

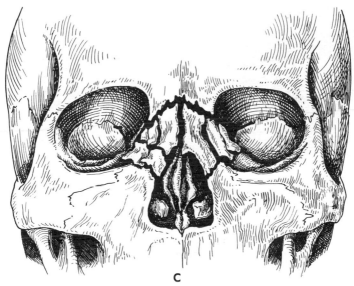

Figure 20. (Continued) C, Severe naso-orbital fracture with lateral displacement of the nasal and frontal processes of the maxillary bones. (From Leone, C. R., Jr., American Family Physician, 5:102, 1972.)

diameter. These lenses usually can be identified by reflection from an edge on lateral illumination.

2. **"Soft."** These extend onto the sclera; usually they are 12 to 14 mm. in diameter.

Removal may be necessary in an emergency situation since either type may cause serious irritation if retained for more than 12 hours.

METHODS

1. **Removal by suction.** With the eyelids separated, press a small suction cup (Fig. 21) against the middle of a "hard" lens and lift it out.

2. **Removal by irrigation.** With the patient supine and the head turned toward the side to be irrigated, float the lens out by gentle lavage with normal saline solution, using a soft-tipped rubber bulb syringe.

3. **Removal by pinching** ("soft" lens only). With the eyelids separated, pinch the lens out by gentle pressure between the thumb and fore-

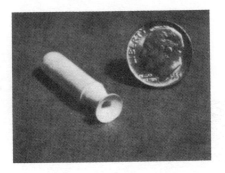

Figure 21. A new item for the physician's emergency kit: suction cup for removing corneal contact lenses. (From Halberg, G. P., Hospital Physician, Vol. 8, No. 8, p. 17, August, 1972.)

finger. Place the removed lenses in normal saline solution at once to prevent dehydration and shriveling.

35 – 14. DIFFERENTIAL DIAGNOSIS OF CONJUNCTIVITIS, GLAUCOMA AND IRITIS

	CONJUNCTIVITIS	GLAUCOMA	IRITIS
Aqueous humor	normal	cloudy	cloudy
Cornea	normal	steamy	clear
Eyeball	normal	hard	soft
Headache	never	frequent, severe	frequent
Iris	normal	muddy	muddy
Nausea	never	frequent	occasional
Pain	slight	very severe	severe
Pupil	normal	dilated	small
Redness	marked	variable	circumcorneal
Vision	normal	marked to complete loss	some loss

36. FOREIGN BODIES

See also **48 – 29.** *Foreign Bodies in Children.*

36 – 1. IN THE EARS

Examine with an otoscope. Children frightened from previous attempts at removal often require sedation by a pentobarbital sodium (Nembutal) suppository before examination. If superficial, and if swelling of the wall of the external auditory meatus has not resulted from previous attempts at removal (usually at home), most foreign bodies can be removed with forceps or by carefully inserting a curved probe behind the object and gently working it outward. Gravity may help. Dry, firm foreign bodies can sometimes be removed by pressing a cotton applicator tip moistened with collodion against the surface.

Substances which will not absorb moisture can sometimes be removed by syringing. Do not attempt irrigation for beans, peas, candy, etc.; absorption of moisture and subsequent swelling can cause serious and permanent damage. Do not irrigate if there is suspicion or evidence of drum perforation.

Foxtails can usually be removed with forceps without difficulty. A few drops of any glycerin or petrolatum base ear drops instilled into the ear will result in immediate relief of discomfort and spontaneous evacuation if the patient sleeps with the affected ear against the pillow.

Hot slag particles usually are loose in the canal and can be removed with a cotton applicator. If particles are firmly adherent to the drum or if there is evidence of severe drum damage, treatment by an otolaryngologist should be arranged.

Insects alive and buzzing in the external auditory canal will often fly or crawl out toward a flashlight held close to the external auditory meatus. If this maneuver is unsuccessful, removal by syringing may be necessary.

Referral to an otolaryngologist generally is required if there is damage to or perforation of the drum, if the foreign body cannot be removed on 1 or 2 gentle attempts or if the cooperation of the patient cannot be obtained.

36 – 2. IN THE EYES See **35 – 31.** *Injuries to the Conjunctiva;* **35 – 32.** *Injuries to the Cornea;* **35 – 38.** *Sympathetic Ophthalmia*

36 – 3. IN THE NOSE

Foreign bodies in the nose are frequently encountered in small children; often, the person giving emergency care cannot obtain sufficient cooperation to permit removal of the object with forceps, a small wire probe or an ear curette with the tip bent into a scoop. Sedation by means of a pentobarbital sodium (Nembutal) suppository may be tried; however, if the child struggles or resists examination, hospitalization in order to use general anesthesia should be considered. If the parents are reasonable, postponement until care by an otolaryngologist can be arranged will result in no danger to the patient.

In some instances, foreign bodies will be expelled from the nares in infants and small children by sneezing. Small children will sometimes sneeze if a puff of cigarette smoke is blown suddenly against the nose while the mouth is kept covered. An alternative method consists of blowing into the child's mouth with the uninvolved nostril closed by pinching. Preliminary shrinking with Neo-Synephrine may be helpful.

36 – 4. IN THE LARYNX, TRACHEA OR BRONCHI (See also 48 – 29. *Foreign Bodies in Children;* 48 – 44. *Obstruction of Breathing Apparatus – Localization Chart*)

If a patient has a history of swallowing a foreign body, and if cyanosis, air hunger and dyspnea are present, then immediate action on the part of the physician may be required as a lifesaving measure. If the patient is markedly cyanotic or moribund, mouth-to-mouth respiration (11 – 1) should be started (unless prevented by obstruction) and the following procedures done without hesitation:

1. Have the parents, relative or friends leave the room unless their assistance will be needed.

2. Attempt dislodgment of the foreign body by concussion, utilizing the pull of gravity. If this procedure results in increased airway obstruction, an emergency tracheostomy (14 – 12) must be considered.

3. Give oxygen inhalations under positive pressure by face mask and rebreathing bag or through the tracheostomy tube.

If signs and symptoms of irritation or obstruction are less severe, x-ray films (anteroposterior and lateral) of the chest should be taken after examination of the posterior pharynx. If a radiopaque foreign body is lodged in the trachea, its greater surface will appear in the lateral film; if in the esophagus, the anteroposterior film will show the greater width. Small pointed or irregularly shaped nonradiopaque foreign bodies can sometimes be demonstrated by x-ray films taken after the patient has swallowed a small cotton pledget saturated with contrast media.

Foreign bodies lodged in the larynx, trachea or bronchi which cannot be located with a laryngoscope and removed with long forceps require that the patient be transferred to a hospital as soon as possible. If the airway obstruction is acute, an emergency tracheostomy should be done before transporting the patient.

36 — 5. IN THE ESOPHAGUS, STOMACH AND GASTROINTESTINAL TRACT (See also 48 — 29. *Foreign Bodies in Children*)

If the object is small enough to pass through the esophagus into the stomach and does not have any extremely sharp points, it will generally pass through the small and large bowel without difficulty. Smooth-edged foreign bodies can sometimes be removed from the esophagus by passing a No. 12 Foley urethral catheter beyond the obstruction (under sedation and fluoroscopic control if necessary), inflating the reservoir and withdrawing the catheter gently with the foreign body in front of it. The patient should be on his right side to prevent aspiration. Great care should be used to prevent perforation of the esophagus.

Nonradiopaque foreign bodies in the stomach can sometimes be visualized by x ray films taken immediately after a few swallows of a cold carbonated beverage. Any space-occupying object will cause a defect in the gas shadow caused by the released carbon dioxide.

Sharp-pointed objects should be watched, and watched for, carefully. If careful screening of all stool specimens for 3 days indicates that the foreign body has not passed through the gastrointestinal tract, then further x-ray studies should be made. If signs suggestive of perforation or acute obstruction develop, immediate hospitalization for operative intervention must be arranged.

36 — 6. IN THE MUSCULOSKELETAL STRUCTURES

Whether the foreign bodies are wood (splinters), plastic (spicules of plastic toys), steel or other metals (industrial accidents, household and auto accidents, bullets, needles), dirt, gravel or rock (explosions, falls, auto accidents), glass (household injuries, auto accidents) or semisolid (graphite, grease), the general principles of treatment are the same.

1. Careful cleansing and irrigation.

2. Exploration to determine the extent of penetration. This should be done with great care under direct vision if possible and with extension of the entrance tract under local anesthetic if necessary.

3. X-ray films (AP and lateral). Skin markers should be placed for reference before the films are taken if the presence of an easily overlooked radiopaque foreign body which cannot be located by direct vision or palpation is suspected.

4. If the foreign body is superficial and easily accessible, it should be removed by splinter forceps or a pointed scalpel. Deeper foreign bodies require sharp dissection and debridement, followed by thorough irrigation and primary closure if within 6 hours of injury; after a longer period, the wound should be debrided but should not, as a general rule, be sutured. See **55 — 20**. *Lacerations.*

Deeply embedded foreign bodies should be treated conservatively [tetanus-immune globulin (TIG) or toxoid (**16**), local treatment of point of entry and observation]. Antibiotic therapy may be indicated.

Musculoskeletal foreign bodies require hospitalization:

1. When there is severe or persistent bleeding which cannot be controlled by pressure.

2. If the location of the foreign body or its point of entry or course, together with clinical examination, indicates perforation of the pleura, pericardium, peritoneum or viscera.

3. If the foreign body lies within the skull.

4. If there is evidence of severe or extensive bone damage.

5. When evidence of nerve pressure or severance is present.

6. If x-ray or clinical examinations indicate that the foreign body lies within a joint.

36 — 7. IN THE URETHRA See **38 — 8**. *Urethral Injuries;* **48 — 29**. *Foreign Bodies in Children*

36 — 8. IN THE VAGINA

1. Retained pessaries, tampons, etc., may require use of a speculum for localization and removal.

2. A variety of metallic or other objects inserted into the vagina or cervix in attempts to induce an abortion or by mentally deranged persons may require removal. A thorough examination to rule out perforation should be made.

36—9. IN THE VENOUS SYSTEM

Runaway broken intravenous catheters (and occasionally intravenous needles) present a true emergency. As soon as the condition is recognized, the following steps should be taken:
1. Prevent any motion of the extremity.
2. Apply a tourniquet proximal to the site of entry.
3. Take scout x-ray films. If the catheter is not radiopaque, a venogram should be done.
4. Immediate removal of the foreign body by cutdown under local anesthetic if in an available site, usually in an extremity. If more central, immediate arrangements should be made for operative removal under general anesthesia.

37. GASTROINTESTINAL EMERGENCIES

See also **48—30.** *Gastrointestinal Tract Emergencies in Children.*

37—1. NEONATAL CONDITIONS

Neonatal conditions, often associated with severe feeding problems, respiratory distress, abnormal elimination and signs of obstruction, may require emergency care. Among these are diaphragmatic hernia, imperforate anus, intestinal atresia, megacolon, pyloric stenosis and tracheoesophageal fistula. All require immediate hospitalization for surgical evaluation and possible intervention.

37—2. OBSTRUCTION

MECHANICAL

Intraluminal
1. Fecal impaction. If the patient is in acute discomfort from partial or complete obstruction, and rectal examination demon-

strates a mass of hard-packed feces, an attempt may be made to remove the mass with the gloved finger. In elderly women, posterior and downward digital pressure through the vagina may cause sufficient dilation of the sphincter ani to allow the impacted mass to pass. These procedures are usually very painful and often unsuccessful. Premedication with rapid-acting barbiturates or pentazocine lactate (Talwin) is essential. Morphine sulfate and other opiates contract the sphincter ani and, therefore, are contraindicated. Hospitalization for general anesthesia may be necessary if an attempt at digital removal is unsuccessful or is too painful to be tolerated. In less severe cases in which obstruction is not complete, the patient can be sent home with instructions regarding warm oil enemas and diet.

    2. Foreign bodies. See **36 — 5; 48 — 29.** *Foreign Bodies in Children.*
    3. Gallstones (**37 — 8.** *Cholecystitis*).

Extraluminal
    1. Adhesions, usually postoperative.
    2. Hernia, incarcerated (**37 — 5; 48 — 35.** *Hernias in Children*).
    3. Malignancies. See **37 — 4.** *Hemorrhage;* **42 — 22.** *Rectal Bleeding.*
    4. Pyloric stenosis (**48 — 38.** *Intestinal Obstruction in Children*).
    5. Volvulus (**48 — 38.** *Intestinal Obstruction in Children;* **48 — 61**).

NONMECHANICAL

Nonmechanical obstruction may be the result of inflammation (enzymes, organisms, poisons), of ischemia (mesenteric or vascular occlusion) or of reflex action following surgery or trauma. It is characterized by repetitious, sometimes fecal, vomiting, abdominal distention, diffuse tenderness, high-pitched bowel sounds, decreased elimination and progressive dehydration.

TREATMENT
    1. No food by mouth.
    2. Antiemetics parenterally.
    3. Hydration parenterally and rectally (**6.** *Fluid Replacement*).
    4. Treatment of shock (**53 — 7**).
    5. Referral for hospital care.

37 — 3. PERFORATION

Esophageal. Breaks in the walls of the esophagus may be caused by corrosives (**49 — 26.** *Acids;* **49 — 39.** *Alkalies;* **49 — 432.** *Lye*), foreign bodies (**36 – 5**) or instrumentation, and may result in severe abdominal pain, shock (**53**) and mediastinitis.

Intraperitoneal (gallbladder, intestines, spleen, stomach).

Intraperitoneal perforation may be caused by foreign bodies (**36 – 5**), medications such as phenylbutazone (Butazolidin), reserpine and steroids, trauma and ulcerative processes. Abdominal pain and rigidity, local or generalized tenderness and shock (**53**) usually are present. X-ray films may demonstrate free air in the abdomen.

TREATMENT
1. Nothing by mouth.
2. Treatment of shock (**53 – 7**).
3. Analgesics after the diagnosis has been established.
4. Hospitalization for definitive care, usually surgical.

37 – 4. HEMORRHAGE (See also **42 – 22**. *Rectal Bleeding;* **42 – 25.** *Bleeding from the Stomach*)

Severe bleeding from any point along the enteric tract can present a serious life-threatening situation. Gastrointestinal tract bleeding may be frankly evident from blood in the emesis or stool or may be occult with the patient initially presenting in a state of hypovolemic shock (**53**).

TREATMENT
1. Start therapy for shock (**53 – 7**).
2. Obtain a rapid history from patient and relatives to determine causes contributing to hemorrhage that should receive immediate treatment, i.e., use of anticoagulants or steroids, familial conditions such as hemophilia, improper diet, etc.
3. Hospitalize for thorough clinical and laboratory investigation, observation and treatment, even when bleeding and anemia appear to be mild. Immediate endoscopy (e.g., endoscopy, gastroscopy, sigmoidoscopy) and radiologic examination with barium are of value for establishing correct diagnosis and treatment.
4. Institute iced water gavages for gastrointestinal bleeding.
5. For esophageal bleeding, give oxytocin (Petocin), 20 clinical units by intravenous drip over a 20 minute period.

Rectal Bleeding (See also **42 – 22**.)

Cryptitis. Inflammation of the crypts of Morgagni may cause anal spasm and pain, pruritus and frequent bowel movements in addition to bleeding. Treatment consists of sitz baths, dilation of the sphincter and administration of antibiotics.

Hemorrhoids. Loss of blood may be enough to cause anemia or shock (**53**). (See also **37−6**. *Anorectal Conditions;* **42−22**. *Rectal Bleeding.*)

Malignancies. All cases of rectal bleeding of undetermined cause, especially in persons over 50, should be considered as possible malignancies until proved otherwise.

Poisons. Many substances which can be ingested, absorbed or inhaled can cause severe gastrointestinal and rectal bleeding. See listing under **49**. *Poisons.*

Ulceration, infection and inflammation. This group of pathologic conditions may be manifested clinically by anorexia, fever, nausea, vomiting, abdominal pain and tenderness and may be compounded by alteration of normal evacuation and fluid/electrolyte balance and by hemorrhage.

37−5. ANATOMIC DEFECTS

Achalasia

Persons with an atonic esophagus may develop sudden distress with dysphagia or respiratory difficulty from aspiration of gastric overflow or regurgitated food.

TREATMENT
1. Insurance of an adequate airway.
2. Evacuation of the esophagus with an Ewald tube or by use of an esophagoscope.
3. Reference to a gastroenterologist for evaluation and treatment.

Hernia (See also **48−35**. *Hernias in Children*)

Although congenital or developmental structural weaknesses usually are the underlying causes of all types of herniae, direct or indirect trauma often precipitates symptoms severe enough to require emergency attention.

Diaphragmatic (Hiatal) Hernia. See **48−35**. *Hernias in Children.*
This condition may be responsible for a variety of symptoms severe enough to cause the patient to request emergency therapy, including dyspnea, cyanosis, chest pain and bleeding from the gastrointestinal tract. The diagnosis usually cannot be made in an emergency setting.

TREATMENT

1. Symptomatic and supportive care.

2. Hospitalization for complete investigation and definitive therapy.

Femoral Hernia

Incarceration and strangulation is rare but does occur, usually in infants and children. See **48 – 35.** *Hernia in Children.*

Hiatal Hernia. See *Diaphragmatic Hernia* (above); **48 – 35.** *Hernia in Children.*

Inguinal Hernia

Failure of support of the lower abdominal wall in the inguinal regions represents the underlying reason for the majority of hernias. Congenital structural weaknesses of the supporting structures are almost invariably present. Herniation of bowel or other intraabdominal contents may occur spontaneously or be precipitated by lifting, straining, coughing or any other mechanism which increases intraabdominal pressure.

TREATMENT

1. Strangulation is an urgent condition requiring immediate hospitalization for surgical intervention.

2. Incarceration. Reduction can sometimes be accomplished by sedation and gentle manipulation with the patient supine. If reduction cannot be done or if incarceration recurs after reduction, the patient should be referred for surgical consultation.

3. All other patients should be advised regarding surgical repair and application of support and warned of the possible development of incarceration or strangulation.

Umbilical Hernia. See **48 – 35.** *Hernia in Children.*

Ventral Hernia

Herniation of fat, omentum or abdominal contents through a weakness in the abdominal wall may be congenital or the result of penetrating injuries; however, usually it is at the site of previous operative procedures. For treatment, see *Inguinal Hernia.*

Industrial Hernias. (See also **75.** *Workmen's Compensation [Industrial] Cases*)

History. At the first visit a thorough and complete history *must* be taken on every case of claimed hernia when the condition is alleged to have arisen out of or to have been caused by the patient's work. This history should include details regarding the exact effort which the patient was exerting when he first felt subjective symptoms, the position of the patient while lifting or straining, weight of the object lifted, type of pain and presence or absence of nausea, vomiting and general malaise. A statement regarding the type of work usually performed and any variation from the normal routine at the time of the alleged injury should be included with a detailed interval history covering the period between the time of the alleged injury and medical examination.

A specific statement should be obtained from the patient regarding previous signs and symptoms, such as pain, swelling or bulging in the affected area. If the patient has had previous operative repairs at the site of complaints or on the opposite side, full details of the onset of the original condition, with operative findings and industrial status, should be determined.

Physical examination

1. Presence or absence of a defect in support or a bulge on inspection and/or palpation, especially while coughing or straining.

2. Size of the inguinal rings *on both sides* by digital examination.

3. Presence or absence of an impulse in the inguinal canal or at the site of the palpable defect on coughing or straining.

4. Tenderness on digital examination.

Treatment and management

Industrial Cases (arising out of or caused by employment and covered by state or federal compensation laws). All strangulated hernias and some incarcerated hernias are acute surgical emergencies and should be hospitalized for immediate care. All other cases should be examined in detail and a First Report of Injury (**75**) made out, *but no treatment of any kind given.* This includes recommendations for any type of home therapy and/or the purchase of an athletic supporter or truss. Instead, the patient should be referred to the compensation insurance carrier or employer for disposition. He should be warned to report immediately for medical care if severe discomfort, marked enlargement or irreducibility should develop.

Prolapse of the Rectum

In infants and children this condition is fairly common. It is probably the result of congenital defects in the firmness of the connective tissue between the muscular layers of the rectum.

TREATMENT

1. Preliminary sedation.

2. *Reduction at once* by manual replacement. The sooner this is accomplished, the easier the procedure. Delay results in shutting off the blood supply by sphincter spasm, with resultant extreme edema.

3. Elevation of the foot of the bed.

4. Application of cold packs to decrease edema.

5. Tight strapping of the buttocks.

6. Immediate hospitalization for reduction under general anesthesia if the measures given above are unsuccessful.

In adults prolapse generally results from lesions (hemorrhoids, proctitis, polyps) which cause excessive straining at stool. Reduction by the methods outlined above is generally much more difficult in adults than in children, and recurrence is more common. The patient should be hospitalized if replacement cannot be obtained on 1 or 2 attempts, if there is discoloration of the prolapsed structures indicative of circulatory embarrassment, if marked edema is present or if the prolapse recurs spontaneously after reduction.

37 – 6.   ANORECTAL CONDITIONS (See also 42 – 22. *Rectal Bleeding*)

This area of the body is particularly prone to develop inflammatory conditions which are extremely painful and likely to be accompanied by bleeding.

Cryptitis (37 – 4)

Fissures

A small break in the continuity of the mucous membrane of the rectum or of skin around the anus may cause itching, pain and bleeding on defecation. See **54 – 12.** *Pruritus Ani.*

TREATMENT

1. Sitz baths.

2. Fecal softeners.

3. Low residue diet.

4. Sedation as necessary.

5. Referral to a proctologist if symptoms are severe or persistent.

Hemorrhoids (Piles) (See also 42 – 22. *Rectal Bleeding*)

Not thrombosed. If not thrombosed but prolapsed or protruding, replacement using a lubricated gloved finger should be attempted.

If this cannot be done because of acute pain or strangulation, inject 100 TRU (turbidity reducing units) of hyaluronidase in 2 ml. of 0.5% procaine into the swollen tissues at 3 or 4 different points. After a short wait, painless and complete replacement can usually be accomplished. Ethyl aminobenzoate (Benzocaine) suppositories and sitz baths at home should be prescribed. The patient should be instructed to arrange for further care if the symptoms persist or recur.

Thrombosed. If thrombosed, severe pain can be relieved by injection of a small amount of 1% procaine or lidocaine (Xylocaine) into the mucous membrane and evacuation of the clots through a small incision. Suturing is not necessary. The patient should be advised to take sitz baths until the acute inflammation subsides and to obtain further medical care if not completely relieved.

Prolapse. See **37 − 5.** *Anatomic Defects − Achalasia.*

Pruritus Ani. See **37 − 6.** *Fissures;* **54 − 12.**

Stricture of the rectum may occur following rectal surgery; more often, it results from infections such as lymphogranuloma venereum (**60 − 4**). No emergency treatment is indicated unless acute infection is present or complete obstruction has occurred. For acute infection, antibiotics and hot sitz baths may give relief; for complete obstruction the patient should be hospitalized.

37 − 7. APPENDICITIS (Acute)

Hospitalization for close observation and possible surgical intervention is indicated whenever the clinical picture suggests the possibility of acute appendicitis.

37 − 8. CHOLECYSTITIS (Acute)

Frequently, a history of prior gallbladder complaints will be obtained. Obstruction of the biliary tract from choleliths, from inflammation following passage of a stone or from infection may precede involvement of the gallbladder. Generally, pain is present in the right upper quadrant of the abdomen. The gallbladder itself may or may not be palpable.

TREATMENT
Referral for hospitalization and decision regarding immediate surgical evaluation.

37—9. DIARRHEA (See also 48—21. *Diarrhea in Children*)

Diarrhea may present as an emergency situation with moderate or marked dehydration, incipient or frank shock (**53**), watery and bloody stools, high fever, tenesmus and toxic state. Specific bacteria (Shigella and Salmonella), amebae, exogenous toxins or acute fulminant ulcerative colitis may be the cause. Initially, emergency treatment is massive general supportive measures; diagnostic procedures and specific therapy follow.

Determination of the specific cause of the diarrhea is indicated even in mild cases.

37—10. DIVERTICULITIS

In adults acute inflammation of diverticuli may cause signs and symptoms difficult to differentiate from an acute surgical abdomen. If perforation should occur, the treatment is emergency surgery; however, subacute inflammatory conditions characterized by pain, mild fever and bleeding are more common. Diverticulitis is one of the common causes of rectal bleeding in children.

TREATMENT

1. In mild cases, control of the infection by antibiotics and administration of a bland, low residue diet and fecal softeners may give relief.

2. Acute cases require immediate hospitalization.

37—11. ESOPHAGITIS AND GASTRITIS

TREATMENT

1. Treatment as under peptic ulcer. See **37—4**. *Hemorrhage from the Gastrointestinal Tract,* **42—25**. *Bleeding from the Stomach.*

2. Topical Xylocaine, 15 to 30 ml. orally, may give dramatic relief of symptoms.

37—12. FECAL IMPACTION See **37—2**. *Obstruction, Mechanical*

37—13. FISSURE-IN-ANO See **37—6**. *Anorectal Conditions*

37—14. HEMORRHOIDS See **37—6**. *Anorectal Condition;* **42—22**. *Rectal Bleeding*

37 – 15. HERNIA See **37 – 5; 48 – 35.** *Hernia in Children*

37 – 16. IMPACTION (Fecal) See **37 – 2.** *Obstruction, Mechanical*

37 – 17. INTUSSUSCEPTION See **48 – 38.** *Intestinal Obstruction in Children*

37 – 18. ISCHIORECTAL ABSCESS. (See also **20 – 15.** *Ischioanal Abscesses*)

Complete disability from severe local pain and tenderness may be present together with generalized abdominal distress and distention.

TREATMENT

1. Administration of broad spectrum antibiotics.
2. Application of local heat by sitz baths.
3. Analgesics or sedation.
4. Referral to surgeon or proctologist for hospitalization and drainage under general anesthesia when the abscess has localized.

37 – 19. PANCREATITIS (Acute) (See also **55 – 25.** *Traumatic Pancreatitis*)

This condition may come on suddenly, although it is frequently preceded by symptoms of gallbladder disease, peptic ulcer or high intake of alcohol. Pain in the midabdomen with penetration to the back or flanks may be severe. Vomiting and paralytic ileus are common. Shock (**53**) may develop and is an ominous early sign.

TREATMENT

1. Treatment of shock (**53 – 7**).
2. Hospitalization for definitive care. General treatment is similar to the treatment for acute cholecystitis, except that surgical intervention need not be considered.

37 – 20. PARASITIC INFECTIONS

Many parasites may cause signs and symptoms involving the gastrointestinal tract which are severe enough to require emergency medical care. See table (Common Intestinal Parasites) on pages 230–231.

37 — 21. PILES See **37 — 6.** *Anorectal Conditions—Hemorrhoids;* **42 — 22.** *Rectal Bleeding*

37 — 22. POLYPS

Polyps (ulcerative) may be mistaken for internal hemorrhoids if located near the anus; if in the rectum, they may cause recurrent rectal prolapse (**37 — 5**).

TREATMENT

1. Control of infection and edema by sitz baths, ethyl amino-benzoate (Benzocaine) suppositories and antibiotics.

2. Referral to a surgeon or proctologist for examination and treatment. These lesions may be premalignant.

37 — 23. PROLAPSE OF RECTUM See 37 — 5.

37 — 24. ULCERATIVE COLITIS See 37 — 9. *Diarrhea.*

37 — 25. VASCULAR PROBLEMS

Either arterial or venous pathologic conditions may be responsible for several types of gastrointestinal emergencies.

Esophageal varices. See **37 — 4; 42 — 22.** *Rectal Bleeding.*

Mesenteric artery occlusion from thrombosis or embolism causes acute severe midabdominal pain with minimal or no abdominal tenderness and hyperactive bowel sounds. Ileus, shock and blood in the peritoneal space and stool are later manifestations. Peritoneal aspiration (**14 — 8**) may aid in diagnosis.

TREATMENT

1. Treatment of shock (**53 — 7**).

2. Referral for surgical resection of the involved bowel.

Rectal bleeding. See **37 — 6.** *Anorectal Conditions;* **42 — 22.**

COMMON INTESTINAL PARASITES

COMMON NAME	SCIENTIFIC NAME (Synonyms or Varieties)	DISTRIBUTION	PORTAL OF ENTRY
FLUKES Blood	Schistosoma japonicum	Orient	Skin
	S. mansoni	Africa Latin America	Skin
Intestinal	Fasciolopsis buski Heterophyes, Echinostoma	Orient, tropics, U.S.A. (rare)	Mouth
PROTOZOA Dysentery ameba	Entamoeba histolytica (E. dysenteriae, E. histolytica)	World-wide, especially in moist climates	Mouth
Giardia	Giardia lamblia	World-wide, in warm climates	Mouth
ROUNDWORMS Hookworm	Ancylostoma duodenale, Necator americanus	Warm, moist climates	Skin, especially of feet
Intestinal round worm	Ascaris lumbricoides	World-wide	Mouth
	Capillaria filippinensis	Northern Philippines	Mouth
Pinworm (Seat worm)	Enterobius vermicularis (oxyuris vermicularis)	World-wide, especially in children	Mouth
Threadworm	Strongyloides stercoralis	Southern U.S.A., moist tropics	Skin, usually of the feet
Whipworm	Trichuris trichiura (Trichocephalus trichiuris)	Gulf coast, U.S.A., warm moist climates	Mouth
TAPEWORMS Beef	Taenia saginata	World-wide	Mouth
Dwarf	Hymenolepis nana	Southern U.S.A.	Mouth
Fish	Diphyllobothrium latum (Bothriocephalus latus)	Minnesota and Michigan in U.S.A., Canada	Mouth
Pork	Taenia solium	Latin America, U.S.A. (rare)	Mouth

SOURCE OF INFECTION	COMMON SYMPTOMS	THERAPEUTIC AGENTS
Water containing larvae of snail hosts	Dysentery, intestinal and hepatic cirrhosis	Antimony potassium. tartrate; stilbophen
Same	Same	Same
Vegetation, fresh water snails and fish	Intestinal toxemia and obstruction	Aspidium, hexylresorcinol, tetrachloroethylene
Feces – contaminated water, food and fomites	Abdominal pain, dysentery, hepatitis	Oxytetracycline, diiodohydroxyquin, chloroquine phosphate, emetine hydrochloride
Human feces	Abdominal pain, mucous diarrhea, weight loss	Quinacrine hydrochloride
Fecal contamination of soil	Melena, anemia, retarded growth	Hexylresorcinol, tetrachloroethylene, bephenium hydroxynaphthoate
Fecal contamination of soil	"Acute abdomen," colicky pain, diarrhea, obstruction of bile or pancreatic duct, intestinal blockage	Dithiazanine iodide, hexylresorcinol, piperazine
Fecal contamination of soil	Diarrhea, marasmus, emaciation	Dithiazanine iodide, thiabendazole
Eggs from contaminated fomites	Perianal itching, convulsions in children	Piperazine
Fecal contamination of soil	Severe radiating gastric pain, diarrhea	Dithiazanine iodide
Fecal contamination of soil	Nausea, vomiting, diarrhea, retarded growth	Dithiazanine iodide, hexylresorcinol
Raw or incompletely cooked infected beef	"Acute appendix," severe abdominal pain, systemic toxemia	Quinacrine hydrochloride
Eggs contaminating environment	Abdominal pain, diarrhea, dizziness, inanition	Hexylresorcinol, quinacrine hydrochloride
Infected fresh water fish	Bowel obstruction, intestinal toxemia – may cause severe anemia	Aspidium, quinacrine hydrochloride
Incompletely cooked infected pork	Acute abdominal pain, guarding, rigidity, systemic toxemia	Quinacrine hydrochloride

38. GENITOURINARY TRACT EMERGENCIES

TRAUMATIC CONDITIONS

If injury to any part of the urogenital tract is suspected, the attending physician should perform a thorough physical examination of the abdomen, lower back, flanks and scrotum or perineum, followed by gross and microscopic examination of the urine for blood cells. Catheterization (14—3) may be necessary but should be avoided whenever possible; a "clean-catch" or second glass specimen is usually satisfactory. If there is blood in the urine or if there is any reasonable doubt as to the nature or extent of the injury, the patient should be hospitalized for urologic examination and treatment.

38—1. BLADDER INJURIES

Ruptures of the bladder may vary in degree from tears of a few fibers of the muscular wall with microscopic hematuria to large rents with extensive extravasation of urine, hemorrhage, peritonitis and shock. The most common causes are:

Fracture of the pelvis with perforation or laceration of the bladder wall by sharp bone ends.

Direct trauma over a distended bladder. Gross and microscopic examination of a "clean-catch" or second glass specimen of urine should be done if the type of injury suggests possible bladder damage. Cystograms may be indicated to confirm the diagnosis.

TREATMENT

All cases of proved or suspected bladder damage should be transferred at once for hospitalization. Shock must be treated (53—7) immediately.

38—2. KIDNEY INJURIES

A severe blow over the flank or paralumbar muscles may cause a contusion or rupture of a kidney. Suspected cases should be hospitalized for observation, diagnosis and treatment. Severe shock is common and must be treated (53—7) at once.

38 — 3. ORCHITIS

Direct blows to the scrotum, as well as straddling injuries, may cause traumatic orchitis with extreme pain, rapid swelling, nausea and vomiting and complete temporary prostration. Hospitalization is rarely indicated, although it may be several hours before the acute discomfort and reflex nausea and vomiting decrease enough to allow any type of physical activity.

TREATMENT

1. Control of pain and anxiety by sedatives, anodynes and narcotics. Chlorpromazine hydrochloride (Thorazine) will often help to control reflex nausea and vomiting.

2. Application of cold compresses.

3. Support by a T binder or athletic supporter until swelling subsides.

38 — 4. PENIS INJURIES

Abrasions. Cleanliness will promote rapid healing.

Contusions. No special care is required; the profuse blood supply will cause rapid recovery.

Dislocation from external trauma may result in displacement of the base of the corpus beneath the symphysis pubis or into the adjacent abdominal wall or scrotum.

TREATMENT

1. Replacement in normal position by manipulation and traction under general anesthesia as soon as possible.

2. Application of a tight fitting athletic supporter.

3. Hospitalization if there is evidence of urethral damage or if the reduced position is not stable.

"Fracture" of the shaft of the penis may be caused by direct trauma or coitus. Treatment consists of sedation and cold packs. Hospitalization may be necessary if pressure from deep bleeding interferes with urination or if a hematoma beneath Buck's fascia is present and does not absorb spontaneously.

Frenal injuries may cause severe bleeding requiring control by suturing.

Lacerations. Because of the redundant loose skin and abundant blood supply of the penis, surgical repair of lacerations usually can be performed without difficulty. Debridement should be minimal. The patient should be informed in advance that scarring following healing may result in irreparable contractures and deformity, especially curvature during erections (chordee). If a large amount of skin or soft tissue has been lost, hospitalization for grafting usually is necessary.

Necrosis of the portion of the penis distal to a constricting band (usually applied in an attempt to control urinary incontinence or to improve sexual performance) may occur. If swelling (sometimes tremendous) or the type of constricting object will not allow severance by use of a ring cutter or scissors or removal of the round-and-round constriction with the aid of a lubricant, wrapping with package cord, starting just distal to the constriction should be tried. If this is unsuccessful, removal under general anesthesia may be necessary. Extreme distal urethral edema may require use of a retention catheter. Because of the profuse blood supply, complete and rapid recovery is the general rule unless actual gangrene is present.

Zipper injuries. See 48—66.

38—5. POSTCIRCUMCISION BLEEDING

Improper operative technique, especially in the use of the Gomco clamp, may result in bleeding, coming on from a few minutes to several days after circumcision.

TREATMENT

Mild bleeding or oozing generally can be controlled by pressure. Gelform or Oxycel held snugly over the bleeding area may be necessary. Severe bleeding requires immediate surgical control by properly placed mattress sutures.

38—6. SCROTAL INJURIES

Direct blows or straddling injuries may cause extensive bleeding into the areolar tissue of the scrotum, as well as injury to the penis and the scrotal contents. Rupture of the membranous urethra must be ruled out by careful examination including digital rectal examination, since even a suspicion of urethral rupture requires immediate hospitalization for operative repair before extensive extravasation of urine has occurred.

TREATMENT
1. Bed rest until the swelling subsides.
2. Sedatives and anodynes.
3. Support by a T binder, suspensory or athletic supporter.

4. Reference to a surgeon or urologist; evacuation of a hematoma or of extravasated urine may be necessary.

5. Hospitalization in severe cases; however, most patients do well on home care, provided the urethra is intact.

38 – 7. TESTICULAR TORSION

Testicular torsion usually occurs in children and requires immediate hospitalization if the position and circulation cannot be improved by gentle manipulation. Surgical stabilization will prevent recurrence. Differentiation from inguinal hernia, epididymitis, hydrocele and hematocele may be difficult.

38 – 8. URETHRAL INJURIES

Characterized by urethral bleeding, pain and difficulty in urination, injury to the urethra may be caused by:

Severe scrotal injuries (38 – 6), especially those caused by straddling some hard object, with compression of the membranous urethra against the symphysis pubis.

Displaced or comminuted fractures of the pelvis near the symphysis pubis.

Dislocation or "fracture" of the penis (38 – 4) by direct trauma.

Introduction of foreign bodies into the urethra by children (48 – 31) and mentally deranged persons.

Inexpert or injudicious attempts at catheterization (14 – 3).

TREATMENT

1. Sedation by intravenous barbiturates. Pain may be severe enough to require a narcotic.

2. Treatment of shock (53 – 7).

3. Immediate hospitalization for urologic care.

38 – 9. VAGINAL AND VULVAL INJURIES

Marked swelling and profuse bleeding may result from tears at delivery, blows, straddling injuries, forcible intercourse, attempted rape (9), insertion of foreign bodies (36 – 8) and caustic burns. Thorough examination after cleansing and hemostasis is always indicated.

TREATMENT

1. Repair of small lacerations under local anesthetic.

2. Hospitalization if large hematomas are present, if lacerations

enter or closely approximate the bladder or rectum or if blood loss has been excessive.

3. Reduction of swelling and pain by cold compresses, subcutaneous hyaluronidase (Wydase) or oral enzyme tablets (Chymoral).

NONTRAUMATIC CONDITIONS

38 — 10. CYSTITIS

Characterized by dysuria and bladder tenderness, cystitis rarely causes severe systemic reactions except in children, especially girls. It is one of the common causes of sudden temperature rise in small children. If suspected, a "clean-catch" or second glass urine specimen should be examined microscopically for pus and blood. Cultures and sensitivity tests should be done.

TREATMENT

1. Force fluids orally and intravenously.

2. Give appropriate antibiotics or sulfonamides as indicated by cultures and sensitivity tests.

3. Recommend bed rest until afebrile.

4. Prescribe bladder sedation.

In adults. A mixture of tincture hyoscyamus and potassium citrate may give subjective relief from the burning and scalding sensation.

In children. Mandelic acid preparations often give relief, provided fluids are restricted for at least 12 hours.

5. Refer to a urologist for further care. Severe cases may require hospitalization.

38 — 11. EPIDIDYMITIS

The discomfort of an acute epididymitis is often severe enough to bring the patient for emergency care, frequently with the story that the pain developed following lifting or a strain. Investigation will generally disclose a nontraumatic etiology, although straddling injuries with contusion of the scrotum (**38 — 6**) and traumatic orchitis occasionally are associated with traumatic epididymitis. Testicular torsion (**38 — 7**) must always be ruled out.

TREATMENT

1. Bed rest until the acute signs and symptoms subside.

2. Cold compresses.

3. Support by an athletic supporter or T binder.

4. Analgesics. Morphine sulfate in small doses may be required to control severe pain.

5. Administration of broad-spectrum antibiotics.

6. Reference for urologic care and hospitalization as needed.

38 — 12.   HYDROCELE

Even though the patient may insist that the excess fluid in the scrotal sac is very uncomfortable, drainage as a rule is not an emergency procedure. The patient should be advised to consult a urologist. In children, testicular torsion (**38 — 7**) must always be ruled out by careful examination, even if the transillumination test is positive.

38 — 13.   HYDRONEPHROSIS

Diagnosis of this condition cannot be made from an emergency examination. All that can be done is to attempt to give symptomatic relief and to combat infection as outlined under *Cystitis* (**38 — 10**), followed by referral to a urologist.

38 — 14.   NEPHRITIS (Bright's Disease)

If glomerular, degenerative or arteriosclerotic kidney disease is present or suspected, the only emergency measures required are:

1. Treatment of convulsions (**31.** *Convulsive Seizures;* **29.** *Coma*).

2. Treatment of congestive heart failure (**26 — 8**).

3. Arrangement for immediate hospitalization for medical work-up and care.

38 — 15.   PARAPHIMOSIS

Retraction of the foreskin can usually be reduced by application of cold compresses and steady constant manual compression of the glans penis for 10 to 15 minutes, followed by gentle traction on the prepuce. If this is unsuccessful, infiltration around the constricting ring of 150 turbidity reducing units (TRU) of hyaluronidase dissolved in 2 ml. of normal saline may make reduction possible. In rare instances hospitalization for use of a general anesthetic may be necessary.

38-16. PERIRENAL (Perinephric) ABSCESS

If this condition is suspected, immediate hospitalization for care by a urologist is indicated.

38-17. PERIURETHRAL ABSCESSES See 20-23.

38-18. PHIMOSIS

Basically due to chronically tight structures covering the glans penis, acute symptoms are usually brought on by trauma but occasionally may develop without known precipitating cause. If the acute swelling of the glans cannot be controlled by sedation and cold compresses, and if the constriction cannot be released by gentle manipulation, the patient should be hospitalized for surgical relief. Dorsal slits or other surgical procedures should *not* be done as emergency measures unless there has been prolonged constriction and delay in surgical treatment is anticipated.

38-19. RETENTION OF URINE

This very uncomfortable condition is a common and legitimate emergency. If any difficulty is encountered during catheterization (**14-3**), the patient should be given an anodyne and referred to a urologist unless the bladder is grossly distended. In this case suprapubic drainage (**14-3**) should be done at once. In any case, acute urinary retention is a sign of underlying pathology requiring urologic investigation.

Passage of sounds, filiform catheters or stylet-stiffened catheters should not be attempted unless the attending physician is familiar with and skilled in their use. Nonbreakable catheters (never glass!) should be used in females. For technique of catheterization, see **14-3**.

38-20. STONE IN THE URINARY TRACT

The severe radiating, often agonizing, pain caused by passage of a stone down a ureter is a legitimate emergency requiring immediate relief, However, because the clinical picture is chiefly subjective, it can be simulated convincingly by narcotic addicts. A careful history supplemented by review of any available previous records and by examination of a urine specimen (obtained in the presence of an attendant) for red blood cells is essential before narcotics are administered or prescribed. In questionable cases, x-ray films of the abdomen may be necessary. A negative x-ray, however, does not rule out the presence of calculi; many are not radiopaque.

TREATMENT

1. Bed rest, with application of hot stupes to the abdomen.

2. Morphine sulfate, 15 mg., with atropine sulfate, 0.4 mg. subcutaneously, or, if the pain is very severe, intravenously. Meperidine hydrochloride (Demerol), 50 to 100 mg., or pentazocine lactate (Talwin), 15 to 30 mg., may be substituted if the pain is of moderate intensity.

3. Methantheline bromide (Banthine), 25 mg. intravenously.

4. Nitroglycerin in tablet form, 0.4 to 0.6 mg. sublingually.

5. Papaverine hydrochloride, 30 to 60 mg. intravenously.

6. Adiphenine hydrochloride (Trasentine), 0.25 mg. by mouth, or 0.12 gm. subcutaneously.

Sudden and complete subsiding of the acute pain indicates that the stone has passed through the ureter into the bladder. When this occurs, reference to a urologist on a nonurgent basis is all that is indicated. If the pain persists, or if there is any question regarding the validity of subjective complaints and objective findings, hospitalization for observation, evaluation and treatment should be suggested. Narcotic addicts will usually suddenly remember a number of apparently good reasons for refusing hospitalization, particularly if it has been suggested, directly or indirectly, that a method of hospital treatment without use of narcotics is planned.

38—21. URETHRITIS

Specific. See **60—3.** *Gonorrhea.*

Nonspecific. Acute urethritis is a very common condition, especially in young females, and is often overlooked as a cause for urinary complaints. Prescription of a mild sedative for symptomatic relief is all that is required. Thorough pediatric or medical investigation should be recommended.

39. GYNECOLOGIC CONDITIONS

39-1. ABORTIONS See 47-1.

39-2. AMENORRHEA (Absence of Menses)

No emergency treatment is required.

39-3. BARTHOLIN GLAND ABSCESSES

Bartholin gland abscesses may require incision and drainage if acute or fluctuant, but whenever possible the patient should be referred to a gynecologist for this procedure.

39-4. DYSMENORRHEA (Painful Menstruation)

TREATMENT
1. Application of hot stupes to the abdomen.
2. Administration of antispasmodics:
   Phenobarbital sodium, 0.06 gm. intramuscularly.
   Atropine sulfate, 0.4 mg. subcutaneously or intravenously.
   Adiphenine hydrochloride (Trasentine), 75 mg., or adiphenine hydrochloride, 50 mg., combined with phenobarbital, 20 mg. by mouth every 4 to 6 hours.

39-5. ECTOPIC PREGNANCY See 47-2.

39-6. MENORRHAGIA (Abnormally Profuse Menstruation)

TREATMENT
1. Severe cases require plasma volume expanders intravenously followed by hospitalization.
2. In mild cases the patient may be sent home for bed rest and given a prescription for ergonovine maleate (Ergotrate), 0.2 mg. orally every 4 hours. Gynecologic examination in 1 or 2 days should be recommended.

39-7. METRORRHAGIA (Bleeding Between Periods)

TREATMENT
If excessive, hospitalize at once.

If mild
1. Limited activity; preferably bed rest.
2. Ergonovine maleate (Ergotrate), 0.2 mg. orally every 4 hours.
3. Examination by a gynecologist as soon as possible.

39—8. MITTELSCHMERZ (Pain Midway Between Periods)

Differential diagnosis from an acute surgical condition may require hospitalization for laboratory studies and observation. Sedation and analgesics will control milder cases.

39—9. PELVIC INFLAMMATORY DISEASE (Salpingitis, Tubo-ovarian Abscess)

If febrile, hospitalize at once; if afebrile, prescribe sedation, bed rest and broad spectrum antibiotics in large doses. The patient should be referred to a gynecologist for examination and care.

39—10. POSTPARTUM BLEEDING

Mild cases
TREATMENT
1. Limited activity; preferably bed rest.
2. Ergonovine maleate (Ergotrate), 0.2 mg. by mouth 3 times a day for 3 days.
3. Antibiotics for prevention of secondary infection.
4. Gynecologic examination if bleeding persists.

Severe cases, especially those with fever, require immediate hospitalization. Treatment of shock (**53—7**) may be necessary. Intravenous injection of 1 ml. of oxytocin (Pitocin) in 500 ml. of 5% dextrose solution will control hemorrhage in some instances. Fibrinogen level and other blood clotting factors should be determined.

39—11. PRURITUS VULVAE

Topical anesthetics such as dibucaine (Nupercaine) ointment, with sedation, will usually control symptoms until the patient can be seen by a gynecologist. Cellulitis of the external genitalia from fingernail excoriations may be severe enough to warrant hospitalization. Fungal infections and diabetes mellitus should be considered as causative factors and treated if present.

39–12. SALPINGITIS See **39–9.** *Pelvic Inflammatory Disease*

39–13. TORSION OF THE PEDICLE OF AN OVARIAN CYST

This condition requires surgical correction at once. The diagnosis is usually made at exploratory laparotomy for acute abdominal pain.

40. HAND INJURIES

Adequate treatment of injuries to the hand requires specialized knowledge, skill and experience – not only in the proper care of soft tissue injuries but also in traumatic orthopedics, peripheral nerve repair and plastic surgery, especially skin grafting. If the emergency physician is not sure of the proper procedures, even though the injuries appear to be minor, he should arrange for treatment as soon as possible by a surgeon experienced in hand injury care. Nerve and tendon function should always be determined on initial examination and recorded in detail in the emergency chart before any debridement or repair is begun. Except in minor injuries involving other parts of the hand than the digit upon which the ring is worn, rings should always be removed, using a ring cutter or compressive centripetal wrapping if necessary.

40–1. ABRASIONS OF THE HAND

1. Cleanse thoroughly with a mild detergent such as pHisoHex or with nonmedicated soap and water. Remove any superficially embedded foreign materials by sharp dissection under local anesthesia.

2. Inspect carefully, using magnification such as an eye loupe if necessary. Remove any firmly adherent or deeply imbedded foreign bodies by sharp dissection under local anesthesia.

3. Irrigate thoroughly; repeat 2 (above) if necessary.

4. Apply a petrolatum gauze dressing. Bacitracin (Parentracin) gauze may be used in place of petrolatum gauze if infection is apparent or suspected. Dressings should be snug and securely anchored but not tight enough to interfere with circulation. Allowance should be made for the inevitable posttraumatic swelling.

5. Give tetanus-immune globulin (TIG) or toxoid (**16**) and broad spectrum antibiotics if warranted by the circumstances of the injury, if gross contamination has been present or if more than 6 hours have elapsed since injury.

6. Impress on the patient the fact that the original dessing *must* be checked by a physician within 24 hours.

40 – 2. CELLULITIS OF THE HAND

Any evidence of severe infection of any part of the hand calls for immediate treatment to preserve maximal function and minimize permanent damage.

1. Elevation and partial immobilization by a splint and sling.
2. Control of pain. Narcotics may be required.
3. Administration of antibiotics in large amounts, preferably after cultures and sensitivity tests.
4. Administration of tetanus-immune globulin (TIG) or toxoid (**16**).
5. Incision and drainage of small superficial abscesses with insertion of a small rubber dam drain if necessary. Spraying with ethyl chloride is usually adequate for anesthesia. The necessity of redressing in 24 hours should be stressed to the patient.

Incisions should always be made in the "safe areas" of the palm and digits (Fig. 22) to avoid severance of essential structures and development of function-limiting scarring.

6. Hospitalization is usually indicated if a general anesthetic or forearm, brachial or axillary block will be required, if the deep palmar spaces or flexor tendon sheaths are involved or if the patient is not making satisfactory progress under conservative ambulatory treatment.

40 – 3. CONTUSIONS OF THE HAND

Mild contusions require no emergency treatment. Cold compresses for the first 12 to 24 hours, followed by hot soaks, will accelerate recovery. If extensive hematomas are present, the hand or digit should be immobilized on a padded splint, elevated, anodynes given and surgical or orthopedic follow-up care arranged. Severe crushing injuries may require hospitalization. Traumatic aneurysms of the palmar arteries have been reported following localized contusions.

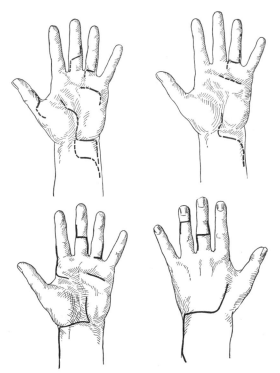

Figure 22. Certain general principles apply to the location of incisions on the hand. Incisions should avoid the midline; they should not cross flexion creases, but should parallel them as closely as possible and should be planned so as to produce flaps of skin and subcutaneous tissue to overlie the operative area. The same principles apply to enlargement of accidental wounds, which should be incorporated as well as possible into the general pattern of ideal incisions. (From Davis, L., *Christopher's Textbook of Surgery*, 9th ed., Philadelphia: W. B. Saunders Company, 1968.)

SUBUNGUAL HEMATOMAS

1. Small hematomas should be evacuated only if severe throbbing is present. Painless removal of the blood beneath the nail by burning a small hole through the nail with a red-hot paper clip gives complete relief. As a rule, no return visit is necessary.

2. Hematomas with associated external wounds are potentially infected and require free drainage. A small section of the nail should be removed with sharp-pointed scissors after a preliminary drainage hole has been made (see step 1), and the blood evacuated. A dressing should be applied and protected by an aluminum or plastic fingertip guard. Recheck in 24 hours is essential.

3. Incomplete avulsion of the proximal end of the nail may require completion of the avulsion under digital block anesthesia. Using sterile technique, the proximal portion, usually about one third of the nail, should be excised, blood removed from beneath the nail and soft tissue folds by irrigation and a stay suture of No. 40 cotton inserted through the nail and soft tissue on each side. A Telfa dressing and protective guard should be applied, tetanus-immune globulin (TIG) or toxoid given (**16**) and follow-up care in 24 hours arranged.

Contusions of the joints of the fingers usually require prolonged splinting to minimize permanent limitation of motions from fibrosis of the joint capsule. *If there is pain on motion, splint!* Persistent gentle massage (inunction) of the bruised area with an ointment of hydrocortisone acetate (2½%) in neomycin sulfate (Neo-Cortef) will often decrease swelling and pain.

40—4. FRACTURES OF THE HAND

SIMPLE (CLOSED) FRACTURES

Scaphoid (Navicular) Fractures (see also **44—40**) require immobilization in a short arm plaster cast with the wrist in slight cock-up (grasping) position and the thumb in extreme abduction. The cast should extend to the metacarpophalangeal joints of the fingers and include the distal joint of the thumb. Small chip or avulsion fractures of the carpal bones require splinting in plaster in a position which will relax ligamentous or tendon pull.

Semilunar (Lunate) Fractures are often associated with partial or complete dislocation which may be difficult to recognize on routine x-rays (**44—16.** *Lunate Dislocations;* **44—19.** *Perilunar Dislocations*). If dislocation is present, hospitalization is indicated; if not, a short arm cast (elbow to metacarpophalangeal joints) should be applied, with recheck by an orthopedist in 24 to 48 hours.

Metacarpal Fractures (See also **44—42**)

All undisplaced metacarpal fractures should be immobilized in plaster. A gauntlet cast is usually adequate.

Displaced fractures with angulation, overriding or comminution usually require hospitalization. An exception is the so-called "boxer's fracture" of the distal ends of the 2nd to 5th metacarpals (usually the 5th).

After injection of a local anesthetic into the hematoma, correction of the volar angulation of the distal fragment of the metacarpal can usually be obtained by firm pressure dorsally, using the proximal phalanx flexed to 90 degrees as a lever. If x-ray or fluoroscopic examination shows satisfactory reduction, the hand should be flexed over a roller bandage and immobilized with tape or plaster of Paris. The position should be confirmed by post-reduction x-rays. Recheck examination in 24 hours, preferably by an orthopedist, should be arranged.

Fractures of the medial angle of the proximal end of the metacarpal of the thumb (Bennett's fracture) are unstable from muscle pull and usually require special orthopedic care to prevent a large permanent disability from shortening, instability and decrease in grip.

Proximal and Middle Phalanx Fractures

If multiple, hospitalization is advisable. Single fractures, even though considerably displaced, usually can be manipulated into satisfactory position without difficulty under local anesthesia. A pin inserted through the pulp of the ball of the injured digit on the volar side of the distal phalanx, with traction by rubber bands attached to a banjo splint, may be necessary to maintain satisfactory position and alignment. Frequent adjustments of the amount of tension may be necessary. The attachments and pull of the flexor tendons should be kept in mind when splinting and applying traction; acute flexion at the proximal interphalangeal joint is required if the fracture is distal to the attachment of the flexor digitorum sublimis tendon.

All proximal and middle phalangeal fractures should be immobilized in plaster or on aluminum splints. Recheck in 24 hours, preferably by an orthopedist, should be arranged.

Distal Phalanx Fractures

Fractures of the tuft require no treatment except protection with an aluminum or plastic splint. Fibrous union, with no deformity or dysfunction, usually occurs.

Fractures of the proximal lip of the dorsal aspect of the distal phalanx at the attachment of the extensor tendon (baseball finger, mallet finger) should be taped or splinted in plaster of Paris, or an

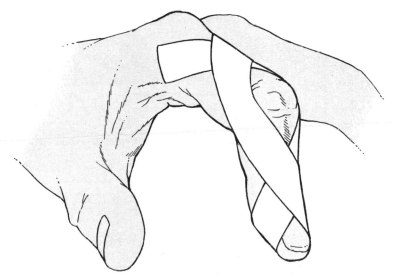

Figure 23. A single strip of adhesive tape holds an acute baseball finger in optimal position. (Modified from Lissner, B., Emergency Medicine, Vol. 5, No. 4, p. 260, April, 1973.)

individually fitted aluminum splint should be applied, with the proximal interphalangeal joint in about 40 degrees flexion and the distal joint in hyperextension to obtain maximum relaxation of the extensor tendon. For optimal position, see Figure 23. Secondary surgical pinning of the fragment may be necessary.

COMPOUND (OPEN) FRACTURES

Compound (open) fractures of any portion of the hand should be referred for hospital care, with the following exceptions:

Shattering Fractures of the Tuft

These should be irrigated, debrided and closed, saving as much length as possible and avoiding suture lines on the tactile surface of the ball. Small, loose fragments of bone should be removed but larger pieces left in situ. Fibrous union often occurs, with no loss of function.

Multiple Crushing Fractures of the Digits Associated with Loss or Maceration of Soft Tissues

A plastic amputation should be performed, saving as much length as possible, especially of a thumb. Amputated portions can sometimes be filleted and used as full thickness grafts. Every precaution should be taken to insure satisfactory shape and thickness, with minimal scarring of the tactile surface of the stump. Digital nerves should be identified, clipped off and allowed to retract to prevent formation of neuromas. If the amputation is through the base of the nail, all nail matrix cells should be removed by sharp dissection and curetting.

40–5. LACERATIONS OF THE HAND (See also 55–20)

In order to prevent limitation of function, all possible measures to prevent infection must be taken.

PRINCIPLES OF TREATMENT

1. **Repair** within 6 hours if possible. This limit may be extended to 12 hours if the wound is not deep or extensive and if there is no evidence of gross contamination or infection. Lacerations more than 12 hours old should be irrigated and debrided (below) *but not sutured.*

2. **Preliminary washing and irrigation before debridement,** using copious amounts of bland nonmedicated soap and water, followed by normal salt solution. If very painful, this preliminary washing may be done under a local anesthetic.

3. **Application of sterile drapes** after preliminary irrigation and cleansing of the wound and surrounding skin.

4. **Observation of sterile operating room technique.** All persons, including the patient, should be masked. Cap, mask and sterile gloves should be worn by the surgeon, with a sterile gown if an extensive or lengthy procedure is contemplated.

5. **Application of a tourniquet** to obtain a relatively bloodless field. A rubber band around the base of the digit is adequate in most finger cases.

6. **Anesthesia**

Local infiltration of digital block with 1 or 2% procaine or lidocaine (Xylocaine) is usually sufficient. Nerve blocks (forearm, elbow, brachial, axillary) give excellent results. Local anesthesia should be used unless the patient is comatose or in such a condition that pain perception is markedly decreased, a very short procedure (for instance, 1 or 2 stitches) is planned or there is reason to believe that the patient is sensitive to procaine or other local anesthetics.

Administration of a general anesthetic should be postponed until *at least 6 hours* after the last intake of food or liquids.

7. **Examination of the wound** under local anesthesia for severance of large blood vessels, muscles, nerves or tendons; fractures, dislocations, epiphysial displacements; foreign bodies; hematomas; and openings into or contamination of joints, tendon sheaths or fascial spaces. If unexpectedly severe damage is encountered, the tourniquet should be removed (or loosened and reapplied if indicated), a sterile pressure bandage applied and the patient transferred *at once* to an adequately equipped hospital. Administration of a sedative may be advisable.

8. **Debridement**

The object of debridement is to convert an area of traumatized and potentially infected tissue into a surgically clean wound. With a small toothed forceps, sharp scalpel and small curved scissors, sharp dissection should be used to remove any damaged structures to a depth of 1 to 2 mm., starting with the skin and working toward the depths of the wound. If necessary for adequate exposure, the surface laceration should be extended, bearing in mind the areas of safe incisions in the hand (Fig. 22). Nerves, tendons, blood vessels and articular surfaces should be preserved.

All dead spaces should be eliminated by application of mattress sutures after careful evacuation of blood clots. Bleeding not controllable by pressure should be stopped by clamping and tying with No. 000 plain catgut. Buried suture material, however, should be kept to an absolute minimum.

Completely severed small sections of soft tissue (for instance, fingertips) which are not badly macerated, in some instances (especially in small children) can be carefully cleaned and sutured back in place as full thickness grafts. The quicker this suturing is done, the better the chance of a "take." Intact skin from amputated parts which are to be discarded can be used for grafting denuded areas.

No antibiotics, antiseptics, disinfectants, sulfonamides or other substances of any type should be painted, sprayed, insufflated or sprinkled into the wound.

9. **Closure**

Bony surfaces, joints, nerves and tendons must be completely covered, using skin grafts or relaxing incisions if necessary. A pedicle graft with the base proximally can be transferred from the

page 249

immediate neighborhood and the resultant defect covered with split thickness grafts. All dead spaces should be obliterated by mattress sutures of 4-0 plain catgut.

Careful approximation of skin edges without inversion or undue tension is essential, using nonabsorbable sutures. Cotton (No. 40 or 50) and Dermalin are satisfactory. Interlocking adhesive "butterflies" or SteriStrips result in an excellent skin closure but must be inspected frequently to detect slippage which can be minimized by preliminary application of tincture of benzoin.

10. **Dressings**

A small strip of sterile petrolatum gauze or a nonadherent dressing such as Telfa should be placed over the sutures and a pressure bandage applied to control oozing. Collodion dressings should never be placed directly over a wound because of the possibility of promoting growth of anaerobic organisms, and because of the difficulty in removal. Collodion, however, can be used very satisfactorily to hold the edges of the outer dressings in place, especially on persons sensitive to adhesive tape.

Except in very small lacerations, the following measures should be routine:

Splinting to limit motion and prevent tension on repaired structures.

Application of a sling; elevation.

Administration of large doses of penicillin or other antibiotics as indicated by sensitivity tests if the wound was grossly contaminated or surgical repair was delayed beyond the safe time limit.

Protection against tetanus by tetanus-immune globulin (TIG) or toxoid (**16**).

Control of apprehension, anxiety and pain by acetylsalicylic acid (aspirin), barbiturates or narcotics.

11. **Postoperative care.** Small superficial lacerations as well as more serious wounds require *removal of the original bandage in 24 hours* for inspection and to allow for swelling. Failure to stress to the patient the need for this recheck examination constitutes negligence (**68 − 1**).

40 − 6. NERVE INJURIES IN THE HAND (See also **46 − 10.** *Peripheral Nerve Injuries*)

Primary versus secondary (delayed) nerve suturing. Unless the emergency physician has had neurosurgical training, he should not attempt a primary nerve suture. If immediate referral for care by a neurosurgeon is not possible, careful debridement (**40 – 5**) should be performed and the ends of the severed nerve identified and "tagged" with a small knot of black silk or very fine stainless steel wire. Closure should then be done in the usual manner. The procedure should be explained to the patient (or parents, spouse or legal guardian) and secondary nerve suture by a neurosurgeon recommended. The optimum wait before secondary suture is generally accepted to be 21 days. Whenever possible, a basal electromyogram should be made since, as a rule, denervation potentials do not develop until about 21 days after injury.

Evaluation of motor and sensory deficits. Localized pressure from crushing injuries, or from a too tight tourniquet, may result in motor and/or sensory loss distal to the point of pressure. Before any treatment is given, motor function and sensation should be carefully evaluated and noted in detail on the emergency chart. Slow recovery of complete function usually occurs if pressure is the only causative factor in the motor or sensory deficit.

40 – 7. PUNCTURE WOUNDS OF THE HAND

The treatment of puncture wounds requires the exercising of good judgment and common sense by the attending physician. The method of injury, chance of infection and possibility of buried foreign bodies must be considered. All puncture wounds should receive tetanus-immune globulin (TIG) or toxoid (**16**).

Enlargement of the wound tract, thorough irrigation, careful debridement and suturing (**40 – 5**) are indicated for gross contamination, possible foreign bodies embedded in the soft tissue (**36 – 6**), human bites (**24 – 13**) and indelible pencil wounds, whether or not the lead is still present. These require extensive excision of all discolored tissue as soon as possible. See **49 – 74**. *Aniline dyes.*

40 – 8. TENDON INJURIES IN THE HAND

In the palm or dorsum of the hand. If inspection or tests of function show evidence of complete severance of a flexor or extensor tendon proximal to the metacarpophalangeal joints, immediate referral for specialized care is indicated. Partial severance without separation or loss of continuity can be repaired after irrigation and debridement, using fine silk or cotton for suturing.

In the digits

Flexors. Refer for specialist care.

Extensors. Severed extensor tendons (except in the thumb) retract very little and no true pulleys or tendon sheaths are present; therefore, repair can usually be accomplished at the time of emergency debridement and closure. Fine cotton or silk should be used, employing the Bunnell double-right-angle stitch and splinting for 3 weeks in full extension. The specialized flexible pull-out wire technique recommended by Bunnell should not be attempted as an emergency procedure unless the emergency surgeon has had adequate training and experience in this method. Extensor tendon injuries requiring special handling are avulsion of the extensor tendon attachment to the proximal lip of the dorsal aspect of the distal phalanx, usually associated with tearing off of a small flake of bone — the so-called "baseball" or "mallet" finger. For treatment, see **40 — 4.** *Distal Phalanx Fractures.* Buttonhole longitudinal splitting of an extensor tendon at the proximal interphalangeal joint, causing "paradoxical flexion." After debridement, the longitudinal split in the tendon can be repaired easily using interrupted sutures of fine cotton or silk. Splinting in full extension for 3 weeks followed by gradually increasing active (no passive) motion usually results in recovery of full function.

Traumatic tendinitis. See **44 — 61.**

Acute tenosynovitis. See **44 — 61.**

Stenosing tenovaginitis (De Quervain's Disease)

Thickening and narrowing of the sheath of the abductor pollicis longus (and sometimes of the extensor brevis) causes severe pain and loss of function which can be relieved by longitudinal splitting of the sheath under local anesthesia.

41. HEAD INJURIES

See also **29 — 17.** *Coma of Undetermined Etiology;* **34 — 4.** *Excitement States;* **48 — 9** to **48 — 11.** *Brain Injuries in Children;* **48 — 32.** *Head Injuries in Children.*

41 — 1. THE GENERAL CONDITION

The general condition of the patient is the primary consideration in all head injuries. Blood pressure, pulse, pulse pressure, respiration, color and especially *degree or state of consciousness* are rapid and accurate indices of the patient's condition. All should be checked as soon as possible and at frequent intervals thereafter. *Changes in condition* are the most important factors in the evaluation of head injuries. Rapid or progressive deterioration may indicate a serious condition, such as an epidural hemorrhage from the middle meningeal artery (**41 – 19**), requiring immediate surgical intervention as a lifesaving measure (**17.** *Urgency Evaluation – Triage*).

41 – 2. INITIAL EXAMINATION

Initial examination is all-important and should be done first with the patient clothed (**29 – 17**) and later completely undressed. The following points should be covered in detail and recorded in the patient's record, giving negative as well as positive findings:

Temperature, pulse, respiration and blood pressure.

General appearance – position, condition of clothing, etc., when first seen.

Evidence of severe or multiple injuries requiring immediate attention (**17.** *Urgency Evaluation – Triage*).

Examination of the head for evidence of trauma (wounds, hematomas, depressions, bleeding from the ears, nose or throat, etc.).

State of consciousness and mental status:

Clear. Presence or absence of retrograde amnesia, disorientation as to time and place and aphasia (perceptive and expressive) should be determined.

Semicomatose. Response to commands and painful stimuli, delirious, restless.

Comatose. No response to painful stimuli.

Eyes. Size and quality of pupils, reaction to distance and light, nystagmus, diplopia, coordination of extraocular movements, funduscopic examination.

Motor power. Ability to move the facial muscles equally on both sides; weakness or paralysis (flaccid, spastic) of an extremity.

Rectal sphincter tone.

Sensation. Variations in perception of pin prick and light touch on the face, arms, legs and trunk.

Special senses. Vision, hearing, smell, taste; position and vibratory sense.

Reflexes. Superficial (corneal, gag, abdominal, cremasteric); deep tendon (biceps, triceps, radial, knee jerks, ankle jerks).

41 – 3. SHOCK IN HEAD INJURIES

Pathologic reflexes. Babinski response on each side – positive (extensor) or negative (flexor); Hoffman; clonus.

41 – 3. SHOCK

Shock does not usually accompany head injuries in adults but may be encountered in children (**48 – 51**). If present, it must be controlled (**53 – 7**) before definitive treatment for other conditions is begun. Injuries elsewhere should always be looked for and treated in order or urgency (**17**). A gradually decreasing pulse pressure may be the only evidence of increasing intracranial pressure. Intensive treatment of gross cerebral edema (**41 – 22**) may be lifesaving.

41 – 4. ADEQUACY OF THE AIRWAY

Adequacy of the airway is essential. Removal of mucus and blood by postural drainage and suction should be begun at once and continued as needed. If the patient is vomiting, his head should be lowered and turned to the side and frequent suction utilized to minimize the danger of secondary lung infection from aspirated vomitus. Emergency tracheostomy (**14 – 12**) may be lifesaving.

41 – 5. PROPHYLACTIC INJECTIONS

Prophylactic injections (tetanus-immune globulin, toxoid, antibiotics) may contribute additional insult to an already critically embarrassed organism and, therefore, should be postponed until the patient's condition has stabilized.

41 – 6. SEDATION

Sedation should be avoided unless extreme restlessness or excitement (**34 – 4**) is present, but should be used without hesitation if forcible manual or mechanical restraint would otherwise be necessary. Parenteral administration of rapid-acting drugs whose effect is of short duration is preferable, although rectal administration may be advisable in some circumstances – for instance, if a properly signed treatment permit (**69 – 19**) cannot be obtained. The oral route should never be used; it may cause vomiting which, in turn, may cause increased intracranial pressure with extension of intracranial damage.

EFFECTIVE SEDATIVES

Chlorpromazine hydrochloride (Thorazine), 25 to 50 mg. intramuscularly.

Prochlorperazine dimaleate (Compazine), 10 to 25 mg. intramuscularly.

Paraldehyde, 5 to 10 ml. intramuscularly.

Phenobarbital sodium, 120 to 180 mg. intramuscularly.

Chloral hydrate, 1 to 2 gm. by retention enema.

41–7. CONTROL OF PAIN

Opiates and synthetic narcotics are definitely contraindicated in the presence of head injuries because of the possibility of loss or modification of pupillary signs, depression of respiration or masking of signs of developing intracranial pressure. If serious injuries elsewhere in the body cause severe pain, pentazocine lactate (Talwin) intramuscularly or intravenously in 15 to 30 mg. doses may be given for relief.

41–8. UNRELATED CONDITIONS

The clinical picture of acute head injury can easily be confused with certain endocrine disorders (**33**), intoxications from alcohol (**34–1; 49–315.** *Ethyl Alcohol*) or drugs (**29–13**), diabetes (**29–3**) and heat stroke (**57–4**). If the history or physical findings suggest the possibility of head injury, the patient should be kept under close observation and control until the picture has clarified.

41–9. CONCUSSION OF THE BRAIN (See also **48–9.** *Concussion in Children;* **48–32.** *Head Injuries in Children*)

If details of the history or neurologic findings suggest the possibility of concussion, the patient should be kept under close observation for at least 2 hours after his condition has stabilized before release from control. If unrelated conditions (**41–8**) which might confuse the picture are present, close observation until the possibility of brain damage can be ruled out is mandatory. Frequent examinations for changes in condition (**41–2**) should be made and recorded chronologically in the patient's record. X-rays may be indicated to rule out fracture or for medicolegal purposes (**18–1**);

but unless they are necessary for determination of emergency therapy, they should not be taken until the patient's condition has stabilized. If, in the considered opinion of the attending physician, it is safe to send the patient home, specific instructions regarding observation for posttraumatic symptoms and signs should be given by the physician personally to responsible members of the family. These instructions should be in simple nonmedical language and cover the following points:

Development of any difference in size of the pupils.

Increasing or recurring headaches.

Development of any facial asymmetry or of muscle weakness anywhere in the body.

Development of persistent vomiting.

Increasing sleepiness or stupor, or variations from the usual personality or behavior pattern.

These oral instructions should be supplemented by a printed form (Fig. 24) given to a responsible person accompanying the patient.

41 – 10. ACUTE EXCITEMENT STATES

Acute excitement states (**34 – 4**), sometimes even mania (**50 – 1**), can follow brain concussion. Rapid-acting barbiturates, chloral hydrate, chlorpromazine hydrochloride (Thorazine), paraldehyde or prochlorperazine dimaleate (Compazine) should be used for sedation in doses large enough to make physical restraint unnecessary.

41 – 11. FRACTURES OF THE SKULL See **41 – 12** through **41 – 18**; **48 – 32.** Head Injuries in Children

41 – 12. LINEAR FRACTURES WITHOUT DEPRESSION

Linear fractures without depression are surprisingly well tolerated, especially by children, provided the middle meningeal artery or its branches are not damaged (see **41 – 19.** Extradural Hemorrhage).

The location, not the extent, of the fracture and the condition of the patient are the most important factors to be considered in disposition. All patients with proved or suspected skull fracture should be kept under close observation for at least 6 hours; patients without neurologic signs can be allowed to go home with instructions to responsible members of the family as outlined under **41 – 9.** Concussion. If the general and neurologic pictures indicate that the pa-

Date _____

Time _____

EMERGENCY DEPARTMENT

INSTRUCTIONS FOR PATIENTS WITH HEAD INJURIES

Although no evidence of any serious injury is found at this time, careful attention for the next 24–48 hours is advised.

Patients should return to Emergency Department at once, day or night, if there is:

(1) Increased drowsiness

(2) Difficulty in rousing the patient (the patient should be awakened every two hours during the first night)

(3) Vomiting

(4) Slowing of pulse

(5) Continued headache

(6) Stiffness of neck

(7) Bleeding or clear fluid dripping from the ears or nose

(8) Weakness of facial muscles or of either leg or cither arm

(9) Development of convulsions (fits)

Figure 24. Printed instructions form for persons accompanying patient with head injury. Modified from an instruction sheet given to patients with head injuries as they are released by emergency room physicians at the Hamilton and Henderson Hospitals in Hamilton, Ontario, Canada. (From Angel, J., and McFarlane, A. H.: Patient Care, Vol. 5, No. 13, p. 118, July 15, 1971. Copyright © Miller & Fink Corporation, Darien, CT. All rights reserved.)

tient's condition is deteriorating, immediate hospitalization under the care of a neurosurgeon should be arranged.

41–13. DEPRESSED FRACTURES

Depressed fractures can easily be confused with the edge of a scalp hematoma. Palpation may be misleading and tangential x-ray films or direct observation is necessary to establish the diagnosis. Conservative treatment ordinarily is carried out. Elevation of depressed fragments is not an emergency procedure unless signs of rapidly increasing intracranial pressure are present. All patients with proved or suspected depressed skull fractures should be hospitalized for close observation under the care of a neurosurgeon.

41−14. COMPOUND (OPEN) DEPRESSED FRACTURES

TREATMENT
1. Immediate hospitalization for neurosurgical care is indicated after superficial cleansing and application of a turban-type head dressing.
2. If the condition is noted during or after debridement, the galea and scalp should not be closed. Instead, after control of gross hemorrhage, a sterile dressing should be applied and the patient transferred at once to a hospital by ambulance for neurosurgical evaluation and treatment.

41−15. BASAL SKULL FRACTURES

Basal skull fractures have a high mortality rate. Diagnosis usually depends upon the clinical picture since this type of fracture often cannot be demonstrated by x-ray films.

41−16. ANTERIOR FOSSA FRACTURES

TREATMENT
1. Place in a position of maximal drainage, usually on the side or face down.
2. Caution the patient against blowing his nose.
3. Give sedation as needed but avoid opiates and synthetic narcotics (**41−7**).
4. Hospitalize by ambulance as soon as possible. Do not attempt to control rhinorrhea or nasal hemorrhage by packing or intranasal medication of any type.

41−17. MIDDLE FOSSA FRACTURES

Blood or a mixture of spinal fluid and blood from an undamaged ear canal may be diagnostic.

TREATMENT
1. Warn the patient against blowing his nose.
2. Cover the ear with sterile gauze and apply a turban-type head dressing.
3. Give sedatives as needed but avoid opiates and synthetic narcotics (**41—7**).
4. Hospitalize by ambulance as soon as possible.
Do not attempt to cleanse the external auditory canal.

41—18.   POSTERIOR FOSSA FRACTURES

Unless the fracture is compound (open), the diagnosis of fractures in this area of the skull can be made only by x-rays. Anteroposterior, posteroanterior, basilar, Towne, and lateral views usually are required. No emergency measures except supportive therapy and hospitalization for observation are indicated.

41—19.   EXTRADURAL (EPIDURAL) HEMORRHAGE (See also **48—26.** *Extradural Hemorrhage in Children;* **59—2.** *Intracranial Bleeding*)

Tearing of the middle meningeal artery or its branches may cause collection of blood between the dura mater and the skull. Direct trauma, sometimes very slight, is the usual cause; persons between 20 and 50 years of age represent the majority of cases.

SIGNS AND SYMPTOMS. Disturbances of consciousness of varying degrees of length, an asymptomatic "lucid interval" lasting from one half hour to several days (not always present), and rapid deterioration of condition with symptoms and signs of cerebral compression (headache, vomiting, increasing stupor, decreased respiration and pulse rate, deep coma, contralateral hemiplegia, terminal vasomotor collapse). Unilateral dilation of the pupil occurs in about 75% of cases but may be transient. Funduscopic examination is of no value.

TREATMENT
If the patient's condition is deteriorating rapidly, *immediate* evacuation of the hematoma may be a lifesaving measure (**17.** *Urgency Evaluation—Triage*). This should be done if possible in a properly equipped hospital; but if a delay in hospitalization is unavoidable, it should be performed in an emergency setting. Delay will result in irreversible brain damage from pressure. As soon

as the acute compression of the brain is released, the acute emergency is over. Hospitalization for postoperative care should, of course, be arranged as soon as possible.

41−20. SUBDURAL HEMORRHAGE

The bleeding in this condition usually comes from a tear in one of the cerebral veins entering the dural sinuses, the result of direct trauma to the frontal or occipital regions. This hemorrhage is venous, and its pressure less than in extradural hemorrhage (**41−19**); hence, signs of brain damage are much slower−sometimes weeks−in developing.

TREATMENT
Hospitalization for localization and definitive care is indicated as soon as signs and symptoms suggestive of increased intracranial pressure are noted.

41−21. LACERATIONS OF THE SCALP

TREATMENT
1. After a careful history and thorough examination for evidence of intracranial damage, the area should be prepared by thorough cleansing of the surrounding scalp. Shaving is not necessary for small clean lacerations but should be done if the laceration is jagged or extensive. Under 1% procaine or lidocaine (Xylocaine) anesthesia, the skull should be palpated with the gloved finger and, if possible, inspected. If a depression or defect can be felt or seen, a sterile nonradiopaque dressing should be applied, with x-ray studies (including tangential views) made before closure of the laceration. Negative x-ray films do not rule out the presence of a fracture; therefore, if an apparent defect or variation from normal has been noted, the patient should be kept under close observation for at least 8 hours. Palpation and direct observation are often more accurate than x-rays, especially if a nondepressed linear or stellate fracture is present. Neurologic findings suggestive of brain injury, with or without evidence of skull damage, call for hospitalization for close observation and frequent determination of vital signs (**41−1**). It should be remembered that thickening of scalp layers by blood or fluid may simulate a fracture (**41−13**) and that the location of the lesion (**41−12**) is of great value in prognosis.
2. After irrigation with sterile saline and careful debridement,

closure should be done with a single row of interrupted sutures of No. 40 or No. 50 cotton using a large curved needle and including, if possible, the galea and full thickness of the scalp. Pressure usually will control bleeding, but mattress sutures may be necessary. After closure, a pressure bandage should be applied to control oozing.

3. Tetanus-immune globulin (TIG) or toxoid (**16**) and antibiotics should be administered if gross contamination is present or if treatment has been delayed.

4. Hospitalization is not necessary unless excessive blood loss has occurred, examination has indicated the possibility of a depressed fracture, or signs of increased intracranial pressure (**41 – 9**) have been noted or develop.

5. All patients should be told to report to a physician for recheck examination in not more than 2 days. The patient or a responsible member of the family should be instructed in detail orally by the attending physician regarding signs and symptoms of increased intracranial pressure (**41 – 9**) and given a printed head injury instructions form (Fig. 24).

41 – 22. MANAGEMENT OF PATIENTS WITH SERIOUS HEAD INJURIES AWAITING TRANSFER FOR HOSPITAL CARE

ROUTINE THERAPY AND HANDLING

1. Insistence on absolute rest in a position most suitable for adequate drainage. Visiting, even by members of the family, should be discouraged.

2. Insurance of an adequate airway by support of the angles of the jaw, positional drainage and application of suction as needed.

3. Administration of oxygen under positive pressure by face mask and rebreathing bag as needed for dyspnea and cyanosis.

4. Avoidance of oral medications; they may induce vomiting.

5. Limitation of fluids.

6. Frequent checking of state of consciousness, pulse, blood pressure, respiration, temperature and neurologic findings. These findings should be recorded on the patient's emergency chart and a summary, together with any x-rays, sent with the patient on transfer.

7. Use of gentle restraint and sedation as needed. Forcible physical restraint should be kept to a minimum; if it is necessary,

sedation is not adequate. An able-bodied attendant should be present at all times.

8. Use of cooling measures (ice bags, cold compresses, blower, iced saline enemas, etc.) if the patient's temperature is higher than 39°C. (102.2°F.).

9. Treatment of gross cerebral edema with 15 to 25 mg. of dexamethasone (Decadron) intravenously and 15 to 25 grams of 25% mannitol intravenously.

10. Tactful and sympathetic handling of the patient's family, friends or other interested persons, with avoidance of specific statements concerning extent of injuries, condition, type and duration of further treatment, possible complications and prognosis.

41 – 23. AXIOMS IN EMERGENCY CARE OF HEAD INJURIES
(Modified from Metcalf, S.)

Axiom 1. Initial impression of the severity of any head injury must never be regarded as final. Within 12 hours the apparently trivial head injury may become surgical, the closed head injury may turn out to be trivial.

Axiom 2. Any force of sufficient magnitude to produce either skull fracture or concussion may also have caused a cervical spine fracture. *Cross-table lateral cervical spine x-rays using a portable x-ray machine should always precede a skull series.*

Axiom 3. Except for infants and young children, if a patient with head injury is in shock, he will be found to have injuries elsewhere to account for his shock. Treatment of shock takes precedence over all other diagnostic and therapeutic measures.

Axiom 4. Never send a patient to the ward with diagnosis other than *"Head Injury."* A specific diagnosis can more safely be made when the patient leaves the hospital.

Axiom 5. Never give narcotics or sedatives to head injury patients. Thorazine may be used for excessive restlessness.

Axiom 6. Avoid general anesthesia whenever possible in head injury patients.

Axiom 7. Lumbar punctures should *not* be done in cases of recent head injury. The information so gained is useless, and a lumbar puncture can be lethal if the patient has an unrecognized clot.

Axiom 8. Early tracheostomy may save more lives from head injury than any other therapeutic step.

Axiom 9. If a neurosurgeon is not available, a burr hole to let out an intracranial hematoma made within minutes by an inexperienced physician is better than one made too late by a neurosurgeon.

Axiom 10. When discharging a patient with head injury from the hospital, always inform the family (not the patient) of the possibility of a delayed intracranial clot and its manifestations — namely, progressively severe headache, weakness of one side, visual disturbances, undue drowsiness, and unequal pupils. For written form, see Figure 24.

42. HEMORRHAGE

42 – 1. CONTROL OF BLEEDING

Control of bleeding as soon as possible is one of the chief functions of the physician in an emergency situation (**17.** *Urgency Evaluation – Triage*). For hemorrhage from an accessible part of the body, one or more of the following local measures may be used:

1. Digital or manual pressure over the bleeding area or vessel.
2. Proper application of a tourniquet (above systolic arterial blood pressure) to an extremity. Too loose an application may cause increase in or continuation of bleeding. If dangerous hemorrhage has been controlled, a tourniquet should *not* be loosened until facilities are available for surgical control.
3. Clamping and tying or insertion of mattress sutures incorporating the bleeding vessels.
4. Application of topical hemostatics or packing with sterile gauze.

42 – 2. GENERAL MEASURES

1. Absolute rest in a position of comfort; prevention of chilling.
2. Treatment of hypovolemic shock (**53 – 7**).
3. Morphine sulfate, 10 to 15 mg. intravenously, to control pain, restlessness and apprehension unless intracranial damage (**41.** *Head Injuries;* **59 – 2.** *Intracranial Bleeding*) or intrathoracic injuries (**28.** *Chest Injuries*) are causative factors, or extreme respiratory depression is present. Pentazocine lactate (Talwin), 15 to 30 mg. intramuscularly or intravenously, is an effective anodyne without marked respiratory depressive effect.

4. Hospitalization if blood loss has been excessive, if extensive surgical repair is needed or if damage to a major blood vessel (especially an artery) is evident or suspected (**59 – 1**).

5. Presence of any clotting defects should be assessed initially by history, presence of petechiae or purpura, bleeding and clotting time, quality of clot (firmness, retraction, lysis), platelet number by smear and count, prothrombin and partial thromboplastin time and fibrinogen level.

HEMORRHAGE FROM SPECIAL SITES

42 – 3. BLEEDING FROM ADENOID FOSSA

Severe hemorrhage following adenoidectomy can usually be controlled by proper insertion of a posterior nasal pack (**14 – 6**). Enough blood may be lost to require transfusion.

42 – 4. BLEEDING FROM MAJOR ARTERIES See 59 – 1.

42 – 5. BLEEDING FROM EARS

Following trauma to the head, bleeding from an ear is pathognomonic of skull fracture (**41 – 12**), provided there are no lacerations of the external auditory canal.

TREATMENT

Hospitalize *at once* for head injury care. No attempt should be made to cleanse the canal. A sterile pad may be applied over the ear, but nothing should be inserted into the external auditory canal.

42 – 6. EPIDURAL HEMORRHAGE See 41 – 19; 48 – 26. *Extradural Hemorrhage in Children*

42 – 7. EPISTAXIS See 45 – 3.

42 – 8. ESOPHAGEAL BLEEDING See 37 – 4.

42 – 9. EXTRADURAL HEMORRHAGE See 41 – 19; 48 – 26. *Extradural Hemorrhage in Children*

42 – 10. BLEEDING IN AND AROUND THE EYES See 35 – 29 through 35 – 32. *Eye Injuries*

42 – 11.   GASTROINTESTINAL TRACT See **37 – 6.** *Anorectal Conditions;* **42 – 25.** *Bleeding from the Stomach;* **42 – 22.** *Rectal Bleeding*

42 – 12.   HEPATIC BLEEDING See **55 – 1.** *Abdominal Injuries*

42 – 13.   INTRAABDOMINAL BLEEDING See **42 – 22.** *Rectal Bleeding;* **55 – 1.** *Abdominal Injuries*

42 – 14.   INTRAALVEOLAR BLEEDING See **28.** *Chest Injuries;* **42 – 17.** *Bleeding from the Lungs*

42 – 15.   INTRACRANIAL HEMORRHAGE

NONTRAUMATIC See **59 – 2.** *Subarachnoid Hemorrhage.*

TRAUMATIC See **41 – 19.** *Extradural Hemorrhage;* **41 – 20.** *Subdural Hemorrhage;* **48 – 32.** *Head Injuries in Children;* **59 – 2.**

42 – 16.   INTRAPERICARDIAL HEMORRHAGE See **26 – 22.** *Hemocardium with Tamponade*

42 – 17.   BLEEDING FROM THE LUNGS. (See also **28 – 3.** *Contusions of the Lungs*)

Gross hemorrhage from the lungs from any cause requires immediate hospitalization. Morphine sulfate may be given subcutaneously or intravenously to allay the characteristic acute apprehension. Treatment of hypovolemic shock (**53 – 7**) may be necessary before and during transportation to a hospital. Bleeding following therapeutic pneumothorax can sometimes be controlled by diluting 1 ml. of surgical Pituitrin to 10 ml. with normal salt solution and administering it intravenously slowly – no faster than 1 ml. per minute.

42 – 18.   BLEEDING FROM MAJOR BLOOD VESSELS See **17.** *Urgency Evaluation – Triage;* **42 – 1.** *Local Measures;* **42 – 2.** *General Measures*

42 – 19.   MEDIASTINAL BLEEDING See **28.** *Chest Injuries*

42 – 20. HEMORRHAGE FROM THE NECK

Knife slashings and glass cuts (accidental, suicidal or homicidal) may cause hemorrhage from the large superficial neck vessels and must be controlled immediately to prevent exsanguination. Digital pressure or pinching of the bleeding vessels or clamping with hemostats may be necessary. No attempt should be made to tie off the vessels in severe cases; blood loss should be countered by the measures outlined for hypovolemic shock (**57 – 3**) and the patient transferred by ambulance to a hospital with the clamps in place, accompanied if possible by a physician, nurse or trained attendant. If the patient is in profound hypovolemic shock, 5% dextrose in saline, 1/6 molar lactate or normal salt solution intravenously en route may be necessary to support the circulation until whole blood can be administered. Morphine sulfate, 10 to 15 mg., should be given, preferably intravenously, before transportation to allay the patient's typical extreme anxiety and apprehension and to control restlessness and pain.

42 – 21. BLEEDING FROM THE NOSE See 14 – 6. *Nasal Packing;* 45 – 3. *Epistaxis*

42 – 22. RECTAL BLEEDING

Blood in the stool, whether bright red or changed, represents a potential emergency until its source (Fig. 25) can be determined. If gastrointestinal tract hypermobility is present, blood from the respiratory and upper gastrointestinal tract may appear unchanged in the rectum. Conversely, retention of blood from the colon may cause alteration falsely suggestive of a lesion of the upper portion of the tract. In addition, ingestion of brightly colored substances – beets, red ink or paint, Jello, strawberries, etc. – can mimic bright red blood in the stool. For treatment see the area involved.

42 – 23. BLEEDING FROM THE SCALP See 41 – 21. *Lacerations of the Scalp*

42 – 24. SPLENIC BLEEDING See 55 – 1. *Abdominal Injuries;* 55 – 31.

42 – 25. BLEEDING FROM THE STOMACH

Vomiting of grossly bloody, blood-stained or coffee-ground material and passage of tarry or red stools (**42 – 22**) are specific indica-

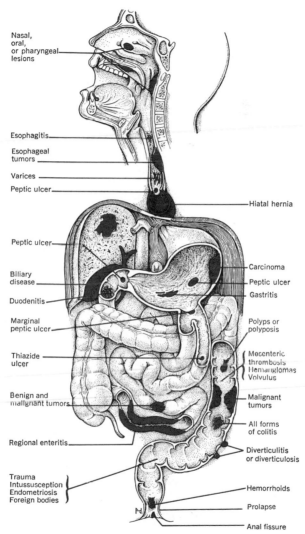

Nasal,
oral,
or pharyngeal
lesions

Esophagitis

Esophageal
tumors

Varices

Peptic ulcer

Hiatal hernia

Peptic ulcer

Biliary
disease

Duodenitis

Marginal
peptic ulcer

Carcinoma

Peptic ulcer

Gastritis

Polyps or
polyposis

Thiazide
ulcer

Mesenteric
thrombosis
Hemangiomas
Volvulus

Benign and
malignant tumors

Malignant
tumors

All forms
of colitis

Regional enteritis

Diverticulitis
or diverticulosis

Trauma
Intussusception
Endometriosis
Foreign bodies

Hemorrhoids

Prolapse

Anal fissure

Figure 25. Some important causes of blood in the stool. (Modified from Turell, R.: Hosp. Med., Vol. 4, No. 6, 1968.)

tions for hospitalization for immediate thorough clinical and laboratory investigation. Preliminary treatment for hypovolemic shock (**53 — 7**) may be necessary. Vomiting can usually be controlled by intramuscular injection of dimenhydrinate (Dramamine), 50 mg. every 4 to 6 hours.

42 — 26. **SUBDURAL HEMORRHAGE** See **41 — 20; 48 — 32.** *Head Injuries in Children*

42 — 27. **THROAT**

In the absence of evidence of local injury to the nose (**45**) or throat, bleeding from the posterior wall of the nasopharynx following severe trauma should be considered as indicative of basal skull fracture (**41 — 15**). For post-tonsillectomy bleeding, see **42 — 43.**

42 — 28. **UMBILICAL STUMP HEMORRHAGE**

This condition usually occurs during the first 2 weeks after birth.
TREATMENT
1. Mild cases can be controlled by direct pressure.
2. Severe cases require hospitalization after control of hemorrhage by clamping or ligatures.

42 — 29. **URETHRAL BLEEDING** See **38.** *Genitourinary Tract Emergencies, Traumatic Conditions*

42 — 30. **VAGINAL BLEEDING** See **38; 38 — 9.** *Vaginal and Vulval Injuries;* **39 — 4.** *Dysmenorrhea;* **39 — 6.** *Menorrhagia;* **39 — 7.** *Metrorrhagia*

In certain cases, examination for rape or criminal assault (**9**) must be performed.

42 — 31. **BLEEDING FROM VARICOSITIES** See **59 — 12.** *Varicose Veins*

HEMORRHAGE FROM SPECIFIC CONDITIONS

42 — 32. **ABORTIONS** See **47 — 1.**

42—33. ANEURYSMS See **59—2.** *Saccular Aneurysm;* **59—3.** *Dissecting Aneurysm*

42—34. ANTICOAGULANT THERAPY (See also **49—79.** *Anticoagulants*)

1. If caused by Dicumarol (**49—265**), give 5 to 15 mg. of an aqueous solution of vitamin K_1 (AquaMephyton) intravenously, or 5 to 10 mg. of phytonadione (Konakion) intramuscularly; repeat as necessary. Severe cases require blood transfusions.

2. If caused by heparin (**49—363**), inject 50 mg. of protamine sulfate intravenously very slowly and repeat every 15 minutes until the desired effect has been obtained. Neutralization of the effects of long-acting depot heparin may require several injections of protamine sulfate. Transfusions of whole blood may be necessary.

42—35. BLOOD DYSCRASIAS

Leukemia, hemophilia, purpura, sickle cell anemia and other blood dyscrasias can cause severe intractable bleeding. Hospitalization for thorough study, transfusions and other therapy is always indicated.

42—36. CORTICOSTEROID THERAPY (See also **49—227.** *Cortisone*)

Gross hemorrhage from softening of scars may occur, usually in the gastrointestinal tract. Immediate hospitalization after treatment of hypovolemic shock (**53—7**) is indicated.

42—37. ECTOPIC PREGNANCY See **47—2.**

42—38. HEPATIC DISEASE

Hospitalization for control of hemorrhage—usually from esophageal varices (**37—4**)—and treatment of the underlying cause are essential.

42—39. MENORRHAGIA See **39—6.**

42—40. METRORRHAGIA See **39—7.**

41—41. POSTOPERATIVE BLEEDING

Mild bleeding or oozing usually can be controlled by absolute rest, application of pressure locally or over "pressure points" if accessible, sedation by rapid-acting barbiturates or paraldehyde, control of restlessness and anxiety by small doses of morphine sulfate subcutaneously or intravenously or by packing, clamping, tying or suturing after exposure of the bleeding vessel.

Severe hemorrhage may require heroic measures.

1. Control of the hemorrhage by whatever means are available may mean the difference between life and death to the patient. If necessary, the following measures should be used promptly and without waiting for preparation of a sterile operating field:

Digital pressure or pinching of the hemorrhaging vessel.

Application of a tourniquet if on an extremity (**42—1**).

Packing with gauze.

Clamping.

Ligation.

2. Treatment of hypovolemic shock (**53—7**).

3. Transportation by ambulance for hospitalization as soon as the patient's condition has stabilized, preferably to the hospital where the surgery was done. Intravenous supportive therapy should be continued in the ambulance. Every possible effort should be made to get in touch by telephone with the surgeon who performed the original surgical procedure. If this is not possible, a résumé outlining all emergency treatment given should be sent with the patient. In all cases, the hospital to which the patient is being sent should be notified in advance so that there will be no delay in treatment on the patient's arrival.

42—42. POSTEXTRACTION HEMORRHAGE

Postextraction hemorrhage can result in loss of a large amount of blood.

TREATMENT

1. Have the patient bite firmly on a small pad of gauze.

2. Pack the area with sterile cotton moistened with 1:1000 epinephrine hydrochloride (Adrenalin) solution.

3. Inject sodium estrone sulfate (Premarin Intravenous), 20 mg. intravenously. Repeat in 1 hour if necessary.

4. Place a small piece of oxidized cellulose (Gelfoam or Oxycel)

in the bleeding socket and hold firmly in place with a pad of gauze held between the teeth.

5. Give acetaminophen, with or without codeine sulfate, for pain.

6. If severe bleeding persists, suture the gums over the bleeding socket.

7. Instruct the patient not to eat solid foods of any kind until he has received further dental care.

8. If possible, refer the patient back to the dentist who performed the extraction.

42—43. POST-TONSILLECTOMY BLEEDING

Post-tonsillectomy bleeding may be delayed, profuse and difficult to control. Hospitalization for suturing under general anesthesia often is required. To prevent swallowing blood, the patient should sit up during transportation unless signs of severe shock (**53**) are present. Morphine sulfate subcutaneously to allay anxiety and to quiet the patient may be necessary.

42—44. POSTPARTUM BLEEDING See 39—10.

42—45. SPONTANEOUS HEMORRHAGE

Although trauma is the most common cause of severe hemorrhage, spontaneous onset of bleeding of various degrees of severity may be caused by:

1. Congenital structural blood vessel weakness (**59—2; 59—3.** *Dissecting Aortic Aneurysm*).

2. Degenerative disease processes involving the blood vessel walls (**59—2**).

3. Erosion of a blood vessel by pressure from an adjacent space-consuming or invasive tumor.

4. Drugs or other agents which interfere with normal coagulation of the blood (**42—34; 49—79.** *Anticoagulants*) or cause softening of previously formed scars (**49—227.** *Cortisone;* **49—593.** *Phenylbutazone*).

5. Familial or acquired blood dyscrasias (**42—35**).

The known or suspected presence of any of these factors requires hospitalization after treatment of hypovolemic shock (**53—7**) for thorough investigation and treatment of the underlying condition.

43. METABOLIC DISORDERS

See also **33**. *Endocrine Emergencies.*

43−1. ACIDOSIS

Formation or accumulation of acid products in the body more rapidly than removal or neutralization can take place results in a characteristic train of symptoms. This disturbance in metabolism may be caused by interference with respiration by asthma, bronchitis, pneumonia, emphysema or other pulmonary conditions, cardiac decompensation, high concentration of carbon dioxide in the air or deep narcosis. The same effect may be caused by alkali deficiency, excessive acid production or decreased acid urine excretion as seen in diabetes mellitus or kidney failure.

SIGNS AND SYMPTOMS. All may be modified, masked or intensified by the causative condition but in general consist of headache, drowsiness, generalized weakness, pain in the abdomen and extremities, tachycardia, rapid respiration (later becoming weak and shallow), fruity odor to the breath, progressive stupor and coma. Acetone and diacetic acid are present in the urine. Arterial pH and Pco_2 determinations are of assistance in determining the type and severity of acidosis.

TREATMENT

1. Keep the patient warm but not overheated.
2. Give caffeine sodiobenzoate, 0.5 gm. intramuscularly.
3. Inject 50 ml. of sodium bicarbonate solution (44.6 mEq. of sodium) intravenously, repeated as necessary; in severe cases this should be followed by an infusion of 500 ml. of 1/6 molar sodium lactate solution.
4. Start treatment of the underlying causative condition as soon as identified.
5. Hospitalize for acid-base balance determinations and definitive therapy. (See also **14−9**. *Peritoneal Dialysis;* **29−3**. *Diabetic Coma;* **48−20**. *Diabetic Coma in Children;* **52−1**. *Asthma;* **48−6**. *Asthma in Children.*)

43−2. ADDISONIAN CRISES See **33−1**. *Adrenal Insufficiency*

43−3. ADRENAL INSUFFICIENCY, ACUTE (Addisonian Crisis) See **33−1**.

43—4. AIR SICKNESS

This is due not to changes in atmospheric pressure but to motion. See **43—18.** *Motion Sickness.*

43—5. ALKALOSIS

Alkali excess in the blood may be due to hyperventilation (**34—6**) caused by high temperature—body or external (**57—2** through **57—4**), hysteria (**50—6** and **11**), encephalitis (**62—5**), hyperpnea due to high altitudes (**23—1.** *Altitude Sickness;* **23—6.** *Mountain Sickness*) and anesthesia (second stage). In addition, excessive loss of acid-chloride ions from prolonged vomiting or gastric suction, overzealous administration of alkaline substances or congenital metabolic variations from normal may cause a similar clinical picture.

Signs and Symptoms. Restlessness, irritability, excitability, slow deep respiration (the rate may be as low as 5 per minute) and signs of neuromuscular irritability: *Erb's sign* (muscular response to a very weak galvanic current); *Chvostek's sign* (twitching of the facial muscles brought on by tapping the skin just anterior to the external auditory meatus); *Trousseau's sign* (an "obstetrical position" of the hand and fingers brought on by constriction of the arm above the elbow).

Treatment

If due to hyperventilation, see **34—6.**

If due to excess alkali:

1. Discontinue alkali therapy.
2. Force fluids by mouth or give 500 to 1000 ml. of normal saline intravenously. In severe cases, ammonium chloride intravenously may be required.
3. Give calcium gluconate, 10 ml. of 10% solution intravenously.
4. Hospitalize for laboratory studies and treatment.

43—6. ALTITUDE SICKNESS See **23—1; 23—6.** *Mountain Sickness*

43—7. CAISSON DISEASE (*Bends,* Compressed Air Sickness, Decompression Sickness) See **23—3.**

43—8. CAR SICKNESS See **43—18.** *Motion Sickness*

43 – 9. COMPRESSED AIR SICKNESS See **23 – 3.** *Caisson Disease*

43 – 10. DIABETIC COMA See **29 – 3; 48 – 20.** *Diabetic Coma in Children*

43 – 11. GOUT

Acute totally disabling swelling and pain in the joints, especially of the feet, may occur with gouty arthritis and represent a true emergency.

TREATMENT

1. Codeine sulfate, 0.06 gm. subcutaneously, or pentazocine lactate (Talwin), 15 to 30 mg. intramuscularly. Administration of morphine or other addictive narcotics should be avoided.

2. Colchicine, 4 ml. (0.2 mg.) intravenously, followed in 4 hours by 0.5 mg. by mouth every hour for 8 doses or until nausea or diarrhea becomes troublesome.

3. Dextrose 5% in saline, 500 to 1000 ml. intravenously.

4. Referral for complete medical check-up after relief of acute symptoms and signs. Hospitalization is rarely necessary.

43 – 12. HYPERCALCEMIA

High serum calcium levels may occur from excessive prolonged intake of vitamin D and in conditions such as metastatic malignancy, sarcoidosis, multiple myeloma and hyperparathyroidism (**33 – 3.** *Acute Parathyroid Intoxication*). Manifestations are usually headache, nausea, vomiting, dryness of the mucous membranes of the nose and mouth, pruritus and urinary distress.

TREATMENT

1. Antinauseants as required.

2. Correction of dehydration (**6**).

3. Consideration of the need for corticosteroid therapy. In severe cases, intravenous injection of 100 to 300 mg. of hydrocortisone may be indicated.

4. Hospitalization for evaluation and treatment of the primary cause may be required.

43 – 13. HYPERINSULINISM See **29 – 3.** *Diabetes Mellitus*

43 – 14. HYPERPARATHYROIDISM See **33 – 3.** *Acute Parathyroid Intoxication*

43—15. HYPERTHYROID CRISES (See also **33—5.** *Hyperthyroid Emergencies*)

Two types which may require emergency therapy are recognized:
The activated type, characterized by restlessness increasing to delirium, tachycardia, vomiting, diarrhea, dehydration, occasional jaundice and high temperature, sometimes as high as 41°C. (105.8°F.).
TREATMENT
1. Physical restraint until adequate sedation can be accomplished.
2. Oxygen inhalations by face mask and rebreathing bag.
3. Cold packs and antipyretics.
4. Immediate hospitalization.
The apathetic type, characterized by extreme prostration with muscular hypotonia, mental apathy and a relatively low temperature rise, usually not above 38.3°C. (101°F.).
TREATMENT
1. Administration of oxygen under positive pressure if cyanosis is present, preferably by face mask and rebreathing bag.
2. Treatment of shock (**53—7**).
3. Immediate hospitalization.

43—16. HYPOGLYCEMIA

Although often used synonymously with *hyperinsulinism* (**29—3**), hypoglycemia is a much broader term. Among its causes are abnormal functioning of the islets of Langerhans (**33—2**); liver, pituitary and suprarenal disorders (**33—4**); severe head injuries (**41**); "dumping syndrome" after gastric resection (**33—2**); and administration of excessive amounts of insulin, or inadequate food intake after the usual dose of insulin. Occasionally, oral hypoglycemic agents may cause an acute picture. Other causes may be pregnancy; extreme muscular fatigue; sympathetic nervous system disorders, often functional; renal glycosuria; and idiopathic hypoglycemia of infancy.

SIGNS, SYMPTOMS AND TREATMENT are the same as outlined for *Hyperinsulinism* (**29—3.** *Diabetes Mellitus*).

43—17. HYPOPARATHYROID CRISES

Hypoparathyroid crises are caused by atrophy, degeneration, fibrosis or surgical removal of the parathyroid glands. See **33—3.** *Hypoparathyroidism.*

43—18. MOTION SICKNESS

Certain individuals who are particularly prone to air, sea or train sickness do not follow the usual course of rapid complete recovery following cessation of the motion. Nausea, vomiting and dizziness may be severe or persistent enough to bring the patient for emergency treatment. Any normal human being can be made sick by motion. The exact causal mechanism is not as yet fully understood, although labyrinthine vestibular stimulation undoubtedly plays a part. Vertical (rise and fall—elevators, ships, planes, buses, cars), linear (forward and backward, stop and go—cars, buses, planes, playground and carnival swings, etc.) or angular acceleration (the normal rhythmic pitch and sway of moving vehicles) or any combination of all three may be the precipitating agent which may be reinforced, facilitated and enhanced by special sense stimuli such as sound, sight, taste, smell and perception of vibration. Undoubtedly psychologic and emotional states contribute to and exaggerate motion sickness, although they cannot cause it.

SIGNS AND SYMPTOMS. Restlessness, general malaise, hypersensitivity to sensory stimuli, lassitude, yawning, pallor and difficulty in breathing. Waves of nausea and vomiting may be present followed by acute depression, apathy and generalized prostration. Vague and inconstant objective signs, such as increased pulse rate and blood pressure, are transient only.

TREATMENT (Prophylactic, symptomatic and definitive)

1. Avoidance of eating or drinking just before starting a trip.

2. Proper selection of a vehicle and location therein:

As large a vehicle as possible.

A central seat or cabin to minimize roll (sideways motion) and pitch (end-to-end, up-and-down motion).

Smoothly driven vehicles—a bus is more stable than a passenger car, a jet more stable than a propeller-driven aircraft.

Focusing the eyes on a distant object, especially while traveling by air.

Avoidance of a seat over the rear axle in a bus or passenger car—the site of maximum up-and-down motion.

3. Belladonna alkaloids prophylactically as preliminary tranquilizers, sometimes combined with barbiturates or chloral hydrate.

4. Antinauseants. Repeated tests conducted by the U.S. Armed Services have resulted in the conclusion that the following are the most effective drugs for prevention and treatment of motion sickness of any type (air sickness, car sickness, sea sickness):

Meclizine hydrochloride (Bonine), 25 to 50 mg. orally once daily.

Cyclizine hydrochloride (Marezine), 50 mg. orally 3 or 4 times daily; 50 mg. intramuscularly, 3 times a day; or 100 mg. by rectal suppository, every 4 to 6 hours. For children the dosage must be adjusted according to age (**4**).

Dimenhydrinate (Dramamine), 50 mg. orally or intramuscularly 3 times a day, or 100 mg. by rectal suppository twice a day.

Prochlorperazine dimaleate (Compazine), 10 mg. orally 3 or 4 times daily, or 10 mg. intramuscularly (deep in buttocks) 3 times a day. In children the oral dosage should be adjusted as follows:

Under 9 kilograms of body weight — not to be used.

9 to 12 kilograms of body weight — 2.5 mg. not more than twice a day.

13 to 18 kilograms of body weight — 2.5 mg., not to exceed 3 times a day.

19 to 40 kilograms of body weight — 3 mg. twice a day.

5. Amphetamine or dextroamphetamine orally to combat depression.

6. Replacement therapy (**6.** *Fluid Replacement*).

PROGNOSIS. Complete recovery without residual ill-effects always takes place after cessation of motion, although symptoms may persist for several days.

43-19. PANCREAS See **29-3**. *Diabetes Mellitus;* **33-2**.

43-20. PARATHYROID CRISIS See **33-3**. *Acute Parathyroid Intoxication*

43-21. PITUITARY See **33-4**.

43-22. PORPHYRIA

Acute intermittent porphyria may cause signs and symptoms requiring emergency care in adults of both sexes. Abdominal pain, often severe enough to be mistaken for an acute surgical abdomen, may be the presenting complaint, but a wide variety of neurologic complaints of extreme severity may be confused with poliomyelitis (**30-21; 46-9; 48-49**), encephalitis (**48-24; 62-5**) or acute poisoning (**49**). The characteristic laboratory findings are the change in color of the urine to dark red or even black on exposure to sunlight and increased urinary porphyrins.

Treatment

1. Control of severe pain by meperidine hydrochloride (Demerol).
2. Assistance with respiration (**11 – 1**). In severe cases tracheostomy (**14 – 12**) may be necessary.
3. Sedation by chloral hydrate, paraldehyde or chlorpromazine hydrochloride (Thorazine). *Barbiturates should never be used.*
4. Hospitalization during the usually prolonged recovery from acute episodes.

43 – 23. RADIATION SICKNESS See **18 – 7.** *X-ray Burns;* **63 – 4.** *Ionizing Radiation Effects*

43 – 24. SEA SICKNESS See **43 – 18.** *Motion Sickness*

43 – 25. TETANY

ACTIVE

Signs and Symptoms of acute tetany are spectacular and consist of carpopedal spasm; spasm resulting from involvement of the autonomic nerve supply of the iris, bronchi, diaphragm, heart, gastrointestinal tract and bladder; and convulsions of varying degrees of severity. These convulsions may be generalized or unilateral or confined to isolated muscle groups.

Treatment

1. Treatment of the underlying condition.
2. Carbogen inhalations or paper bag rebreathing if tetany is due to hyperventilation (**34 – 6**).
3. Calcium gluconate, 10 ml. of 10% solution intravenously.
4. Hospitalization for blood studies unless hyperventilation (**34 – 6**) is the causative condition.

LATENT

Caused by hypocalcemia, alkalosis or occasionally hyperphosphatemia, and characterized by neuromuscular excitability; this condition is rarely encountered as an emergency. Erb's, Chvostek's and Trousseau's signs (**43 – 5**) are pathognomonic. No emergency treatment is required. The patient should be referred for medical evaluation and treatment.

43—26. THYROID See **33—5; 43—15.** *Hyperthyroid Crises*

43—27. TRAIN SICKNESS See **43—18.** *Motion Sickness*

44. MUSCULOSKELETAL DISORDERS

44—1. ARTHRITIS

Although the numerous conditions grouped under this general heading usually cause chronic symptoms, acute discomfort caused by fulminating infections (especially viral) or by traumatic aggravation of the underlying condition may require emergency care or hospitalization. Use of a bed board, home application of cold or heat, local massage and large doses of salicylates by mouth may give relief in some types of arthritis. Muscle relaxants such as 5 mg. of diazepam (Valium) or 350 mg. of carisoprodol (Rela, Soma) orally 3 times a day, and 2 ml. (60 mg.) of orphenadrine citrate (Norflex) intramuscularly, or 1 tablet orally 2 or 3 times a day, may be effective. Corticosteroids and phenylbutazone (Butazolidin), although effective, as a rule are not utilized for emergency therapy since their safe use requires controlled follow-up care. For treatment of gout, see **43—11.**

44—2. BACK INJURIES

Back injuries vary markedly in intensity and type from slight muscular strains to fracture-dislocation of the spine with cord damage and partial or complete motor and sensory paralysis. For treatment, see under the specific type of injury.

44—3. FRACTURES See under the bone or area involved.

44—4. SOFT TISSUE DAMAGE

Soft tissue damage (contusion, sprains, strains) may cause acute symptoms which often can be relieved by one or more of the following means:
1. For control of this type of pain acetylsalicylic acid (aspirin)

with or without codeine sulfate by mouth is very effective. In extreme cases morphine sulfate can be given subcutaneously in the smallest possible effective doses.

2. To decrease muscle spasm, cold packs often are of value, as are skeletal muscle relaxants (**44 – 1**).

3. Application of local heat and gentle massage improves circulation and may decrease pain.

4. Infiltration of "trigger points" with 0.5 to 1.0% procaine or lidocaine (Xylocaine).

5. To lessen skin sensitivity, spraying of the painful areas with ethyl chloride.

6. Limitation of movement and support in the cervical area may be accomplished to some extent by snug application of a Thomas collar if the patient is ambulatory; severe injuries require careful handling and transportation in the supine position, sometimes with sandbags and manual traction, preferably applied by the attending physician. A lumbrosacral or sacroiliac support or tight adhesive strapping may give relief if the injury is to the soft tissues of the low back.

44 – 5. BURSITIS (See also **44 – 59**. *Peritendinitis*)

Inflammation of any of the numerous bursae of the body is very painful and may be totally disabling. Anodynes, including narcotics, should be given as needed to control the acute pain until the patient can receive definitive treatment. If the bursa is hot, red and swollen, 600,000 units of penicillin intramuscularly, or tetracyclines in adequate doses orally, may be of benefit, as may be immobilization and spraying the skin over the affected part with ethyl chloride. Infiltration of the painful area with 1% procaine or lidocaine (Xylocaine) may give spectacular relief, although the patient should be warned of the possibility of a temporary flare-up when the effect of the local anesthetic wears off. Slower relief may follow daily intramuscular injection of 1 ml. (1000 mcg.) of vitamin B_{12}. Hot compresses are contraindicated; cold sometimes decreases the acute discomfort.

Injection of 1 ml. (25 mg.) of hydrocortisone acetate preceded by a local anesthetic directly into the affected bursa sometimes is of benefit, although there may be a temporary increase in discomfort when the local anesthetic effect is dissipated. All patients should be instructed to make arrangements for follow-up care.

44 — 6.   CERVICAL INJURIES See **44 — 58**. *Neck Injuries;* **46 — 8**. *Whiplash Injuries;* **46 — 11**. *Spinal Injuries with Cord Compression*

44 — 7.   DISLOCATIONS (See also **14 — 10**. *Reduction of Dislocations*)

General principles of emergency care.   X-rays should always be taken before reduction of a dislocation is attempted. If a fracture is present, especially in the region of the shoulder or hip, reduction should be postponed until the patient has been hospitalized. If no fracture is present, reduction may be attempted by any of the approved methods (**14 — 10**). Morphine sulfate should be given 20 minutes before manipulation except in small children. Dislocated small joints or epiphyses can sometimes be reduced under a local anesthetic injected directly into the joint or into the hematoma caused by the injury. *Before and after reduction,* the circulation and nerve supply should be checked carefully and x-rays taken to verify correct position and alignment. If 1 or 2 attempts at reduction by any method are unsuccessful, no further manipulation should be attempted; instead, the patient should be hospitalized for possible general anesthesia.

DISLOCATIONS REQUIRING SPECIAL HANDLING

44 — 8.   ACROMIOCLAVICULAR SEPARATIONS

Complete acromioclavicular separations are clinically apparent, but more often lesser degrees of separation can be demonstrated only by comparative x-rays of the shoulder girdles taken with a heavy weight in each hand.

TREATMENT

1. Mild cases require only support for 2 or 3 weeks with a Velpeau bandage.

2. Severe cases require hospitalization for operative repair.

44 — 9.   ANKLE DISLOCATIONS

Ankle dislocations of any degree usually do not occur without accompanying fractures, especially of the avulsion type, and gross ligamentous damage. To prevent subsequent instability, hospitalization for surgical repair of the damaged ligamentous structures is usually necessary even if reduction of the dislocation has been accomplished as an emergency measure.

44 – 10.   CARPAL DISLOCATIONS See **44 – 16.** *Lunate Dislocations;*
44 – 19. *Perilunar Dislocations*

44 – 11.   CERVICAL SPINE DISLOCATIONS (See also **44 – 58.** *Neck Injuries;* **46 – 11.** *Spinal Injuries with Cord Compression*)

Immediate hospitalization with the head and neck immobilized by sandbags is imperative. Manual neck traction during transportation may be necessary.

44 – 12.   ELBOW DISLOCATIONS (See also **44 – 21.** *Radial Head Subluxations*)

Provided no fractures are present, dislocations of the elbow can sometimes be reduced under heavy sedation but without anesthesia by the following method:
1. Have the patient lie face down on a narrow table with the injured arm hanging down.
2. Make gentle downward traction on the wrist.
3. When the olecranon slides distally on the humerus with wrist traction continued, lift the humerus laterally.
4. Check for complete reduction by palpation, comparison with the uninjured side and x-rays.
5. Immobilize with a Velpeau bandage.
6. Arrange for a check-up on circulation and sensation in 24 hours. If reduction cannot be obtained in 2 attempts, the patient should be hospitalized for reduction under general anesthetic.

44 – 13.   EPIPHYSIAL DISLOCATIONS See **44 – 30.**

44 – 14.   FINGER DISLOCATIONS See **44 – 20.** *Phalangeal Dislocations*

44 – 15.   HIP DISLOCATIONS

Hospitalization for reduction under general anesthetic is always required.

44 – 16.   LUNATE DISLOCATIONS (See also **44 – 19.** *Perilunar Dislocations*)

Severe direct trauma to the wrist may cause rupture of the ligamentous structures at the distal end of the lunate with subsequent partial or complete rotatory displacement. Hospitalization is usually indicated because reduction may be difficult and operative fixation of the distal end of the bone may be necessary.

44—17. NASAL BONE AND CARTILAGE DISLOCATIONS See 45—5.

44—18. PATELLAR DISLOCATIONS

Direct trauma or violent contraction of the quadriceps femoris can cause lateral dislocation of the patella, especially if the lateral parapatellar ridge is lower than normal or genu valgus is marked. Medial dislocations are very rare. Reduction can usually be obtained without anesthetic by a sudden forcible thrust medially with the palm of the hand.

Recurrent dislocations may require operative transference of the tibial tuberosity medially or other revision of quadriceps pull as an elective procedure.

44—19. PERILUNAR DISLOCATIONS OF THE CARPUS

In this type of dislocation the lunate remains in normal relationship to the radius and ulna while all of the other carpal bones are displaced. Routine x-rays may be misinterpreted, especially if associated fractures of the scaphoid or cuneiform are present. Reduction is usually difficult and requires regional block or general anesthesia, followed by immobilization for 6 to 8 weeks in a plaster of Paris short arm cast.

44—20. PHALANGEAL (CARPAL) DISLOCATIONS

Limited almost exclusively to the metacarpophalangeal joint of the thumb and the proximal interphalangeal joints of the other digits, these dislocations can usually be reduced easily by traction and manipulation, often without anesthesia. If necessary, 1% procaine or lidocaine (Xylocaine) can be injected into the joint before manipulation. By determining that the finger flexes normally into the palm, lateral or medial deviation (or slight degrees of rotation) can be avoided. After reduction, a short plaster cast should be applied and the position confirmed by x-rays.

Immobilization for 3 weeks, followed by institution of active motion, will usually result in regaining full function, although

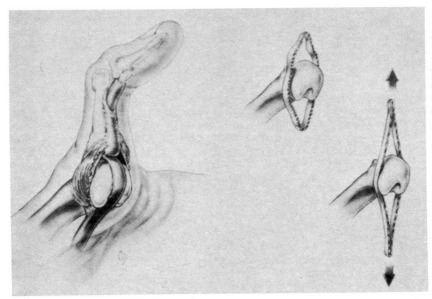

Figure 26. **A locked thumb dislocation:** The metacarpal head (left) pushes forward through a "buttonhole" on the capsule's palmar aspect, shown in schematic (middle). Reduction attempts using longitudinal traction won't work, but merely tighten the slit (right). Surgical reduction is necessary. (From Flatt, A. E.: Consultant, Vol. 12, No. 4, p. 23, April, 1972.)

some permanent thickening of the capsule may result. Compressive centripetal wrappings (**59–14**) are of value in reduction of local edema. A dislocation of the metacarpophalangeal joint of the thumb may become locked due to anterior protrusion of the metacarpal head through a rent in the capsule (Fig. 26). Operative reduction is necessary.

44–21. RADIAL HEAD SUBLUXATIONS

Partial subluxation of the proximal end of the radius from the sling formed by the orbicular ligament occurs almost exclusively in small children in the toddling age, although it may occur in injudiciously handled infants. The mechanism of injury is usually a sudden jerk on the outstretched arm by an adult leading or lifting the child by the hand.

SIGNS AND SYMPTOMS. Severe pain which is difficult to localize, with refusal of the patient to fully extend the forearm, is characteristic. The child usually holds the arm with the elbow slightly flexed and the forearm pronated and resists any attempts at examination or motion. X-rays are of no value in diagnosis except to rule out associated conditions, especially displacement of the epicondylar or radial epiphyses (**44 – 30**).

TREATMENT

If the injury is recent, complete reduction can usually be accomplished without anesthesia by:

1. Gentle traction on the forearm.
2. Pressure over the radial head with the thumb.
3. Gradual extension and supination of the forearm. A palpable (sometimes audible) click or snap indicates reduction.
4. Application of a sling. The parents should be instructed to encourage use of the arm as soon as the pain subsides.

44 – 22. SHOULDER DISLOCATIONS

Whenever possible, x-rays should be taken and tests for neurologic deficits done before reduction of a dislocated shoulder is attempted. If the films show a fracture – usually of the rim of the glenoid – hospitalization is indicated. If no fracture is demonstrated, reduction may be attempted by one of several methods (**14 – 10**). Pain and apprehension should be controlled by a preliminary injection of morphine sulfate.

44 – 23. SPINAL DISLOCATIONS

These usually occur in the cervical or upper dorsal regions. See **44 – 11.** *Cervical Spine Dislocations;* **44 – 58.** *Neck Injuries;* **46 – 11.** *Spinal Injuries with Cord Compression.*

44 – 24. STERNOCLAVICULAR DISLOCATIONS

These injuries are uncommon and usually heal satisfactorily if partially immobilized by tight adhesive strapping over a pressure pad and use of a sling. Severe cases require operative repair as an elective procedure.

44–25. TARSAL DISLOCATIONS

Slipping between the tarsal bones is usually of small degree but can be very painful and cause complete disability, especially in professional athletes. Careful comparative x-ray studies are essential for diagnosis.

TREATMENT

Treatment consists of manipulative or open reduction with plaster cast immobilization.

44–26. TEMPOROMANDIBULAR DISLOCATIONS

These dislocations are usually unilateral and, because of spasm of the powerful muscles controlling the jaw, are difficult to reduce. If heavy pressure downward and backward (with the operator's thumbs well padded) does not cause reduction, the patient should be referred to a dental surgeon. General anesthetic may be necessary for reduction.

44–27. TOE DISLOCATIONS

Toe dislocations are easily reducible by gentle traction followed by strapping to adjacent toes for 2 or 3 weeks.

44–28. ULNAR SHAFT FRACTURES (Monteggia)

Ulnar shaft fractures with radial head dislocation usually require open reduction in adults, closed manipulation in children.

44–29. EPICONDYLITIS

The acute pain from this condition (probably a localized viral fascitis or fibrositis) can sometimes be relieved by spraying with ethyl chloride. Temporary (sometimes permanent) relief follows infiltration of the painful area with a local anesthetic. Local heat may be of benefit in some cases; it may make others worse. Application of a splint or cast to control rotation of the forearm as well as elbow and wrist motion may be necessary. Since the discomfort is often acute, anodynes are indicated until the patient can receive definitive orthopedic care.

44 — 30. EPIPHYSIAL DISPLACEMENTS

Many of these displacements or slips reduce spontaneously. Examination for localized tenderness or guarding muscle spasm, fluoroscopic examination for excess mobility and comparative x-rays of the uninjured side, are often necessary to establish the diagnosis. With certain exceptions (see below), if a loose epiphysis is in satisfactory position, a well-padded plaster of Paris cast should be applied and the position confirmed by periodic x-rays through the cast — slippage may occur when a decrease in swelling results in loosening of the cast.

Application of a temporary splint, control of pain and immediate transfer for orthopedic care are indicated if:

1. Associated fractures are present.

2. There is marked displacement of the epiphysis.

3. Any of the epiphyses around the elbow joint are involved. Special orthopedic evaluation is indicated in all injuries of this type.

4. The capital epiphysis of the femur is loose or displaced even slightly; this condition practically always requires operative reduction and fixation.

5. Reduction is unstable.

6. Sufficient cooperation to allow proper reduction and application of a cast cannot be obtained.

44 — 31. FRACTURES

All severe bone injuries require control of pain and shock (53 — 7) as soon as possible. If a case is too difficult or too lengthy for the attending physician to handle on an emergency basis, a splint, support or cast should be applied and arrangements made for care by an orthopedist at once; *do not splint and tell the patient to report the following day* — in 24 hours, swelling and spasm are maximal, use of local anesthesia unsatisfactory and adequate reduction much more difficult.

Morphine sulfate, 8 to 15 mg., should be given subcutaneously at least 15 minutes before any attempt at reduction. In children 2 years of age or younger, a 30 to 60 mg. pentobarbital sodium (Nembutal) suppository should be substituted. In older children, the dose of narcotic should be adjusted carefully to the age or weight (4).

The following fractures can often be treated in an emergency setting, with follow-up orthopedic care in 24 hours.

44 – 32.   FRACTURES OF THE NASAL BONES OR CARTILAGES See 45 – 5

44 – 33.   FRACTURES OF THE UPPER OR LOWER JAW WITHOUT DISPLACEMENT OR DISTURBANCE OF DENTAL OCCLUSION

These require only control of pain and application of a four-tailed bandage, with reference to a dental surgeon for definitive care.

44 – 34.   FRACTURES OF THE CLAVICLE

Reduction of closed transverse or diagonal fractures of the medial three-quarters, even with considerable displacement or overriding, can generally be obtained by proper application of a clavicular cross or figure-eight bandage. Fractures of the distal quarter require only a Velpeau bandage or a snug sling. Check x-ray films should be taken in 24 hours and should be followed by any modifications in immobilization necessary to improve the position. Compound (open) and severely comminuted clavicular fractures may require hospitalization.

44 – 35.   AVULSION FRACTURES (NONDISPLACED) OF THE GREATER TUBEROSITY OF THE HUMERUS

A Velpeau bandage plus anodynes for control of pain is all that is necessary.

44 – 36.   GREENSTICK FRACTURES

In these cases misalignment and angulation is minimal and can generally be corrected without difficulty by manipulation after injection of 1% procaine or lidocaine (Xylocaine) into the hematoma at the fracture site. Position after reduction and application of plaster should always be checked by x-rays. Circulation and sensation should always be rechecked in 24 hours.

44 – 37.   FRACTURES OF TRANSVERSE PROCESSES

Fractures of transverse processes of the lumbar vertebrae are always painful but rarely serious, although injury to underlying intraabdominal organs (**55 – 1**) must always be ruled out. Partial immobolization by strapping or application of a lumbosacral belt or snug fitting plaster body jacket may decrease the pain. The site of the fracture may be infiltrated with 1% procaine or lidocaine (Xylocaine). The patient should be instructed to sleep on a non-sagging bed. Anodynes as needed are in order, since any motion of the back may be very painful for 7 to 10 days after injury. Excessive application of local heat should be avoided. Cold may be beneficial.

44 – 38.   FRACTURES OF THE RIBS AND STERNUM

Linear fractures of the sternum or fractures of 1 or 2 ribs without displacement usually require nothing but heat and anodynes. Strapping of the chest is ineffective and may result in the development of pneumonitis. Infiltration of the hematoma at the site of the fracture with 1% procaine or lidocaine (Xylocaine) will lessen discomfort on breathing, as will blocking of the intercostal nerves proximal to the fractures.

Marked displacement, multiple fractures (**28 – 2**), severe pain or evidence of traumatic pneumothorax (**28 – 4**) requires immediate hospital care.

44 – 39.   FRACTURES INVOLVING THE WRIST JOINT [Colles,' Reversed Colles' (Smith's)]

If comminution, angulation, displacement, misalignment or distortion of the articular surface of the radius is present, accurate reduction is essential for a satisfactory functional result. Injection of 1% procaine or lidocaine (Xylocaine) into the joint and into the hematoma usually gives satisfactory anesthesia. Restoration of the correct angle of the articular surface and length of the radius is necessary; if not obtained under local anesthesia and confirmed by post-reduction x-rays, the patient should be transferred at once to an orthopedist for possible reduction under general anesthesia. If a satisfactory reduction (checked by x-ray) is obtained, a long-arm plaster cast (with pressure points well padded) extending from the upper third of the humerus to the proximal interphalangeal joints (including the base of the proximal phalanx of the thumb) should be applied with the elbow at 90 degrees and the forearm in neutral position. If an adequate, stable reduction has been obtained, the wrist should be immobilized in optimum grasping position (slight dorsiflexion and slight ulnar deviation). After the cast has set, sensation and circulation should be checked carefully and x-rays taken. Tests of sensation and circulation should be repeated in 24 hours. In all cases, follow-up care should be arranged so that in adults the cast can be shortened in 7 to 10 days to allow active motion of the thumb and fingers after pain, spasm and swelling have subsided. Shortening the cast is not necessary in children.

44-40. FRACTURES OF THE CARPAL (NAVICULAR) SCAPHOID

If marked comminution or displacement is present, a temporary volar splint should be applied and the patient referred at once for orthopedic care. If the position is satisfactory, a padded plaster short arm cast extending from just below the elbow to the metacarpophalangeal joints of the fingers and to the distal joint of the thumb should be applied with the wrist in slight cock-up position and the thumb fully abducted. Follow-up orthopedic care for a lengthy period is indicated because of the possibility of aseptic necrosis and nonunion.

44-41. FRACTURES OF THE OTHER CARPAL BONES

Immobilization by a padded arm and hand cast is all that is necessary unless comminution or displacement of fragments or associated dislocations (see **44-16.** *Lunate Dislocations;* **44-19.** *Perilunar Dislocations*) and soft tissue damage make hospitalization for orthopedic care in order.

44-42. FRACTURES OF THE METACARPALS

Without displacement. Apply a padded plaster cast, take check x-rays, check for sensory and circulatory changes and refer for orthopedic care in 24 hours. Exception: Bennett's fractures, (**40-4.** *Metacarpal Fractures*).

With displacement. Multiple fractures, angulation, overriding and comminution generally require orthopedic care for reduction. Fractures of the distal ends of the 2nd to 5th metacarpals (usually the 5th) are the exception. These "boxer's" fractures can usually be reduced without difficulty under local anesthesia injected into the hematoma, with correction of the volar angulation of the distal fragment by firm dorsal pressure, using the proximal phalanx flexed to 90 degrees as a lever (**40 – 4.** *Metacarpal Fractures*). Direct traction in the long axis of the metacarpal is useless in fractures of this type.

44 – 43. FRACTURES OF THE CARPAL PHALANGES

Proximal or middle phalanges. Apply an aluminum or plaster splint in corrected position (after reduction under local anesthesia if necessary) and refer for orthopedic care in 24 hours. Flexion is required if a fracture of a middle phalanx is distal to the attachment of the tendon of the flexor sublimis.

Distal phalanges. A protective aluminum guard is all that is necessary. A throbbing subungual hematoma may require evacuation (**40 – 3**). For treatment of avulsion of the extensor tendon attachment (baseball finger), see **40 – 4.**

44 – 44. FRACTURES INVOLVING THE KNEE

Avulsion fractures due to partial tearing loose of the attachments of the collateral ligaments should be casted in a position which will relax the injured ligament, using a padded cast from the groin to the toes, with the knee slightly flexed and the ankle at 90 degrees. Follow-up orthopedic care is essential.

Plateau fractures without displacement: same as avulsion fractures.

Patellar fractures without separation or displacement of fragments require a well-padded, skin-anchored walking cast (groin to 2 inches above the ankle), with the knee in full extension.

Tibial tubercle fragmentation (Osgood-Schlatter disease) is characterized by pain over the tibial tubercle on local pressure or contraction of the quadriceps femoris. X-rays of this condition may show the characteristic "crow beak" deformity but more often only epiphysial fragmentation is seen. Treatment consists of application of a long leg cylinder cast with the knee in full extension.

44 – 45. TIBIAL SHAFT FRACTURES

If the fracture is relatively transverse (not spiral or oblique) and there is no displacement or misalignment, a long leg cast – groin to toes – should be applied with the knee in slight flexion and the ankle and foot at 90 degrees. Check x-rays must be taken and the patient referred for orthopedic care in 24 hours.

44 – 46. FRACTURES AROUND THE ANKLE JOINT

Avulsion or sprain fractures should be immobilized in a plaster short leg cast with felt pressure pads over the injured area and other pressure points and the foot in 7 to 10 degrees plantar flexion. The foot should be inverted or everted to relax the injured collateral ligament.

Malleolar fractures without displacement of fragments or distortion of the ankle mortise may be treated by a short leg cast. Bimalleolar or trimalleolar fractures require hospitalization for reduction, as do any fractures resulting in distortion of the normal shape or width of the ankle joint.

44 – 47. OS CALCIS FRACTURES

Incomplete or linear fractures without displacement should be placed in a padded, well-molded, short leg cast and referred for orthopedic care within 12 hours. Any comminution, subastragaloid involvement or change in Boehler's angle makes hospitalization for manipulation and reduction necessary.

44 – 48. TARSAL AND METATARSAL FRACTURES

If the bones are in good position with preservation of the normal arch, a padded plaster short leg cast with the foot plate molded to the arch should be applied. If there is overriding or malposition of the fragments, or if several fractures are present, referral for orthopedic care is in order.

44 – 49. FRACTURES OF THE GREAT TOE

Proximal phalanx. These fractures often require hospitalization, since rotation and displacement of the distal fragment, which is very difficult to reduce and control, may be present. If the fragments are stable and alignment is satisfactory, a short leg cast with a heavy platform sole may be applied and arrangements made for orthopedic care within 2 to 3 days.

Distal phalanx. A cut-out shoe and metatarsal bar generally are all that is necessary. Fibrous union often occurs.

44 — 50. FRACTURES OF THE PHALANGES OF THE SECOND TO FIFTH DIGITS OF THE FOOT

Strapping of the injured digit to its neighbor, a cut-out shoe and a metatarsal bar will generally allow the patient to continue with normal activity.

44 — 51. SACRAL AND COCCYGEAL FRACTURES

Sacral and coccygeal fractures may require hospitalization for a few days for control of acute pain. Usually, however, strapping the buttocks together or prescription of a rubber chair ring or a cut-out sponge rubber cushion will allow home care. Sitz baths may be of benefit.

44 — 52. IMMEDIATE TRANSFER TO A HOSPITAL FOR CARE

Immediate transfer to a hospital for orthopedic care [after treatment of shock (**53 — 7**) and application of a splint if necessary] is required in the following types of fractures:

1. All compound (open) fractures except those of the distal phalanges of the fingers (**40 — 4**) and toes.

2. All fractures with marked comminution, angulation, displacement or overriding.

3. All skull fractures, suspected from history or clinical findings or proved by x-rays, in adults (**41 — 12**). In children (**48 — 32**), home care of linear or nondepressed fractures may be feasible if neurologic signs are absent and if the parents can be depended upon to recognize and report at once any changes in condition (Fig. 24).

4. All cervical spine fractures, with or without evidence of spinal cord damage, suspected or proved (**46 — 11**).

5. All fractures of the dorsal and lumbar spine except transverse processes (**44 — 37**).

6. Rib fractures if multiple, comminuted, markedly displaced or associated with signs of pleural perforation or lung damage (**28 — 2**).

7. Sternal fractures with depression of fragments or evidence of mediastinal bleeding (**28 — 2**).

8. All fractures involving the head, neck, shaft or distal end of the humerus except incomplete or nondisplaced avulsion fractures of the greater tuberosity (**44 — 35**) and greenstick fractures without misalignment (**44 — 36**).

9. All pelvic fractures, with or without comminution, displacement or signs of bladder, urethral or intraabdominal damage.

10. Bennett's fracture of the thumb (**40 — 4**).

11. Multiple carpal or metacarpal fractures with comminution, displacement or overriding (**44 — 40** through **44 — 42**).

12. Fractures of the shafts of both the radius and ulna, with displacement or overriding.

13. Shattering fractures of the radial head with depression or loss of contour of the articular surface. Small chip fractures require only use of a sling for 2 to 3 weeks with active motion within painless limits.

14. Olecranon fractures with comminution or separation of the fragments.

15. All fractures in and around the hip joint or acetabulum.

16. All fractures of the neck, shaft or condyles of the femur. These fractures have a tendency to cause severe, sometimes delayed, shock. Supportive measures (**53 — 7**) before and during transportation are always indicated, whether or not signs and symptoms of shock are present.

17. All complete oblique, spiral or other unstable fractures of the shaft of the tibia even though there may be no displacement or overriding.

18. Plateau fractures of the tibia with depression or distortion of the articular surface.

19. All fractures around the ankle resulting in mortise widening or distortion [avulsion fractures ("sprain-fractures"), fracture-dislocations, bimalleolar and trimalleolar fractures].

20. Multiple tarsal or metatarsal fractures with comminution, displacement or overriding.

21. Fractures of the great toe which are displaced or unstable [except the distal phalanx (**44 — 49**)].

22. Comminuted or displaced fractures of the upper or lower jaws or facial bones.

44 — 53. MYALGIA (See also **44 — 1**. *Arthritis*)

Muscle pain severe enough to require emergency treatment may be the result of a large number of conditions, including direct or indirect trauma, metabolic disturbances, postural strain, acute infections (especially viral) and certain poisons (**49**).

TREATMENT

1. Treatment of poisoning, if a toxic substance is the causative agent (**49**). Slow intravenous injection of 10 ml. of 10% calcium gluconate solution is often effective in controlling this type of myalgia.

2. Control of pain by salicylates, codeine, or pentazocine (Talwin) orally.

3. Local application of heat or, if better tolerated, cold.

4. Spraying of the skin over the pain areas with ethyl chloride.

5. Infiltration of painful myofibrositic nodules with 1% procaine or lidocaine (Xylocaine).

6. Administration of muscle relaxants.

7. Referral for investigation and treatment of the underlying cause.

SPECIAL TYPES OF MYALGIA

44 – 54. NOCTURNAL CRAMPS ("Jumpy Legs")

Cramping in the leg muscles severe enough to interfere with sleep may occur in any age group but is more common in children and persons beyond 50. Fatigue probably is a causative factor. Treatment of severe cases consists of slow intravenous administration of 10 ml. of 10% calcium gluconate. In milder cases the patient should be instructed to take 0.6 gm. of calcium lactate by mouth 3 times a day. Methoxyphenamine hydrochloride (Orthoxine), 100 mg. by mouth at bedtime, may give relief, as may 300 international units of Vitamin E (tocopherol) once daily.

44 – 55. SHIN SPLINTS

"Shin splints" occur in athletes, especially sprinters and hurdlers, and may cause severe pain, probably from a combination of tendinitis and myofascitis.

TREATMENT

1. Anodynes and sedatives for severe pain.

2. Limited activity – complete rest if practical.

3. Application of an elastic bandage.

4. Reference to an orthopedist for physical therapy and instructions concerning strapping during exercise.

44−56. MAGNESIUM DEFICIENCY

Magnesium deficiency, usually seen in chronic alcoholics and asthenic persons, may cause leg cramps, tremors and acutely painful paresthesias, especially burning sensations in the feet.

TREATMENT

Magnesium sulfate, 2 gm. intramuscularly 3 or 4 times a day, usually gives rapid and complete relief.

44−57. MYOFIBROSITIS (See also 44−53. *Myalgia*)

Both acute myofibrositis, characterized by spasm, limitation of motion and muscle tenderness, and chronic myofibrositis, characterized by loss of normal elasticity, a "doughy" feeling on palpation and "trigger nodules" in the substance of the muscle, can cause severe discomfort.

TREATMENT

1. Immobilization if muscle spasm is acute. In the cervical area a Thomas collar is effective; in the low back a lumbosacral belt will often relieve discomfort.

2. Anodynes. Propoxyphene (Darvon), codeine, or pentazocine (Talwin) may be required.

3. Muscle relaxants orally or, in severe cases, intramuscularly.

4. Local application of heat or cold, depending upon tolerance.

5. Injection of "trigger nodules" with a local anesthetic.

6. Reference for physical therapy. Ultrasonic therapy is effective after the acute stage.

44−58. NECK INJURIES

Severe injury to the neck should always be suspected and ruled out by careful clinical and x-ray examination whenever:

1. There is a history of direct trauma to the head or neck, especially when the neck was flexed at the time of injury.

2. The patient was riding in a moving or stationary vehicle which was involved in a collision.

3. Any story is obtained of pain or sensory disturbances, no matter how transient, in the back of the head or in the neck, shoulders or arms following a sudden jerking strain or a blow on the head severe enough to cause even transient loss of consciousness.

Fractures and dislocations of the neck must be ruled out by careful clinical and x-ray examination before the patient is allowed to move his head or neck or to sit up. Cross-table lateral views of the cervical spine, using a portable x-ray, may give valuable information. All questionable cases should be taken to the hospital by ambulance if clinical examination suggests the possibility of cervical fracture or dislocation even if x-rays are negative. The patient's head should be supported in a neutral position by the physician or a trained attendant when the patient is moved from or to a stretcher. Ambulance transportation with the patient flat on his back—his head immobilized by sandbags—is relatively safe. The ambulance crew should be told that smoothness, not speed, is essential.

Severe strains ("whiplash" injuries) of the neck. A sudden jerk to the neck may cause extensive soft tissue damage and acute symptoms, often deferred for 12 to 24 hours, which apparently are all out of proportion to the trauma alleged to have been sustained. Acute soft tissue injuries often cannot be differentiated from fracture or dislocation and may require hospitalization for observation and special x-ray studies. Mild cases can be treated by partial immobilization by a Thomas collar, with application of heat (or cold) and gentle massage at home. Traction by means of a Sayre sling may be beneficial. The pain is often severe enough to require codeine or morphine sulfate hypodermically and muscle relaxants for relief.

Posttraumatic symptoms (neck pain, limitation of cervical and shoulder girdle motion, headache, dysphagia, dizziness) persist for a lengthy time after posterior cervical strains and require prolonged treatment for relief.

44—59. PERITENDINITIS (See also 44—5. *Bursitis*)

Whether or not x rays show amorphous calcification in the affected area (usually the shoulder or hip), palliative treatment is all that can be given as an emergency measure. When the pain is extremely acute, hospitalization for treatment is indicated, but relief (or, at least, decrease in acute discomfort) can often be obtained by:

1. Hot or cold packs. Heat is beneficial in the majority of cases but occasionally is unbearable.

2. Spraying with ethyl chloride.

3. Codeine sulfate, 0.03 to 0.06 gm., and acetylsalicylic acid (aspirin), 0.6 gm., orally every 2 to 4 hours usually will control pain; occasionally parenteral use of pentazocine (Talwin) or morphine may be necessary.

4. Infiltration with 1% procaine or lidocaine (Xylocaine) with or

without hydrocortisone acetate. The patient should be warned that this procedure may result in a temporary flare-up of symptoms after the local anesthetic effect has worn off.

5. Application of a Velpeau bandage (a sling is usually not enough) if the shoulder is involved. Crutches may be necessary if the structures around the hip, ankle or heel are affected.

44−60. SPRAINS

Sprains vary in intensity from tearing of a few fibers of a ligamentous structure to complete severance and loss of support. For common sites of ankle sprains, see Figure 27.

Mild sprains. Patients with relatively minor ligamentous and soft tissue damage often request treatment after 24 to 48 hours because increased edema and pain have developed. In many cases involving the extremities, instructions regarding limitation of activity, compresses or soaks at home (cold if within 24 hours, hot if later) and the application of an elastic bandage are all that is required. Ad-

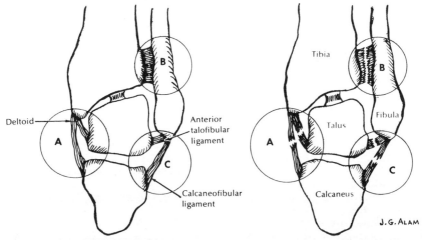

Figure 27. Normal ankle. A, Medial collateral ligament; B, anterior tibiofibular ligament; C, lateral collateral ligament. On the right is a corresponding diagram showing the ligaments that are most frequently sprained in the ankle. (From Novich, M. M.: Consultant, Vol. 12, No. 9, p. 73, September, 1972.)

hesive strapping should be used only for temporary support. Round-and-round strapping should never be applied.

Severe sprains. These require casting in a position which relaxes the damaged ligaments for a minimum period of 6 weeks. Stress x-ray films (with the uninjured side for comparison) should be taken when the cast is removed, but not at the time of original treatment.

Unless there is a specific indication for the procedure (63−12), ambulation after injection of the structures around a weight-bearing joint with a local anesthetic should be prohibited because healing of the damaged ligaments in a lax position will often result in an unstable joint and recurrent sprains and strains.

Avulsion type fractures should be ruled out by x-ray (with the opposite side in exactly the same position for comparison) especially in industrial injuries (75) and potential public liability cases (67).

Splinting by bias-cut stockinette or elastic bandages, metallic trough splints or plaster of Paris may be indicated. The patient should be given crutches if a severe strain involves a lower extremity and weight bearing causes pain.

If a cast is applied, it should not be done until acute swelling has been controlled by elevation and application of cold. The circulation and sensation of the casted part should be checked in 24 hours and follow-up orthopedic care arranged.

If operative repair of damaged ligamentous structures is considered necessary, it should if possible be done within 24 hours of the injury.

44−61. TENDON INJURIES (See also 40−8. *Tendon Injuries in the Hand*)

All lacerations, stab wounds and puncture wounds should be checked carefully for tendon damage by tests of function. A severe contusion may cause severance by compression of a tendon against a bony prominence. Tendons (especially the biceps in the arm, the supraspinatus in the shoulder, the soleus in the calf and the tendo Achillis near its insertion) may rupture as a result of sudden severe muscle strain.

TREATMENT

All cases of suspected or proved tendon severance should be referred for hospitalization and surgical care with the exception of:

1. Incomplete severances—these can usually be treated by immobilization or repaired under local anesthesia, depending on the location and extent of damage.

2. Extensor tendons of the fingers without retraction (**40—8**).

3. Extensor tendons (dorsiflexors) of the 2nd to 5th digits of the foot without retraction. These can easily be repaired under local anesthesia using the Koch or Bunnell technique.

4. Severance of the palmaris longus tendon. No repair is necessary because this tendon is vestigial and serves no useful function in the wrist or hand.

5. Severance of the flexor tendons of the 2nd to 5th digits of the foot. These do not require repair.

6. Rupture of the soleus tendon. Application of a plaster cast from the knee to the toes with the ankle in moderate plantar flexion is usually required, with referral to an orthopedist for follow-up care.

TRAUMATIC TENDINITIS

TREATMENT

1. Application of cold compresses to decrease edema and lessen acute pain.

2. Limitation of motion by strapping, splinting or casting.

3. Anodynes.

4. Reference for follow-up care.

ACUTE TENOSYNOVITIS

Ambulatory treatment consisting of splinting, anodynes and antibiotics may be tried. Hospitalization is indicated if:

1. The infection is extending in spite of conservative therapy.

2. The patient will not cooperate in limitation of activity.

3. Incision and drainage are indicated.

STENOSING TENOVAGINITIS (De Quervain) See **40—8.** *Tendon Injuries in the Hand.*

45. NASAL CONDITIONS

45—1. AEROSINUSITIS (Sinus Squeeze)

Common in sports divers (**23—5**), this painful condition, characterized by collection of bloody exudate within the sinuses, is due to the effect of increased barometric pressure on partially blocked ostia.

TREATMENT

1. Avoidance of diving until all evidence of infection and edema have disappeared – usually 4 to 6 weeks.

2. Insurance of adequate sinus drainage by frequent use of decongestant nose drops. Sinus washing or drainage should not be done. Ultrasonic therapy to the affected areas may be beneficial. Antibiotics may be used for secondary infection.

45 – 2. CONTUSIONS

TREATMENT

1. Rule out fractures of the skull, nasal cartilages or nasal bones by thorough clinical and x-ray examination. Injection of 150 TRU of hyaluronidase in 1% procaine or lidocaine (Xylocaine) into the swollen areas will decrease edema and allow more accurate evaluation.

2. Instruct the patient to apply cold compresses or an icebag at frequent intervals during the first 24 hours; after 24 hours local heat should be substituted.

3. Refer the patient to an otolaryngologist if the swelling persists or if crepitation of the soft tissues is present.

45 – 3. EPISTAXIS (Nosebleed)

Nontraumatic epistaxis may be caused by varicosities, telangiectasis, hypertension, nasal polyps, abrasions from nose-picking, tuberculosis, malignant disease, hemophilia, acute infectious diseases, etc. For the location of major blood vessels, see Figure 28. The emergency treatment is the same for all conditions:

1. Upright position to allow drainage.

2. Pressure on the nostrils with the fingers.

3. Avoidance of blowing the nose.

4. Cautious cauterization with a silver nitrate stick of observed bleeding points.

5. Wedging of a pad of gauze, cotton or paper tissue between the upper teeth and the upper lip.

6. Insertion of a gauze strip saturated with 1:1000 epinephrine hydrochloride (Adrenalin) solution into the bleeding nostril.

7. Packing of the anterior nares with a sterile gauze strip or petrolatum gauze (**14 – 6**). *Do not* use iodoform or other medicated gauze.

8. Insertion of a posterior nasal pack. For technique, see **14 – 6**. Since any type of nasal packing results in nasopharyngeal obstruc-

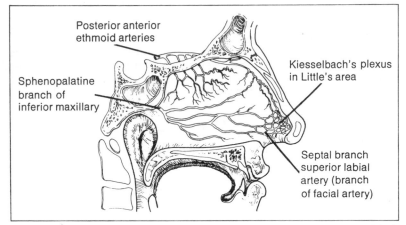

Figure 28. Landmarks in the nose: the location of vessels most often responsible for both anterior and posterior nosebleeds are illustrated here. (From Norman, F. W.: Patient Care, January, 1972. Copyright © Miller & Fink Corporation, Darien, CT. All rights reserved.)

tion and edema, alteration of airway resistance in the entire pulmonary system occurs with Po_2 depression. Therefore, administration of oxygen is indicated for as long as a nasal pack is in place.

9. Intravenous injection of 20 mg. of sodium estrone sulfate (Premarin) if oozing is present. Repeat in 1 hour if necessary.

10. Hospitalization if the bleeding cannot be controlled by the measures given above. Blood loss may be sufficient to require treatment of shock (**53−7**) before transportation.

Traumatic epistaxis. If there is any possibility that the drainage from the nose following injury is a mixture of blood and spinal fluid, no packing or medication of any type should be inserted into the nostrils. The case should be treated as a skull fracture and the patient hospitalized at once. The presence of rhinorrhea can sometimes be confirmed by placing a drop of the bloody fluid on a white blotter; the presence of a light pink area around a darkened center indicates the presence of spinal fluid. For treatment, see **45−3**.

45−4. FOREIGN BODIES IN NOSE. See 36−3

45-5. FRACTURES OF THE NASAL BONES AND CARTILAGES

TREATMENT

1. Simple displaced fractures can usually be restored to normal alignment by digital manipulation. If depression is present, the fragment can be elevated by pressure with a blunt padded instrument within the nostrils.

2. Comminuted, compound (open) or depressed fractures, especially those which result in marked septal deviation or distortion, should be referred to an otolaryngologist for reduction and follow-up care.

45-6. HEMATOMAS

If untreated or if treatment is delayed, hematomas may result in permanent saddling of the bridge. The patient should be referred to an otolaryngologist as soon as presence of a hematoma (usually septal or between the lateral cartilages and the nasal bone) is recognized. If a delay in treatment is anticipated, prophylaxis against tetanus (**16**) and antibiotics are indicated.

45-7. LACERATIONS

See **55-20** for general principles of treatment. Since the nose is in the "danger zone," prophylaxis against tetanus (**16**) and antibiotics should be given routinely.

45-8. SEPTAL INJURIES

All cases with septal deviation or distortion require care by an otolaryngologist.

46. NEUROLOGIC DISORDERS

46-1. COMA OF UNDETERMINED ORIGIN See 29-17

46-2. COMA DUE TO SPECIFIC CAUSES

Acidosis (**43-1**).
Acute infectious diseases (**29-1; 30.** *Contagious and Communicable Diseases;* **48.** *Pediatric Emergencies;* **62.** *Viral Infections*).

46 – 3. MENIERE'S DISEASE

MILD CASES

TREATMENT
1. Sedation through barbiturates.
2. Control of pain during attacks by analgesics and anodynes. Pentazocine lactate (Talwin), 15 to 30 mg. intramuscularly every 4 hours, may be effective. Addictive opiates and synthetic narcotics should be avoided.
3. Administration of dimenhydrinate (Dramamine), 50 to 100 mg. by mouth 3 times a day.
4. Low sodium diet and diuretics may be helpful.
5. Reference to an otolaryngologist.

SEVERE CASES

TREATMENT
1. Control of severe pain by morphine sulfate subcutaneously, provided the patient has none of the stigmata of addiction (**2 – 4**).
2. Hospitalization at once.

46—4. MENINGITIS See **30—16; 48—41.** *Meningitis in Children;* **62—1.** *Arboviral Infections;* **62—5.** *Viral Encephalitis*

46—5. MENINGOCOCCEMIA See **48—42; 48—63.** *Waterhouse-Friderichsen Syndrome*

46—6. MIGRAINE See **27—21.** *Migraine Headaches;* **48—43.** *Migraine in Children*

46—7. MYASTHENIA GRAVIS

Progressive paresis of facial, oculomotor, pharyngeal and respiratory muscles may occur. Skeletal muscles are involved in advanced states. Marked fatigability is common, with aggravation of symptoms by mental as well as physical stress. Symptoms requiring emergency care are usually related to acute infections, aspiration of food or respiratory failure.

TREATMENT
1. Place the patient in the recumbent position.
2. Clear the airway and support ventilation (**11—1**).
3. Give neostigmine methylsulfate, 1 ml. of 1:2000 solution (0.5 mg.) intramuscularly, unless the patient is a known myasthenic or neostigmine overdosage is suspected.
4. Inject edrophonium chloride (Tensilon), 10 mg. intravenously, or 25 mg. intramuscularly. As a diagnostic measure 3 mg. intravenously will cause improvement in a myasthenia gravis crisis but will cause no significant lasting change in symptoms caused by neostigmine overdosage.
5. Improvement with large doses of steroids during crises has been noted.

46—8. NEURITIS (Neuralgia)

Although many conditions (infections, trauma, toxins, viruses, poisons, pressure, etc.) may cause irritation and pain along the course and distribution of various nerves, the discomfort in most cases is not severe enough to bring the patient for emergency treatment. The chief exceptions are as follows:

46—8. NEURITIS

ALCOHOLIC NEURITIS

Occurring mostly in female chronic alcoholics, the extreme discomfort caused by toxic neuritis from alcohol often requires emergency care, followed by prolonged hospital therapy. Control of pain and sedation as indicated under **34—3.** *Delirium Tremens* is all that is indicated as an emergency measure.

ARSENICAL NEURITIS See **49—90.** *Arsenic.*

BELL'S PALSY (Peripheral Facial Nerve Paralysis)

The clinical picture (inability to close the eye, wrinkle the forehead or elevate the corner of the mouth on the affected side and drooling of saliva from the mouth) usually develops following chilling or injury of the involved side.

TREATMENT
1. Oral administration of 20 mg. of prednisone 3 times a day for 2 or 3 days, then gradual tapering off over a 7 to 10 day period.
2. Application of an eye patch with a bland ophthalmic ointment.
3. Protection of the involved side from wind and cold.
4. Instruction in measures to prevent loss of facial muscle tone (upward massage, taping, etc.). Electrical stimulation may be indicated.

CAUSALGIA

Severe causalgia following trauma probably has a reflex neuritic component. Relief of severe discomfort can sometimes be obtained by oral administration of tolazoline hydrochloride (Priscoline), 25 to 50 mg. every 4 hours, but pentazocine lactate (Talwin), 15 to 30 mg. intramuscularly, or opiates may be necessary. Severe cases may require sympathetic blocks or serial amputations.

HERPES ZOSTER (For eye involvement, see **35—14.** *Herpes Zoster Ophthalmicus*).

TREATMENT
1. Protection of lesions from infection by petrolatum gauze or dibucaine (Nupercaine) ointment dressings or dusting with thymol iodide (not in eyes!).
2. Control of pain, if moderate, by sedation and analgesics; if severe, by pentazocine lactate (Talwin) intramuscularly or intravenously, or codeine or morphine sulfate subcutaneously.

3. Administration of antibiotic therapy if bacterial infection is a complicating factor.

4. Hospitalization if the pain is severe or the lesions extensive.

PERIPHERAL NEURITIS DURING PREGNANCY See 47 — 10.

This condition is usually associated with pernicious vomiting (**47 — 9**).

RETROBULBAR NEURITIS

SIGNS AND SYMPTOMS. Headache and discomfort in the eye on the affected side with increase of ocular pain on eye motion or pressure and rapid impairment of vision — blurring and central scotomata. There is a slow temporary constriction of the affected pupil in response to light. Injection and blurring of the disk margins is a late development.

TREATMENT

1. Prednisone, 60 mg. orally in a loading dose, and then daily in divided doses, tapering the dosage downward as soon as improvement begins.

2. Referral to an ophthalmologist.

SCIATICA

Pain along the course of the sciatic nerve may be severe and totally disabling. Causative orthopedic pathology in the low back is usually present.

TREATMENT

1. Local application of heat or cold as tolerated. Massage usually causes an increase in discomfort.

2. Application of a lumbosacral belt.

3. Muscle relaxants in large doses every 4 hours by mouth or parenterally for relaxation of spasm.

4. Salicylates, propoxyphene (Darvon) and codeine sulfate by mouth for pain. Pentazocine lactate (Talwin), 15 to 30 mg. intramuscularly, may give relief. In severe cases, morphine sulfate, 10 to 15 mg. subcutaneously, may be required. The patient should be checked carefully for evidence of addiction (**2 — 4**) before any narcotic is given.

5. Hospitalization if the pain is intractable and severe for determination and treatment of the causative condition, which is usually orthopedic in nature.

TRIGEMINAL NEURALGIA (Tic Douloureux)

TREATMENT
1. Control of pain by pentazocine lactate (Talwin), 15 to 30 mg. intravenously or intramuscularly, or by the smallest possible effective dose of morphine sulfate intramuscularly. Sedatives, hypnotics and muscle relaxants are of no value. Because of its extreme toxicity, trichlorethylene therapy should not be attempted as an emergency procedure.
2. Referral to a neurologist.

"WHIPLASH" INJURIES OF THE NECK (See also **44 — 58**. *Neck Injuries;* **46 — 11**. *Spinal Injuries with Cord Compression*)

Severe neuritis of the cervical nerves supplying the neck, head, shoulders, arms and hands may follow sudden jerking motions of the neck. In addition, irritation of the nervi vasorum may cause apparently unrelated pain through reflex mechanisms. Development of neuritic pain is often delayed for several days after injury.

TREATMENT. See **44 — 58**. *Neck Injuries.*

46 — 9. PARALYSIS

Loss of muscle power, partial or complete, sudden or progressive, usually results in a situation requiring emergency management. No matter what the etiology may be, persons showing evidence of recent, progressive or extensive paralysis (except those who respond to simple emergency measures) should be hospitalized as soon as possible and receive appropriate supportive therapy en route.

Acute involvement of the muscles of deglutition may be caused by:

Botulism (**49 — 141**).
Brain injuries (**41**. *Head Injuries;* **48 — 9** through **48 — 11**. *Brain Injuries in Children;* **48 — 32**. *Head Injuries in Children*).
Diphtheria (**30 — 4**).
Myasthenia gravis (**46 — 7**).
Poliomyelitis, bulbar (**30 — 21; 48 — 49**).
Tetanus (**30 — 31**).
High cervical injuries (**44 — 58**. *Neck Injuries*).
Involvement of the muscles of respiration may occur in:
Anterior poliomyelitis (**30 — 21; 48 — 49**).
Cervical fractures and dislocations (**44 — 58**. *Neck Injuries*).
Head injuries involving the respiratory center in the medulla (**41; 48 — 32**. *Head Injuries in Children*).

Guillain-Barré syndrome.
Acute intermittent porphyria (**43 – 22**).
Familial periodic paralysis (see below).
Tick bites (**24 – 22**).
Electric shock (**25 – 11.** *Electrical Burns;* **29 – 5**).
Acute poisoning (**29 – 13; 49**).

TREATMENT

Expired air respiration or mechanical ventilation (**11 – 1**), often followed by tracheostomy (**14 – 12**), may be necessary as a life-saving measure. Neck injuries must be immobilized.

Paralysis of central nervous system origin may result from:

Brain infarction or increased intracranial pressure resulting from cerebrovascular accidents (**59 – 2**).
Space-consuming intracranial or cord tumors.
Head injuries (**41; 48 – 9** through **48 – 11.** *Brain Injuries in Children;* **48 – 32.** *Head Injuries in Children*).
Vertebral fractures (**44 – 3**).
Partial or complete dislocation of any portion of the spine (**44 – 7; 44 – 11.** *Cervical Spine Dislocations*).

Paralysis due to peripheral neuropathy may be caused by herniated intervertebral disk, discogenic disease, neuritis (metabolic, toxic or traumatic) of cauda equina syndrome.

Familial periodic paralysis. This rare disorder of electrolyte metabolism is characterized by recurrent episodes of profound paralysis and weakness, usually associated with low serum potassium levels.

TREATMENT

1. Supportive therapy, particularly ventilatory assistance.
2. Restriction of sodium intake.
3. Potassium chloride, 5 to 10 gm. by mouth.
4. Correction of severe hypokalemia by slow (not to exceed 5 ml./min.) intravenous infusion of 500 ml. of 5% dextrose in water containing 3 gm. of potassium chloride. Intermittent electrocardiographic monitoring is desirable.

Hysterical paralysis (**50 – 6**) must always be considered if the findings are bizarre and the exact causative factor cannot be determined.

46 – 10.   PERIPHERAL NERVE INJURIES IN THE EXTREMITIES (See also **40 – 6.** *Nerve Injuries in the Hand*)

An injured peripheral nerve can be recognized by impairment or loss of motor function or sensory perception in areas innervated by that nerve. The location of injury can often be determined by overlying soft tissue trauma or adjacent bone fracture and displacement.

TREATMENT

1. Splint the involved extremity.
2. Control pain by anodynes or narcotics.
3. Treat soft tissue injuries.
4. Refer to a neurosurgeon for end-to-end anastomosis of completely severed nerves or decompression of severely compressed nerves.
5. If possible, obtain an electromyogram in all cases of peripheral nerve injury as soon as possible after injury to rule out preexistent pathology. Degenerative changes do not develop until about 21 days after injury. This is particularly important in workmen's compensation cases (**75**) and potential public liability cases (**67**).

46−11. SPINAL INJURIES WITH CORD COMPRESSION (See also 44−3. *Fractures;* 44−11. *Dislocations;* 44−58. *Neck Injuries*)

All cases of obvious or suspected head or back injury, with or without a history of severe direct trauma, should be considered as possible spinal cord injuries until the condition has been ruled out by careful general, x-ray and neurologic examination. The following points should be checked at first examination of the patient:

1. Determine if possible the probable type and mechanics of injury. Although relatively minor accidents may cause contusion or edema of the cord without fracture or dislocations, acute flexion and hyperextension injuries are more likely to result in cord damage, especially in the neck (**44−58.** *Neck Injuries*).
2. Ask the patient where he hurts. Radicular pain is common with cord injuries, and careful localization of pain is very important.
3. Carefully palpate the spine, working downwards from the base of the skull, for deformity (especially prominence of a spinous process), muscle spasm, guarding, fibrillation or tenderness on pressure or percussion over the spinous processes.
4. Test for motion and strength of extremities.
5. Check for reflex changes and abnormal reflexes.
6. Determine the condition of the sphincters. Digital rectal examination is very important and is often omitted.
7. Examine for sensory changes—test light touch, pain and position and vibratory sense.

8. If possible, take x-ray scout films of suspected areas, moving the patient as little as possible. As a general rule, compression frac tures are less likely to cause severe cord damage than fracture dislocations and displaced fractures through the laminae or pedicles. Serious cord embarrassment may follow contusion and compression as well as partial or complete severance; therefore, careless handling during examination or transportation may result in irreparable damage.

TREATMENT

1. Immobilize the spine as much as possible by means of sandbags on each side of the head and body. Manual or head halter cervical traction may be necessary.

2. Treat for shock (**53 – 7**).

3. Transfer for hospitalization with immobilizing measures (sandbags, traction, etc.) in place. *The attending physician should personally supervise lifting the patient to and from the ambulance stretcher.* The ambulance crew should be instructed specifically and emphatically that smoothness, not speed, is essential.

46 – 12. CORD COMPRESSION WITHOUT DIRECT TRAUMA

Evidence of acute spinal cord compression may occur without any evidence of direct trauma. Spontaneous compression in these cases may be related to epidural abscess (**20 – 12**), collapse of a pathologic vertebra due to advanced osteoporosis or a malignant process and, occasionally, to spontaneous hemorrhage. Treatment is as outlined under **46 – 11.** *Spinal Injuries with Cord Compression,* with transfer for hospitalization and evaluation for appropriate surgical intervention.

PROGNOSIS.   No estimate of the amount of damage, or of the permanence thereof, should ever be given based on emergency examination alone.

46 – 13. VERTIGO

Vertigo may be objective (the environment seems to spin) or subjective (the body seems to float or revolve in space) and may be caused by any disturbance in any of the structures (brain or end organs) concerned with transmission of the impulses. Vertigo should be distinguished from dizziness, which is merely an unsteadiness caused by a sensation of motion within the head.

TREATMENT

Removal or treatment of the cause of the vertigo is the most important therapeutic measure. Although in some instances hospitalization is required, in many cases the following symptomatic measures will give relief:

1. Bed rest.
2. Sedation by barbiturates or paraldehyde orally or intramuscularly.
3. Cyclizine hydrochloride (Marezine), 50 mg. orally or intramuscularly, or 100 mg. by rectal suppository.
4. Dimenhydrinate (Dramamine), 50 to 100 mg. by mouth.
5. Chlorpromazine hydrochloride (Thorazine), 25 to 50 mg., or prochlorperazine dimaleate (Compazine), 5 to 10 mg. orally or intramuscularly.
6. Atropine sulfate, 0.4 to 0.6 mg. subcutaneously.
7. Intravenous administration of hypertonic dextrose solution.
8. Vitamin B_6 (pyridoxine hydrochloride), 25 to 50 mg. intravenously.

47. OBSTETRICAL EMERGENCIES

Many conditions during pregnancy may require emergency care.

47 — 1. ABORTIONS For definition, see **65 — 5.**

Suspected early or threatened. These patients should be hospitalized at once if bleeding is excessive — by ambulance if necessary. Sedation by barbiturates and control of pain and uterine contractions by opiates or meperidine hydrochloride (Demerol) are in order. Intravenous administration of plasma volume expanders may be necessary before transfer if the patient is in shock (**53 — 7**).

Incomplete. Hospitalization as soon as possible is essential if bleeding is excessive and equipment for vacuum curettage is not available in the emergency department. If a delay in arranging hospitalization is anticipated, small doses of morphine sulfate subcutaneously may be necessary to control restlessness and anxiety. Excessive bleeding can sometimes be controlled by ergonovine maleate (Ergotrate), 0.2 mg. intramuscularly. Treatment for shock (**53 — 7**) should be given before transfer if blood loss has been excessive.

Complete. If the attending physician is sure that no tissue has been retained and that bleeding has been controlled, home or office treatment may be feasible after antibiotics have been given.

Any case in which the history or physical examination suggests the possibility of a criminally induced abortion must be reported at once to the proper authorities.

47 – 2.   ECTOPIC PREGNANCY

Ruptured ectopic pregnancy is an acute surgical emergency requiring immediate hospitalization for operative treatment after treatment of hypovolemic shock (**53 – 7**).

47 – 3.   MISCARRIAGE See **47 – 1.** *Abortions*

47 – 4.   PREMATURE SEPARATION OF THE PLACENTA

SIGNS AND SYMPTOMS. Sudden onset, during the latter months of pregnancy of sharp abdominal pain associated with a hard firm uterus, evidence of fetal distress and signs of acute blood loss and shock (**53**).

TREATMENT

Immediate transfer by ambulance to a hospital after control of restlessness and anxiety, by a small dose of morphine. Measures to combat hypovolemic shock (**53 – 7**) may be necessary en route.

47 – 5.   TOXEMIAS OF PREGNANCY

True toxemia of pregnancy is characterized by lassitude and general malaise, severe headaches, generalized edema, albuminuric retinitis and increasing hypertension, with convulsions and coma.

TREATMENT

1. Mild cases without convulsions or coma need no special emergency treatment but require careful prenatal care.
2. Severe cases with convulsions and coma require immediate hospitalization after symptomatic supportive therapy.

47 – 6.   ACUTE YELLOW ATROPHY OF THE LIVER

SIGNS AND SYMPTOMS. Acute headache, usually with a subnormal temperature, nausea, vomiting, diarrhea, acute onset of severe convulsions which may be mistaken for eclampsia or acute poisoning (**49**), jaundice, mild or pronounced, and decreased urinary output with high specific gravity. Albumin and casts of all types may be present.

TREATMENT

1. Protection from injury during convulsions.
2. Insurance of an adequate airway.
3. Control of convulsions by intravenous injection of rapid-acting barbiturates in large doses, intragluteal injections of paraldehyde or inhalations of ether.
4. Intravenous administration of 500 ml. of 5% dextrose in saline.
5. Immediate hospitalization for probable emptying of the uterus.

47−7. ECLAMPSIA

Limited almost exclusively to the second half of pregnancy, an eclamptic convulsion coming on without premonitory signs or symptoms may be severe enough to require emergency care. Generally, however, signs and symptoms of preeclamptic toxemia can be elicited on careful questioning and examination.

TREATMENT

1. Insurance of an adequate airway.
2. Protection against injury, especially tongue biting and musculoskeletal damage.
3. Immediate injection of meperidine hydrochloride (Demerol), 50 to 100 mg. subcutaneously, or pentazocine lactate (Talwin), 15 to 30 mg. intramuscularly or intravenously.
4. Administration of oxygen under positive pressure by face mask or endotracheal tube.
5. Transportation to a hospital at once, with an attendant in the ambulance if possible. Inhalations of ether to control convulsions, or of oxygen to combat cyanosis, may be necessary en route.

47−8. PREECLAMPTIC TOXEMIA

Preeclamptic toxemia should be suspected whenever a patient in the second half of pregnancy complains of headache, lassitude or edema, or whenever examination shows an elevated blood pressure with diminished urine containing albumin. In severe cases, epigastric pain, impaired vision and hallucinations may be present.

TREATMENT

1. Mild cases need no emergency treatment but should be referred to an obstetrician without delay. Bed rest, sedation and a milk diet may be prescribed in the interim.

2. Severe cases require the same treatment as eclampsia (**47 — 7**).

47 — 9. PERNICIOUS VOMITING OF PREGNANCY

Pernicious vomiting of pregnancy may be toxemic or neurotic in origin. Either type may result in extreme dehydration, malnutrition, and cachexia — even death — unless controlled.

TREATMENT OF MILD CASES

Administration of sedatives and/or antispasmodics and reference to an obstetrician for care. Any of the following drugs may be tried:

1. Atropine sulfate, 0.5 to 1.0 mg. by mouth 3 times a day.

2. Amphetamine sulfate (Benzedrine), 5 mg. 3 or 4 times daily by mouth.

3. Adiphenine hydrochloride (Trasentine), 30 mg. orally 3 or 4 times a day.

4. Cyclizine hydrochloride (Marezine), 50 mg. orally or intramuscularly, or 100 mg. by rectal suppository — repeated every 6 hours if necessary.

5. Dimenhydrinate (Dramamine), 50 to 100 mg. by mouth every 6 hours.

6. Meclizine hydrochloride (Bonine), 25 mg. orally every 8 hours either in the form of tablets or as medicated chewing gum.

7. Pyridoxine hydrochloride (Vitamin B_6), 25 to 50 mg. intramuscularly once a day. Bendectin — a combination of pyridoxine hydrochloride, 10 mg., dicyclomine hydrochloride (Bentyl), 10 mg., and doxylamine succinate (Decapryn), 10 mg. — one tablet 3 or 4 times a day by mouth is often effective.

8. Chlorpromazine hydrochloride (Thorazine), 25 to 50 mg. orally or intramuscularly every 6 hours. Promazine hydrochloride (Sparine), 10 to 15 mg., or prochlorperazine maleate (Compazine), 5 to 10 mg., may be substituted for chlorpromazine hydrochloride.

9. Perphenazine (Trilafon), 4 mg. orally, intramuscularly or by rectal suppository, not more than 3 times a day.

10. Pentazocine lactate (Talwin), 15 to 30 mg. intramuscularly every 6 hours.

TREATMENT OF SEVERE CASES

1. Control of acute dehydration by intravenous administration of 500 to 1000 ml. of 5% dextrose in saline.

2. Administration of antinauseants intramuscularly or intravenously.

3. Hospitalization for definitive care.

47 – 10. PERIPHERAL NEURITIS

Peripheral neuritis is sometimes associated with vomiting of pregnancy. The pain from this condition may be severe enough to cause the patient to seek emergency care.

Palliative symptomatic treatment by sedation and anodynes, occasionally opiates, is indicated, with referral for thorough investigation to an obstetrician or internist.

47 – 11. DECISIONS TO BE MADE BY EMERGENCY PHYSICIAN WHEN THE PATIENT IS AT OR NEAR TERM

Is the patient in true labor? This can generally be determined by consideration of the following criteria:

1. History regarding months of gestation. (If a prenatal chart is available, this should be reviewed.)

2. Type, duration, strength and frequency of uterine contractures.

3. Bloody show.

4. Rupture of the membranes.

5. Position of the presenting part and dilation of the cervix by rectal or vaginal examination. If a vaginal examination is done, the patient should be warned in advance of the possibility of slight bleeding.

Is there time for transportation to a hospital for delivery?

Primiparae. It is generally safe to transport primiparae in labor to a hospital for delivery unless the cervix is fully dilated or the presenting part lies on the perineum.

Multiparae

1. In many cases women who have had children are able to tell with surprising accuracy when delivery is near. Before arranging for transportation to a hospital, the physician should question the patient regarding previous precipitate labors and, if possible, review the prenatal record. Rectal or vaginal examination is essential but can often be misleading. In making his decision regarding transfer, the physician should be guided more by the time since onset of pains, the frequency, strength and length of uterine contractions and the patient's opinion regarding the time available before delivery than by his examination.

2. All patients should be instructed to breathe through the mouth and warned against bearing down during transportation to the hospital. However, if delivery en route becomes imperative, it is much better for both the mother and the baby to avoid all delaying procedures.

3. Narcotic drugs, natural or synthetic, should never be given under emergency conditions in an attempt to stop or slow up delivery. Their effect may be the opposite; in addition, their use may result in marked depression of the child's respiratory center.

Is emergency delivery necessary? If, in the opinion of the attending physician, sufficient time for transfer to a hospital for delivery is not available, delivery should be effected using the best possible technique that time and circumstances will allow.

48. PEDIATRIC EMERGENCIES

Infants and children represent a relatively large proportion of emergency cases. In these age groups, under certain circumstances some conditions require a change from or modification in emergency therapy suitable for adults. Treatment for these conditions, and for some emergencies peculiar to children, is outlined in the subheadings under this topic. If the emergency treatment for any condition is the same for children and adults, or if treatment in children has been covered elsewhere, the topic number only is given for reference.

In all cases, drug dosages *must* be modified by weight, age or skin surface area (**4**) unless specific doses are given in the text.

48 — 1. ACCIDENTS

The home, especially the kitchen, is the most dangerous place in the world for children in the preschool age group. The highest accident rate is in children who are under the parents' "direct supervision." During the first years of life absolute protection of the child by the parents is essential; from then on, progressive education is necessary regarding the pull of gravity, the effects of heat, the inedibility of certain substances and the unpleasant effects of water in the breathing apparatus. In one year in the United States alone, 15,000 children are killed, 50,000 are permanently injured and at least 1,000,000 receive medical treatment for the results of home accidents, in most instances resulting directly from parental ignorance, carelessness or neglect.

For treatment, see under the type of injury sustained.

48—2. ACIDOSIS (See also 43—1)

Prolonged vomiting from any cause, starvation or metabolic abnormalities may result in acidosis.

TREATMENT

1. Control of vomiting as outlined under **48—3.** *Alkalosis.*

2. Insurance of adequate oxygenation if dyspnea or cyanosis is present.

3. Hypodermoclysis or intravenous fluids as given under **48—3.** *Alkalosis.*

4. Immediate hospitalization of severe cases for laboratory evaluation and replacement therapy (**6**).

48—3. ALKALOSIS (See also 43—5)

Alkalosis may result in severe convulsions in children. Causes are as follows:

ALKALI EXCESS IN THE BLOOD

TREATMENT

Hospitalization for laboratory tests essential for determination of the therapy needed to restore the normal fluid-electrolyte balance (**6**).

CHLORIDE LOSS DUE TO PERSISTENT VOMITING

TREATMENT

1. Nothing by mouth except cracked ice, or sips of a cold carbonated beverage.

2. Complete rest. Sedation by a pentobarbital sodium (Nembutal) suppository may be necessary.

3. Chlorpromazine hydrochloride (Thorazine) intramuscularly, dose 0.5 mg. per kilogram of body weight. The effects of Thorazine in accentuating and prolonging the effects of sedatives and analgesics should be given due consideration.

4. Dextrose ($2\frac{1}{2}\%$) in $\frac{1}{2}$ normal saline solution intravenously or by hypodermoclysis, 30 ml. per kilogram of body weight.

5. Hospitalization for laboratory determinations and correction of fluid-electrolyte imbalance (**6**).

HYPERVENTILATION See 34 — 6.

METABOLIC ABNORMALITIES (See also 43. Metabolic Disorders)

TREATMENT

1. Administration of oxygen under positive pressure by oxygen tent or face mask and rebreathing bag.

2. Immediate hospitalization. Complex disturbances of sodium, potassium and chloride ions requiring careful replacement therapy (**6**) are usually present.

48 — 4. ANGIOEDEMA (See also 21. Allergic Reactions)

TREATMENT

1. Epinephrine hydrochloride (Adrenalin), 0.2 ml. of 1:1000 solution subcutaneously, repeated at $\frac{1}{2}$ hour intervals if necessary.

2. Diphenhydramine hydrochloride (Benadryl), 1 to 2 mg. per kilogram of body weight subcutaneously.

3. Insertion of an endotracheal tube or performance of an emergency tracheostomy (**14 — 12**) if the edema involves the upper respiratory tract and is sufficient to prevent adequate aeration. If either procedure is done, hospitalization for follow-up care is indicated.

48 — 5. ASPHYXIA NEONATORUM

Mild cases are characterized by embarrassment of respiration, normal or rapid heart rate and normal muscle tone.

TREATMENT

1. Insurance of a clear airway by postural drainage, suction of the pharynx and trachea and support of the angle of the jaw after ruling out the presence of foreign bodies (**36 — 4**).

2. Mouth-to-mouth respiration (**11 — 1**) if necessary, followed by administration of oxygen by tent or face mask.

Moderate or severe cases show extreme embarrassment or absence of respiration, heart rate rapid at first, then slowing terminally, poor muscle tone, livid or pale skin and diminished or lost gag reflex.

TREATMENT
1. Insurance of a clear airway by postural drainage, suction of the pharynx and trachea and support of the jaw after examination for obstructive foreign bodies (**36—4**).
2. Direct inspection of the larynx. If the pharyngeal reflex is present and the vocal cords move, oxygen under positive pressure by face mask and rebreathing bag is indicated; if the pharyngeal reflex is absent, immediate endotracheal intubation or tracheostomy (**14—12**) must be done, with administration of oxygen under positive pressure through the tube.
3. Immediate hospitalization.

48—6. ASTHMA (See also **52—1**)

TREATMENT
1. Rule out mechanical blockage from foreign bodies (**36—4**).
2. Start intravenous administration of 5% dextrose in saline as soon as possible.
3. Relieve dyspnea by subcutaneous injections of 1:1000 aqueous solution of epinephrine hydrochloride (Adrenalin). Repeated small injections are more effective and less dangerous than a single massive dose. The dosage should be as follows:

> Under 2 years, 0.1 ml.
> 2 to 3 years, 0.15 ml.
> 3 to 6 years, 0.2 ml.
> 6 to 12 years, 0.3 ml.
> 12 to 15 years, 0.4 ml.

If necessary these doses may be repeated every $1/2$ hour for 3 doses. In older children occasional use of 1:100 epinephrine hydrochloride (Adrenalin) solution in a nebulizer may give relief. Frequent or excessive use, however, is dangerous.
4. Give oxygen inhalations under positive pressure by face mask and rebreathing bag. In mild cases an oxygen tent may give relief.
5. Prescribe theophylline ethylenediamine (aminophylline) suppositories, provided vomiting is not present. Aminophylline may also be given intravenously very slowly in 20 ml. of 10% dextrose solution, 4 mg. per kilogram of body weight. Oral and intramuscular methods of administration are not satisfactory.
6. Give ephedrine sulfate or phenylpropanolamine hydrochloride (Propadrine), 12 to 25 mg. by mouth in older children.
7. Refer all cases to a pediatrician. Severe cases must be hospital-

ized. Penicillin or other antibiotics, as a rule, should not be administered as an emergency measure unless facilities allow obtaining cultures and sensitivity tests before the antibiotic is given.

48 — 7. BATTERED CHILD SYNDROME

Abuse of children by parents or other custodians is common, so much so that special laws have been enacted in many localities, including all 50 states of the United States, aimed not only at protection of children but also at protection of the attending physician, who has a moral obligation to report cases of child abuse to the proper law enforcement agencies. Evidence of the battered child syndrome is usually incidental to examination for an acute condition for which the child is brought to medical attention.

The attending physician should have a high index of suspicion when examination of an infant or child discloses any of the following conditions:

1. Any instance in which there is a discrepancy between the condition found and the history of onset given by the parents or other interested persons. An attempt should be made to distinguish between an accidental and an induced injury. The possibility of a contrived or prearranged accident should also be considered.

2. All cases in which the history of onset given by the parents differs from that given by neighbors or other witnesses.

3. All "crib deaths" [**48 — 57.** *Sudden Infant Death Syndrome (SIDS)*]. Recent studies seem to indicate that a few of these deaths are in fact infanticide.

4. X-ray demonstration of multiple fractures in varying stages of healing. This finding is usually considered to be conclusive evidence of child abuse.

5. Severe head injuries (fractures, subdural hematomas, etc.), especially if repeated.

6. Multiple bruises in different stages of healing.

7. Burns, especially a series of burns with an indefinite or unconvincing history of how they occurred.

8. Recurrent subluxations, especially of the elbows and shoulders.

9. Malnutrition and skin infections indicative of severe neglect.

The responsibilities of the attending physician are primarily the same as for any other type of case — adequate diagnosis and proper treatment. Every effort should be made to keep good rapport with the persons concerned with care of the injured child, avoiding an accusatory or punitive approach. Secondarily, however, the attending physician has the direct responsibility of reporting the condition to the proper authorities and of assisting in measures for evaluating the personality of the child's attendants by a special examiner trained and skilled in this field. Lastly, the attending physician should be prepared and willing to testify in court in case a legal action should ensue.

48 — 8. BITES See 24; 56. *Stings;* 61. *Venoms*

48 — 9. BRAIN CONCUSSION

Brain concussion (41 — 9) is characterized by complete loss of consciousness for a period which may be very brief and fleeting or prolonged. Children tolerate brain concussion much better than adults — the younger the child, the greater the chance of rapid and complete recovery. Unless definite localizing signs of increased intracranial pressure are present, hospitalization usually is not necessary, provided the parents can be made to understand the importance of limiting the child's activity and of keeping a close watch for changes in condition. These changes, indicative of increased intracranial pressure (41 — 9), should be specified in detail in simple nontechnical language to the persons responsible for the child's care.

48 — 10. BRAIN CONGESTION (Edema)

Brain congestion (edema) is caused by swelling of the brain substance within its nonelastic bony case and is characterized by slow development of signs and symptoms of pressure. Early physical and neurologic examination usually discloses no abnormalities. Early signs and symptoms are severe headache or persistent vomiting, or both; hypersensitivity and irritability; drowsiness, apathy and other variations from the normal behavior pattern. Late signs are papilledema, increased initial spinal fluid pressure and localizing neurologic signs (rare).

TREATMENT

Hospitalization for close observation and symptomatic treatment based on changes in condition noted on frequent recheck examinations. Spinal puncture rarely gives important information and may be dangerous.

48–11. BRAIN CONTUSION

Brain contusion predicates brain substance damage. The clinical picture depends upon the location and extent of damage. A history of transient unconsciousness may or may not be obtained. Common signs and symptoms are retrograde amnesia; acute excitement, sometimes maniacal; heavy breathing, occasionally of Cheyne-Stokes type; rapidly shifting and changing focal signs; convulsions, usually generalized; stupor or coma.

TREATMENT

1. Provided the child's condition has stabilized and the parents are reasonably intelligent and sensible, mild cases can be sent home with specific, detailed and well-understood instructions to the parents, or persons responsible for the child, to report any changes in condition immediately (41–12).

2. Severe cases require immediate hospitalization. Sedation by phenobarbital sodium subcutaneously or a pentobarbital sodium (Nembutal) suppository [dosage according to age (4)] may be necessary before transfer but should be avoided whenever possible.

No opiates or synthetic narcotics should ever be administered or prescribed because of their respiratory depressant effect and because of the possibility of masking important clinical signs (41–7).

48–12. BRAIN HEMORRHAGE See 41–19. *Epidural (Extradural) Hemorrhage; 41–20. Subdural Hemorrhage; 48–26*

48–13. BRONCHITIS See 48–48. *Respiratory Infections; 52–2*

48–14. BURNS (See also 25)

Many common household articles are hazards to children and may cause burns of varying extent and severity. Hot coffee, tea, foods and grease, stoves, fireplaces, steam kettles and unguarded electrical outlets all lie in wait for the unwary and curious toddler. Scalding bath water, burns from playing with matches, even sunburn (25–28), can be fatal.

The treatment and prognosis in burns in children depend upon the five factors outlined in **25 – 1**, with some modifications for age.

Per cent of body surface affected. This can be roughly calculated by a modification for age of the "Rule of Nines" (**25 – 1**).

PART OF BODY	PER CENT OF BODY SURFACE				
	At Birth	1 Year	5 Years	10 Years	Adults
Head, face and neck	21	19	15	13	9
Right arm, forearm and hand	9	9	9	9	9
Left arm, forearm and hand	9	9	9	9	9
Thorax – front	9	9	9	9	9
Thorax – back	9	9	9	9	9
Abdomen – ribs to inguinal creases	9	9	9	9	9
Back – ribs to subgluteal creases	9	9	9	9	9
Right thigh, leg and foot – front	6	$6^{1/2}$	$7^{1/2}$	8	9
Right thigh, leg and foot – back	6	$6^{1/2}$	$7^{1/2}$	8	9
Left thigh, leg and foot – front	6	$6^{1/2}$	$7^{1/2}$	8	9
Left thigh, leg and foot – back	6	$6^{1/2}$	$7^{1/2}$	8	9
Genitalia	1	1	1	1	1
	100	100	100	100	100

Depth of burn (25 – 1). Accurate estimation of the depth is impossible on first examination, even in superficial (first degree) burns with slight erythema.

Location of burn (25 – 1). Involvement of head, hands, genitalia and feet requires careful evaluation because of the tendency of burns in these areas to cause severe shock in 24 to 48 hours from "burn edema" or expansion of the extracellular fluid spaces.

Time elapsed since the burn (25 – 1).

Age and general physical condition (25 – 1). In children up to 5 years of age, severe shock may be caused by a partial skin thickness burn involving as little as 10% of the total skin surface. Older children will usually tolerate damage of as much as 20 to 25% of the total skin surface without serious complications. If the child is below normal in nutrition, development or general resistance, even smaller burned areas may have serious sequelae.

TREATMENT (See also **25 – 2**)

Minor burns (first degree or superficial, involving less than 25% of the body surface).

1. Place infants and small children under sedation with a pentobarbital sodium (Nembutal) suppository, 0.03 to 0.06 gm. In children 6 years old or older, small doses of codeine sulfate or, if the pain

is very great, morphine sulfate, subcutaneously [dosage according to age or weight (**4**)] may be necessary. Morphine should never be used for control of pain in infants.

2. Remove all contamination – especially the numerous materials which may be applied as "first aid" by inexperienced persons – by gentle sponging with a mild detergent, followed by warm, sterile saline solution.

3. Apply a petrolatum gauze dressing.

4. Administer tetanus-immune globulin (TIG) or toxoid (**16**).

Severe burns (second or third degree, involving more than 25% of the total body surface).

1. Cover the burned areas with sterile towels or clean sheets.

2. Control severe pain by small doses of barbiturates or, in older children, narcotics, in the smallest possible effective doses (**4**).

3. Institute supportive therapy at once by intravenous plasma volume expanders and electrolyte solutions (**6**), avoiding excessive chloride intake. (Note: Before intravenous administration of synthetic plasma volume expanders, 20 ml. of blood should be collected so that typing, cross-matching and other necessary tests can be performed more easily and accurately.) Saline solution should be given by mouth after vomiting has stopped. Tap water should not be used.

4. Use aseptic technique while cleansing the burned areas with a mild detergent and sterile saline solution. All surface contamination should be removed. Loose flaps of charred or devitalized tissues should be trimmed off with sterile scissors. Blebs should not be opened or extensive debridement attempted.

5. Apply an occlusive dressing of petrolatum gauze or fine mesh gauze, held in place by bias-cut stockinette.

6. Elevate burned extremities and splint damaged joints.

7. Hospitalize at once. A detailed summary of all treatment must accompany the patient to the hospital. Sulfamylon cream therapy should be instituted as soon as the child is hospitalized.

For treatment of burns requiring special management, see **25**. *Burns*.

48 – 15.   CARDIAC EMERGENCIES IN CHILDREN

Except for cardiac arrest (**26 – 7**), the common heart conditions requiring emergency handling which occur in adults (**26**) are relatively rare in infants and children. However, certain cardiac conditions in infants and children do require immediate recognition and treatment, sometimes as a lifesaving measure.

CONGENITAL CYANOTIC HEART DISEASE WITH ACUTE HYPOXEMIA

There is no satisfactory explanation for this acute oxygen want, usually occurring in infants but occasionally in older children. The hypoxemia may last for a few minutes or persist for several hours with complete spontaneous recovery, or death may occur from cardiac arrest (**26 – 7**).

SIGNS AND SYMPTOMS. Irritability, vigorous crying followed by progressively increasing dyspnea and cyanosis, loss of consciousness from lack of adequate oxygenation and cardiac failure.

TREATMENT

1. Expired air respiration (**11 – 1**) until administration of oxygen under positive pressure by face mask or endotracheal catheter and rebreathing bag can be substituted.

2. Morphine sulfate, 0.2 mg. per kilogram of body weight subcutaneously; or in extreme cases, 0.1 mg. per kilogram of body weight intravenously. (Do not use in infants or children under 3 years of age.)

3. Knee-chest position.

CONGESTIVE FAILURE (ACUTE) (See also **26 – 8.**)

SIGNS AND SYMPTOMS. Restlessness and irritability, cough, dyspnea, cyanosis, vomiting, edema (especially of the face) and enlargement of the liver.

TREATMENT

1. Oxygen under positive pressure by face mask or endotracheal catheter.

2. Short-acting barbiturates intramuscularly or by rectal suppository or retention enema – dosage according to age or weight (**4**).

3. Digoxin intramuscularly in divided doses (if not already digitalized). The total digitalizing dose for infants and children under 2 years of age is 0.03 to 0.04 mg. per kilogram of body weight; for children who are 2 years of age and older, the dose is 0.02 to 0.03 mg. per kilogram of body weight.

Paroxysmal tachycardia. (See also **26 – 13.** *Nodal Paroxysmal Tachycardia.*) The cause of this condition is unknown, although congenital heart disease, drug sensitivity and acute infections seem to play a part. It is characterized by rapid breathing, grayish pallor, irritability, sleepiness, vomiting and very rapid, often uncountable, pulse. Electrocardiograms show a regular rapid rate with absence of normal P waves and P-R intervals. Enlargement of the heart and liver may be present.

TREATMENT

1. Digital pressure over the carotid sinus — *one side only* (**26–13**).

2. Induction of vomiting by oral administration of 4 to 8 ml. of syrup of ipecac.

3. Administration of oxygen under positive pressure by face mask or endotracheal catheter and rebreathing bag.

4. Subcutaneous injection of morphine sulfate, 0.2 mg. per kilogram of body weight, for extreme restlessness but not in infants or children under 3 years of age.

5. Immediate hospitalization if steps 1 and 2 (above) are not successful. Detailed studies may be required to distinguish between ventricular and supraventricular tachycardia.

Pericardial tamponade may be due to acute pericardial effusion or bleeding (**26–22**). Any overwhelming infection or injury to the heart or pericardium may be responsible.

SIGNS AND SYMPTOMS. Dyspnea, pulsations of the veins of the neck; paradoxical pulse and enlargement of the heart and liver.

TREATMENT

1. Administration of oxygen by face mask if extreme dyspnea is present.

2. Immediate hospitalization for evacuation of the excess pericardial fluid unless rapid degeneration in condition requires immediate aspiration (**14–7**).

Stokes-Adams Syndrome. (See also **26–20**.) Congenital heart disease, rheumatic fever and diphtheria may cause partial or complete heart block. It also may be caused by poisoning from certain drugs, especially metacholine (Mecholyl) (**49–444**) and potassium salts.

SIGNS AND SYMPTOMS. Sudden collapse, cyanosis, convulsions and very slow or absent pulse, with absence of any perceptible heart beat by auscultation. Death usually occur in a few minutes unless the heart beat becomes reestablished.

TREATMENT

The treatment available under emergency conditions rarely influences the outcome, but the following measures may be tried:

1. Expired air respiration (**11–1**) and closed cardiac massage (**11–2**).

2. Intravenous or intracardiac injection of small doses (0.1 to

0.5 ml.) of a 1:1000 solution of epinephrine hydrochloride (Adrenalin), repeated at 5 to 10 minute intervals.

3. Subcutaneous or intravenous injection of atropine sulfate, 0.25 to 0.6 mg.

4. Immediate hospitalization with heart-lung resuscitation (**11**) continued en route. If equipment is available, stimulation by an artificial pacemaker may result in life-saving reestablishment of the normal heart beat.

48 – 16. CONCUSSION OF THE BRAIN See 48 – 9. *Brain Concussion*

48 – 17. CONTAGIOUS DISEASES See 30. *Contagious and Communicable Diseases*

48 – 18. CONVULSIONS (See also 31. *Convulsive Seizures*)

CAUSES. Convulsions are much more frequent in children than in adults. Hyperpyrexia caused by acute infections is by far the most common etiologic factor. Among other causative conditions are:

Alkalosis (**48 – 3**) from prolonged vomiting or hyperventilation (**34 – 6**).
Allergic reactions (**21**).
Brain abnormalities (congenital, developmental or traumatic).
Breath holding (occasionally).
Cerebral degenerative diseases.
Encephalitis (**48 – 24**).
Epilepsy (**29 – 7**).
Extradural hemorrhage (**41 – 19**).
Head injuries (**41**).
Hypocalcemia from tetany (**43 – 25**), rickets or hypothyroidism.
Hypoglycemia (**43 – 16**), with or without diabetes.
Hysteria (**50 – 6**).
Intracranial blood vessel abnormalities (**59 – 2**).
Kernicterus in erythroblastotic infants.
Lead encephalopathy (**49 – 420**).
Meningitis (**48 – 41**).
Otitis media (**32 – 13**).
Parasitic infection (**37 – 20**).
Pneumonia (**48 – 45; 52 – 14; 62 – 11**. *Interstitial Pneumonia*).
Poisoning from ingestion, inhalation of fumes or absorption

through the skin or mucous membranes of many drugs and other substances.

Among the more common are:

Amphetamines (**49 – 64**)
Arsenic salts (**49 – 90**)
Aspirin (**49 – 101**)
Atropine (**49 – 104**)
Bromates (**49 – 143**)
Caffeine (**49 – 157**)
Camphor (**49 – 163**)
Carbon tetrachloride (**49 – 173**)
Castor beans (**49 – 177**)
Chokecherry (**49 – 206**)
Codeine (**49 – 219**)
Ephedrine (**49 – 300**)
Ethyl alcohol (**49 – 315**)
Fluorides (**49 – 336**)
Gasoline (**49 – 349**)
Kerosene (**49 – 408**)
Lead salts (**49 – 420**)
Metaldehyde (**49 – 462**)

Methyl salicylate (**49 – 486**)
Moth repellents (**49 – 497**)
Mushrooms (**49 – 502**)
Naphthol (**49 – 511**)
Nicotine (**49 – 523**)
Opiates (**49 – 545**)
Organic phosphates (**49 – 546**)
Phenol (**49 – 590**)
Phenothiazines (**49 – 592**)
Picrotoxin (**49 – 606**)
Quinine (**49 – 642**)
Saccharin (**49 – 658**)
Salicylates (**49 – 664**)
Silver nitrate (**49 – 688**)
Snake venom (**24 – 19; 61.** *Venoms*)
Tetrachlorethane (**49 – 758**)
Thiocyanates (**49 – 774**)
Tobacco (**49 – 790**)

Septicemia and bacteremia (**48 – 41.** *Meningitis;* **48 – 42.** *Meningococcemia*).

Subdural hemorrhage (**41 – 20**).

Temper tantrums (**34; 48 – 25.** *Excitement States*).

Tetanus (**30 – 31**).

Tetany (**43 – 25**).

TREATMENT

Convulsions, as a general rule, are self-limiting and of short duration and do not require heroic measures for control. The causative factor should be determined as soon as possible. Any or all of the following measures may be indicated if the convulsions are prolonged or repeated, and as protection against injury:

1. Prevention of self-injury, such as tongue-biting or injuries to the musculoskeletal structures (strains, dislocations, fractures).

2. Insurance of an adequate airway by positioning, removal of mucus and secretions by suction, and support of the jaw.

3. Administration of oxygen by face mask if cyanosis is present.

4. Reduction of high fever by sponging with alcohol or tepid water, application of cold compresses, or cold water enemas.

5. Sedation by:

Suppositories or capsules of:

Pentobarbital sodium (Nembutal), 0.03 gm. for children under 2 years of age; 0.06 gm. for children over 2 years of age.

Secobarbital (Seconal) according to the following dosage table:

Under 1 year, 50 mg.
1 to 2 years, 50 to 100 mg.
2 to 3 years, 100 to 200 mg.
3 to 5 years, 200 to 250 mg.
Over 5 years, 250 to 330 mg.

Subcutaneous administration of phenobarbital sodium, 4 to 5 mg. per kilogram of body weight. In children over 5 years the doses should be adjusted according to age or weight (**4**).

Amytal sodium, 60 to 120 mg.

Pentothal sodium given only by or under the direct supervision of an anesthesiologist. The intravenous route should be used only in severe or protracted convulsions.

Rectal instillation (by retention enema) of:

Pentothal sodium, 0.4 ml. of 10% solution per kilogram of body weight.

Paraldehyde in olive oil, 0.4 ml. of 10% solution per kilogram of body weight.

Inhalations of ether by the open drop method if the convulsions cannot be controlled within 30 to 45 minutes by other means.

6. Determination of causative factors. If signs and symptoms suggestive of meningitis (**48 – 41**) or intracranial hemorrhage (**41 – 19.** *Extradural Hemorrhage;* **41 – 20.** *Subdural Hemorrhage;* **59 – 2**) are present, or if the convulsions are severe and no extracranial cause can be found, spinal puncture (**14 – 11**) as an emergency diagnostic procedure is indicated provided preliminary examination of the fundi shows no evidence of choked disks. The spinal fluid pressure and appearance (clear, turbid, bloody or xanthochromic), together with the presence or absence of block, should be noted.

NORMAL SPINAL FLUID IN CHILDREN

Cell count	0 to 5 per cu. mm. (mostly lymphocytes). More than an occasional polymorphonuclear leucocyte or red blood cell in an atraumatic tap is abnormal.
Chlorides	120 to 130 mEq. per L.
Glucose	50 to 70 mg. per 100 ml.
Protein	15 to 40 mg. per 100 ml.
Pandy test	Negative

7. Hospitalization in all cases except uncomplicated, easily controlled, febrile convulsions.

Do not

Allow the child to injure himself during a convulsion.

Delay anticonvulsive treatment. If the convulsion is prolonged, death may occur from exhaustion, high fever or cerebral accident.

Give chloroform by the drop method for control of convulsions; the margin of safety between the effective and lethal doses is too small.

Administer opiates or synthetic narcotics of any type.

Send a child home when the cause of severe or protracted convulsive seizures has not been determined. Hospitalization for thorough study is a *must*.

48–19. CROUP

Croup is a symptom complex (not a disease entity) caused by narrowing of the epiglottic aperture by edema or swelling. It is characterized by stridulous cough, usually preceded by or associated with mild respiratory infection, and has a notorious tendency to develop without warning during sleep and to become worse suddenly. Usually there is little temperature rise. As the child coughs, his voice becomes progressively hoarse.

Home treatment may be tried.

1. Position of comfort; most children are more comfortable sitting up.

2. Increase of moisture content of the air by:

Cold vaporizers

Hot steam devices, placed where they cannot be upset.

Running a hot shower in a closed bathroom.

Use of a steam kettle if other means are not available. Every precaution should be taken to prevent burning the patient or other children if a steam kettle must be used.

3. Antipyrine by mouth, 0.06 gm. per year of age up to 3, repeated if necessary every 4 hours for 4 doses.

4. Syrup of ipecac, 4 ml. by mouth every 15 minutes until vomiting occurs (not more than 6 doses).

5. Sedation by a pentobarbital sodium (Nembutal) suppository, 0.03 to 0.06 gm., or by camphorated opium tincture (paregoric) in small doses by mouth, provided the child is over 1 year of age.

Hospital treatment is definitely indicated if the measures given above do not result in a decrease in signs and symptoms or if there is any suspicion of loss of airway patency.

48 – 20. DIABETIC COMA (See also 29 – 3. *Diabetes Mellitus*)

Coma may develop in diabetic children with astonishing rapidity. Vomiting, acute infections or refusal of food for any reason may be the precipitating factor. Whenever possible, a blood sugar determination should be obtained before treatment is begun.

For signs, symptoms and differential diagnosis of diabetic coma, see **29 – 3**.

TREATMENT

1. Intravenous injection of 25 ml. of the following sterile hydration solution per kilogram of body weight (**6**):

0.9% sodium chloride	200 ml.
Molar lactate	20 ml.
Distilled water q.s. ad	500 ml.

2. Intravenous injection of plasma volume expanders, 10 ml. per kilogram of body weight.

3. Subcutaneous injection of regular insulin, 1 to 1½ units per kilogram of body weight. Any potassium imbalance should be corrected (**6**).

4. Hospitalization for further care. A detailed summary of findings and treatment *must* accompany the patient to the hospital.

48 – 21. DIARRHEA

ACUTE TOXIC DIARRHEA

TREATMENT

Mild Cases

1. Discontinue all food or liquids by mouth if vomiting is present. When vomiting has been controlled (**48 – 62**), start on sips of boiled water or weak tea, supplemented in 8 to 12 hours by barley or rice water and boiled skim milk; later, add gelatin preparations and crushed ripe bananas.

2. Give tincture of opium (laudanum) or camphorated tincture of opium (paregoric) by mouth provided the child is over 6 months old [dosage according to age or weight (**6**)], and provided there is not excessive mucus in the stool.

3. If infection is present, and the offending organism and its sensitivity are known, give the appropriate antibiotic (**30 – 41**.

Antimicrobial Drugs of Choice); otherwise, avoid antibiotic therapy, which in itself may cause diarrhea.

4. Refer to a pediatrician for follow up care.

Severe Cases

1. Stop intake of all fluids and foods by mouth if vomiting is present.

2. Combat shock and dehydration by intravenous electrolytes and/or dextrose (**6**).

3. Give oxygen under positive pressure by face mask and re-breathing bag if cyanosis or air hunger is present.

4. Arrange for transportation at once to a hospital equipped for blood chemistry determinations and replacement therapy (**6**). A detailed summary of all emergency treatment must go with the patient to the hospital.

ACUTE INFECTIOUS DIARRHEA

This type may require immediate hospitalization for isolation and treatment.

48–22. DROWNING (See also 22–3)

In children, the most efficient methods of resuscitation, after insurance of a clear airway by postural drainage and suction, are:

1. Expired air respiration, with or without alternating gentle chest compression (**11–1**).

2. The prone tilting visceral shift teeter-board method (Rickard), for infants only. For technique, see **11–1**.

All patients, particularly those who have undergone immersion in fresh or brackish water, should be hospitalized for at least 48 hours for observation and treatment of delayed symptoms.

48–23. ELECTRIC SHOCK See 25–11. Electrical Burns; 29–5

48–24. ENCEPHALITIS, ACUTE (See also 62–5)

CAUSES. Acute encephalitis with high fever, restlessness, head-ache, delirium, convulsions and coma may be caused by many con-ditions in children. Among these are:

Choriomeningitis.

Contagious diseases, especially chickenpox (**30–3**), measles (**30–15**), Coxsackie and ECHO viruses, mumps (**30–17**) and poliomyelitis (**30–21**).

Epidemic and equine encephalitis (**62—5**).

Herpes simplex (**62—9**).

Lymphopathia venereum (**60—4**).

Poisoning due to ingestion, inhalation of fumes or dust or absorption through the skin or mucous membranes of many substances. Notorious offenders are:

Alkyl mercury compounds (**49—42**)

Arsenic compounds (**49—90**)

Carbon monoxide (**49—172**)

Iodoform (**49—394**)

Isopropyl alcohol (**49—403**)

Lead and its salts (**49—420**)

Morphine and other opiates (**49—495**)

Sulfathiazole (**49—731**)

Tetraethyl lead (**49—761**)

Thallium (**49—768**)

Polioencephalitis (**30—21**).

Smallpox vaccination (very rare—practically never occurs in children under the age of 3).

Toxoplasmosis (usually chronic but occasionally acute).

TREATMENT

Symptomatic

1. Alcohol or tepid water sponges to reduce fever.

2. Sedation as given under *Convulsions* (**48—18**).

3. Acetylsalicylic acid (aspirin) to relieve headaches and to lower the temperature.

4. Treatment for poisoning as outlined under the specific poison (**49**).

5. Immediate transfer to a hospital equipped for adequate investigation and definitive therapy.

48—25. EXCITEMENT STATES (See also **34**)

CAUSES. Acute excitement states in children may be caused by fear, high fever, psychologic conflicts at home or elsewhere, or trauma, especially chest injuries (**28**) and head injuries (**41; 48—32**). Since there seems to be some relation between extreme excitement and cardiac arrest (**26—7**), children should be under sedation when they are taken to the operating room and should be watched carefully by an anesthesiologist during any surgical procedure.

TREATMENT

1. Restraint—gentle manual restraint if possible, mechanical if necessary.

2. Sedation by:

Barbiturates. A pentobarbital sodium (Nembutal) suppository,

0.03 to 0.06 gm., is generally adequate in small children. In older children phenobarbital sodium, 6.5 mg. per kilogram of body weight intramuscularly, may be required.

Chloral hydrate by mouth in orange juice or a carbonated beverage, 0.4 ml. of 10% solution per kilogram of body weight; total not over 10 ml.

Paraldehyde by retention enema or intramuscularly, 0.15 ml. per kilogram of body weight.

Chlorpromazine hydrochloride (Thorazine) orally, rectally or intramuscularly in children over 2 years of age.

DOSAGE BY AGE
2 to 4 years, 5 mg.
4 to 6 years, 8 mg.
6 to 8 years, 10 mg.
8 to 15 years, 15 mg.

DOSAGE PER KILOGRAM OF BODY WEIGHT
Orally or intramuscularly, 0.5 mg.
Rectally, 1.0 mg.
Note: If Thorazine or allied drugs are used, the dosage of barbiturates or narcotics should always be reduced by at least one-half because of the potentiating effect of phenothiazines (**49 – 592**).

3. Hospitalization if a chest injury (**28**) or head injury (**41; 48 – 32**) is present or suspected. Acute excitement may be the only indication of severe intrathoracic or intracranial damage in children.

4. Referral to a pediatrician for investigation and treatment of the causative factors.

48 – 26. EXTRADURAL (EPIDURAL) HEMORRHAGE (See also 41 – 19)

This condition is relatively uncommon in infants and children.

SIGNS AND SYMPTOMS

A history of a fall or of a blow on the head, sometimes apparently very minor.

A period of unconsciousness of varying length followed by a lucid interval. This, however, is not always present; coma may persist from the time of injury, or coma may develop without previous impairment of consciousness.

Dilation of the pupil on the injured side.

Twitching or progressive weakness of the muscles of the face or of the extremities on the side opposite the head injury, followed by a convulsive seizure.

Aphasia, with progressively increasing stupor; then coma, with slow pulse and labored respiration.

Terminal rapid pulse and temperature elevation.

TREATMENT

1. Sedation by intravenous or rectal barbiturates (**48 — 18.** *Convulsions in Children*).

2. *Immediate* hospitalization. Surgical exploration and control of the bleeding vessel, usually the middle meningeal artery or one of its branches, must be performed as quickly as possible. This is one of the few instances in which speed in transportation to a hospital equipped for brain surgery is essential in order to prevent irreparable brain damage.

48 — 27. EYE INJURIES AND INFECTIONS See 35.

48 — 28. FALLS (See also **48 — 1.** *Accidents in Children*)

Since children must learn about the effects of gravity by experience, it is not surprising that the incidence of injuries caused by falls is quite high, especially in the 6 months to 3 years age group. Carelessness of the parents is, of course, the most important factor. The distance the child falls may be of importance, but a severe, even fatal, injury may occur from what is apparently a minor incident. Conversely, a fall of many feet may result in little, if any, injury, especially in small children. Careful physical examination and close observation over at least 8 hours for changes in the state of consciousness and development of localizing neurologic signs is essential (**41 — 2**). Treatment of the different types of injuries resulting from falls is covered under their respective headings.

48 — 29. FOREIGN BODIES (See also **36**)

Contrary to general belief, unless actual obstruction or danger of perforation is present, foreign bodies, especially in the respiratory and alimentary tracts, do not always represent urgent emergencies.

In the ears. See **36 — 1.**

In the eyes. See **35 — 31.** *Conjunctiva;* **35 — 32.** *Cornea;* **35 — 38.** *Sympathetic Ophthalmia.*

In the nose. See **36 — 3.**

In the throat (see also **36 — 4; 48 — 44.** *Localization Chart*). If the child is cooperative, removal of small sharp objects (fish bones, splinters, sucker sticks, toy arrows, etc.) imbedded in the gums, hard palate, posterior nasopharynx or tonsillar fossae may be possible. In many cases, particularly after unsuccessful attempts at removal at home, a general anesthetic is necessary.

In a bronchus (see also **36—4**). Immediate hospitalization for bronchoscopic examination, localization and removal is indicated. Emphysema, caused by the ball-valve action of the foreign body, and aspiration pneumonia may develop if the obstruction is not removed. Peanuts are especially dangerous due to the action of an absorbable alkaloid, arachine.

In the esophagus (see also **36—5**). Hospitalization is required if x-rays at 6 to 8 hour intervals show no progress in 24 hours, if severe pain is present or if there is clinical evidence of obstruction or perforation.

In the stomach (see also **36—5**). Rounded objects under 1½ inches in size will usually pass through the stomach and intestinal tract without complications unless the child is very small. No changes in diet should be made or laxatives or cathartics given. Sharp objects (straight pins, open safety pins, needles, large glass fragments, etc.) require close clinical and x-ray observation, preferably in the hospital. Lack of progression and clinical evidence suggestive of perforation are indications for gastroscopic or surgical exploration and removal.

In the intestinal tract (see also **36—5**). Close observation is usually all that is required. Any object which will enter and leave the stomach will almost always go the rest of the way. Severe pain, abdominal rigidity and clinical and x-ray signs of obstruction or perforation are indications for hospitalization for possible surgical removal (**36—5**).

In the soft tissues or skeletal structures. See **36—6**.

48—30. GASTROINTESTINAL TRACT EMERGENCIES (See also 37)

Diarrhea. See **48—21**.

Infectious. Immediate hospitalization for isolation and treatment is mandatory.

Toxic. See **48—21**.

Foreign bodies. See **36—5; 48—29**.

Hemorrhage (see also **37—6.** *Anorectal Conditions;* **42—22.** *Rectal Bleeding;* **42—25.** *Bleeding from the Stomach*). Persistent or recurrent bleeding of any degree from any part of the gastro-intestinal tract in any child in any age group requires immediate thorough investigation and treatment, preferably in a hospital. In severe cases with extensive blood loss, intravenous plasma volume expanders and replacement fluids (**6**) and support of the circulation by vasopressor drugs (**53 — 7**) may be necessary before and during transfer to the hospital.

Poisoning. See **48 — 47** and listings under the appropriate heading in section **49**.

Rectal prolapse. See **37 — 5**.

Surgical abdominal conditions (see also **19**. *Abdominal Pain*). In infants and children acute abdominal conditions requiring surgical intervention are most commonly due to:

Appendicitis (**37 — 7**).

Foreign bodies (**36 — 5; 48 — 29**).

Hernia, strangulated or incarcerated (**37 — 5; 48 — 35**).

Malformation of the large or small bowel (**48 — 38**. *Intestinal Obstruction*).

Peptic ulcer with perforation (**37 — 3**. *Perforation, Intraperitoneal*).

Pyloric stenosis (**48 — 38**. *Intestinal Obstruction*).

Trauma — especially rupture of the spleen (**55 — 31**. *Splenic Injuries*).

Volvulus (**48 — 61**).

All require immediate hospitalization for careful differential diagnosis, usually followed by laparotomy.

48 — 31. GENITOURINARY TRACT EMERGENCIES (See also 38)

ANURIA

Sudden decrease in output or complete shutting off of urine may be caused by:

Obstruction of the Urethra with Resultant Distended Bladder from Inflammation or Edema

TREATMENT

1. Hot compresses or baths.

2. Gentle dilatation with a small catheter. Insertion of an indwelling catheter, using sterile technique (**14 — 3**), may be necessary.

3. Antibiotic therapy after determination of the offending

organism and its sensitivities (**30 – 41.** *Antimicrobial Drugs of Choice*).

4. Hospitalization in severe cases for care by a urologist.

Obstruction from Insertion of Foreign Bodies into the Urethra

TREATMENT

1. Gentle "milking" of the male urethra from the base of the penis toward the glans sometimes allows removal through the meatus.

2. Surgical removal with the aid of a urethroscope. This procedure requires hospitalization.

Kidney Diseases

Acute and chronic glomerulonephritides are the conditions most frequently found in children. Both require hospitalization for pediatric care.

Extrarenal Conditions (especially cardiac decompensation)

TREATMENT. Hospitalization for pediatric care is usually indicated.

Central Nervous System Disease or Injury

TREATMENT. Hospitalize for diagnosis and treatment, preferably under the care of a neurologist.

Overdosage of Sulfonamides (See also **49 – 731**)

TREATMENT

1. Check the urine for sulfa crystals; if present, stop the offending drug at once.

2. Force fluids by mouth.

3. Give sodium lactate, 250 to 500 ml. of 1/6 M solution, intravenously (**6**).

4. Hospitalize for pediatric care if the anuria is complete or if the history indicates or suggests excessive intake of, or sensitivity to, sulfonamides (**49 – 731**).

BLADDER INJURIES See 38 – 1.

CYSTITIS (See also 38 – 10)

Infections of the bladder are very common in girls and should be ruled out by urinalysis in all cases of unexplained high fever or abdominal pain in young females.

KIDNEY INJURIES See 38 – 2.

PARAPHIMOSIS See **38 − 15.**

RENAL COLIC See **38 − 20.** *Stone in the Urinary Tract*

TESTICULAR TORSION (See also **38 − 7**)

This condition must always be differentiated from incarcerated hernia (**37 − 5; 48 − 35**), epididymitis (**38 − 11**) and orchitis (**38 − 3**). If gentle manipulation under sedation does not correct the torsion, *immediate* referral for operative relief is indicated.

URETHRAL INJURIES See **38 − 8.**

48 − 32. HEAD INJURIES (See also **34 − 4.** *Excitement States;* **41;** **48 − 9** through **48 − 12.** *Brain Injuries in Children;* **48 − 26.** *Extradural Hemorrhage*)

Head injuries are far better tolerated by children, especially infants, than by adults. Neurologic examination often is not satisfactory or reliable in determining the extent of the injury, no matter what the age of the child. Neither is the history, as the severity of the accident often has little, if any, relation to the amount of intracranial damage. All children with known or suspected head injuries should be examined *at frequent intervals* for signs and symptoms of increased intracranial pressure (**41 − 2**). Changes in condition are the most important factors in evaluation and prognosis.

State of consciousness. A prolonged acute excitement state (**34;** **48 − 25**) often indicates a poor prognosis.

Shock (**53**) is unusual following head injuries in adults, but severe, sometimes terminal, shock may occur in children following head injuries which appear to be comparatively mild.

Pupillary signs

Pinpoint pupils are usually considered to be indicative of severe brain stem damage.

Dilated fixed pupils may indicate extensive brain damage.

Unilateral dilation of the pupil usually is transient and of little importance; if persistent, it may indicate severe brain damage.

Reflex changes

Hyperactive deep tendon reflexes in children may indicate severe brain contusion (**48 − 11**) with a poor prognosis for complete recovery.

Complete loss of deep tendon reflexes may follow severe brain stem injury. The prognosis is poor.

Hyperactivity of deep tendon reflexes or clonus on one side only suggests local brain damage on the opposite side of the head with a favorable prognosis following adequate therapy. A positive Babinski sign ("up-going toe") is indicative of the same condition.

TREATMENT. See **41.** *Head Injuries.*

Transient blindness following head trauma. Total blindness lasting from a few minutes to a few hours may follow apparently trivial head injuries, especially contusions over the temporoparietal areas, in children — usually without other ocular abnormalities or impairment of consciousness. Electroencephalograms may show temporary cerebral dysfunction. In the absence of other signs of brain damage, recovery is usually spontaneous and complete.

48 — 33. HEAT EMERGENCIES See **57 — 2.** *Heat Cramps;* **57 — 3.** *Heat Exhaustion;* **57 — 4.** *Heat Hyperpyrexia;* **57 — 6.** *Iatrogenic Heat Stroke;* **57 — 7.** *Low Salt Syndrome*

48 — 34. HEMORRHAGE IN CHILDREN See **41.** *Head Injuries;* **42.** *Hemorrhage;* **48 — 32.** *Head Injuries in Children;* **59 — 1** and **59 — 2.** *Vascular Emergencies*

48 — 35. HERNIA (See also **37 — 5**)

Diaphragmatic (hiatal). Diagnostic signs and symptoms (progressive dyspnea, cyanosis, shift of the heart to the right) result from encroachment of the stomach and small bowel into the chest, the so-called "upside down stomach." This condition is usually the result of congenital weakness, but trauma may be the precipitating factor.

TREATMENT

Immediate hospitalization for evaluation and possible surgical exploration and repair. The sooner this is accomplished, the better the prognosis.

Femoral. Protrusion of a loop of bowel through a femoral ring is rare in infants and children but occasionally does occur. Surgical repair as soon as possible is indicated if the hernia cannot be reduced by gentle manipulation; if reduction is possible, repair becomes an elective procedure.

Hiatal. See *Diaphragmatic* (above).

Inguinal. In children, these hernias are almost always direct and represent a surgical emergency only if strangulation or irreducible incarceration is present. Support by a tight-fitting binder is often all that is necessary until operative repair can be done as an elective procedure.

Umbilical. This is by far the commonest type of infantile hernia. Incarceration and strangulation practically never occur. Repeated reassurance of the parents is often the most important part of therapy. Spontaneous closure without treatment usually occurs.

48−36. HICCUPS

In infancy, gentle pressure over the upper abdomen after each feeding is usually all that is necessary. For treatment of hiccups in older children, see **52−7**.

48−37. HYPOGLYCEMIA (See also **29−3**. *Coma;* **43−16**. *Metabolic Disorders*)

Blood sugar levels below 40 mg. per 100 ml. from any cause may cause signs and symptoms requiring immediate therapy. These include restlessness, hunger, dilated pupils, increased pulse rate and convulsions followed by coma.

TREATMENT

1. Orange juice or sugar-containing carbonated beverages by mouth are usually all that is necessary in mild cases without unconsciousness or vomiting. If vomiting is present, 500 ml. of 5% dextrose in water should be given intravenously.

2. Severe cases should be hospitalized at once after intravenous administration of 10% dextrose in saline. Convulsions (**48−18**) should be controlled before transfer.

3. All cases should be placed under pediatric supervision as soon as possible.

48−38. INTESTINAL OBSTRUCTION (See also **37−2**)

Early recognition of obstruction is essential for successful therapy. Among the many causes are:

Annular pancreas with compression of the duodenum.

Foreign bodies. See **36−5; 48−29**.

Hernia with strangulation (usually inguinal). See **48−35**.

Ileus—from meconium or following abdominal injury.

Imperforate anus, intestinal atresia at any level, megacolon, and other congenital or developmental abnormalities (**37 — 1**).

Intussusception and volvulus (**48 — 61**).

Pyloric stenosis (**37 — 1**).

TREATMENT

No matter what the cause, suggestive or conclusive evidence of intestinal obstruction in children requires immediate hospitalization for diagnosis, localization and possible surgical treatment.

48 — 39.   KETOSIS

Children store a relatively small amount of glycogen in the liver; hence, in the absence of adequate insulin therapy, or in the presence of an acute infection, unconsciousness may develop very rapidly in diabetic children.

TREATMENT

See **48 — 20**. *Diabetic Coma in Children.*

48 — 40.   LACERATIONS See **55 — 20**.

48 — 41.   MENINGITIS (See also **30 — 16**, **48 — 42**. *Meningococcemia;* **48 — 63**. *Waterhouse-Friderichsen Syndrome*)

Among the many organisms which may cause meningitis are:

Arboviruses (**62 — 1**)	Meningococcus
E. coli	Pneumococcus
Friedlander's bacillus	Staphylococcus
Fungi	M. tuberculosis
Hemophilus influenzae	

All may cause identical clinical pictures — stiff neck, high fever, convulsions, and coma — and all may be fatal if not treated promptly and energetically.

TREATMENT

1. Prevention of injury during convulsions (**31**. *Convulsive Seizures;* **48 — 18**. *Convulsions in Children*).

2. Insurance of an adequate airway by postural drainage and suction.

3. Reduction of high fever by sponging, ice packs and other available means.

4. Spinal puncture (**14 — 11**) under isolation technique for deter-

mination of pressure, appearance and chemical findings, with identification of the causative organism. Disposition will depend upon the established diagnosis, since isolation precautions not available in many general hospitals may be required.

5. Immediate institution of treatment while awaiting arrangements for disposition. (See **30—41.** *Antimicrobial Drugs of Choice.*)

48—42. MENINGOCOCCEMIA (See also 48—41. *Meningitis;* 48—63. *Waterhouse-Friderichsen Syndrome*)

Development of signs and symptoms suggestive of this very serious condition—especially rapid development of petechiae—requires *immediate* massive antibiotic therapy (see **30—41.** *Antimicrobial Drugs of Choice*), preferably intravenously, while transfer for hospitalization is being arranged.

48—43. MIGRAINE (See also 27—21. *Migraine Headaches*)

Migraine may occur in infancy but is more common in children between 5 and 10 years of age. Although there is a strong hereditary tendency toward the condition, attacks may be precipitated by allergic conditions, acute or chronic infections, errors in refraction, psychogenic disturbances, fatigue, lack of sleep or other breaks in the normal habit pattern. Nausea and vomiting, with abdominal pain severe enough to be mistaken for an acute surgical condition, are the main symptoms in children under 12 years of age; over 12, headaches are predominant. Vertigo, scintillation and scotomata are common; hemianopsia is rare. Edema of the face and eyelids, cardiac symptoms ("precordial migraine") and disturbances in smell may occur. Headaches apparently become more severe and more frequent as the child grows older (possibly because it is difficult to determine whether or not a small child has a headache).

TREATMENT

1. Acetylsalicylic acid (aspirin) will control mild cases.

2. Ergotamine tartrate, 1 mg. by mouth for a child of 6, repeated in 1 hour, usually will give some relief.

3. Codeine sulfate intramuscularly or orally, or pentazocine lactate (Talwin) intramuscularly may be necessary in severe cases [dosage according to age (**4**)], but neither should be prescribed for children under ten years of age. Morphine sulfate, meperidine hydrochloride (Demerol) and other narcotics should never be used because of their addictive tendencies.

4. Antihistaminics, barbiturates, epinephrine hydrochloride, ephedrine sulfate and diphenylhydantoin (Dilantin) are of little, if any, permanent value, although transient relief may be obtained. Methysergide maleate (Sansert) is of value as a preventive agent but has many undesirable side effects.

5. Referral to a pediatrician for follow-up care is always indicated.

48—44. OBSTRUCTION OF THE BREATHING APPARATUS

Dyspnea of varying degrees of severity is the one characteristic sign of obstruction of the respiratory tree. Obstruction may occur at any level; therefore, effective treatment depends upon accurate and rapid localization (see localization chart, p. 346).

CAUSES OF RESPIRATORY OBSTRUCTION

Allergy
Allergic edema associated with acute tracheobronchitis (**48—48**).
Angioedema (**48—4**).
Asthma (**48—6**).

Developmental Abnormalities
Tracheoesophageal fistula.

Infections
Croup (**48—19**).
Diphtheria (**30—4**).
Pneumonia (**48—45; 52—14**).
Poliomyelitis (**30—21; 48—49**).
Tracheobronchitis (**48—48**)

Mechanical
Foreign bodies (**36—4; 48—29**).
Swallowing the tongue. This may occur following severe direct trauma to the head or face, during convulsions or while in coma.
TREATMENT
Pulling the tongue back into normal position by whatever instruments are available (it is almost impossible to do this manually, even in a small child) and support of the angles of the jaw. If these measures are unsuccessful, tracheostomy (**14—12**) must be done immediately as a lifesaving measure.
Pressure from outside the respiratory tract.

LOCALIZATION CHART – RESPIRATORY OBSTRUCTION

SIGN OR SYMPTOM	LEVEL OF OBSTRUCTION			
	Pharynx	*Larynx*	*Trachea*	*Bronchi*
Voice changes	Slurred or thick	Hoarse or absent	Decreased volume	Decreased volume
Cough	Persistent, scratchy	Stridulous, "croupy"	Reflex irritative	Reflex irritative
Swallowing	Difficult	Difficult	Usually normal, but occasionally painful	Normal
Dyspnea	Positional	Inspiratory	Inspiratory	Often present with wheezing
Cyanosis	May be present – relieved by position changes	May be present	May be present	Often present
Intercostal retraction	Usually absent	Inspiratory	Inspiratory	If a large bronchus is blocked
Breath sounds	Normal	Roughened – coarse	Coarse râles and rhonchi	Rhonchi; absent over collapsed lung
Restlessness, excitement, apprehension	Intermittent; acute during episodes of dysphagia and dyspnea	Often acute	Rarely occur	Acute if a large bronchus is blocked

TREATMENT
Supportive and palliative measures awaiting determination and treatment of the cause.

48–45. PNEUMONIA (See also 52–14; 62–11)

SIGNS AND SYMPTOMS.   Persistent cough with high fever, and grunting respiration with dilation of the alae nasi with each breath. The respiration rate is often increased to 50 or more per minute. The characteristic dyspnea and cyanosis is caused by reduced vital capacity and pain on breathing, not by obstruction. Characteristic x-ray changes are present—involvement by lobes if due to pneumococcal infection; patchy infiltration if due to other organisms (including viruses).

TREATMENT
1. Insurance of an adequate airway.
2. Oxygen inhalations by face mask or tent.
3. Hospitalization for pediatric care.

48–46. PNEUMOTHORAX (See also 28–4. Traumatic Pneumothorax; 28–5. Tension Pneumothorax)

This condition is uncommon in children but may occur from birth injury, pneumonia (48–45) or injuries to the chest (28). Because of the elasticity of the chest wall in children, there may be no external evidence of trauma, but through the "accordion-action" of direct force, severe damage may occur. Spontaneous (nontraumatic) rupture of an emphysematous bleb, usually apical (52–16), is extremely rare in children.

SIGNS AND SYMPTOMS.   Dyspnea, cyanosis, absent breath sounds and mediastinal shift—demonstrable clinically and by x-ray films.

TREATMENT
1. Insurance of an adequate airway by postural drainage and suction. Insertion of a chest tube, with water-seal drainage, may be indicated for a traumatic or extensive pneumothorax.
2. Oxygen inhalations by tent. A face mask and rebreathing bag may be necessary if dyspnea and cyanosis are severe.
3. Aspiration of the air using a medium bore needle and gentle suction. (See also 28–5. Tension Pneumothorax.)
4. Bed rest at home under the care of a pediatrician is all that is required in mild cases; severe cases with massive collapse or

signs of tension pneumothorax (**28 — 5**) require hospitalization until reexpansion of the lung has taken place and until any infection has been controlled.

48 — 47. POISONING

More than 500,000 American children receive medical treatment every year for poisoning; more than 500 a year die.

It is conceivable that any of the substances listed under **49. *Poisoning, Acute,*** and many more, might cause acute toxic signs and symptoms. Children are taught from earliest infancy that in order to live and grow they must put substances into their mouths. As a result of negligence, carelessness and ignorance of parents and other adults, children have access in and around their homes to an almost endless list of toxic substances. Ninety per cent of reported cases of poisoning occur in children under the age of 5; the substances most frequently ingested are aspirin (**49 — 101**), cleaning and polishing agents (**49 — 216**), pesticides (**49 — 241.** *DD Compounds;* **49 — 546.** *Organic Phosphates*), turpentine paints (**49 — 559**), petroleum products (**49 — 585**) and cosmetics (**49 — 228**).

For the general principles of treatment of acute poisoning, refer to **49 — 3**. In all instances, the doses of medicines recommended in various treatments should be adjusted to the age, weight or skin surface area of the child (**4**).

For signs and symptoms and treatment of toxicity from specific poisonous substances, see under alphabetical arrangement (**49 — 7** to **49 — 857**); for poisonous cultivated or garden plants, see **49 — 858** to **49 — 1000**.

48 — 48. RESPIRATORY INFECTIONS

BRONCHITIS

Bronchitis in children, especially infants, almost invariably involves the terminal bronchioles. It may be associated with acute laryngotracheobronchitis (below) and with a patchy pneumonia (**48 — 45**). The child generally has a toxic appearance; a temperature of 38.8 to 40.6°C. (102 to 105°F); a persistent cough with coarse rales and rhonchi on auscultation; dyspnea and occasionally cyanosis. Febrile convulsions are a common occurrence.

TREATMENT

1. Insurance of an adequate airway by postural drainage and suction. Tracheostomy is almost never necessary.

2. Oxygen by face mask or tent if cyanosis is acute. Moisture often is beneficial.

3. Control of convulsions (**48 — 18**).

4. Strict pediatric supervision with administration of ampicillin and other antibiotics as indicated by culture and sensitivity tests. Hospitalization may be necessary in severe cases.

CROUP See **48 — 19**.

DIPHTHERIA

Infections from this specific organism (*Corynebacterium diphtheriae*) are now fortunately relatively rare. Immediate treatment must be given if the condition is even suspected (**30 — 4**).

LARYNGOTRACHEOBRONCHITIS

Acute infections of these sections of the respiratory tract must be distinguished from croup (**48 — 19**), diphtheria (**30 — 4**) and obstruction (**48 — 44**). They are often associated with and complicated by capillary bronchitis (bronchiolitis) (**52 — 2**) and patchy pneumonia (**48 — 45**). Symptoms similar to croup (**48 — 19**) often persist in spite of treatment and are associated with extreme toxicity with a high temperature, acute dyspnea and cyanosis.

TREATMENT

1. Insurance of an adequate airway. This includes performance of an emergency tracheostomy (**14 — 12**) if necessary.

2. Oxygen inhalations by tent or face mask if extreme dyspnea and/or cyanosis is present.

3. Warm, moist air inhalations. Many varieties of very efficient and safe patented devices are on the market, but the old-fashioned steam kettle (with precautions against burning the patient or other members of the family) is often the only means available in the home for producing warm moisture.

4. Antibiotic therapy based upon cultures and sensitivity studies (**30 — 41**. *Antimicrobial Drugs of Choice*).

Ampicillin, dosage according to age (**4**).

Erythromycin orally. Tetracyclines should be avoided in children under 5 years of age because of the possibility of tooth staining.

5. If there is evidence of allergic edema, epinephrine hydro-

chloride (Adrenalin), 1:1000 solution, may be given subcutaneously provided there is no tachycardia or evidence of impending heart failure.

DOSAGE
Under 2 years, 0.1 ml.
2 to 3 years, 0.15 ml.
3 to 6 years, 0.2 ml.
6 to 12 years, 0.3 ml.
12 to 15 years, 0.4 ml.

6. Hospitalization for pediatric care in severe cases with evidence of respiratory tract obstruction (**48 — 44**).

NASOPHARYNGITIS

Blocking of the nostrils of infants by crusts of thick secretion may require emergency care. The clinical picture of nasopharyngitis may simulate the prodromal picture of more serious conditions such as poliomyelitis (**30 — 21; 48 — 49**), otitis media (**32 — 13**) or (rarely) mastoiditis (**32 — 10**).

TREATMENT
1. Removal of the obstructing crusts from the nostrils in infants.
2. Shrinking of the nasal mucous membranes with 0.25% phenylephrine hydrochloride (Neo-Synephrine) drops or spray.
3. Administration of antihistaminics if an allergic factor is suspected.
4. Antibiotic therapy as indicated by cultures and sensitivity tests (**30 — 41.** *Antimicrobial Drugs of Choice*).
5. Home care, especially complete bed rest and copious fluids. Hospitalization is practically never necessary.

OTITIS MEDIA See **32 — 13**.

PNEUMONIA See **48 — 45; 52 — 14; 62 — 11.** *Interstitial Pneumonia*.

TONSILLITIS

Acutely inflamed and swollen tonsils, sometimes sufficient to cause dysphagia and dyspnea, are common in childhood.

TREATMENT
1. Aspirin for pain.
2. Throat cultures and sensitivity tests as soon as possible.
3. Soft or liquid diet.
4. Icebags or cold compresses to the throat.

5. Penicillin, 200,000 to 600,000 units intramuscularly, or other antibiotics based on the results of the cultures and sensitivity tests.

6. Acute cases with extreme toxicity or edema require hospitalization and strict pediatric supervision.

TRACHEOBRONCHITIS. See *Laryngotracheobronchitis* (p. 349)

48—49. RESPIRATORY PARALYSIS IN ANTERIOR POLIOMYELITIS
(See also **46—9.** *Paralysis*)

Emergency tracheostomy (**14—12**) is an absolute necessity if signs and symptoms indicating airway obstruction cannot be cleared by postural drainage and suction. No patient in the acute stage of infantile paralysis should be transported until a tracheostomy has been performed if there is any possibility of the development or progression of respiratory paralysis requiring ventilatory assistance.

48—50. SERUM REACTIONS (See also 21—4)

TREATMENT
1. Epinephrine hydrochloride (Adrenalin), 1:1000 solution, subcutaneously.

DOSAGE
Under 2 years, 0.1 ml.
2 to 3 years, 0.15 ml.
3 to 6 years, 0.2 ml.
6 to 12 years, 0.3 ml.
12 to 15 years, 0.4 ml.

2. Tripelennamine hydrochloride (Pyribenzamine) or diphenhydramine hydrochloride (Benadryl) subcutaneously, 5 to 7 mg. per kg. of body weight.

3. If the above methods are unsuccessful, hospitalize at once.

48—51. SHOCK (See also 53)

The chief difference between shock in children and shock in adults is that in children the changes in condition described under **53** may develop and become irreversible very rapidly. Identification of these early changes depends upon frequent and careful observation and examination. In children a slowly falling rectal temperature is often indicative of incipient shock. As a general rule, treatment of shock (**53 – 7**) takes precedence over all other emergency procedures except control of gross hemorrhage (**42 – 1**) and restoration of respiration (**11 – 1**).

48 – 52.   SKULL FRACTURES See **41 – 12** to **41 – 18; 48 – 32.** *Head Injuries*

48 – 53.   SMOKE INHALATION (See also **22.** *Asphyxiation*)

The dangers of inhalation of smoke by infants and children are often unrecognized. Acute carbon monoxide poisoning (**49 – 172**) may occur. The onset of secondary, serious signs and symptoms may be delayed for 1 to 5 hours after exposure.

TREATMENT

1. Insurance of an adequate airway by postural drainage and suction.

2. Relief from dyspnea and anoxia by expired air respiration (**11 – 1**), followed by oxygen inhalations under positive pressure by face mask and rebreathing bag.

3. Control of pain and restlessness by barbiturates rectally or intramuscularly, or, in severe cases in older children, by morphine sulfate subcutaneously or intravenously (dosage according to age or weight [**4**]).

4. Hospitalization for at least 48 hours for treatment of the inevitable edema of the respiratory tract. Steroids may relieve edema.

48 – 54.   STINGS See **56; 61.** *Venoms* (also **24.** *Bites*)

48 – 55.   SUBARACHNOID HEMORRHAGE (See also **59 – 2**)

This condition is rare in infancy and childhood unless other severe head injuries are present. Hospitalization for diagnostic and therapeutic measures is usually indicated if subarachnoid bleeding is suspected.

48 – 56.   SUBDURAL HEMORRHAGE See **41 – 20; 48 – 32.** *Head Injuries in Children*

48 – 57.   SUDDEN INFANT DEATH SYNDROME (SIDS) – "Crib deaths"

Every year about 25,000 infants, usually between one week and two years of age, in good health when put to bed, are found dead in bed in the morning. Death is invariably silent, and occurs during sleep. At postmortem, examination usually indicates that death was the result of acute laryngospasm and interstitial pneumonitis. No cause for these conditions is usually found.

Crib deaths have been blamed in the past on numerous conditions. Among these are suffocating from bedclothes, battered child syndrome (**48—7**), hypertrophy of the thymus, parathyroid abnormality, acute overwhelming bacterial or viral infections, hypersensitivity to cow's milk, deficient levels of immunoglobulins, and toxic agents. More recently, deficits in magnesium and selenium in the diet have been suspect.

It is now recognized that SIDS is a definite clinical entity of unknown etiology. This should always be explained to the parents to prevent the development of guilt complexes.

48—58. SUNSTROKE See 57—8.

48—59. TETANUS (See also 16. *Tetanus Immunization*; 30—31)

Immunization. Of all reported cases of tetanus, 50 to 70% occur in children. Because immunity is not derived from the mother, active immunization of all children at an early age by a series of toxoid injections is very important. Fluid or aluminum hydroxide toxoid is preferable to alum-precipitated toxoid because it produces a faster rise in antitoxin titer. In badly contaminated wounds, tetanus-immune globulin (TIG) should be given (**16**).

48—60. TETANY See 43—25.

48—61. VOLVULUS (See also 48—38. *Intestinal Obstruction*)

Twisting of the small bowel usually results from improper developmental rotation of the duodenum and may cause signs and symptoms of high intestinal obstruction developing during the first few hours of life or months or years later. The diagnosis cannot be made on symptoms and physical findings alone but requires thorough x-ray studies.

TREATMENT

Hospitalization is indicated whenever volvulus is suspected. Operative untwisting of the distal portion of the duodenum or of other involved areas may be lifesaving.

48—62. VOMITING

Prolonged and persistent vomiting, no matter what its cause, results in acute dehydration, acidosis or alkalosis and complete collapse from exhaustion. Occasional regurgitation or vomiting in infants and children is of no clinical importance.

Control of prolonged vomiting depends on 4 factors:

1. Physiologic rest of the stomach.

2. Correction of any water-electrolyte imbalance by administration of appropriate fluids intravenously or by hypodermoclysis (**6**).

3. Identification and treatment of the cause.

4. Gradual resumption of a normal diet.

TREATMENT

1. Give nothing by mouth except ice chips.

2. Insist on complete rest. Sedation by means of a pentobarbital sodium (Nembutal) suppository may be necessary.

3. In children accustomed to chewing gum, meclizine (Bonine) gum, 25 mg., chewed for 5 or 10 minutes, often gives lasting relief.

4. Administration of $2\frac{1}{2}\%$ dextrose in water and $\frac{1}{2}$ normal saline solution intravenously (or, in less severe cases, by hypodermoclysis), 25 ml. per kilogram of body weight.

5. Intramuscular injection of chlorpromazine hydrochloride (Thorazine), 0.6 mg. per kilogram of body weight.

6. Hospitalization for supportive therapy, laboratory studies, correction of fluid-electrolyte imbalance (**6**) and determination and treatment of the underlying cause is essential if the procedures outlined above do not result in cessation of vomiting.

48—63. WATERHOUSE-FRIDERICHSEN SYNDROME (See also
48—42. *Meningococcemia*)

Acute adrenal insufficiency with bacteremia (usually meningococcic) represents a true emergency. Early recognition of the clinical picture and immediate appropriate treatment may be life-saving.

SIGNS AND SYMPTOMS are often dramatic and include sudden onset of acute malaise, chills and high fever, dyspnea, cyanosis, gradually decreasing blood pressure with a gradually increasing pulse rate, rapid development of petechiae and acute respiratory and circulatory collapse—often terminal.

TREATMENT

1. Start oxygen under positive pressure immediately.

2. Begin massive penicillin G therapy without waiting for the results of cultures and sensitivity tests. The adult dose (20,000,000 units per day intravenously divided into 4 doses or 1,000,000 units every 2 hours intramuscularly) must be adjusted according to the child's weight or age (**4**). Ampicillin (150 to 175 mg. per kilogram of body weight per day in divided doses) is a satisfactory alternate to penicillin. In penicillin-sensitive children, chloramphenicol (chloromycetin), 25 to 50 mg. per day per kilogram of body weight in divided doses, may be used with close observation for adverse reactions, particularly those involving the hematopoietic system. The drug must be discontinued if any evidence of an adverse reaction is noted.

3. Give plasma volume expanders or 5% dextrose in saline intravenously, 25 ml. per kilogram of body weight.

4. Support the blood pressure in children over 5 by intravenous or intramuscular caffeine sodiobenzoate [dosage according to age or weight (**4**)].

5. Arrange for immediate hospitalization for isolation, laboratory studies, determination of the causative organism and sensitivity tests. If hospitalization is delayed for any reason, aqueous adrenal cortical extract therapy should be begun. As an emergency measure, 2.2 ml. of aqueous adrenal cortical extract per kilogram of body weight is safe. Heparin therapy may be indicated if intravascular clotting (purpura, low platelet count and low fibrinogen level) occurs.

48 – 64.   WHEEZING (See also **48 – 44.** *Obstruction of the Breathing Apparatus*)

Development of acute wheezing in a child is an urgent medical emergency until the cause has been determined.

CAUSES

1. Bronchial asthma – allergic (most common) (**48 – 6; 52 – 1**).

2. Foreign bodies (**48 – 29; 36 – 4.** *Foreign Bodies in the Larynx Trachea or Bronchi*).

3. Pulmonary or vascular tree abnormalities – congenital.

4. Congestive heart failure (**26 – 8; 48 – 15**).

5. Bronchiolitis (**48 – 48**).

6. Pancreatic pathology – usually cystic fibrosis.

7. Mediastinal tumors.

TREATMENT

Treatment depends upon causative factors. Persistent acute wheezing for which the cause cannot be determined is an indication for hospitalization.

48 – 65. WRINGER INJURIES

The advent of the household spin-dry washer has resulted in definite decrease in this serious type of injury. Such injuries are confined almost exclusively to children of run-about age and can result in extensive permanent disability and deformity. Severe crushing and avulsion of soft tissues, abrasions, lacerations, friction burns, and nerve and blood vessel damage may occur. Fractures and epiphysial damage, usually of the hand, wrist or elbow, may be demonstrable by x-ray films but are surprisingly rare.

Danger Signs in Children with Wringer Injuries

Massive edema	Skin pallor or poor color return on pressure and release. Pulse may be obscured.
	Digital or radial pulse absent or difficult to palpate
Discolored abrasions	Deep red to purple color with no blanching on digital pressure
Avulsion of skin with a distally based flap	Skin rolled distally
	Flap discoloration (cyanosis or pallor)
Pain	Ischemic variety unrelieved by splinting; aggravated by repeatedly opening and closing hand
	Crying, fretfulness
Anesthetic skin	Possible nerve severance or contusion or loss of arterial supply
	Absent sweating
	Diminished or absent pinprick and discriminatory sensation
Absent pulses in fingers or major arterial trunks	Possible diminished or absent blood flow due to internal pressure

TREATMENT

1. Control of panic and pain by pentobarbital sodium (Nembutal) suppositories in children under 4 years of age. Morphine sulfate subcutaneously may be indicated in older children [dosage according to age, weight or skin surface (**4**)].

2. Splinting, followed by x-ray films.

3. Repair of soft tissue damage by:

Cleansing of abrasions and superficial lacerations; application of petrolatum or bacitracin (Parentracin) gauze dressings. Debridement, evacuation of hematomas, obliteration of dead spaces and suturing of gaping, deep or extensive lacerations (**40 – 5.** *Lacerations of the Hand;* **55 – 20**) under general anesthesia is usually necessary.

4. Reduction of any fractures, followed by application of a removable type of splint or plaster shell.

5. Administration of tetanus-immune globulin (TIG) or toxoid (**16**).

6. Streptokinase-streptodornase (Varidase), 0.5 ml. (5000 units) intramuscularly twice a day, accompanied by a broad spectrum antibiotic.

7. Arrangement for observation within 24 hours. Extreme edema, common following crushing injuries, often requires loosening of dressings, especially around the digits and elbow. Hospitalization is advisable in severe cases, especially those with suspected or known circulatory impairment.

8. Explanation to the parents or legal guardian of the injured child of the potential seriousness of the injury and of the possible need for secondary skin grafting, tendon suture or nerve repair at a later date.

48 – 66. ZIPPER INJURIES (See also **38 – 4.** *Lacerations of the Penis*)

Although other redundant loose soft tissues may occasionally be involved, zipper injuries to the penis – especially the prepuce – are by far the most common. Proper removal under emergency conditions may prevent marked deformity. Removal is usually easy if the cooperation of the patient can be obtained. Small children should be quieted by a pentobarbital sodium (Nembutal) suppository; older children should receive a small subcutaneous injection of morphine sulfate, dosage according to age or weight (**4**). The zipper – its supporting fabric cut from the clothing by scissors, *but not bent or cut with wire cutters* – should be held firmly by both ends, and closed a short distance further, then gently disengaged. A short inhalation anesthesia sometimes must be used, but dibucaine (Nupercaine) ointment rubbed gently on the skin is generally adequate. After removal, apply an antiseptic ointment dressing and suggest cold compresses for 12 hours. In older male patients recommend use of a suspensory.

Do not

1. Inject a local anesthetic. The resultant edema makes removal more difficult. In addition, acute toxic reactions (**49 – 72.** *Anesthetics, Local*) may occur because of extreme vascularity of the tissues and subsequent rapid absorption.

2. Cut through the zipper with a metal-cutting instrument; this may lock the teeth so that the slide cannot be pulled back.

3. Use sharp dissection. A gaping laceration requiring surgical closure may result in scar tissue and irreparable deformity (chordee).

49. POISONING, ACUTE

49—1. DEFINITION (Sollmann)

"A poison is any substance which, acting directly through its inherent chemical properties, and by its ordinary action, is capable of destroying life or of seriously endangering health, when it is applied to the body externally, or in moderate doses (to 50 gm.) internally." This definition specifically excludes injurious physical, mechanical and bacterial agents, and substances which are toxic only in very large doses.

49—2. CLASSIFICATION

Irritant Poisons

Simple irritants.
Corrosives—produce direct destruction of tissues.

Nerve Poisons (Neurotoxins)

Convulsants—cause spasms and convulsions.
Somnifacients—cause sleep and coma.
Cardiac poisons—embarrass, and eventually stop, heart action.

Blood Poisons (Hematoxins)

Alter the oxygen-carrying ability of the hemoglobin and/or blood corpuscles, with resultant cyanosis.

49—3. GENERAL PRINCIPLES OF TREATMENT

Removal of the toxic substances as soon as possible
From the skin and mucous membranes. Wash with large amounts of water to which has been added the appropriate chemical antidote; i.e., for acids, magnesium, chalk, baking soda or soap; for alkalies, acetic acid, lemon juice or vinegar. (For exception, see **49—787.** *Titanium Tetrachloride.*).
From wounds or following hypodermic administration
Limit activity.
Apply a tourniquet to limit diffusion of the poison by vascular and lymphatic channels if the wound is on or the injection has been made into an extremity.
Apply suction, excise or cauterize.
Induce hypothermia.
From the lungs. After removing the patient from further exposure and determining that the airway is patent, start artificial respiration by expired air or mechanical methods at once. Direct administration of air or oxygen under positive pressure is the most effective method and should be substituted for any of the other methods at the earliest possible opportunity. See **11.** *Resuscitation.*
From the alimentary and gastrointestinal tract. Swallowed poisons should be evacuated as soon as possible by emetics or lavage unless definite evidence of mucous membrane corrosion is present even though the patient has vomited and several hours have passed since ingestion. If it is known or suspected that the poison has been swallowed with the intent of self-destruction (**13.** *Suicide*), other body cavities should be examined and evacuated if necessary. Specimens should be saved for possible chemical analysis.

Household Measures to Induce Vomiting:

1. Insertion of a finger as far as possible into the throat, with a prop (preferably wood) between the teeth to prevent finger injury.

2. Gargling with soapsuds (nondetergent). Table salt should not be used.

3. Swallowing of large amounts of household mustard in warm water (often ineffective).

Emetics. Measures to cause vomiting are indicated whenever a poisonous substance has been swallowed, except when the vomiting center is paralyzed, the poison is a corrosive, or the patient is extremely depressed or comatose. Vomiting will often result in removal from the stomach of food or other large particles which will not pass through a stomach tube. If emetics are ineffective, lavage is indicated because emetic drugs in themselves have some toxicity.

Administration of syrup of ipecac: This is the method of choice in children. An oral dose of 15 ml. followed by large amounts of water should be given, and repeated in $1/2$ hour (once only) if necessary. If emesis does not take place within one hour, the ipecac should be removed from the stomach by gastric lavage. Parents of children given syrup of ipecac should be informed of its delayed depressant side action, which may last for 2 to 3 hours after an emetic dose. This depressant action is only temporary and does not require any treatment.

Fluidextract of ipecac is 14 times stronger than syrup of ipecac and should never be used – deaths have been reported from confusion of the two preparations.

Injection of apomorphine hydrochloride: Apomorphine, in a dose of 5 mg. subcutaneously for an adult (for children see **4**), is the most effective of all emetics because of its direct action on the vomiting center. Do not give following corrosive poisons. Its secondary depressant action can easily be neutralized by injection of naloxone hydrochloride (Narcan), 0.01 mg. per kilogram of body weight.

Gastric Lavage. Emptying of the stomach by washing is indicated if the vomiting center is paralyzed (as in deep morphine or chloral hydrate poisoning) and in many cases of known or suspected ingestion of acutely toxic substances, provided that the danger from the toxic substance is considered to be greater than the risk of possible aspiration during lavage. The danger of aspiration can be decreased by careful positioning, by use of a cuffed tube, and by pinching off the tube during removal. Lavage should not be used if a corrosive poison (see **49 – 26.** *Acids;* **49 – 39.** *Alkalies;* **49 – 432.** *Lye*) has been swallowed, in advanced strychnine poisoning (**49 – 729**), or if an acute excitement state (**34**) is present. For technique of gastric lavage, see **14 – 4.**

Cathartics. Many toxic substances are absorbed by or cause irritation of the small and large bowel. Saline cathartics, especially magnesium sulfate (Epsom salts), are usually given by mouth or instilled through the stomach tube after lavage. For some poisons, oily cathartics (castor oil) result in more complete elimination.

From the peritoneal cavity. Peritoneal dialysis is a method of removal of toxic doses of many substances from the body, which is highly effective in the treatment of certain poisons. Among these poisons are acetone (**49 – 17**), amanita toxins (**49 – 502**), ammonia (**49 – 59**), amphetamines (**49 – 64**), aniline (**49 – 73**), barbiturates (**49 – 111**), bromides (**49 – 144**), carbon tetrachloride (**49 – 173**), chlorates (**49 – 187**), diphenylhydantoin (**49 – 276**), Doriden (**49 – 295**), ethyl alcohol (**49 – 315**), ethylene glycol (**49 – 320**), isopropyl alcohol (**49 – 403**), lithium (**49 – 428**), methyl alcohol (**49 – 475**), salicylates (**49 – 664**), sulfonamides (**49 – 731**), and thiocyanates (**49 – 774**). For technique, see **14 – 9.**

From the circulating blood. This may be accomplished by hemodialysis or by replacement or exchange transfusions of properly matched blood (**14 – 13**).

Neutralization of the poison by antidotes. With a few exceptions, this method is relatively ineffective, and should only be used in conjunction with other methods of treatment.

Acids (**49 – 26**). Give alkalies by mouth – magnesium, soap, chalk, baking soda. Chalk and baking soda should not be used if there is danger of perforation of the stomach wall by the production of gas.

Alkalies (**49−39**). Give weak acids by mouth−vinegar, lemon juice, orange juice, tartaric acid.

Organic poisons [alkaloids (**49−40**), glucosides, etc., and phosphorus (**49−602**)]. Give oxidizing agents such as ½ strength hydrogen peroxide, or potassium permanganate, 0.12 gm. to 200 ml. of water by mouth, followed by gastric lavage with instillation of activated charcoal in water through the lavage tube.

Hydrocyanic acid (**49−377**). Give potassium permanganate, ½ strength hydrogen peroxide; or 5% sodium thiosulfate ("hypo") solution by mouth, followed by gastric lavage with 1:2000 potassium permanganate solution. For intravenous therapy (5% sodium thiosulfate and sodium nitrite), see **49−235**. *Cyanides*.

Narcotics (natural or synthetic). Give naloxone hydrochloride (Narcan) intravenously, 0.01 mg. per kilogram of body weight, repeated as necessary. Naloxone has no respiratory cardiac depressant effect. See **49−495**. *Morphine* and **49−366**. *Heroin*.

Organic phosphate (phosphate ester) *pesticides* (**49−546**). Give atropine sulfate intravenously in large doses, preferably with 2-PAM (**49−546**).

Precipitation of the poison

Tannic acid, 4 ml. in 100 ml. of water, or 1 cup of strong tea, is harmless and may be of some benefit as a first aid measure in poisoning from the following substances:

Antipyrine (**49−82**)	Iron salts (**49−399**)
Apomorphine (**49−85**)	Mercury (**49−455**)
Cinchona alkaloids (**49−211**)	Silver (**49−688**)
Colchicine (**49−220**)	Strychnine (**49−729**)
Copper (**49−223**)	Veratrine (**49−824**)
Digitalis (**49−272**)	Zinc (**49−850** to **49−855**).

Alkaloids (**49−40**). Give tincture of iodine, 1 ml. in 100 ml. of water.

Arsenic (**49−90**). Ferric hydrate with magnesia has a questionably beneficial effect.

Barium (**49−112**). Magnesium sulfate (Epsom salts) by mouth may form a less toxic compound.

Mercuric salts. (See also **49−455**. *Mercury;* **49−128**. *Bichloride of Mercury*.) Give raw eggs followed by sodium thiosulfate or sodium formaldehyde sulfoxylate by mouth.

Metals. Give raw eggs. Egg albumin may be effective against mercury salts (**49−455**).

Opiate-containing substances. (See also **49−219**. *Codeine;* **49−366**. *Heroin;* **49−495**. *Morphine*.) Give calcium (lime water, chalk), followed as soon as possible by intravenous naloxone hydrochloride (Narcan).

Pentazocine (Talwin). Give naloxone hydrochloride (Narcan) intravenously, dose 0.01 mg. per kilogram of body weight−repeated at 3 to 5 minute intervals as necessary.

Phosphorus (**49−602**). Give cupric sulfate by mouth.

Propoxyphene (Darvon). Give naloxone hydrochloride (Narcan) intravenously, 0.01 mg. per kilogram of body weight.

Absorption of the poison by activated charcoal and demulcents (raw eggs, boiled starch, flour, milk), followed by a saline cathartic.

49−4. SYMPTOMATIC TREATMENT

Respiratory failure

1. Insurance of an adequate airway by positioning, suction and support of the angles of the jaw.

2. Artificial respiration by expired air or mechanical methods (**11−1**), followed by administration of air or oxygen under positive pressure by face mask or endotracheal catheter and rebreathing bag.

3. Temporary reflex respiratory stimulation. Give 2 ml. of spirits of ammonia in 200 ml. of water orally.

Circulatory failure. See **11−2**. *Cardiac Compression;* **26−7**. *Cardiac Arrest;* and **53**. *Shock*.

Pain. Control by codeine sulfate, meperidine hydrochloride (Demerol) or morphine sulfate intramuscularly or intravenously in the smallest possible effective doses, provided respiratory depression will not be harmful to the patient. Pentazocine lactate (Talwin) is a valuable nonnarcotic anodyne. Calcium gluconate (10% solution) injected slowly intravenously will relieve some types of acute muscle pain.

Cooling or chilling. The body temperature should be raised by application of warmed blankets, clothing, or by use of a cast dryer or bed warmer. Do not use hot water bottles if other means of keeping the patient warm are available.

Convulsions. See **31.** *Convulsive Seizures;* **48 – 18.** *Convulsions in Children.*

Coma. Symptomatic and supportive therapy should take precedence over attempts to determine the causative condition. See **29.** *Coma.*

49 – 5. UNIVERSAL ANTIDOTE VERSUS ACTIVATED CHARCOAL

The universal antidote referred to in many texts on treatment of toxic materials is made up as follows:

CHEMICAL CONSTITUENTS	HOUSEHOLD EQUIVALENTS
2 parts activated charcoal	2 parts burned toast
1 part magnesium oxide	1 part milk of magnesia
1 part tannic acid	1 part strong tea

Fifteen milliliters of this mixture given in 200 ml. of warm water formerly was recommended whenever the exact nature of the poison had not been determined or a delay in instituting lavage was anticipated.

During the last few years, use of this extraordinarily unattractive mixture has been supplanted by pure activated charcoal, 50 to 100 mg. in water, preferably given through the lavage tube. Among the available preparations are Norit A, Darco G, and Nuchar C. All have the ability to adsorb toxic chemicals [except cyanides (**49 – 235**)] and to retain them tenaciously while they are being passed through the bowel.

Activated charcoal should not be given before, or with, an emetic or a specific antidote – it may adsorb the emetic or neutralizing drug and decrease its effect.

49 – 6. LETHAL BLOOD LEVELS OF COMMONLY USED DRUGS

AGENT	LETHAL BLOOD LEVEL (estimated)	AGENT	LETHAL BLOOD LEVEL (estimated)
Acetaminophen (**49 – 12**)	150 mg.%	Desipramine (**49 – 805.** *Tricyclic antidepressants*)	0.3 mg.%
Ammonia (**49 – 59**)	0.1 mg./%		
Amphetamines (**49 – 64**)	0.2 mg.%	Diphenylhydantoin (**49 – 276.** *Dilantin*)	10 mg.%
Arsenic (with BAL) (**49 – 90**)	0.1 mg.%		
Aspirin (**49 – 101**)	140 mg.%	Ethanol (**49 – 315.** *Ethyl Alcohol*)	400 mg.%
Barbiturates (**49 – 111**)			
Long-acting	8 mg.%	Ethchlorvynol (**49 – 311**)	15 mg.%
Intermediate-acting	5 mg.%	Ethylene glycol (**49 – 320**)	100 mg.%
Short-acting	3.5 mg.%	Glutethimide (**49 – 295.** *Doriden*)	3 mg.%
Boric acid (**49 – 138**)	50 mg.%		
Bromides (**49 – 144**)	20 mEq./L.	Isopropyl alcohol (**49 – 403**)	80 mg.%
Chloral hydrate (**49 – 184**)	25 mg.%	Magnesium (**49 – 436.** *Magnesium Sulfate*)	5 mEq./L.
Chlorpromazine (**49 – 203**)	1 mg.%		

AGENT	LETHAL BLOOD LEVEL (estimated)	AGENT	LETHAL BLOOD LEVEL (estimated)
Meprobamate (**49—448**)	20 mg.%	Propoxyphene (**49—629**)	6 mg.%
Methanol (**49—475.**		Quinine (**49—642**)	1.2 mg.%
Methyl Alcohol)	100 mg.%	Salicylates (**49—664**)	
Methamphetamine		(For single dose levels,	
(**49—64.** *Amphetamines*)	4 mg.%	see Fig. 29)	140 mg.%
Paraldehyde (**49—568**)	50 mg.%	Thiocyanates (**49—774**)	20 mg.%

TREATMENT OF SPECIFIC POISONS

The alphabetic list (**49—7** to **49—1017**) on the following pages includes substances which may give toxic signs and symptoms from inhalation of fumes or from skin absorption as well as by ingestion. Unless otherwise specified, ingestion is the mode of entry.

Whenever the substances listed in this alphabetical list are drugs used medicinally for their therapeutic effect, reference is suggested to a standard pharmacology text, or to the brochures furnished by the manufacturers, for more detailed accounts of recommended dosages, toxicities and side effects.

49—7. ABRUS PRECATORIUS L.

The seeds of this ornamental plant, originally from Africa but now common in the West Indies, Central America and Florida, contain a toxalbumin, abrin. Ingestion of the seeds, called "crab-eyes," jequirity beans, jumbo beans and rosary beads, results in generalized weakness, a rapid weak pulse, extreme and persistent nausea, coarse tremors and severe colicky diarrhea.

TREATMENT

1. Emptying of the stomach by emetics or gastric lavage followed by activated charcoal in water by mouth.

2. Administration of saline cathartics.

3. Symptomatic care as required, especially combatting of dehydration. For signs and symptoms resulting from inhalation of dust from the dried seeds, see **49—406.** *Jequirity Beans.*

49—8. ABSINTHE (Wormwood)

The dried leaves and flowers of this plant, formerly used as a medicine and liqueur, especially in France, contain a toxic substance, thujone. The signs and symptoms of toxicity are a clammy skin, severe gastric pain, convulsions (tonic and clonic) and cardiac failure.

TREATMENT

1. Emptying of the stomach by emetics and gastric lavage followed by activated charcoal in water.

2. Control of convulsions by intramuscular or intravenous barbiturates.

3. Cardiac support.

49—9. ACACIA (Gum Arabic)

Derived from a gum exuded by the stems and branches of an African tree, this substance is utilized in medicine as a colloid in intravenous solutions in the treatment of shock and kidney disease. Occasional severe reactions, with dyspnea, rapid pulse, acute anxiety and terminal circulatory collapse, have been reported, as well as cases of hypersensitivity and anaphylactoid shock (**21.** *Allergic Reactions*).

TREATMENT. Symptomatic and supportive.

49 – 10. ACEDON (Dihydrocodeinone Cholactate)

This synthetic analgesic and narcotic has approximately the same toxic effects and addictive tendency as the opium derivatives. See **2 – 3.** *Addiction (Narcotics);* **49 – 219.** *Codeine;* and **49 – 495.** *Morphine.*

49 – 11. ACETALDEHYDE

Used in silver plating and industrial chemistry, acetaldehyde fumes in moderate concentration may cause intense mucous membrane irritation, characterized by conjunctivitis, photophobia, corneal injury, rhinitis and anosmia. Removal from exposure usually results in complete clearing of symptoms. High concentrations give a toxic picture similar to acute alcoholic intoxication (**49 – 315.** *Ethyl Alcohol*).

49 – 12. ACETAMINOPHEN (Paracetamol)

Liver and kidney damage have been reported not only from overdosage of this drug but also from repeated therapeutic doses. There is no known antidote. Inductance of vomiting, followed by activated charcoal, 50 to 100 mg. in water, and appropriate treatment of symptoms as they develop usually result in full recovery.

49 – 13. ACETANILID (Antifebrin)

SIGNS AND SYMPTOMS.   Nausea, vomiting, cyanosis (especially of the face), cold clammy skin and feeble rapid pulse with slow respiration.

TREATMENT

1. Emetics and/or gastric lavage with 500 ml. of 1:2000 potassium permanganate solution, followed by activated charcoal in water orally or through the lavage tube.

2. Application of external heat.

3. Oxygen therapy by face mask and rebreathing bag.

4. Methylene blue (1% solution in 1.8% sodium sulfate solution), 50 ml., intravenously very slowly if evidence of acute methemoglobinemia is present.

5. Hospitalization if a large amount has been ingested or cyanosis is extreme.

49 – 14. ACETARSONE

This arsenic derivative is used orally under a large number of trade names for treatment of dysentery, and locally for treatment of trichomonal infections. By either route it may cause the toxic effects of arsenicals. For signs and symptoms of toxicity and treatment, see **49 – 90.** *Arsenic,* and **49 – 96.** *Arsphenamine and Neoarsphenamine.*

49 – 15. ACETIC ACID

The most common cause of acute acetic acid poisoning is ingestion of "essence of vinegar," a common household flavoring agent. The toxic picture is characterized by severe pain in the upper alimentary tract; grayish white ulcers in the mouth and throat;

profuse vomiting; cold, clammy skin; subnormal temperature; rapid, shallow respiration; acute dyspnea; sometimes pulmonary edema (**51**) with terminal collapse.

TREATMENT

1. Demulcents; milk is the most effective.

2. Gastric lavage with warm lime water, followed by activated charcoal in water through the lavage tube.

3. Oxygen inhalations under positive pressure by face mask or intranasal catheter and rebreathing bag.

4. Metaraminol bitartrate (Aramine), 2 to 10 mg. intramuscularly, or 0.5 to 5 mg. intravenously, or 4 ml. of a 0.2% solution of arterenol bitartrate (Levophed) in 1000 ml. of 5% dextrose in saline, preferably through a plastic intravenous catheter, to support the blood pressure for lengthy periods. The rate of injection must be regulated by frequent blood pressure determinations.

5. Treatment of pulmonary edema (**51**).

6. Hospitalization in severe cases.

49—16. ACETOARSENITES

These compounds are powerful pesticides and extremely toxic. For treatment see **49—90.** *Arsenic.*

49—17. ACETONE (Dimethylketone, Propanone)

Inhalation of fumes or ingestion may cause severe toxic manifestations, characterized by a fruity odor on the breath; severe gastrointestinal symptoms (nausea, vomiting, abdominal pain); and rapid fall in temperature, pulse, respiration and blood pressure.

TREATMENT

1. Emetics or gastric lavage followed by activated charcoal.

2. Oxygen under positive pressure.

49—18. ACETONE CYANOHYDRIN

This extremely toxic liquid used in industry can cause death if a few drops are splashed on the skin. The signs, symptoms and treatment are as outlined under **49—235.** *Cyanides.*

49—19. ACETOHEXAMIDE (Dymelor)

Excessively large doses of this recently introduced oral hypoglycemic drug have caused coma lasting for several days in spite of large amounts of intravenous glucose. All reported cases have made complete recoveries under energetic supportive care.

49—20. ACETONITRILE (Methylcyanide)

Exposure to this commercial solvent causes severe chest pain, cough with bloody sputum, convulsions and coma.

TREATMENT

1. Removal from exposure—supportive care.

2. Severe cases require treatment as outlined under **49—235.** *Cyanides.*

49—21. ACETOPHENETIDIN (Phenacetin)

Too large or too frequent doses of this analgesic and antipyretic drug may cause a weak and feeble pulse, extreme cyanosis, excessive perspiration, hematuria and respiratory and circulatory collapse. Prolonged use may result in severe agranulocytosis.

TREATMENT
See **49—13.** *Acetanilid.*

49—22. ACETYLCARBROMAL (Abasin)

Therapeutic doses of this sedative drug may cause hemorrhagic purpura and thrombocytopenia.

TREATMENT
1. Discontinue use of the drug.
2. Treat thrombocytopenia.

49—23. ACETYLCHOLINE

SIGNS AND SYMPTOMS.   Sweating, salivation, dyspnea, tightness in chest, excessive micturition and collapse.

TREATMENT
1. Atropine sulfate, 1 mg. intramuscularly, repeated as necessary until signs of atropinization (**49—104**) develop.
2. Oxygen therapy under positive pressure.
3. Arterenol bitartrate (Levophed) given intravenously in 1000 ml. of 5% dextrose in saline may be necessary if marked hypotension is present. Metaraminol bitartrate (Aramine) can be given subcutaneously, intramuscularly or intravenously for a similar vasopressor effect.

49—24. ACETYLENE (Ethine, Narcylene)

Inhaled in strong concentrations, this commonly used commercial gas causes rapid onset of deep narcosis. Inhalation of lower concentrations causes dizziness and mental confusion, usually transient.

TREATMENT
1. Stop exposure.
2. Give oxygen inhalations under positive pressure by face mask or intranasal catheter with rebreathing bag.
3. Watch for complications, usually due to impurities, such as hydrogen sulfide (**49—380**) or phosphine (**49—600**).

49—25. ACETYLSALICYLIC ACID See **49—101.** *Aspirin;* **49—664.** *Salicylates*

49—26. ACIDS [Acetic, Acetic Anhydride, Carbolic (Phenol), Hydrochloric (Muriatic), Lactic, Nitric, Sulfuric (Oil of Vitriol), Trichloracetic]

For exceptions to the therapy outlined below, see **49—378.** *Hydrofluoric Acid;* **49—552.** *Oxalic Acid;* **49—634.** *Pyrogallic Acid;* and **49—742.** *Tannic Acid.*

TREATMENT OF EXTERNAL CONTACT.
Repeated flooding with large amounts of water, followed by application of a paste of sodium bicarbonate.

TREATMENT OF INGESTION

1. Do not use stomach tube or emetics if concentrated acid has been swallowed.

2. Neutralize with aluminum hydroxide, magnesium oxide, milk of magnesia, milk, chalk, egg white or soap solution. Do not use sodium bicarbonate because of possible stomach distention and subsequent rupture of an eroded area.

3. Give olive oil, 200 ml. (1 glass), by mouth for relief of gastric distress.

4. Apply external heat.

5. Inject morphine sulfate, 8 to 15 mg. intravenously, for severe pain.

6. Perform a tracheostomy (**14—12**) if edema of the glottis is severe.

7. Hospitalize if there is any evidence or suspicion of corrosion.

49—27. ACONITE (Aconitine)

Known as blue rocket, monkshood, Wolfsbane, friar's cowl and mousebane, this flowering plant is common in gardens. Ingestion of the flowers, foliage or stems by children may cause severe toxic symptoms. Acute poisoning also may result from mistaking the aconite plant for horseradish or from ingestion of medicinal compounds containing aconite. It is characterized by a burning sensation in the mouth and throat, acute dysphagia, impairment of speech, vertigo and eye signs (lacrimation, muscle imbalance and diplopia). Paresthesias, generally starting with the fingers but sometimes involving the whole body, may develop. Nausea, vomiting and diarrhea are common, as are marked hypotension and tonic and clonic convulsions. Fatalities are usually due to respiratory failure.

TREATMENT

1. Emptying of the stomach by emetics and/or gastric lavage with 1:2000 potassium permanganate solution, provided convulsions have not developed.

2. Application of external heat.

3. Control of convulsions (**31.** *Convulsive Seizures*).

4. Immediate institution of oxygen inhalations under positive pressure by face mask and rebreathing bag.

5. Intramuscular injection of caffeine sodiobenzoate, 0.5 gm., in mild cases; or of arterenol bitartrate (Levophed) or metaraminol bitartrate (Aramine) in 1000 ml. of 5% dextrose in saline intravenously if the blood pressure is very low.

PROGNOSIS   Poor in most cases. Fatalities have been reported from ingestion of 20 ml. of the tincture and from as little as 2 mg. of aconitine. Twice as much is rapidly and invariably fatal.

49—28. ACRIDINE (Acrylaldehyde)

This coal tar derivative causes yellow discoloration of the skin and mucous membranes, tracheobronchitis and asthma, all of which clear when exposure is terminated.

49—29. ACROLEIN

This commercial solvent, used in the resin industry, may cause acute toxic symptoms through inhalation of fumes as well as by ingestion. The usual signs and symptoms consist of a sensation of tightness in the chest, drowsiness, nausea, vomiting and diarrhea. Vertigo, occasionally syncope, may occur.

TREATMENT

1. Removal from exposure.

2. Oxygen inhalations under positive pressure, preferably by a face mask and rebreathing bag.

3. Symptomatic therapy as required.

PROGNOSIS. Complete recovery in a short time unless severe irritation of the respiratory tract has occurred.

49-30. ACRYLONITRILE (Ventox)

Used as an insecticide and in the rubber industry, this inflammable liquid may give an acute toxic picture following inhalation of the fumes or absorption through the skin. This picture is characterized by acute conjunctivitis, vomiting and diarrhea. Restlessness and irritability are evident at first, then are supplanted by somnolence and coma. Respiratory arrest may be terminal.

TREATMENT

Mild cases

1. Remove from exposure and give respiratory support (11-1) as needed.
2. Give strong, black coffee by mouth.

Severe cases

1. Remove contaminated clothing at once.
2. Treat as outlined above and under **49-235.** Cyanides.

49-31. AGROSTEMMA GITHAGO (Corn Cockle, Corn Campion, Corn Rose)

Ingestion of cereal grains contaminated by the saponin-containing seeds of this widespread weed can result in nausea, vomiting, diarrhea, severe headache, pain in the spine, impaired locomotion, respiratory collapse, coma and death.

TREATMENT

1. Discontinuance of contaminated food.
2. Gastric lavage followed by activated charcoal in water by mouth or through the lavage tube.
3. Saline cathartics.
4. Respiratory support.

49-32. ALCOHOL See 49-315. Ethyl Alcohol; 49-403. Isopropyl Alcohol; 49-475. Methyl Alcohol; 49-33. Alcohols (Higher)

49-33. ALCOHOLS (Higher)

The aliphatic liquid alcohols (amyl, butyl, ethylhexyl, isoamyl, etc.) are used extensively in industry as solvents. All are extremely toxic if ingested. For signs and symptoms of toxicity and treatment, see **49-67.** Amyl Alcohol.

49-34. ALDEHYDES See 49-340. Formaldehyde

49-35. ALDRIN

This complex insecticide is similar in actions and toxicity to dieldrin (**49-267**).

49-36. ALFALFA

Decoctions of the seeds of this extensively cultivated fodder have an undeserved reputation as a remedy for arthritis. In some individuals, intense dermatitis results from ingestion. This clears when oral intake is stopped.

49—37. ALIPHATIC HYDROCARBONS

These petroleum derivatives are widely used as cleaners, fuels and solvents. For toxic symptoms and treatment, see **49—349.** *Gasoline;* and **49—408.** *Kerosene.*

49—38. ALIPHATIC THIOCYANATES (Lethanes) See **49—774.** *Thiocyanates*

49—39. ALKALIES

TREATMENT OF EXTERNAL CONTACT
Flood with large amounts of water; then wash with vinegar or weak acetic acid. Use weak boric acid solution in the eyes after prolonged irrigation with tap water.
TREATMENT OF INGESTION
1. Neutralize with vinegar or acetic acid in water.
2. Give demulcents—white of egg, olive oil and absorbents such as activated charcoal (Norit A).
3. Hospitalize if evidence of erosion or corrosion is present or if ingestion of a large amount of a strong alkali is known or suspected to have occurred.
Do not use a stomach tube or give emetics if a concentrated solution has been swallowed or if marked erosion of the mucous membranes of the mouth or throat is apparent or suspected.

49—40. ALKALOIDS

TREATMENT
1. Tincture of iodine, 1 ml. in 100 ml. of water, by mouth.
2. Gastric lavage with large amounts of 1:5000 potassium permanganate solution followed by activated charcoal in water by mouth or through the lavage tube.
3. Application of external heat.
4. Symptomatic care.

49—41. ALKAVERVIR (Veriloid)

Use of this mixture of alkaloids derived from *Veratrum viridi* as a hypotensive agent has caused esophageal and substernal burning, dysphagia, blurred vision, bradycardia and extreme hypotension.
TREATMENT
1. Discontinue medication.
2. Give pressor substances (epinephrine, ephedrine) until blood pressure regains a safe level.
For symptoms and treatment following nonmedical ingestion, see **49—825.** *Veratrum Viride.*

49—42. ALKYL MERCURY COMPOUNDS

These compounds, especially the chlorides and phosphates, are widely used commercially as seed fungicides. Inhalation of fumes, or ingestion, causes fatigue and myalgia, headache and vertigo, sometimes associated with hyperactive reflexes and ataxia. There may be some decrease in visual fields and delirium and hallucinations.
TREATMENT
If symptoms follow ingestion, emetics and gastric lavage are indicated. If from fumes, oxygen inhalations after removal from exposure will result in rapid and complete recovery.

49—43.   ALKYL SODIUM SULFATES

These complex compounds are the active agents in many household detergents. Their toxicity is very slight. Emetics, followed by a saline cathartic, should be given if large amounts have been ingested.

49—44.   ALLETHRIN (Allyl Cinerin)

Allethrin is similar in use and toxicity to *Pyrethrum* (**49—631**).

49—45.   ALLIUM SATIVUM L. (Garlic)

The cloves may cause burning and blistering of the skin, with formation of indolent ulcers.

49—46.   ALLYL DIBROMIDE

Inhalation of fumes results in nausea, bradycardia, conjunctivitis, blurred vision and strabismus—all transient.

49—47.   ALOIN

This irritant laxative acts only on the large bowel and has no serious systemic effects.

49—48.   ALPHA NAPHTHYL THIOUREA See 49—83. *Antu*

49—49.   ALUM See 49—50. *Aluminum and Its Salts*

49—50.   ALUMINUM AND ITS SALTS [Aluminum Ammonium Sulfate (Alum), Aluminum Acetate, Aluminum Chloride]

All of the soluble salts of aluminum may cause gastroenteritis if ingested; the only treatment needed is demulcents. Aluminum oxide and hydroxide are insoluble and harmless.

49—51.   AMANITA POISONING See 49—502. *Mushroom Poisoning*

49—52.   AMINOAZOTOLUENE (Toluazotoluidine) See 49—672. *Scarlet Red*

49—53.   AMINOPHYLLINE (Theophylline Ethylenediamine)

In adult patients this dangerous drug is often injected intravenously in the treatment of asthma and coronary disease by physicians who are not cognizant of its toxicity or of the marked variation in reactions of different individuals (or of the same individual at different times). The smallest size suppositories commercially available (0.25 gm.) can cause acute toxic symptoms (irritability, restlessness, vomiting, convulsions and respiratory depression) in children under 3 years of age. Too rapid injection may result in cardiac palpitation, mydriasis, syncope and death from respiratory and circulatory collapse.

TREATMENT
1. Prophylactic – slow injection.
2. Oxygen inhalations by face mask and rebreathing bag.
3. Caffeine sodiobenzoate, 0.5 gm. subcutaneously in mild cases. Severe cases may develop severe shock and require use of vasoconstrictor drugs (53–7) for a lengthy period.
4. Immediate hospitalization for observation and symptomatic treatment. Although usually rapidly absorbed, aminophylline occasionally has a prolonged and cumulative effect.

49 – 54. AMINOPTERIN

Used in treatment of neoplasms, aminopterin causes acute toxic reactions characterized by glossitis, stomatitis, ulcerative colitis, vaginitis and proctitis. In addition, pancytopenia and aplastic bone marrow changes may occur. Treatment is symptomatic and supportive.

49 – 55. 2-AMINOPYRIDINE

Inhalation of fumes from melting of this industral material results in the delayed appearance (after 2 to 4 hours) of headache, dizziness, dyspnea, convulsions and marked elevation of blood pressure.
TREATMENT
Mild cases clear in a few hours after termination of exposure; severe cases require hospitalization for symptomatic treatment and close observation because of the danger of delayed pulmonary edema (51).

49 – 56. AMINOPYRINE (Amidopyrine, Aminophenazone, Pyramidon)

Common commercial preparations are Aminophen Pulvules, Cibalgine, Felsol Powder and Tablets, Optalidon and Ray-Pyrine. All are sold without prescription except in Denmark, Sweden and the United States. Therapeutic doses recommended by the manufacturer may cause hypersensitivity reactions, especially agranulocytosis.
For signs and symptoms of acute toxicity and treatment, see 49–13. Acetanilid.

49 – 57. 2-AMINOTHIAZOLE

Exposure to this industrial chemical results in deep brown discoloration of the urine; anorexia; nausea and vomiting; a serum sickness-like syndrome (21–4), with large wheals, dependent edema and generalized myalgia and arthralgia.
TREATMENT
1. Removal from exposure.
2. Oxygen under positive pressure by face mask and rebreathing bag.
3. Epinephrine hydrochloride (Adrenalin), 0.3 to 0.7 ml. of 1:1000 solution intramuscularly, repeated at 15 minute intervals as needed.
4. Hospitalization of severe cases for symptomatic care.

49 – 58. AMIZOL (ATA)

The toxicity of this herbicide, used especially for control of poison oak and ivy, is probably low, but following ingestion emetics should be given at once as a precautionary measure.

49 – 59. AMMONIA (Refrigerants, Household Cleansers, Medications) (See also **49 – 653.** *Rocket Fuels*)

TREATMENT OF EXTERNAL CONTACT
Wash the skin or irrigate the eyes with copious amounts of water.
TREATMENT OF INGESTION
1. Have the patient drink large quantities of dilute fruit juices or vinegar.
2. Start artificial respiration or oxygen inhalations at once if dyspnea or cyanosis is present. Tracheostomy (**14 – 12**) may be lifesaving and should be done without hesitation if acute edema·of the glottis is present.
3. Apply external heat by means of warm blankets, bed warmer or cast dryer.
Do not use a stomach tube, or prescribe emetics or respiratory depressants (especially narcotics), or apply hot water bottles for external heat.

49 – 60. AMMONIATED MERCURY

If ingested, this preparation has about the same toxicity as bichloride of mercury. Systemic effects may occur from absorption through the intact skin. For treatment, see **49 – 128.** *Bichloride of Mercury.*

49 – 61. AMMONIUM CHLORIDE (Sal Ammoniac)

In the presence of even slightly impaired liver or kidney function, the usual therapeutic dose of ammonium chloride, continued for a few days, may cause accumulation of toxic amounts of ammonia. See **29 – 10.** *Hepatic Coma.*
Acidosis, hypoproteinemia and coma may develop if long-continued use of ammonium chloride has embarrassed ammonia synthesis in the body. If given at the same time as sulfonamides, the danger of deposit of sulfa crystals in the kidneys is markedly increased.
TREATMENT
Treatment is primarily preventive.
1. Limitation of therapeutic use of ammonium chloride to not more than 3 to 6 gms. for 4 days in persons with normal renal function.
2. Avoidance of administration to persons with impaired liver or kidney function.
3. Avoidance of administration at the same time as sulfonamide therapy.
TREATMENT OF OVERDOSAGE
1. Discontinue medication.
2. Repeated intravenous administration of 5% solution of sodium bicarbonate. As an alternative, a 1/6 molar solution of sodium lactate, 30 ml. per kilogram of body weight, may be used.

49 – 62. AMMONIUM PICRATE (Carbazotate)

This substance is used in explosives and fireworks. For treatment, See **49 – 605.** *Picric Acid.*

49 – 63. AMMONIUM SULFITE

Widely used in metallurgy, photography and as a "cold wave set," ammonium sulfite is extremely toxic if ingested or absorbed through the skin or scalp. The treatment of toxic symptoms is similar to that outlined in **49 – 380.** *Hydrogen Sulfide.*

49–64. AMPHETAMINES (Benzedrine, Dexedrine, Methamphetamine)

Medical use of more than 20 mg. a day, or too frequent use of inhalers, may cause toxic signs and symptoms. Following inhalation, the toxic picture usually develops within 5 to 10 minutes; after ingestion, a time lag of 30 to 45 minutes is common.

Signs and Symptoms of toxicity are acute restlessness, inability to relax, flushed face (later becoming pale), mydriasis, dryness of the mucous membranes of the nose, mouth and throat, rapid pulse, elevated blood pressure, shallow respiration and final collapse. Chronic use – short of acute toxicity – may cause personality changes and increased irritability. Paranoid symptoms, hallucinosis (often prolonged), acute anxiety and exhaustion may develop.

Severe withdrawal symptoms (apathy, psychomotor depression, sleep disturbances, aggravation of previous psychopathology and suicidal tendencies) may require a controlled environment for several weeks.

Treatment

1. Empty the stomach by gastric lavage if ingested, followed by activated charcoal.

2. Inject a rapid acting barbiturate intravenously – watching closely for hypotension. Oral administration of 40 to 80 mg. of diazepam (Valium) during follow-up care usually controls anxiety and hyperactivity. Persistent depression may be controlled by imipramine hydrochloride (Tofranil), 75 to 100 mg. per day. Frequent administration of barbiturates and of chlorpromazine (Thorazine) should be avoided because of their hypotensive effects.

3. Give oxygen by face mask or catheter and rebreathing bag.

4. Acidify the urine by ammonium chloride to accelerate excretion.

5. Hospitalize for observation and treatment for at least 24 to 48 hours. Psychiatric evaluation and treatment usually is indicated. Illicit ("street") use of amphetamines may consist of oral ingestion of a large number of Benzedrine or Dexedrine pills or intravenous injection of Methamphetamine solutions of varying degrees of purity ("speed-balls"). See **49–715.**

49–65. AMYGDALIN

Amygdalin occurs in peach and apricot pits, chokecherries and bitter almonds. For treatment, see **49–235.** *Cyanides.*

49–66. AMYL ACETATE (Banana Oil, Pear Oil) (See also **49–610.** *Plastic Cements and Glues*)

Signs and Symptoms may develop following exposure to fumes as well as ingestion – headache, conjunctivitis, vomiting, muscular incoordination, laryngeal edema with or without dyspnea and cyanosis, pulmonary edema (**51**) and severe central nervous system depression.

Treatment

1. If from inhalation, remove from exposure; if from skin contact, remove all clothing (including shoes and socks) and wash contaminated areas thoroughly with soap and water; if from ingestion, institute gastric lavage immediately using large amounts of water, unless profuse vomiting has occurred.

2. Combat dyspnea and cyanosis by administration of air or oxygen under positive pressure by face mask or intranasal catheter and rebreathing bag.

3. Hospitalize if signs of laryngeal edema, pulmonary edema (**51**) or marked central nervous system involvement are present.

49—67. AMYL ALCOHOL

This alcohol is used extensively as a solvent for lacquer and explosives and is extremely dangerous if ingested or if fumes in high concentrations are inhaled. Both methods of exposure may result in headache, sleepiness, irritation of the throat, nausea, vomiting, anorexia, twitching, coma and death.

TREATMENT

Treatment is outlined in **49—66.** *Amyl Acetate* and **49—315.** *Ethyl Alcohol.*

49—68. AMYLENE HYDRATE (Tertiary Amyl Alcohol)

Excessive amounts of this occasionally used hypnotic are acutely toxic.

SIGNS AND SYMPTOMS.   Severe headache, deep sleep followed by coma, areflexia, flaccid paralysis and circulatory failure.

TREATMENT

1. Discontinue use of drug.
2. Hospitalize—usually for several days—for circulatory and cardiac support.

49—69. AMYL NITRITE

The first evidence of nitrite toxicity is cyanosis, initially of the lips, later spreading to the fingers, toes and remainder of the body. Hypoxemia from methemoglobinemia then develops, followed in severe cases by coma and death from circulatory failure.

TREATMENT

1. Gastric lavage if ingested.
2. Oxygen inhalations under positive pressure, preferably by endotracheal catheter and rebreathing bag.
3. Ephedrine sulfate, 15 mg. intramuscularly.
4. Plasma volume expanders intravenously until whole blood transfusions can be arranged. Either 50 to 200 mg. of metaraminol bitartrate (Aramine), or 4 ml. of 0.2% solution of levarterenol bitartrate (Levophed) in 1000 ml. of 5% dextrose in saline or water (or added to the plasma volume expander), given slowly intravenously may be necessary if shock (**53**) is severe.
5. Methylene blue (50 ml. of 1% solution in 1.8% sodium sulfate solution), given very slowly intravenously. This can be repeated every 45 minutes until 200 ml. have been given.

49—70. ANESTHETICS, INHALATION (See also **49—197.** *Chloroform;* **49—800.** *Trichlorethylene*)

The gases most commonly used for inhalation anesthesia are ether, chloroform, ethyl chloride, ethylene and nitrous oxide. Although there is a marked difference in the margin of safety for each gas, the symptoms of toxicity and treatment are approximately the same for all—deepened unconsciousness, rapid heart beat, loss of reflexes and respiratory and/or cardiac failure.

TREATMENT

1. Stop administration of the anesthetic as soon as any of the signs of incipient cardiac arrest (**26—7**) develop.
2. Start oxygen inhalations under positive pressure at once, preferably by means of an endotracheal catheter and rebreathing bag.
3. Give pentylenetetrazol (Metrazol), 0.2 gm. intramuscularly.
4. If cardiac arrest occurs, the circulation of the blood must be reestablished within 3 minutes if irreversible degenerative changes caused by hypoxemia are to be avoided.

49-71. ANESTHETICS, INTRAVENOUS See 49-580. *Pentothal Sodium*

49-72. ANESTHETICS, LOCAL

Toxicity of usual doses. The widespread use of local anesthesia in present-day medicine and dentistry has resulted in the recognition of 3 important types of toxic reactions to usual therapeutic amounts.

Allergic reactions. (See also **21**.) This type of toxic reaction occurs in persons who are allergic by heredity (atopic), and fortunately is relatively rare. It may be so overwhelming that death occurs in a few minutes, with rapid development of skin wheals and angioedema. Swelling of the soft tissues of the throat may be severe enough to require tracheostomy (**14-12**). Acute bronchospasm (**52-1**) may occur.

TREATMENT

1. The best treatment is prevention. Patients should be questioned regarding any family or personal history of allergy before the local anesthetic is used. In these cases, intracutaneous tests for sensitivity are of absolutely no value. Instead, a small amount of the solution to be used should be applied intranasally by means of an applicator. In an atopic patient, itching, burning and congestion will develop within 10 minutes. If the test is negative, injection of the local anesthetic can be considered as relatively safe; if positive, injection of even a minute amount may be fatal.

2. Maintenance of a clear airway and prevention of hypoxemia by whatever means are necessary.

3. Epinephrine hydrochloride (Adrenalin), 0.5 to 1.0 ml. of 1:1000 solution subcutaneously, intramuscularly or intravenously.

4. Tripelennamine hydrochloride (pyribenzamine), 50 to 100 mg. orally, or 25 to 50 mg. intramuscularly.

5. Hydrocortisone sodium succinate (Solu-Cortef) or methylprednisone sodium succinate (Solu-Medrol), intravenously.

PROGNOSIS. Complete recovery unless the onset has been overwhelming and fatal. The need for avoidance of the offending drug, or of others of similar chemical structure, should be stressed to the patient. Constant wearing of a "dog tag" or wristlet (**21. Allergic Reactions**) specifying the offending substances should be recommended.

Immediate toxic reactions may be caused by accidental injection into a blood vessel, use of too concentrated a solution or extremely rapid absorption through an extremely vascular area. Acute toxic symptoms develop within a few seconds after injection or topical application. If death occurs, it is usually due to complete circulatory and respiratory collapse and occurs within 1 or 2 minutes of the onset of the toxic picture.

TREATMENT

Although in many cases the onset is too overwhelming and death too rapid for any emergency measures to have any effect, the treatment given under *Delayed toxic reactions* (next paragraph) should be attempted.

Delayed toxic reactions are the result of a relatively slow building up of a toxic blood level of a particular agent following injection or topical use. The onset is never less than 5 nor more than 30 minutes after injection or local application. Somnolence, which may progress to coma, develops gradually. This sleepy stage in certain persons may be replaced by marked euphoria, excitement and elation. Generally, the patient feels that there is something wrong and will tell the physician so. There is a progressive decrease in rate and quality of pulse, and development of facial pallor and of a cold, clammy skin. Twitching of the face, hands and feet, with hypotension, syncope and convulsions may occur. Respiratory and circulatory failure may be irreversible and terminal.

TREATMENT

1. Mental changes require no specific treatment; however, these patients should be watched carefully for at least 30 minutes for evidence of more severe reactions.

2. Hypotension, with slow weak pulse, cold, clammy skin, intermittent apnea and dyspnea, should be treated as primary shock (**53 – 7**).

3. Convulsions must be controlled as quickly as possible by rapid-acting barbiturates. Pentothal sodium is the drug of choice. Six ml. of 2½% solution should be injected intravenously, followed by 2 to 3 ml. every 2 minutes until the convulsions have ceased. If pentothal sodium is not available, sodium pentobarbital (Nembutal), 0.12 to 0.25 gm., can be given intramuscularly as an initial dose; after 3 minutes, 60 mg. more can be given.

PROGNOSIS. Good if the early symptoms are recognized and proper treatment given; very poor if extreme hypotension and convulsions are allowed to develop or persist.

Toxicity of excessive amounts. Injection, ingestion or absorption of excessive amounts of any of the local anesthetics may cause extreme excitement, euphoria and laughter, or acute depression and apprehension; pallor followed by dyspnea and cyanosis; tachycardia; convulsions; respiratory and/or cardiac collapse – especially cardiac arrest (**26 – 7**).

TREATMENT

1. If injected in an extremity, apply a tourniquet if time will allow.

2. If ingested, give tannic acid solution by mouth; follow with gastric lavage with large amounts of 1:5000 potassium permanganate solution. Leave 50 mg. of activated charcoal in water in the stomach.

3. In all cases, start oxygen under positive pressure by mask and rebreathing bag as soon as the condition is recognized or suspected. Sedatives and/or analeptics may be necessary but should be used with great caution and only if there is a specific indication for them. Phenobarbital sodium (0.1 gm.) and amytal sodium (0.2 gm.) intramuscularly are effective sedatives. In extreme cases, intravenous pentobarbital sodium may be given cautiously.

4. Treat cardiac arrest (**11 – 2**).

49 – 73.   ANILINE (See also **49 – 74.** *Aniline Dyes*)

Aniline is a powerful and dangerous liquid of wide commercial use, which is also used as a rocket propellant (**49 – 653**). It may cause toxic symptoms and signs by ingestion or absorption through the intact skin. Common household preparations containing potentially toxic amounts of aniline are paints, varnishes, marking inks, stove polishes and shoe polishes.

SIGNS AND SYMPTOMS. Peculiar grayish pallor, amblyopia and decrease in visual fields, photophobia and scotomata, acute dyspnea, hypotension and generalized myalgia, sometimes severe.

TREATMENT

1. Removal from contact or exposure to fumes. To prevent toxic symptoms from absorption through the skin, immediate and thorough washing with dilute vinegar (acetic acid) followed by soap and water in large amounts is indicated.

2. If ingested, immediate gastric lavage with water or 1:5000 potassium permanganate, followed by activated charcoal in water by mouth or through the lavage tube.

3. Cautious administration of ephedrine sulfate and metaraminol bitartrate (Aramine) or levarterenol bitartrate (Levophed) parenterally as required for circulatory support.

4. Oxygen inhalations, preferably by face mask and rebreathing bag.

5. Methylene blue (1% solution), 1 to 2 mg. per kilogram of body weight intravenously. In less severe cases of methemoglobinemia, oral intake of methylene blue, 50 mg. per kilogram of body weight, may be substituted.

6. Calcium gluconate, 10 ml. of 10% solution, slowly intravenously for acute muscle pain – repeated as necessary.

7. Transfusions of whole blood, peritoneal dialysis (**14—9**) or (preferably) extracorporal hemodialysis may be necessary in severe cases.

PROGNOSIS.   Complete recovery after 6 to 8 hours if prompt, energetic and proper therapy has been given.

49—74. ANILINE DYES

Poisoning from the many varieties of aniline dyes is most common in children who have ingested certain types of colored crayons, sucked indelible pencils or drunk or eaten stove or shoe polish. Absorption from colored diapers may cause acute toxic symptoms in infants. The toxic picture (apathy, dyspnea, occasional gastrointestinal upsets and convulsions) is due to methemoglobinemia.

TREATMENT
See **49—73.** *Aniline.*

49—75. ANT PASTES

These may contain arsenic trioxide (**49—90**), calcium arsenate (**49—158**), Chlordane (**49—188**), sodium arsenite (**49—694**) or thallium sulfate (**49—768**). Occasionally antimony salts (**49—81**) are substituted.

49—76. ANT POWDERS See **49—188.** *Chlordane;* Potassium Cyanide (**49—235.** *Cyanides*); Sodium Fluoride (**49—336.** *Fluorides*)

49—77. ANTABUSE (Disulfiram) (See also **49—779.** *Thiram;* **49—848.** *Zerlate*)

Two types of reactions to this drug, which is used in the treatment of chronic alcoholism, may occur.

Side effects from administration of excessive doses. Although there is marked individual variation in tolerance, one 0.5 gm. tablet daily usually is adequate for the desired therapeutic effect; larger doses may cause drowsiness, especially in the morning; headache; loss of appetite, fatigue and psychoses.

TREATMENT
Unless a psychosis has developed, nothing is required except reduction of the size of the dose. If psychotic symptoms are present, disulfiram should be discontinued and symptomatic treatment begun. Complete recovery within 1 to 2 weeks almost invariably occurs if the drug is the causative factor.

Antabuse-alcohol reactions may be brought on by ingestion of alcohol in any form—drinks, foods cooked with wine or medications in alcoholic vehicles. Generally, the amount of alcohol ingested determines the severity of the reaction, but in some individuals even very small amounts may cause severe, even dangerous, toxic manifestations. These usually begin with a flushed skin, severe headache, burning of the eyes, salivation and dyspnea, and nausea and vomiting coming on within $\frac{1}{2}$ hour after ingestion of the alcohol-containing substances. A feeling of tightness in the chest may be severe enough to be mistaken for a cardiac condition. Hypotension, cyanosis and severe shock (**53**) may occur.

TREATMENT
1. Mild cases respond immediately to oxygen inhalations and oral administration of an antihistaminic drug.
2. Severe cases require intravenous administration of diphenhydramine hydrochloride (Benadryl) and immediate shock therapy (**53—7**). Chlorpromazine hydrochloride (Thorazine), 50 mg. intramuscularly, usually controls severe vomiting.

PROGNOSIS.   Complete recovery within a short time. Even if untreated, all except the most severe cases in profound shock will make a complete recovery in 8 to 12 hours.

49—78. ANTIBIOTICS

For a complete listing of adverse reactions or contraindications, see standard current pharmacology texts or the brochures furnished by the manufacturers.

Achromycin (Tetracycline, Polycycline, Steclin, Tetracyn). See Tetracyclines (below).

Aureomycin (Chlortetracycline). See Tetracyclines (below).

Bacitracin (Parentracin). (See also **49—108.**) Acute hypersensitivity reactions (**21**) requiring epinephrine hydrochloride (Adrenalin), oxygen and supportive therapy may result from topical use. In addition, acute renal failure may occur.

TREATMENT

1. Discontinue use of the antibiotic.

2. Symptomatic supportive therapy.

Chloromycetin (Chloramphenicol). In addition to all types of allergic reactions (**21**), this valuable antibiotic in therapeutic doses may cause nausea and vomiting, diarrhea, mucous membrane lesions and aplastic anemia and agranulocytosis.

TREATMENT

1. Discontinue administration at once.

2. Treat acute symptoms due to hypersensitivity (**21**).

3. Prescribe bismuth subcarbonate, 5 gm. by mouth, every 2 to 4 hours.

4. If possible, stop all antibiotics since cross-sensitization may occur.

Neomycin (Mycifradin). Hypersensitivity reactions (**21**) are rare but do occur; they are relatively mild compared with the other commonly used antibiotics.

TREATMENT

1. Discontinue use.

2. Symptomatic and supportive therapy as required.

Penicillin. This may cause severe anaphylactic reactions (**21—1**) characterized by rapid onset of muscular twitching and convulsions, followed by respiratory and cardiac collapse. More common but less serious allergic reactions usually do not appear until from 4 to 7 days after the first injection or oral dose and are characterized by generalized skin rashes often associated with severe, persistent itching, angioedema, severe myalgia and arthralgia and occasional convulsions. Blood dyscrasias may develop.

TREATMENT

1. As a preventive measure, prescribe or administer penicillin in any form *only if there is a definite indication for its use.*

2. Stop administration of the antibiotic.

3. Start antihistaminic agents. In severe cases give diphenhydramine hydrochloride (Benadryl), 5 to 10 mg. in 20 ml. of saline intravenously, or epinephrine hydrochloride (Adrenalin), 0.5 to 1.0 ml. of 1:1000 solution subcutaneously. In milder cases prescribe tripelennamine hydrochloride (Pyribenzamine), 50 to 100 mg. orally 3 times a day.

4. Apply calamine lotion with phenol 1% locally for itching. (Do not compress.)

5. Hospitalize severe cases, especially those with respiratory embarrassment from edema. Marked skin involvement may require referral to a dermatologist for treatment.

PROGNOSIS.   Mild cases usually clear within 12 hours: severe cases may require 5 to 7 days. If administration of penicillin is imperative and the patient gives a history of sensitivity, antihistaminics should be given before, with and after the antibiotic.

Streptomycin (Dihydrostreptomycin). In certain individuals therapeutic doses may cause urticaria and angioedema, varied types of acute skin reactions, acute conjunctival irritation, labyrinthitis and deafness, especially in persons with renal impairment. Acute gastrointestinal symptoms and liver and kidney damage may occur as may severe shock. Cardiac arrhythmias, cardiovascular collapse and progressive anemias and agranulocytosis have been reported.

TREATMENT
1. Stop administration of the drug at once.
2. Treat allergic manifestations (21).
3. Treat shock (53–7).
4. Hospitalize severe cases.

Terramycin (Oxytetracycline). See Tetracyclines (below).

Tetracyclines (Achromycin, Aureomycin, Polycycline, Steclin, Terramycin, Tetracyn). Overenthusiastic employment of these useful antibiotics, especially in futile prophylaxis and treatment of minor ailments, has resulted in increasing numbers of allergic reactions of all types (21), gastrointestinal disturbances (especially persistent diarrhea), vaginal and anal urticaria from monilial infections and staphylococcal enteritis.

TREATMENT
1. Stop use of drug and of all other antibiotics if possible. Cross-sensitization may occur.
2. Give symptomatic and supportive therapy.

49–79. ANTICOAGULANTS

Of the commonly used oral anticoagulant drugs, coumarin derivatives have fewer side effects than those of the indandione group (Danilone, Hedulin). All may cause conjunctivitis, paralysis of ocular accommodation, nausea, vomiting, bloody diarrhea, hematuria, steatorrhea, jaundice, liver damage and agranulocytosis.

TREATMENT
1. Discontinue administration of the drug.
2. Control hemorrhage as outlined in 42–34. *Bleeding from Anticoagulant Therapy.*

49–80. ANTIHISTAMINICS

Use of these commonly prescribed drugs may cause drowsiness, dizziness, headaches, prolonged insomnia, flushing of the skin, dryness of the mouth, dilation of the pupils, gastrointestinal symptoms, and mental confusion—occasionally, visual and olfactory aberrations and hallucinations. Hypotension followed by collapse and unconsciousness may occur. Prolonged use may result in agranulocytosis.

TREATMENT
1. Stop administration of the drug at once.
2. Give amphetamine sulfate (Benzedrine), 5 to 10 mg. by mouth or intravenously.
3. Arrange for adequate follow-up medical supervision.

PROGNOSIS. Complete recovery from acute effects usually occurs within a few hours.

49–81. ANTIMONY

With or without arsenic compounds (49–90), antimony is an active constituent of certain brands of commercial sprays, weed killers, ant killers and snail baits. It is also a constituent of many medicines. Antimony oxide is used in glazing cheap "china" and pottery. Poisoning from antimony compounds is usually delayed from $1/2$ to 2 hours after ingestion.

SIGNS AND SYMPTOMS. Nausea and vomiting, dehydration, extreme thirst, weak rapid pulse, a sensation of choking and tightness in the throat, with difficulty in swallowing, cyanosis, painful profuse watery (sometimes bloody) diarrhea and collapse from severe shock.

TREATMENT
1. Emetics followed by gastric lavage with warm water.
2. Morphine sulfate subcutaneously for colicky pain and diarrhea.
3. Five per cent dextrose in saline, 500 ml. intravenously. Levarterenol bitartrate (Levophed) intravenously, 4 ml. of 0.2% solution in 1000 ml. of 5% dextrose in saline, or metaraminol bitartrate (Aramine), may be necessary in severe cases.
4. Prevention of chilling but avoidance of extreme heat which might cause vasodilation.
5. BAL, 10% solution of dimercaprol in peanut oil and benzyl benzoate, 0.025 ml. per kilogram of body weight intramuscularly.
6. Hospitalization in severe cases because of a definite tendency toward the development of delayed toxicity.

49–82. ANTIPYRINE See **49–56.** *Aminopyrine*

49–83. ANTU (α-Naphthylthiourea)

This rodenticide is of relatively low toxicity to humans, but ingestion of large doses may cause mild respiratory depression.
TREATMENT
1. Emptying of the stomach by emetics or lavage followed by activated charcoal in water orally or through the lavage tube.
2. Oxygen inhalations.
PROGNOSIS.   Complete recovery even after large doses.

49–84. APIOL See **49–811.** *Triorthocresyl-phosphate*

49–85. APOMORPHINE HYDROCHLORIDE

This powerful emetic acts centrally when ingested or injected hypodermically. Doses of not over 5 mg. will cause pronounced vomiting, followed by depression. Larger doses will result in extreme pallor, violent – sometimes projectile – vomiting, irregular, weak respiration, vertigo, sometimes mydriasis, muscle weakness and spasm, and asphyxia.
TREATMENT
1. If injected
  a. Limitation of absorption from an extremity by immediate application of a tourniquet.
  b. Oxygen inhalations, preferably by a face mask and rebreathing bag.
  c. Naloxone hydrochloride (Narcan), 0.01 mg. per kilogram of body weight to combat depressant effects, repeated as necessary.
  d. Caffeine sodiobenzoate, 0.5 gm. intramuscularly.
  e. Fluid replacement by plasma volume expanders or 5% dextrose in saline intravenously.
2. If ingested, gastric lavage with 1:5000 potassium permanganate solution followed by the symptomatic measures given above.
PROGNOSIS.   Good. Even with very large doses, complete recovery usually occurs within a few hours.

49–86. ARECOLINE (Betel Nut)

Ingestion and intravenous injection of this alkaloid has caused nausea and vomiting, extreme diuresis, clonic convulsions and coma. For treatment, see **49–40.** *Alkaloids.*

49—87. ARGEMONE OIL (Prickly Poppy)

Ingestion of preparations of this complex mixture of alkaloids and fatty acids has been reported as causing visual halos and glaucoma, in addition to gastrointestinal irritation and peripheral edema.

TREATMENT
1. Discontinuance of use of the oil.
2. Supportive and symptomatic therapy.

49—88. ARNICA

Extracts of this irritant substance were formerly a common constituent of many "patent medicines." Locally it may cause erysipeloid dermatitis, cutaneous ulceration and gangrene and formation of profuse pus when applied to open wounds. Removal by thorough irrigation is the only treatment required.

Systemically, following ingestion, it may result in severe cephalgia, nausea and vomiting, sometimes associated with severe abdominal pain, extreme pallor, dryness of the skin, rapid weak pulse, irregular (sometimes Cheyne-Stokes) respiration, extreme miosis, sleepiness, unconsciousness and death through respiratory and cardiac collapse.

TREATMENT
1. Gastric lavage with 1:5000 potassium permanganate solution followed by activated charcoal in water by mouth or via lavage tube.
2. Magnesium sulfate (Epsom salts) by mouth.
3. Oxygen inhalations.
4. Hospitalization for supportive care if respiratory or circulatory depression is or has been severe.

49—89. ARSACETIN (Sodium Acetylarsanilate)

This antiluetic and antiprotozoal preparation is extremely toxic and may cause blindness due to retrobulbar neuritis.

For treatment, see **49—96.** Arsphenamine.

49—90. ARSENIC

Arsenic and its compounds are commonly used in medicinal preparations, rodenticides, insecticides, and in metallurgy and the textile and chemical industries.

Methods of absorption are through the intact skin, by inhalation of dust or fumes, by ingestion and by intravenous injection (see **49—96.** Arsphenamine).

SIGNS AND SYMPTOMS of toxicity usually develop in from 15 minutes to 1 hour after ingestion, inhalation of dust or fumes or intravenous injection; or later, if absorbed through the skin. They are characterized by nausea, vomiting (vomitus may have a garlicky odor), acute dysphagia, acute abdominal pain (sometimes severe enough to simulate an acute surgical abdomen), watery diarrhea, cyanosis, weak rapid pulse, cold clammy skin, encephalitis-like symptoms and severe shock (**53**).

TREATMENT
1. If ingested, immediate emptying of the stomach by
    a. Emetics by mouth, followed if necessary by apomorphine hydrochloride, 3 to 5 mg. subcutaneously
    b. Gastric lavage with warm water, with or without 30 mg. of sodium thiosulfate. Activated charcoal should be left in the stomach.
2. Morphine sulfate, 10 to 15 mg. intramuscularly or intravenously, for severe pain and colic. Atropine sulfate, 0.04 mg., may be added.

3. Treatment of shock (**53-7**).

4. Dimercaprol (BAL), 3 mg. per kilogram of body weight intramuscularly, every 4 hours. In severe cases this dosage can be increased to not more than 5 mg. per kilogram.

5. Calcium gluconate, 10 ml. of 10% solution intravenously for abdominal and muscular cramps.

6. Hospitalization for intravenous fluids, continued chelation and possible blood transfusions.

49-91. ARSENIC COLOR PIGMENTS

Auripigment (**49-93.** *Arsenic Trisulfide*), Paris green and Schweinfurt green (**49-223.** *Copper Acetoarsenite*) are used in industry and are extremely dangerous.

TREATMENT

See **49-90.** *Arsenic*.

49-92. ARSENIC TRIOXIDE

This substance is insoluble—hence, has a much lower toxicity than the soluble salts. See **49-90.** *Arsenic*.

49-93. ARSENIC TRISULFIDE (Auripigment)

Arsenic trisulfide is used in yellow and gold paints and may produce symptoms through absorption or ingestion.

TREATMENT

See **49-90.** *Arsenic*.

49-94. ARSINE (Arseniuretted Hydrogens)

This colorless, odorless and dangerous gas may be formed during the burning of lead in industry, from ferrosilicon and from the action of impure sulfuric acid on metals.

SIGNS AND SYMPTOMS of toxicity usually develop 2 to 6 hours after exposure. Severe cases show acute anoxemia; milder cases are characterized by nausea, vomiting, severe epigastric pain, bronze tinting of the skin due to a combination of jaundice and cyanosis, convulsions, delirium and coma.

TREATMENT

1. Morphine sulfate, 10 to 15 mg., or pentazocine lactate (Talwin), 15 to 30 mg., intramuscularly or intravenously for severe pain.

2. Dextrose in saline, 500 to 1000 ml. of 5% solution, intravenously, with or without plasma volume expanders. Use of levarterenol bitartrate (Levophed) or metaraminol bitartrate (Aramine) intravenously may be necessary if hypotension is extreme.

3. Oxygen by face mask and rebreathing bag if cyanosis is pronounced.

4. Hospitalization as soon as the patient's condition permits for possible dialysis and/or exchange transfusions. Dimercaprol (BAL) is of no value in acute arsine poisoning.

49-95. ARSINIMA TRILOBA (Pawpaw)

Contact with the fruit of this North American shrub causes nausea and vomiting and vesicles with acute pruritus. Symptoms clear slowly when contact is avoided, but a brownish discoloration at the site of the vesicles may be permanent.

49–96. ARSPHENAMINE (Salvarsan)

This antibiotic and antitrypanosomal drug and its less irritating and more stable derivative, Neoarsphenamine (Neosalvarsan), may give a variety of toxic symptoms following intravenous injection, most of which are of short duration and rarely fatal. Among these are abscess formation, acute dermatitis, nitritoid reactions similar to anaphylaxis (**21–1**), chills, fever, headache, vomiting, diarrhea and temporary impairment of kidney function.

Serious toxic reactions are neuroretinitis, gangrene of the extremities and hemorrhagic encephalitis. All of these conditions require immediate hospitalization for intensive therapy.

49–97. ARTANE

Dryness of the mouth, blurred vision and hallucinations may follow use of this antiparkinsonian drug. Symptoms clear when the drug is stopped.

49–98. ASARUM EUROPAEUM

Ingestion of a decoction of the roots of this shrub may cause transient vomiting, diarrhea and pelvic congestion. Symptomatic care is all that is required.

49–99. ASBESTOS

Severe cough and chest pain in a person exposed to the dust of this common insulating material may require emergency care followed by referral for thorough investigation, including x-rays, to rule out asbestosis.

49–100. ASPIDIUM (Male Fern)

Even small doses of this anthelminthic may give acute toxic symptoms. Among these are cephalgia, vertigo, amblyopia, yellow vision, rapid pulse, dyspnea, vomiting, diarrhea, transient syncope followed by coma, acute myalgia, trismus and occasional toxic psychoses (**50–1**).

TREATMENT

1. Gastric lavage with warm water, leaving 30 gm. of magnesium sulfate (Epsom salts) in the stomach.
2. Oxygen inhalations by face mask and rebreathing bag.
3. Caffeine sodiobenzoate, 0.5 gm. intramuscularly, and/or ephedrine sulfate, 15 mg. intravenously for circulatory collapse, repeated in 15 minutes if necessary.
4. Hospitalization if gastrointestinal symptoms persist or if shock (**53**) is severe.

PROGNOSIS.   Good. Fatalities are rare, even with relatively large doses.

49–101. ASPIRIN (Acetylsalicylic Acid) (See also **49–664.** *Salicylates*)

Three types of toxic reactions to this widely used antipyretic and analgesic are relatively common.

Allergic sensitivity. This has been reported to occur in as high as 10% of persons with allergic tendencies. For treatment, see **21.** *Allergic Reactions.*

Gastritis and gastric bleeding. This ceases when intake of the drug is stopped.

Toxicity from ingestion of large doses. The minimal lethal dose is usually considered to lie between 0.3 and 0.4 gm. per kilogram of body weight. A blood serum salicylate level of 140 mg.% may be fatal. For qualitative test for salicylate ingestion, see **15–6.** For estimation of peak serum salicylate levels after a single dose see Figure 29.

For signs, symptoms and treatment of acute toxicity, see **49–664.** *Salicylates.*

49–102. ASTEROL DIHYDROCHLORIDE

Especially in children, excessive or prolonged use of this fungicide in treatment of dermatophytoses may cause muscular weakness, incoordination, tremors and ataxia. Symptoms clear slowly when the drug is discontinued.

49–103. ASTHMA REMEDIES

The active agents contained in these proprietary preparations are usually atropine (**49–104**), belladonna (**49–116**), potassium nitrate (**49–525**) or stramonium (**49–724**), although aminophylline (**49–53**), antihistaminics (**49–80**), barbiturates (**49–111**), bromides (**49–144**), ephedrine (**49–300**) and iodides (**49–392**) may be present. Mixed with beer or soft drinks, some of these proprietary preparations have been used as hallucinogens (**49–358**).

The signs and symptoms of toxicity and appropriate treatment depend upon the active agent.

49–104. ATROPINE SULFATE (See also **49–116.** *Belladonna and Belladonna Alkaloids*)

Acute atropine poisoning may be caused by skin absorption from belladonna plasters (**49–116**), by ingestion of jimsonweed berries or by medicinal use–often from mistaking eye drops containing atropine for nose drops. The toxic picture is characterized by dryness of the mouth, difficulty in swallowing, widely dilated pupils, red hot and dry skin, increased body temperature, delirium and collapse.

TREATMENT

1. If ingested, immediate emptying of the stomach by gastric lavage with a weak solution of tannic acid followed by activated charcoal in water through the lavage tube.

2. Physostigmine salicylate (Antilirium), 0.5 to 2.0 mg. subcutaneously, intramuscularly or intravenously, repeated as necessary to reverse the central nervous system affects of atropine.

3. Administration of oxygen by face mask or catheter and rebreathing bag.

4. Control of body temperature by ice bags and alcohol sponging.

5. Sedation by barbiturates in small doses.

6. Hospitalization for close observation for at least 48 hours. Relapses may occur after apparent complete recovery. The patient should be in a darkened room because of photophobia.

49–105. AURAMINE

Auramine is used in veterinary medicine and as a dye. Absorption of auramine through the skin may cause local ulceration, fever, severe pain, headache and yellow vision. Slow spontaneous recovery begins when exposure is stopped.

49–106. AURIPIGMENT (Arsenic Trisulfide) See **49–90.** *Arsenic*

49–107. BABY POWDERS See **49–138.** *Borates;* **49–740.** *Talc;* **49–854.** *Zinc Stearate*

49—108. BACITRACIN (See also 49—78. *Antibiotics*)

Nontoxic if applied locally; intramuscular injection of bacitracin may cause pain at the injection site, skin rashes, petechiae, tinnitus, nausea, vomiting and serious renal damage.

TREATMENT
1. Stop therapeutic use.
2. Give symptomatic and supportive care.
3. Hospitalize if evidence of severe kidney damage is present.

49—109. BAL (British Anti-Lewisite, Dimercaprol, Dithiopropanol)

Originally developed to neutralize the effects of lewisite war gas, BAL at the present time is used for its ability to alleviate toxic symptoms caused by certain heavy metals.

Intramuscular (*not* intravenous) injections of BAL have a definite and effective place in the treatment of poisoning from certain heavy metals [antimony (49—81), arsenic (49—90), gold (49—353), mercury (49—128. *Bichloride of Mercury*), nickel (49—521)] and lewisite war gas (49—832). In some cases of bismuth (49—130), lead (49—420), selenium (49—679) and thallium (49—768) poisoning, it may be of some value. It is ineffective or contraindicated in poisoning from cadmium (49—156), iron (49—399), tellurium (49—752) and zinc (49—849 to 49—855. *Zinc Salts*). The dosage is usually given as 2.5 to 3 mg. per kilogram of body weight every 4 hours for 1 to 2 days, with the first dose as soon as possible after development of toxic effects from the metal, but in extreme cases the initial dose should be increased to 5 mg. per kilogram of body weight. For local effects of lewisite war gas, a 2 to 5% solution or ointment of BAL is recommended.

Toxic effects are almost always caused by excessive dosage (although BAL has a large margin of safety) and develop within 30 minutes of the time of application, injection or ingestion. Most of them can be prevented by premedication with ephedrine sulfate.

SIGNS AND SYMPTOMS OF TOXICITY

From local application—urticaria and wheals with intense pruritus, papular eruptions, mottling and increased pigmentation of the skin.

From ingestion or parenteral administration—severe headache, conjunctivitis, lacrimation, blepharospasm, a burning sensation of gums and pharynx, nausea, vomiting, rapid pulse, elevated blood pressure and tetany-like symptoms with positive Chvostek's and Trousseau signs (43—25).

TREATMENT
1. Discontinue parenteral use.
2. If ingested, empty the stomach by emetics and/or lavage as soon as possible and administer sedation as needed.
3. Give symptomatic and supportive therapy.

PROGNOSIS. Complete recovery within a few hours.

49—110. BANANA OIL See 49—66. *Amyl Acetate*

49—111. BARBITURATES (See also 2—2. *Addiction;* 29—13. *Coma*)

All of the numerous derivatives of barbituric acid act in the same manner, although there is a marked variation in speed and duration of action and in toxicity. Since barbiturates are often prescribed in large amounts, cases of acute poisoning from accidental overdosage and suicide attempts are encountered quite frequently. Toxic effects include severe headache, disturbances in sensation (especially of the extremities), slurred speech and general impairment of coordination. The pupils usually are constricted but may be dilated or nonreactive. In early poisoning, foggy vision, diplopia and color variations may be present. Respirations at first are rapid, then slow and become weak from respiratory center depression. Pulmonary edema (51) from increased capillary permeability may develop. The skin is cold, clammy and cyanotic. A weak, rapid pulse, extreme hypotension and anuria may be present. Acute excitement, hallucinations and delirium followed by increasing sleepiness may progress to coma and death from respiratory failure.

TREATMENT

1. Insurance of an adequate airway by postural drainage, suction, insertion of an endotracheal catheter or tracheostomy (14 – 12).

2. Administration of oxygen under positive pressure by intranasal or endotracheal catheter and rebreathing bag or tracheostomy tube.

3. Gastric lavage with large quantities of warm water, leaving 60 gm. of magnesium sulfate (Epsom salts) dissolved in a glass (200 ml.) of water in the stomach if the drug has been ingested within 6 hours or if the gag reflex is still present. If suicidal intent (13) is suspected, the rectum and vagina should be examined and emptied if indicated.

4. Application of external heat by warm blankets or by a bed warmer or cast dryer. Do not use hot water bottles if other means of applying heat are available.

5. Slow intravenous infusion of 5% dextrose in water or normal salt solution. Monitor the serum potassium level and supplement appropriately.

6. Protection of the eyeballs from drying by taping the eyelids together.

7. Insertion of a retention catheter with careful measurement of intake and output. Furosemide (Lasix) may aid diuresis.

8. Support of the circulation by:
   a. Atropine sulfate, 1 mg. intramuscularly or intravenously.
   b. Ephedrine sulfate, 15 mg. injected slowly intravenously; repeat every 15 minutes if necessary to combat hypotension.
   c. Levarterenol bitartrate (Levophed), 4 ml. of 0.2% solution, or metaraminol bitartrate (Aramine), 50 to 100 mg. in 1000 ml. of 5% dextrose in saline, slowly intravenously, preferably through a plastic intravenous catheter. The average rate of injection should be 0.5 to 1.0 ml. per minute, controlled by frequent blood pressure determinations.

9. Avoidance of the use of all analeptic drugs, including amphetamine sulfate (Benzedrine), pentylenetetrazol (Metrazol) and picrotoxin.

10. Hospitalization of all severe cases, preferably under the care of a competent anesthesiologist or a physician trained in postoperative recovery room care. Peritoneal dialysis (14 – 9) may be lifesaving. Painstaking nursing care is an essential part of therapy.

49 – 112. BARIUM COMPOUNDS

Toxic reactions may follow ingestion of barium carbonate, chloride or sulfide or inhalation of dust of barium carbonate or peroxide. Barium salts are the active ingredient in several brands of commercial rodent poisons (49 – 645). Barium sulfide is used in some depilatories (49 – 248).

Severe toxic effects have been reported following the use in x-ray studies of barium sulfate contaminated with barium carbonate.

SIGNS AND SYMPTOMS.   Dryness and sense of constriction of the mouth and throat, metallic taste, dilated pupils with loss of accommodation, weak, irregular pulse, rapid shallow breathing, cyanosis, nausea, vomiting, severe gastritis with acute watery or bloody diarrhea and gradually increasing sleepiness with mental confusion. Collapse and death from respiratory failure and cardiac arrest may occur.

TREATMENT

1. Oral administration of demulcents and of soluble sulfates (dilute sulfuric acid, alum, magnesium or sodium sulfate), to cause formation of insoluble barium sulfate.

2. Application of external heat.
3. Gastric lavage with 1 to 3% sodium sulfate in warm water.
4. Atropine sulfate, 0.5 to 1.0 mg., to decrease colic. Small doses of morphine may be necessary to control abdominal pain.
5. Oxygen by face mask and rebreathing bag if cyanosis is marked.
6. Control of dehydration by isotonic saline solution intravenously.
7. Intravenous potassium if hypokalemia is present.

49—113. BARRACUDA [See also 49—339 *(Rare Causes of Food Poisoning);* 24—2. *Barracuda Bites*]

During certain seasons, use of this fish as a food may cause acute toxic symptoms coming on many hours after ingestion. The characteristic picture includes paresthesias around the mouth, metallic taste, acute gastrointestinal irritation, severe myalgia and arthralgia and marked hypotension, which may reach shock levels (53).
TREATMENT
See 49—339 *(Rare Causes of Food Poisoning).*

49—114. BEECHNUT

Ingestion of beechnuts may cause facial pallor, severe headache, vomiting, abdominal pain, syncope and lassitude lasting for 5 or 6 hours. If seen early, gastric lavage followed by activated charcoal in water and saline cathartics is indicated. Complete recovery is to be expected.
Beechnut oil is nontoxic.

49—115. BEE VENOM See 56—1. *Bee Stings;* 61. *Venoms*

49—116. BELLADONNA AND BELLADONNA ALKALOIDS

The effects and toxicity of belladonna are approximately the same as those of atropine sulfate (49—104). In certain individuals the use of belladonna plasters may result in acute symptoms through absorption. Children may develop acute toxic symptoms from ingestion of any part of the plant—common in many household gardens.
SIGNS AND SYMPTOMS of belladonna intoxication consist of a dry, hot skin with increased body temperature, dryness of the mouth with difficulty in swallowing, weak rapid pulse, increased blood pressure, dilated pupils, restlessness, confusion, incoordination, speech disturbances, hallucinations (49—358), delirium and convulsions. Elderly arteriosclerotic patients are especially prone to hallucinations. Urinary retention may be acute, especially if prostatic hypertrophy is present. Respiratory and circulatory depression may be extreme.
TREATMENT
See 49—104. *Atropine Sulfate.*

49—117. BENZANTHRONE

Dermatitis, with melanosis of those portions of the skin exposed to light, has been reported following industrial exposure.

49—118. BENZEDRINE See 49—64. *Amphetamines*

49–119. BENZENE (BENZOL) AND ITS DERIVATIVES (Toluene, Xylene, Xylol)

Acute benzene poisoning is usually caused by inhalation of fumes in industry, where it is used as a solvent, cleanser and fuel.

Signs and Symptoms After Inhalation. Acute conjunctivitis, severe headache, general malaise and weakness [sometimes preceded by a brief period of exhilaration ("benzene jag")], nausea, vomiting, facial pallor, cyanosis of the lips and fingertips, weak rapid pulse, unconsciousness and convulsions. Death from respiratory depression may occur.

Treatment
1. Remove from exposure to fumes.
2. Wash the eyes with large amounts of water.
3. Protect against injury during convulsions.
4. Give oxygen inhalations for dyspnea and cyanosis.
5. Inject caffeine sodiobenzoate, 0.5 gm. intramuscularly, for cardiovascular support.

Toxic effects appear more rapidly and are much more severe following ingestion than after inhalation.

Signs and Symptoms After Ingestion. Nausea, vomiting, burning sensation in the epigastrium, headache, dizziness, staggering gait, fixed nonreactive pupils and sleepiness progressing to stupor and loss of consciousness.

Treatment
1. Gastric lavage with warm water or 5% sodium bicarbonate solution, followed by mineral oil through the lavage tube or by mouth. Precautions against aspiration should be taken.
2. Administration of saline cathartics.
3. Oxygen inhalations under positive pressure.
4. Ascorbic acid, 50 to 100 mg. intravenously.
5. Control of convulsions by rapid-acting barbiturates.
6. Correction of fluid-electrolyte imbalance.
7. Continuous ECG monitoring because of the danger of ventricular fibrillation. External cardiac compression (11–2) or defibrillation may be necessary.
8. Treatment of pulmonary edema (51).
9. Hospitalization after control of the acute symptoms. Delayed development of tracheobronchitis, cardiac irregularities, lung infection and severe blood changes may occur.

49–120. BENZENE HEXACHLORIDE (BHC, Benzahex, ChemHex, Lindane, 662, Gammexane)

Acute toxic symptoms from this common insecticide usually follow ingestion or absorption through the intact skin, although inhalation of dust or fumes may cause an acute toxic picture. Commercial preparations contain either a mixture of several isomers in varying proportions or the gamma isomer alone (Gammexane, Lindane). The latter preparations are more dangerous because they are usually in the form of oily sprays which adhere to the skin.

Signs and Symptoms. Extreme hyperirritability to outside stimuli, with intermittent muscular spasm and convulsions, and cyanosis followed by rapidly developing circulatory and respiratory depression.

Treatment
1. Remove all contaminated clothing. Wash the body thoroughly with soap and warm water. Protect from external stimuli.
2. Empty the stomach (if ingested) by gastric lavage, leaving 30 ml. of magnesium sulfate (Epsom salts) in the stomach.

3. Sedate by rapid-acting barbiturates. Calcium gluconate intravenously may be beneficial.

4. Give oxygen under positive pressure by face mask and rebreathing bag.

5. Support the circulation by caffeine sodiobenzoate, 0.5 gm. intramuscularly or intravenously. Severe cases with marked hypotension may require ephedrine sulfate, levarterenol bitartrate (Levophed) or metaraminol bitartrate (Aramine) for circulatory support. *Do not* use epinephrine (Adrenalin) because of the danger of inducing ventricular fibrillation.

6. Hospitalize for close observation. Apparent recovery may be terminated by acute collapse as long as 4 days after initial exposure.

49 – 121.   BENZETHONIUM CHLORIDE (Phemerol, Syntho-San)

Ingestion of a 10% solution may cause nausea, vomiting, respiratory failure and death. Treatment consists of gastric lavage and respiratory support.

49 – 122.   BENZIDINE (Diaminodiphenyl)

Used in the chemical industry and as a laboratory reagent, prolonged exposure to benzidine may cause papillomas of the bladder with secondary carcinomatous degeneration.

49 – 123.   BENZOL See 49 – 119. *Benzene and Its Derivatives*

49 – 124.   BENZPYRENE

Prolonged exposure to this substance may cause warts and epitheliomas.

49 – 125.   BENZYLCHLORIDE

Fumes of benzylchloride may cause severe eye and nose irritation which subsides spontaneously when exposure is stopped.

49 – 126.   BERYLLIUM

Beryllium is widely used in industry, especially as the inside coating of fluorescent tubes and lamps. The metal itself may be the offending agent, but cases of acute poisoning have also been reported from beryllium carbonate, fluoride, hydroxide, oxide, oxyfluoride, silicate and sulfate. Tremendous variation (from a few hours to several months) in the time lag between exposure and the development of acute symptoms has been noted.

Beryllium disease is of 4 main types. Each type may be acute or chronic.

Dermatitis – contact type, usually from solution of beryllium salts. This condition is characterized by itching papulovesicular lesions on exposed parts.

TREATMENT

1. Removal from exposure.

2. Alum and lead acetate compresses (10%).

PROGNOSIS. Good, but reexposure should be avoided.

Skin ulcers – caused by minute lacerations from glass particles carrying beryllium into the skin, with formation of nonhealing ulcers.

TREATMENT

Surgical excision of the ulcers followed by primary closure.

Tracheobronchitis. Rarely seen as an emergency.

TREATMENT

Treatment consists of removal from contact with beryllium. A baseline chest film should be obtained for later reference.

Chemical pneumonitis. This condition must be distinguished from acute miliary tuberculosis. If beryllium pneumonitis is suspected from the history or physical findings, immediate hospitalization is indicated, since the reported mortality varies between 18 and 35%.

49 – 127. BETANAPHTHYLAMINE

Hemorrhagic cystitis, followed by carcinomatous degeneration of polyps of the bladder, may follow inhalation of fumes or absorption through the skin.

49 – 128. BICHLORIDE OF MERCURY (Corrosive Sublimate)

SIGNS AND SYMPTOMS following ingestion of bichloride of mercury consist of metallic taste, whitish tongue, choking sensation, intense esophageal and gastric pain, vomiting, bloody diarrhea, drowsiness, mental confusion, anuria, convulsions and coma.

TREATMENT

1. Administration of egg albumin by mouth.
2. Induction of vomiting at once.
3. Application of external heat.
4. Gastric lavage as soon as possible with large amounts of 5% sodium formaldehyde sulfoxylate solution, leaving about 250 ml. in the stomach. If this solution is not available, a solution of egg white or 2 to 5% sodium bicarbonate may be used, followed by activated charcoal in water through the lavage tube.
5. If seen within 1 hour of ingestion, intravenous administration of 250 ml. of 5% sodium formaldehyde sulfoxylate solution; if over 1 hour has elapsed, 4 ml. of sodium citrate should be given by mouth.
6. Injection of small doses of morphine sulfate subcutaneously or intravenously for control of pain, which may be extremely severe.
7. Support of the circulation by intramuscular injection of 0.5 gm. of caffeine sodiobenzoate.
8. Intravenous infusion of 500 to 1000 ml. of 5% dextrose in saline or water. If signs of collapse are present, 100 to 200 mg. of metaraminol bitartrate (Aramine) or 4 ml. of 0.2% levarterenol bitartrate (Levophed) can be added to each liter.
9. Calcium gluconate, 10 ml. of 10% solution, intravenously for severe myalgia and arthralgia.
10. Dimercaprol (BAL). In moderate cases of bichloride of mercury poisoning, the dose should be 2.5 mg. per kilogram of body weight intramuscularly every 4 hours for 1 to 2 days; in severe cases the initial dose may be increased to 5 mg. per kilogram of body weight.
11. Hospitalization at once for treatment of shock (**53 – 7**) and possible renal insufficiency or failure and for continuation of dimercaprol (BAL) therapy. Follow-up care for possible strictures is essential.

49 – 129. BIRTH CONTROL PILLS

The active ingredients of oral contraceptive pills are usually conjugated estrogens, dimethisterone, ethinyl estradiol, mestranol and norethindrome in varying mixtures. The pills, often in attractive containers, are readily available to children in many households.

Toxic effects are mild and consist primarily of gastrointestinal irritation. Emptying the stomach by emetics or gastric lavage followed by saline cathartics is the only treatment required.

49—130. BISMUTH

Stomatitis, a purplish line on the gums, albuminuria and collapse characterize bismuth poisoning.

TREATMENT

1. Stoppage of administration of the drug.
2. Magnesium sulfate, 30 gm. by mouth.
3. Treatment of shock (53—7).
4. In moderate cases intramuscular injections of dimercaprol (BAL), 2.5 mg. per kilogram of body weight, every 4 hours. In severe cases this can be increased to not more than 3 mg. per kilogram of body weight.
5. Hospitalization for continuation of BAL therapy and for supportive care.

49—131. BISMUTH SUBNITRATE

The toxicity of this commonly used gastrointestinal remedy is due not to bismuth but to reduction of the nitrate radical to nitrites in the intestinal tract. See *Nitrites* (49—528).

49—132. BISMUTH SUBSALICYLATE

Used commercially as a fungicide and medicinally for antiluetic treatment, this practically insoluble salt may give signs and symptoms of bismuth poisoning (49—130) and/or salicylate toxicity (49—664) in the presence of alkalies.

49—133. BITTER ALMONDS, OIL OF See 49—235. *Cyanides*

49—134. BLEACHES (Laundry) See 49—384. *Hypochlorites;* 49—552. *Oxalic Acid;* 49—138. *Sodium Perborate (Borates)*

Contrary to general belief, although nausea and vomiting may be severe, even the most concentrated commercial bleaches do not cause erosion or strictures. In contrast to the effects of caustic alkalies (49—39), complete recovery invariably occurs under symptomatic treatment.

49—135. BLIGHIA SAPIDA

The green and incompletely ripened fruit of this West Indian and Canal Zone tree are acutely toxic if ingested, causing nausea, vomiting, stupor, coma and convulsions. Extreme hypoglycemia is usually present, with death in about 12 hours. Children are especially susceptible.

TREATMENT

1. Emetics or gastric lavage, followed by activated charcoal by mouth or through the lavage tube.
2. Intravenous dextrose.
3. Supportive care.

49—136. BLUE VITRIOL See 49—223. *Copper*

49 – 137. BLUING (Laundry)

This contains minute amounts of aniline dyes (**49 – 74**) and oxalic acid (**49 – 552**).

49 – 138. BORATES, BORIC ACID, BORACIC ACID AND BORON (See also **49 – 653.** *Rocket Fuels*)

Once considered harmless and found in the form of solutions and powder in many household medicine cabinets, boric acid and its salts are now known to be extremely dangerous, especially to infants. Several series of severe poisonings, with some fatalities, have been reported following accidental oral administration of boric acid solution to hospital nursery infants.

SIGNS AND SYMPTOMS. Nausea, vomiting, epigastric pain, diarrhea and collapse may occur. Acute gastroenteritis following skin and mucous membrane absorption has been reported. In severe cases, particularly in children, cyanosis, tachycardia, hypotension and severe shock (**53**) may develop. There is generally an erythematous rash extending over the whole body, sometimes involving the pharynx and tympanic membranes. The temperature may be slightly elevated but usually is subnormal.

Delirium and coma, sometimes delayed for as long as a week, may develop, followed by death from central nervous system depression. Chronic and intractable renal damage may occur.

TREATMENT
1. Application of external heat.
2. Gastric lavage with warm water followed by activated charcoal in water orally or via the lavage tube. A saline cathartic should be administered.
3. Sodium bicarbonate by mouth to alkalinize the urine and prevent metabolic acidosis.
4. Oxygen under positive pressure.
5. Control of convulsions by rapid acting barbiturates.
6. Treatment of dehydration.
7. Hospitalization after treatment of shock (**53 – 7**) because of the danger of severe delayed kidney damage. In severe cases, peritoneal dialysis (**14 – 9**) or hemodialysis may be life-saving.

49 – 139. BORNYL CHLORIDE (Chlorocamphane, "Turpentine Camphor") See **49 – 163.** *Camphor*

49 – 140. BORON ANHYDRIDE (Diborane)

Exposure to fumes of this substance causes an increase in body temperature, shortness of breath, dizziness, double vision and generalized severe myalgia. All symptoms clear when exposure is terminated.

49 – 141. BOTULISM (See also **49 – 339.** *Food Poisoning*)

In many instances a history of eating home-canned or preserved foods can be obtained. A few cases of botulism following puncture wounds have been reported.

TOXIC SIGNS AND SYMPTOMS consist of descending motor paralysis and usually are delayed for 12 to 100 hours after ingestion or exposure, with development in the following order:
1. Nausea and vomiting.
2. Malaise, fatigue, constipation, subnormal temperature.
3. Dizziness, headache and blurring of vision.

4. Difficulty in swallowing and speech.
5. Generalized muscular weakness.
6. Coma and death from respiratory paralysis.

Botulism must be distinguished from basilar artery thrombosis, poliomyelitis (**30—21; 48—49**), Guillain-Barré syndrome, myasthenia gravis (**46—7**) and intoxications such as that due to arsenic (**49—90**).

TREATMENT

Hospitalize at once for treatment with trivalent botulinum antitoxin and symptomatic and supportive care. Since 12 to 100 hours have usually elapsed before post-ingestion toxicity develops, emetics and lavage are of little value. Stimulants and oxygen therapy usually are necessary.

49—142. BRITISH ANTI-LEWISITE (Dimercaprol) See **49—109**. *BAL*

49—143. BROMATES

Deaths from irreversible kidney damage have been reported following ingestion of popular brands of cold-wave hair preparations containing potassium bromate. The sodium salt, used in the processing of gold ores, is also extremely toxic.

TREATMENT

1. Emetics and/or gastric lavage with warm water or 1% sodium thiosulfate solution followed by activated charcoal in water by mouth or via the lavage tube.
2. Control of acute pain by meperidine (Demerol) or pentazocine lactate (Talwin). Morphine should be avoided.
3. Correct dehydration by glucose (5% in water) intravenously.
4. Administer oxygen by face mask and rebreathing bag.
5. Caffeine sodiobenzoate, 0.5 gm. intramuscularly, for circulatory support.
6. Hospitalization because of the tendency of bromates to cause severe kidney damage. Immediate peritoneal dialysis (**14—9**) or hemodialysis may be beneficial. Methylene blue tends to enhance bromate toxicity and should not be used.

49—144. BROMIDES

Sodium bromide as well as other alkaline salts of this halogen cause toxic symptoms by replacement of the chloride radical in the tissues of the body. The toxic picture is quantitative and varies depending upon the degree of intoxication, which, in turn, varies with the tolerance of the individual.

Mild intoxication (from 100 to 200 mg. per 100 ml. of blood) is characterized by general listlessness, malaise, insomnia, inability to concentrate and loss of memory.

TREATMENT

1. Stop administration of bromide-containing medications.
2. Force fluids by mouth.
3. Increase the daily intake of sodium chloride to 4 to 8 gm. daily.

Moderate intoxication (above 200 mg. per 100 ml. of blood, depending on individual tolerance) causes restlessness, irritability, insomnia, generalized myalgia and arthralgia. Severe headache, acute depression and paranoia may occur, as may disorientation, retrograde amnesia and hallucinations (usually visual but sometimes auditory), incoordination and tremors. Vision changes (blurring, diplopia, photophobia, disturbances in color vision) are common. Exophthalmos and ptosis of the lids may be present.

TREATMENT

1. Stop intake of bromides.

2. Because of an apparent synergistic action, all tranquilizers and barbiturates should also be stopped.

3. Normal saline (sodium chloride) intravenously. At least 6 gm. daily–given in divided doses–is required.

Severe intoxication (300 to 500 mg. per 100 ml. of blood) results in dilated fixed pupils, sallow muddy complexion, acneform skin rashes, fetid breath and dehydration. Sexual impotence or menstrual irregularities may be present.

TREATMENT

As given under *Moderate intoxication* (above). Hospitalization is required for prolonged supportive therapy. In extremely severe cases, hemodialysis may be indicated.

49–145. BROMINE

Bromine gives off brown, heavy, irritant fumes. Inhalation of even low concentrations causes lacrimation, conjunctivitis, rhinitis, pharyngitis, glottal spasm and edema, a feeling of suffocation and pulmonary edema (**51**). High concentrations are rapidly fatal.

TREATMENT AFTER INHALATION

1. Removal from exposure to fumes.
2. Inhalation of nebulized 5% sodium bicarbonate solution.
3. Sedation.
4. Hospitalization of severe cases for symptomatic and supportive therapy if glotteal edema is extreme because of the danger of pulmonary edema (**51**).

Swallowing of minute amounts of liquid bromine has been reported as causing stomatitis, esophagitis, gastric hemorrhage and bloody diarrhea.

TREATMENT AFTER INGESTION

1. Gastric lavage followed by activated charcoal in water by mouth.
2. Saline cathartics.
3. Hospitalization because of the danger of delayed pulmonary edema (**51**).

49–146. BROMOFORM (Tribromethane)

Small doses of this sedative drug cause transient listlessness, vertigo and headache.

Large doses may be fatal. The toxic picture is characterized by a burning sensation in the mouth, somnolence, stupor and coma. Areflexia, trismus, convulsions and death from respiratory failure may occur.

TREATMENT

1. Gastric lavage followed by activated charcoal by mouth or through the lavage tube.
2. Saline cathartics.
3. Oxygen by face mask.
4. Analeptics as required.
5. Hospitalization because of the danger of delayed pulmonary edema (**51**).

49–147. BRUCINE

Ingestion of brucine, commonly used as a denaturant, may cause a toxic picture similar to but less serious than strychnine (**49–729**).

49–148. BULAN

Similar in uses and toxicity to DDT (**49–243**).

49—149. BUPHANINE

Derived from a native herb, this alkaloid is used by African medicine men. Its action is similar to scopolamine (**49—676**).

49—150. BUTACAINE

Butacaine sulfate is used as a local anesthetic, particularly on mucous membranes. See *Anesthetics, Local* (**49—72**).

49—151. BUTANE

Inhalation may cause varying degrees of anesthesia. It is very explosive. For toxic effects, see **49—580**. *Pentothal Sodium*.

49—152. BUTANOL (n-Butyl Alcohol)

This alcohol has the same effects as ethyl alcohol (**49—315**) but is much more toxic.

49—153. BUTESIN PICRATE (Butamben Picrate)

Used as an antiseptic ointment, butesin picrate has given rise on many occasions to serious dermatitides. Clearing usually occurs slowly when use of the ointment is discontinued.

49—154. BUTYN See **49—72**. *Anesthetics, Local*

49—155. n-BUTYRALDOXIME

In itself this substance, used in printing inks, is nontoxic, but inhalation of its vapors causes extreme sensitivity to ingestion of small amounts of alcoholic beverages.

49—156. CADMIUM AND ITS SALTS

Acute poisoning occurs in manufacturing and use of cadmium alloys, smelting of ores, coating of bearings and tools with cadmium, electroplating, soldering and welding, process engraving, manufacturing of storage batteries, use of cadmium pigment paints and use of silver polishes containing cadmium carbonate.

Methods of poisoning

Inhalation of fumes, usually from silver-cadmium solder. These fumes are odorless and do not produce immediate irritation; hence, dangerous amounts may be inhaled before acute symptoms occur—usually in 2 to 5 hours. Symptoms are dry throat, cough, headache, nausea, vomiting, a feeling of constriction and pain in the chest, dyspnea and pneumonia. Except for the occasional development of pneumonia, symptoms from inhalation disappear spontaneously in from 12 to 15 hours after onset. Symptomatic treatment only is indicated.

Ingestion. Following ingestion, acute symptoms develop in ½ to 1 hour. Use of cadmium-lined food or drink containers and cadmium-plated eating utensils is banned in some localities because of the tendency of cadmium to dissolve in the acids commonly found in food, thereby producing toxic cadmium chloride. Contamination of the water supply by industrial wastes has been reported from Japan [Itai-itai ("ouch-ouch") disease]. Symptoms consist of salivation, choking, vomiting, abdominal cramps and diarrhea.

TREATMENT FOLLOWING INGESTION

1. Give milk or egg white by mouth.

2. If vomiting is not profuse, gastric lavage with milk or an albumin solution, followed by a saline cathartic.

3. After the gastrointestinal tract has been emptied, give calcium disodium edetate intravenously.

4. Correct dehydration and acid-base imbalance by intravenous fluids.

5. Give supportive therapy for acute renal failure. Use of dimercaprol (BAL) should be avoided. Pulmonary edema (**51**) may be a late complication.

49—157. CAFFEINE

Acute toxic symptoms may be caused by overdoses of medications containing salts of caffeine or by excessive drinking of caffeine-containing beverages (coffee, maté, tea). Infants and small children are peculiarly susceptible to caffeine, and acute toxic symptoms may be caused by ingestion or therapeutic injection of minute amounts.

SIGNS AND SYMPTOMS.   Vomiting, epigastric pain, dizziness, ringing in the ears and eye signs (constricted pupils, decreased visual fields, amblyopia, diplopia and photophobia). Headache, occasionally hallucinations and delirium, palpitation, tachycardia and a tight feeling in the chest may occur, as may trismus, opisthotonus and convulsions.

TREATMENT

1. Emetics or gastric lavage with warm water if due to drinking excessive amounts of coffee.

2. Large amounts of fluids by mouth, or 1000 ml. of 5% dextrose in saline intravenously.

3. Barbiturates for sedation.

PROGNOSIS.   Complete recovery without residual ill effects.

49—158. CALCIUM ARSENATE AND ARSENITE See 49—90. *Arsenic*

49—159. CALCIUM CYANAMIDE

Inhalation of the dust may accentuate the effects of alcoholic beverages. See **49—315.** *Ethyl alcohol.*

49—160. CALOMEL (Mercurous Chloride)

This irritant cathartic is sometimes ingested in relatively large doses, with resultant severe abdominal discomfort and greenish-black diarrhea. Excessive diarrhea can be controlled by tincture opii camphorata (Paregoric), by small doses of morphine sulfate (not in infants or small children) or by atropine sulfate.

49—161. CALTHA PALUSTRIS (Cowslip, Marsh Marigold)

Chewing the leaves of this common plant causes transient burning of the mouth, violent abdominal pain and generalized pemphigus-like skin eruptions. Symptomatic treatment only is needed, with rapid complete recovery.

49-162. CAMBOGIA (Gamboge)

Cambogia is a violent cathartic. Doses of over 3 gm. may cause complete collapse and death.

TREATMENT

Gastric lavage followed by activated charcoal in water, with respiratory and circulatory support as needed.

49-163. CAMPHOR (Camphorated Oil, Spirits of Camphor)

Vicks' VapoRub, Camphor Ice, and other proprietary medical preparations, and some moth repellents, contain camphor as the active ingredient.

SIGNS AND SYMPTOMS. Headache, sensation of warmth, characteristic odor of the breath, weak rapid pulse, convulsions (often epileptiform) and terminal circulatory collapse.

TREATMENT

1. Emetics—apomorphine hydrochloride, 5 mg. hypodermically, is best if seen early.
2. Gastric lavage with warm water, followed by activated charcoal in water by mouth or via the lavage tube. Oils and alcohol enhance absorption and must be avoided.
3. Application of external heat.
4. Oxygen therapy as needed.
5. Caffeine sodiobenzoate, 0.5 gm. intramuscularly—repeated as necessary.
6. Rapid acting barbiturates as needed for prevention and control of convulsions.
7. Hospitalization for supportive care if severe convulsions or deep shock (53) occur. The patient should be protected against external stimuli. Complete recovery usually takes place.

49-164. CANDY CATHARTICS See 49-591. Phenolphthalein.

49-165. CANTHARIDES (Spanish Fly, Russian Fly)

This substance has an undeserved reputation as an aphrodisiac, but its most common use is in hair tonics. Ingestion of small amounts may cause nausea, vomiting, abdominal pain, bloody diarrhea, delirium, coma and death from circulatory collapse.

TREATMENT

1. Administration of demulcents (avoid oils!).
2. Immediate emptying of stomach by emetics or gastric lavage followed by activated charcoal in water by mouth or through the lavage tube.
3. Supportive therapy as required. Shock (53) may be severe.

49-166. CARBARSONE (p-Carbamylaminophenylarsenic Acid)

Used medically in the treatment of amebiasis and Trichomonas vaginalis infection, this substance may cause severe toxic symptoms by absorption through the skin.

TREATMENT

See 49-90. Arsenic.

49-167. CARBIMAZOLE (Neomercazole)

Prolonged use of this antihyperthyroid drug may cause purpura, arthralgia, fever, thrombocytopenia and agranulocytosis.

49 – 168. CARBINOL See **49 – 475.** *Methyl Alcohol*

49 – 169. CARBOLIC ACID See **49 – 590.** *Phenol*

49 – 170. CARBON DIOXIDE (Carbonic Acid Gas, Carbonic Acid Anhydride)

In industry, carbon dioxide, because of its weight, tends to collect in deep enclosures, especially if some fermenting substance is present. Inhalation of concentrations of more than 8% may cause headache, vertigo, apparent inebriation, vomiting, unconsciousness and death from asphyxia.

TREATMENT

1. Removal to fresh air.
2. Oxygen by face mask.
3. Supportive therapy.

49 – 171. CARBON DISULFIDE (Bisulfide)

Carbon disulfide is used as a solvent for fats, oils, waxes, resins and rubber, in the manufacture of rayon and nylon fiber and as an insecticide. Ingestion or inhalation of concentrated fumes may cause respiratory depression, nausea, vomiting, convulsions and death from respiratory failure. Milder toxic symptoms can be caused by absorption through the intact skin.

TREATMENT

1. Respiratory support by expired air methods (**11 – 1**) after removal from exposure and insurance of a clear airway. Oxygen therapy under positive pressure should be substituted as soon as possible.
2. If ingested, immediate gastric lavage with large amounts of warm water followed by 120 ml. of mineral oil.
3. Circulatory support by cautious use of stimulants and analeptics, especially caffeine sodiobenzoate. Amphetamines and reserpine should be avoided.
4. Control of excitement and convulsions by rapidly acting barbiturates (**31.** *Convulsive Seizures*).
5. Large doses of vitamin B_6 parenterally.

PROGNOSIS.   Rapid recovery without permanent ill effects if signs and symptoms are mild; in severe cases the patient may develop severe neuropsychiatric disorders simulating manic-depressive and paranoid states (**50 – 1**).

49 – 172. CARBON MONOXIDE

This colorless, odorless gas, resulting from incomplete combustion, may be inhaled in the presence of improperly functioning or inadequately vented equipment burning heating or illuminating gas, in the presence of automobile exhaust fumes and during the use of open circuit diving apparatus (**23 – 5**). Many deaths credited to smoke inhalation (**22 – 5**) are in fact due to carbon monoxide poisoning.

DIAGNOSIS.   History of exposure, cherry red color to lips (may be absent or transient), peaceful expression, facial twitchings, elevated temperature, pale skin. Brownish red stippling may be present on the arms or trunk.

TREATMENT

1. Immediate expired air respiration after removal from exposure and determining that the airway is clear, followed by 95 to 100% oxygen inhalations under positive pressure using face mask or endotracheal catheter (**11 – 1.** *Resuscitation*).
2. Dextrose solution (50%), 100 ml., slowly intravenously.

3. Prevention of chilling or excitement of any type.

4. Hospitalization for close observation and symptomatic therapy (including transfusions). The patient should be kept on complete bed rest for at least 48 hours. In severe cases, induction of hypothermia should be considered.

Do Not

1. Administer methylene blue solution intravenously.

2. Give morphine, synthetic narcotics or atropine sulfate.

3. Use heart stimulants (analeptics) unless absolutely necessary.

4. Send the patient home after apparent recovery from the acute phase; close observation for and treatment of delayed toxic effects — especially myocardial and neurologic damage — may be lifesaving.

49 — 173. CARBON TETRACHLORIDE

Commercial uses — fire extinguishers, cleaning fluids, plant-forcing preparations and dry shampoos. Toxic effects may arise from inhalation of fumes or skin absorption as well as from ingestion.

TREATMENT

1. *Following inhalation:* Fresh air, expired air or mechanical artificial respiration (**11 — 1.** *Resuscitation*). Administration of air or oxygen under positive pressure may be necessary.

2. *Following ingestion:*

    a. Gastric lavage with potassium permanganate (1:5000 solution) followed by activated charcoal in water by mouth or through the lavage tube.

    b. Magnesium sulfate (Epsom salts) by mouth as a saline cathartic.

3. Caffeine sodiobenzoate, 0.5 gm. intramuscularly, repeated as necessary.

4. Calcium gluconate, 10 ml. of 10% solution intravenously, for control of pain. Small doses of morphine or meperidine (Demerol) may be necessary since abdominal pain may be severe enough to simulate an acute surgical condition.

5. Dextrose, 5% in saline, 500 ml. intravenously.

6. Severe cases require hospitalization for peritoneal dialysis (**14 — 9**), blood transfusions and measures to prevent liver and kidney damage.

Do Not

1. Give fats or oils — they facilitate absorption.

2. Administer epinephrine hydrochloride (Adrenalin) or ephedrine — these increase the danger of ventricular fibrillation.

3. Prescribe or administer alcohol in any form — it tends to increase hepatic damage.

49 — 174. CARBROMAL (Adalin, Bromadal, Uradal, Nyctal)

Used as a sedative and hypnotic, carbromal in large doses (0.5 to 1.5 gm.) produces central nervous system depression, sometimes followed by respiratory arrest.

TREATMENT

1. Gastric lavage followed by activated charcoal in water through the lavage tube.

2. Saline cathartics.

3. Supportive care as outlined in **49 — 111.** *Barbiturates.*

49 — 175. CARDIAZOL See **49 — 488.** *Metrazol*

49 — 176. CASHEW NUTS

The oil from these nuts contains phenols, which resemble in structure and action the irritants in poison oak, poison ivy and poison sumac (**54 — 11**).

49—177. CASTOR BEANS

Commercial extraction of castor oil results in a residual pomace containing a very potent toxalbumin (ricin) which is notorious for causing severe allergic reactions (**21**), especially severe asthma and bronchospasm.

The attractive varicolored beans, which are found on the ornamental shade trees, may be eaten by children with serious results (**49—893**).

49—178. CASTRIX

This insecticide if ingested, may cause severe convulsions. For treatment, see **49—729**. *Strychnine.*

49—179. CAUSTIC ALKALIES See **49—39**. *Alkalies*

49—180. CEDAR OIL

Cedar wood oil has been used as an abortifacient, with development of rapid irregular respiration, cold clammy skin, convulsions and coma.

TREATMENT

1. Gastric lavage followed by activated charcoal by mouth or through the lavage tube.
2. Saline cathartics.
3. Control of convulsions by rapid-acting barbiturates.
4. Supportive therapy.

49—181. CHELIDONINE

This substance is the active principle of a common plant, golden celandine. Chewing the leaves causes burning of the mouth and throat, acute gastric pain, somnolence, diarrhea and collapse.

TREATMENT

1. Gastric lavage followed by activated charcoal in water through the lavage tube.
2. Saline cathartics.
3. Supportive and symptomatic care.

49—182. CHENOPODIUM (Wormseed)

Medicinal use as an anthelmintic may cause acute toxic symptoms even with extremely small doses.

SIGNS AND SYMPTOMS. Nausea, vomiting, abdominal pain, headache, dizziness, impairment of vision and hearing, acute depression, low back and flank pain from kidney damage, delirium and clonic convulsions. Slow weak respirations, sometimes Cheyne-Stokes in type, may occur, with death from respiratory paralysis.

TREATMENT

1. Emetics and/or gastric lavage with 1:5000 potassium permanganate solution. Thirty grams of magnesium sulfate (Espom salts) in a glass (200 ml.) of water should be left in the stomach.
2. Oxygen therapy.
3. Dextrose, 5% in saline, 1000 ml. intravenously.
4. Caffeine sodiobenzoate, 0.5 gm. intramuscularly, for circulatory support.
5. Hospitalization for observation after control of acute symptoms.

PROGNOSIS.   Fair only. Relatively small doses may cause severe symptoms. Sequelae such as polyneuritis, paresis and decreased hearing may persist for a lengthy period.

49 – 183.   CHINIOFON See 49 – 556. *Oxyquinoline Derivatives*

49 – 184.   CHLORAL HYDRATE

"Knockout drops," sometimes administered in alcoholic beverages, usually contain chloral hydrate.

DIAGNOSIS.   History of intake, muscles relaxed, pupils constricted, respiration weak and shallow, pulse barely perceptible, skin cold and clammy, temperature and blood pressure below normal.

TREATMENT

1. Expired air artificial respiration (11 – 1) followed by oxygen under positive pressure by face mask and rebreathing bag.

2. Gastric lavage with warm water or 1:5000 potassium permanganate solution followed by activated charcoal in water through the lavage tube.

3. Stimulants – cardiac and respiratory.

4. Application of external heat.

5. Severe cases with collapse and coma require hospitalization for supportive therapy.

49 – 185.   CHLORAMINE T

Several series of cases have been reported in which severe toxic symptoms have followed accidental ingestion of this commonly used drinking water disinfectant.

SIGNS AND SYMPTOMS.   Rapid onset of respiratory embarrassment, cyanosis, marked hypotension, subnormal temperature, abdominal pain and convulsions. Death from respiratory failure usually occurs within a few minutes if a large amount has been ingested; if the patient survives over 30 minutes, the prognosis is usually good.

TREATMENT

1. Gastric lavage with large amounts of 1:5000 potassium permanganate solution, leaving 30 gm. of magnesium sulfate (Epsom salts) dissolved in 200 ml. (1 glass) of water in the stomach.

2. Oxygen therapy under positive pressure, using a face mask or endotracheal catheter and rebreathing bag.

49 – 186.   CHLORAMPHENICOL (Chloromycetin) (See also 49 – 78. *Antibiotics*)

Usual doses may cause nausea, vomiting, diarrhea, acute skin reactions and vulval and rectal irritation. Prolonged use may result in stomatitis, aplastic anemia and serious liver damage. Children apparently are more susceptible than adults.

TREATMENT

See 49 – 78. *Antibiotics.*

49 – 187.   CHLORATES

Potassium chlorate is used extensively industrially as an oxidizing agent and medicinally as an antiseptic and astringent.

SIGNS AND SYMPTOMS.   Dryness of throat, severe gastric pain, vomiting, diarrhea, yellow sclerae, cyanotic skin due to methemoglobinemia, tendency to hemorrhage (epistaxis, metrorrhagia and purpura hemorrhagica) and respiratory collapse.

TREATMENT

1. Respiratory assistance by expired air respiration (**11–1**) or by oxygen inhalations under positive pressure.

2. Gastric lavage with large amount of warm water followed by activated charcoal in water through the lavage tube.

3. Magnesium sulfate (Epsom salts) by mouth or through the stomach tube.

4. Dextrose, 5% in normal salt solution, 1000 to 2000 ml. intravenously. Methylene blue (intravenously) should not be used.

49–188. CHLORDANE (Compound 1068, Dowklor, Octa-Klor)

This complex substance has wide commercial use as an insecticide spray and dust. Evidences of toxicity may develop following inhalation of the mist or dust, by skin absorption or by ingestion. Convulsions and deep depression, often fatal, may develop.

TREATMENT

1. Removal of contaminated clothing. The skin should be washed thoroughly with large amounts of soap and water. The eyes should be irrigated with tap water.

2. Insurance of an adequate airway.

3. Oxygen inhalations under positive pressure by face mask or endotracheal catheter and rebreathing bag.

4. If ingested, gastric lavage with large amounts of warm tap water followed by activated charcoal in water through the lavage tube.

5. Rapidly acting barbiturates or paraldehyde for sedation, taking care not to deepen the already present respiratory depression.

49–189. CHLORDIAZEPOXIDE (Librium)

In commonly used dosages this sedative-tranquilizer may cause mental confusion, hypotension, extrapyramidal disturbances, edema (especially pretibial) and decreased libido.

TREATMENT

1. Stop the drug.

2. Give symptomatic and supportive treatment for the uncomfortable but not dangerous withdrawal symptoms, which slowly subside without residuals.

49–190. CHLORINATED LIME See 49–384. *Hypochlorites*

49–191. CHLORINE

This irritant gas, when inhaled, causes acute respiratory irritation, which may be followed by pulmonary edema (sometimes delayed) (**51**), pneumonia and circulatory collapse.

TREATMENT

1. Removal from exposure.

2. Removal from the skin by copious use of soap and water.

3. Oxygen under positive pressure.

4. Maintenance of fluid and electrolyte balance (**6**).

5. Control of pain by small dose of morphine sulfate or by inhalation of a mixture of alcohol and ether.

6. Hospitalization because of danger of development of pneumonia (**52–14**) or pulmonary edema (**51**).

49−192.   CHLOROACETOPHENONE (Mace) (See also 49−832. War Gases)

Chloroacetophenone, dissolved in an ether alcohol solution, is the active ingredient in "tear gas" guns. It is emitted, together with paper wadding and synthetic packing, under considerable pressure, usually by a freon propellant. An aerosol preparation containing a 1% chloroacetophenone solution, used by law inforcement officers, is known as "Mace."

Chloroacetophenone is a powerful lacrimator, causing profuse tearing, smarting and burning of the eyes, blurred vision and temporary blindness. The effects are usually transient unless particles have been driven into the tissues by the propellant.

TREATMENT
1. Thorough irrigation, preferably with 2% sodium bicarbonate solution.
2. Protection of the eyes by dark glasses.
3. Instillation 3 times a day of a 1% solution of idoxuridine (IDU). Referral to an ophthalmologist is often indicated if IDU is used.

A few cases of permanent blindness, some requiring enucleation, have been reported.

49−193.   CHLOROANILINE

Absorption of this liquid through the skin may cause immediate or delayed cyanosis and rapid pulse.

TREATMENT
1. Oxygen by face mask and rebreathing bag.
2. Normal saline solution intravenously.
3. Analeptics.

49−194.   CHLOROBENZENE (Monochlorobenzene)

This is used in the dry cleaning industry and in the preparation of coal tar pigments and dyes. It may produce toxic symptoms through skin absorption, inhalation of fumes or ingestion. Evidence of poisoning is usually delayed for 2 to 5 hours after exposure and is characterized by headache, sleepiness deepening into coma, pallor, cyanosis from methemoglobinemia, fibrillary twitching and respiratory and circulatory collapse.

TREATMENT
1. Removal from exposure to fumes; removal from the skin by washing with soap and water; removal from the stomach by gastric lavage and saline cathartics.
2. Oxygen under positive pressure.

49−195.   CHLORODINITROBENZENE

Skin contact with this substance, used in the explosives industry, causes severe dermatitis and acute sensitization. Serious changes (cyanosis, dyspnea, giddiness, staggering gait and liver and spleen enlargement) may follow inhalation of fumes or ingestion. Symptomatic treatment, after stopping exposure, results in a slow clearing of toxic signs and symptoms.

49−196.   CHLOROETHYLENE See 49−173. Carbon Tetrachloride

49−197.   CHLOROFORM (Trichloromethane)

In addition to its use as a general anesthetic, chloroform is used extensively in industry as a solvent for fats and resins. It is not absorbed through the skin but may cause severe erythema and purulent blebs locally.

Three types of acute chloroform poisoning may require emergency treatment.

Inhalation type. Overdosage during chloroform anesthesia or ingestion of large amounts results in sudden dilation of the pupils (terminally, the corneas become dull and cloudy), sudden disappearance of the pulse (good one second, gone the next), complete respiratory failure and death from circulatory collapse and ventricular fibrillation (**26 – 23**).

TREATMENT

1. Stop anesthesia if from inhalation; start gastric lavage immediately if from ingestion.

2. Begin oxygen therapy under positive pressure at once.

3. Inject supportive agents, such as caffeine sodiobenzoate, 0.5 gm. intramuscularly or intravenously. Epinephrine hydrochloride (Adrenalin) is contraindicated; it may cause acute cardiac dilatation or ventricular fibrillation.

4. Hospitalize if the patient survives the often fatal acute stage.

Ingestion type

SIGNS AND SYMPTOMS. Burning sensation in the mouth, throat, esophagus and stomach, nausea, vomiting, cold clammy skin, cyanosis of the extremities and face, gasping irregular respiration, extreme dilation of the pupils and muscular cramping, especially of the masseters. Progressive hypotension from increasing cardiac weakness, peripheral vasodilation and respiratory failure may occur.

TREATMENT

As given for the inhalation type (above). The prognosis, however, is much better. Hospitalization for observation and treatment of possible liver damage is usually indicated.

Delayed toxicity type. Delayed toxic reactions to chloroform usually develop 3 to 5 days after administration of an anesthetic to elderly, rundown or cachectic persons and are characterized by severe liver and kidney damage, gradual development of drowsiness and sleepiness, nausea and vomiting and changes in size of the liver – it is usually enlarged and painful, but may be contracted. Signs of kidney irritation may be present, and the urine may contain acetone and bile pigments. Delirium and coma may develop.

TREATMENT

1. Oxygen inhalations.

2. Circulatory support as required.

3. Hospitalization for supportive care as soon as acute symptoms have been controlled.

49 – 198. CHLORONAPHTHALENE (Halowax)

SIGNS AND SYMPTOMS of toxicity follow absorption through the skin and inhalation of the vapors, fumes and dust; these consist of acute gastrointestinal irritation, jaundice, convulsions and coma. Severe liver damage may occur.

TREATMENT

1. Control of convulsions by ether inhalations or rapidly acting barbiturates.

2. Gastric lavage followed by activated charcoal in water.

3. Oxygen therapy as required.

4. Hospitalization for protective measures against possible liver damage.

49 – 199. CHLORONITROBENZENE See **49 – 529**. *Nitrobenzene*

49 – 200. CHLOROPICRIN

Developed originally as a war gas, chloropicrin (trichloronitromethane) is now used as a fumigant. Vomiting is the chief symptom of toxicity. For treatment, see **49 – 832**. *War Gases.*

49—201.   CHLOROQUINE PHOSPHATE (Aralen Diphosphate)

Blindness and retinopathy have been reported following long-term use of this anti-malarial drug. Accidental ingestion by children of even small amounts has a high mortality rate. Fatalities have been caused by as little as 1 gm.

SIGNS AND SYMPTOMS of toxicity develop rapidly, usually within 30 minutes. Very severe headaches, visual disturbances, and convulsions are common. Respiratory and cardiac arrest (**26—7**) may develop suddenly and without warning.

TREATMENT

1. Emptying of stomach by emetics (**49—3**), followed by gastric lavage after control of convulsions by rapidly acting barbiturates.

2. Oxygen under pressure and, if necessary, closed cardiac compression (**11—2**).

3. Vasopressors as needed.

4. Ammonium chloride by mouth if the patient survives the acute phase, continued for at least 48 hours in the hospital.

49—202.   CHLOROTHIAZIDE (Diuril) See 49—771. *Thiazide Diuretics*

49—203.   CHLORPROMAZINE HYDROCHLORIDE (Thorazine) (See also 49—592)

This valuable drug has multiple actions and may give a wide variety of toxic side effects. Primarily, it is a central nervous system depressant, but it has also a mild anti-spasmodic and antihistaminic action. The amount required to cause undesirable side effects varies markedly in different individuals. These side effects are more uncomfortable than dangerous.

Hypotension. Although the decrease in blood pressure is usually mild and transient, in occasional instances it may be severe enough to require therapy for shock (**53—7**). With even a small initial dose—particularly by injection—the patient should be lying down when the drug is given and kept under observation for at least 20 minutes.

Drowsiness and dizziness. These symptoms are transient but may occur after small oral doses. All patients receiving chlorpromazine hydrochloride (Thorazine) should be warned against driving a motor vehicle.

Transient syncope.

Tachycardia.

Allergic reactions (**21**).

Parkinsonian syndrome symptoms. These may follow large doses but will disappear rapidly on cessation of therapy.

Autonomic nervous system symptoms (nasal congestion, dryness of the mucous membranes, constipation, etc.). These are mild and require no treatment.

Secondary symptoms. These may be caused by the tendency of chlorpromazine to accentuate and prolong the effects of sedatives, narcotics, analgesics and anesthetics.

Jaundice. This is usually transient and benign.

TREATMENT

See **49—592**. *Phenothiazines.*

PROGNOSIS.   Good for rapid complete recovery, unless serious blood changes such as agranulocytosis have occurred. The drug has a wide margin of safety.

49—204.   CHLORTETRACYCLINE HYDROCHLORIDE (Aureomycin) See 49—78. *Antibiotics*

49—205.   CHLORTHION See 49—546. *Organic Phosphates*

49 – 206.   CHOKECHERRY

Sometimes eaten in large quantities by children, campers and tourists, this wild fruit may cause serious and even fatal toxic symptoms. The toxicity is due to the presence of amygdalin (**49 – 65**). The treatment is the same as outlined in **49 – 235**. *Cyanides.*

49 – 207.   CHROMATES, CHROMIC ACID, CHROMIUM TRIOXIDE

Chromic acid and its salts are used medicinally, in paints and in the chemical and leather industries.

Modes of Toxicity

Exposure to dust may cause chronic sloughing of the nasal cartilages, with epistaxis and acute macular dermatitis. Acute allergic reactions (**21**), sometimes severe, may also occur.

Ingestion may cause yellow discoloration of the mouth and pharynx, cold clammy cyanotic skin and dysphagia from corrosion and edema of the posterior pharynx, glottis and esophagus. Severe gastric burning, with vomiting of yellowish and greenish material, followed by watery, bloody diarrhea, often occurs. Generalized myalgia may be acute. Acute kidney damage may cause coma and death.

TREATMENT

1. If ingested, immediate gastric lavage with large amounts of warm water, unless there is evidence of erosion or corrosion.

2. Oxygen under positive pressure by face mask and rebreathing bag for cyanosis.

3. Normal salt solution intravenously.

4. Calcium gluconate, 10 ml. of 10% solution, intravenously, for acute muscular cramps.

5. Morphine sulfate in small doses subcutaneously or intravenously for relief of acute pain.

6. Tracheostomy (**14 – 12**) if swelling of the glottis is progressive and possible interference with breathing is anticipated.

49 – 208.   CHRYSAROBIN

Accidental ingestion of this substance, sometimes used in the treatment of fungous infections, has caused severe nausea, vomiting, gastric pain and diarrhea. It apparently acts only as a simple irritant. Treatment consists of demulcents and emetics by mouth, followed by magnesium sulfate (Epsom salts). Complete recovery without residual ill effects is the rule.

49 – 209.   CICUTA VIROSA (Musquash Root, Spotted Cowbane, Water Hemlock)

The rhizomes of this plant contain a toxic substance, cicutoxin. Ingestion of any part of the root results, after a lapse of about 1 hour, in lassitude (or excitement), nausea, vomiting and convulsions, with trismus and opisthotonus. Loss of consciousness and death from circulatory failure may occur within a few hours.

TREATMENT

1. Gastric lavage with 1:5000 potassium permanganate solution followed by activated charcoal by mouth or through the lavage tube.

2. Oxygen inhalations by face mask.

3. Control of convulsions by rapid acting barbiturates.

4. Circulatory support (53—7).

5. Hospitalization because of the danger of delayed circulatory collapse after apparent recovery.

49—210. CIGARETTES AND CIGARS

Ingestion of cigarette and cigar butts by small children has been fatal. Smoking may result in acute toxic symptoms in nonaccustomed persons. The toxic effects are due to nicotine (49—523). Statistics indicate a direct relationship between chronic smoking and lung cancer, bronchitis and atherosclerotic heart disease.

49—211. CINCHONINE

Cinchonine is one of the alkaloids of cinchona bark which has been used as a bitter tonic. The toxic picture from ingestion of moderate amounts resembles that from strychnine (49—729). The treatment is the same as for strychnine.

49—212. CINCHOPHEN

Cinchophen is used in rheumatism remedies and as an antipyretic.

SIGNS AND SYMPTOMS. Tinnitus, vertigo, deafness, nausea, vomiting, hepatic tenderness and pain and coma. Acute fatty degeneration of the liver is usually present in terminal cases.

TREATMENT

1. Gastric lavage with 1:5000 potassium solution followed by activated charcoal in water orally or through the lavage tube.

2. Caffeine sodiobenzoate, 0.5 gm. intramuscularly.

3. Magnesium sulfate (Epsom salts) by mouth in large doses.

4. Hospitalization if large amounts have been ingested because of possible serious liver damage.

49—213. CINEOL

Cineol is one of the chief toxic substances in oil of cajeput and oil of eucalyptus. (See 49—325. Eucalyptol; 49—543. Oil, Essential.)

49—214. CINNAMON OIL (Oil of Cassia)

Exposure to cinnamon oil in industry may cause acute dermatitis and cheilitis. Hypersensitive persons who use bubble gum, chewing gum, toothpaste or cosmetics containing cinnamon oil may develop similar toxic pictures. Symptoms clear rapidly when exposure is terminated.

49—215. CITRIC ACID

Small amounts of citric acid are harmless. Ingestion of large amounts may cause acute but transient gastrointestinal irritation. Transfusions of citrated blood may cause serious reactions, with tetany-like symptoms (43—25) and serious abnormalities of cardiac function.

TREATMENT

Intravenous administration of 10 ml. of 10% calcium gluconate.

49 – 216.   CLEANING FLUIDS AND COMPOUNDS

These preparations – often attractively packaged – are readily available in most households and account for many cases of severe poisoning in children. Common offenders are ammonia (**49 – 59**), benzene (benzol) and its derivatives [naphtha, toluene, toluol, xylene, xylol (**49 – 119**)], carbon tetrachloride (**49 – 173**), chlorine (**49 – 191**), gasoline (**49 – 349**), hypochlorites (**49 – 384**), kerosene (**49 – 408**), oxalic acid (**49 – 552**), sodium hydroxide (**49 – 701**), Stoddard solvent (**49 – 723**) and trichloro-ethylene (**49 – 800**).

Mixtures of household cleaning agents can be dangerous. Sodium hypochloride (**49 – 394**) and vinegar give off toxic concentrations of chlorine gas (**49 – 191**). Sodium hypochlorite and ammonia-containing preparations give off ammonia gas (**49 – 59**).

49 – 217.   COBALT See **49 – 461**. *Metal Fumes*

49 – 218.   COCAINE ("Snow") (See also **49 – 72**. *Anesthetics, Local*)

Cocaine and its salts may cause severe toxic symptoms in a number of ways.

By absorption from the skin or mucous membranes following topical use. See **49 – 72**. *Anesthetics, Local*.

By use in the eyes

SIGNS AND SYMPTOMS.   Acute conjunctivitis, sometimes with hemorrhage, chemosis, lacrimation, photophobia, edema of the lids, corneal ulceration, keratitis, glaucoma and acute systemic symptoms as outlined below.

TREATMENT

1. Discontinue use of the medication at once.

2. Treat systemic symptoms.

3. Hospitalize if local or general symptoms are severe or if the patient does not respond satisfactorily to treatment.

By self-administration. Cocaine and its salts in certain individuals cause euphoria, elation and increased mental and physical activity. Sniffing of the powder or solution, ingestion, or hypodermic injection may result in toxic effects which will cause the user to be brought for examination and treatment. Tolerance to tremendous doses is rapidly attained, but the remarkable absence of acute withdrawal symptoms results in few, if any, cases of true addiction (**2**). Continued use, however, results in mental and moral deterioration, cachexia, insomnia, diplopia, transient paresthesias, hallucinations, and mania – sometimes homicidal. Self-administration is reportable at once to the proper authorities.

SIGNS AND SYMPTOMS of cocaine intoxication following overdosage by any method, or in hypersensitive persons, consist of widely dilated pupils, weak rapid pulse, severe chills, pale clammy skin, burning and feeling of constriction in the pharynx, dysphagia and vomiting. Gastric pain, with tenesmus and diarrhea, may be severe enough to be mistaken for an acute surgical abdomen. Acute dyspnea (occasionally Cheyne-Stokes respiration) may occur. Central nervous system symptoms (headache, dizziness, excitement, confusion, hallucinations and loss of the senses of taste and smell) are fairly common. Slowly developing coma may be followed by death from respiratory failure.

TREATMENT

1. If cocaine has been recently injected subcutaneously or intramuscularly, absorption sometimes can be controlled to some extent by application of a tourniquet or packing the extremity in ice. If the drug has been injected intravenously, the onset of toxic effects is so rapid that a tourniquet is of no value. If ingested, tannic acid solution (strong tea) or weak potassium iodide solution should be given by mouth, followed by gastric lavage with 1:5000 potassium permanganate solution. If the patient will not cooperate sufficiently to allow safe passage of a stomach tube, 3 to 5 mg. of apo-

morphine hydrochloride should be given subcutaneously followed by as much warm water as the patient will drink. After vomiting has occurred, 50 mg. of activated charcoal in water should be administered orally.

 2. Acute cocaine intoxication, no matter what its cause, should be treated as follows:

  a. Phenobarbital sodium, 0.3 gm. intramuscularly or intravenously. Paraldehyde, 4 ml. in normal saline intramuscularly, may be substituted. Sedatives should be administered only if necessary and with great caution.

  b. Atropine sulfate, 1 mg. subcutaneously or intravenously.

  c. Caffeine sodiobenzoate, 0.5 gm. intramuscularly or intravenously, repeated as necessary.

  d. Hospitalization as soon as the condition permits because of the danger of delayed collapse.

49 – 219.   CODEINE (Methylmorphine)

This widely used narcotic is relatively safe. It practically never causes addiction. Large oral or parenteral doses may cause slowing of the pulse (which usually remains regular and of good quality), flushing of the face, a feeling of tightness in the head (especially in the occipital region), extreme generalized vasodilation, nausea, vomiting, gastric pain, temporary anuria, constipation and fecal impaction. Extreme miosis may occur in early stages, followed by terminal mydriasis. Exophthalmos may be present. Muscle fibrillation, tremors, generalized convulsions and respiratory failure make the prognosis very poor.

TREATMENT

 1. If ingested, gastric lavage with 1:5000 potassium permanganate solution followed by activated charcoal in water by mouth or through the lavage tube.

 2. Magnesium sulfate (Epsom salts) by mouth. Relief of impaction (**37 – 2.** *Gastrointestinal Obstruction*) may be required.

 3. Oxygen therapy under positive pressure.

 4. Naloxone hydrochloride (Narcan) as a narcotic antagonist, repeated as necessary.

 5. Hospitalization in severe cases for symptomatic and supportive therapy.

49 – 220.   COLCHICINE

Colchicine is an active and toxic alkaloid occurring in a common plant, meadow saffron. Ingestion of any part of the plant may cause acute poisoning. Used medicinally as an antigout remedy, overdosage may cause severe toxic signs and symptoms coming on about 2 hours after ingestion.

SIGNS AND SYMPTOMS.   A sensation of suffocation and tightness in the chest, difficulty in swallowing, nausea, violent vomiting and watery or bloody diarrhea may be present. Severe generalized myalgia and arthralgia with twitching of isolated muscle groups – especially in the calves – are common. Late symptoms are cyanosis and dilated pupils, severe shock, hematuria and oliguria, ascending paralysis, delirium and convulsions. The patient is usually fully conscious until death occurs in from 10 to 36 hours from generalized exhaustion and respiratory failure.

TREATMENT

 1. Emetics followed by gastric lavage with 1:5000 potassium permanganate solution.

 2. Treatment of shock (**53 – 7**), which may develop very rapidly.

 3. Respiratory assistance as required.

 4. Correction of fluid-electrolyte imbalance (**6**).

 5. Rapidly acting barbiturates intravenously for sedation.

 6. Calcium gluconate, 10 ml. of 10% solution intravenously for myalgia, reinforced if necessary by small doses of morphine and atropine.

49 – 221. COLOCYNTH (Bitter Apples)

SIGNS AND SYMPTOMS of toxicity following ingestion include visual and auditory disturbances, vertigo, confusion, disorientation, severe abdominal pain, watery or bloody diarrhea, kidney irritation (polyuria, oliguria), liver and pancreas damage and circulatory disturbances (weakness, faintness, clammy skin, etc.), followed by collapse.

TREATMENT

1. Evacuation of stomach contents by emetics if possible; if unsuccessful, by gastric lavage with 1:5000 potassium permanganate solution. In either case, activated charcoal in water should be left in the stomach.

2. Correction of dehydration and electrolyte imbalance (**6**).

3. Hospitalization if signs of kidney, liver or pancreas damage are present.

49 – 222. CONIINE (Hemlock, Horseradish)

The leaves containing this alkaloid may be confused with parsley, celery and parsnip. Ingestion may cause nausea, vomiting, salivation, acute dysphagia, dilated pupils, diplopia, amblyopia, impaired hearing, convulsions and progressive weakening of skeletal musculature with terminal involvement of the respiratory muscles. Complete consciousness usually persists until death from respiratory failure.

TREATMENT

1. Evacuation of stomach contents as soon as possible by emetics or gastric lavage, followed by activated charcoal in water and saline cathartics.

2. Oxygen therapy under positive pressure.

PROGNOSIS. Good unless acute immediate toxicity is overwhelming. If the patient survives for 2 hours, no permanent ill effects are to be anticipated.

49 – 223. COPPER

Chronic copper poisoning gives a toxic picture similar to lead poisoning (**49 – 420. Lead Salts**). Certain soluble copper salts may cause vomiting and acute gastroenteritis:

Copper acetoarsenite (verdigris, Paris green). Arsenic poisoning symptoms (**49 – 90**) are also caused by this pigment.

Copper oxides (see also **49 – 461. Metal Fumes**).

Copper solutions used in the treatment of phosphorus burns (**25 – 22**).

TREATMENT

1. Demulcents – milk, white of eggs.

2. Potassium ferrocyanide, 0.5 gm. in water by mouth.

3. Lavage with 1000 ml. of water containing milk of magnesia, leaving a solution of activated charcoal in the stomach.

4. Treatment with BAL (**49 – 109**) or with penicillamine (Cuprimine).

5. Control severe gastrointestinal pain by small doses of morphine or meperidine (Demerol).

6. Correct any fluid or electrolyte imbalance (**6**).

7. Treat shock (**53 – 7**). Blood transfusions may be necessary.

8. Hospitalize in severe cases for symptomatic and supportive care and because of the danger of renal and hepatic complications.

49 – 224. CORROSIVE ACIDS See **49 – 26.** Acids; **49 – 378.** Hydrofluoric Acid

49 – 225. CORROSIVE SUBLIMATE See **49 – 128.** Bichloride of Mercury

49 – 226. CORTICOTROPIN (ACTH, ACTHAR)

This potent anterior pituitary hormone is a polypeptide which has many adverse physiologic side effects in addition to its main function of stimulating the adrenal cortex to produce and secrete steroids. Any combination of these side effects may result in symptoms severe enough to cause the patient to seek emergency care. The most common are headache, dizziness, transient blurring of vision, bizarre paresthesias, nervousness, insomnia, fatigue, exhaustion, psychoneurosis, signs of fluid balance disturbance (edema, anasarca, polydipsia, etc.) and alkalosis with lowered potassium levels. Acute sensitivity reactions (**21**) may develop in individuals sensitive to porcine proteins.

TREATMENT

Development of any of the symptoms listed above calls for immediate discontinuance of therapy, symptomatic and supportive treatment and hospitalization for thorough investigation, evaluation and restoration of normal fluid balance (**6**).

49 – 227. CORTISONE

This crystalline hormonal substance may cause many types of toxic symptoms, especially through sodium retention and metabolic alkalosis (**43 – 5**). Hypertension, sleepiness, nervousness, extreme weakness, psychosis and pain and hemorrhage from the upper gastrointestinal tract may occur. Except for stopping the cortisone and administering sedation, the only treatment required is arrangement for thorough evaluation, preferably under hospital control.

49 – 228. COSMETICS

Although an almost endless variety of substances are used in cosmetics, antimony (**49 – 81**) and arsenic-containing compounds (**49 – 90**) are the main offenders in the production of acute toxic symptoms. The use of "indelible" lipsticks may cause soreness of the tongue and throat, coryza, sinusitis, dermatitis and urticaria. Patch tests may be necessary to identify the offending substances. Rapid recovery usually takes place when the offending cosmetic is discontinued.

49 – 229. CRAYONS

Most varieties of children's chalk and wax crayons are required by law to be harmless. In spite of this, ingestion of some types of wax crayons – usually red or orange – may cause toxic symptoms from paranitraniline and/or benzidine (**49 – 122**). In addition, toxic symptoms from arsenic salts (**49 – 90**), chromium (**49 – 207**), copper (**49 – 223**) and lead (**49 – 420**) have been reported. Some marking crayons, such as those used by carpenters, contain aniline dyes (**49 – 74**) and may be dangerous if even small amounts are ingested.

49 – 230. CREOLIN

This is a compound containing about 15% cresols. For signs and symptoms of toxicity and treatment, see **49 – 590**. *Phenol.*

49 – 231. CREOSOTE (Wood Creosote, Beech Creosote)

The toxic properties of this substance are the result of its phenol and cresol content. For toxic picture and treatment, see **49 – 590**. *Phenol.*

49—232.   CROTON OIL (See also 49—490)

Acute and dangerous toxic signs and symptoms caused by this potent irritant cathartic and purgative are sometimes encountered following ingestion in an alcoholic drink [the so-called "Mickey Finn" (49—490)] used by bartenders to get rid of offensive or obstreperous customers. There is a burning sensation in the mouth, severe stomach pain, nausea, vomiting, severe purging (often with bloody diarrhea), collapse and coma.

TREATMENT

1. Egg white or flour mixed with water by mouth.
2. Emetics such as mustard in warm water or syrup of ipecac; if unsuccessful, apomorphine hydrochloride, 5 mg. subcutaneously, with neutralization if necessary of the secondary depressant effect of apomorphine by naloxone hydrochloride (Narcan).
3. Stimulants — strong coffee, aromatic spirits of ammonia (4 ml. in water) by mouth or caffeine sodiobenzoate, 0.5 mg. intramuscularly.
4. Artificial respiration (11—1) if necessary.
5. Treatment of shock (53—7).
6. Hospitalization for observation for several hours after apparent recovery.

49—233.   CUBEB

At one time cubeb was commonly used as a urinary antiseptic and in the form of cigarettes for asthma and bronchitis. Inhalation or ingestion of this oleoresin may cause nausea, vomiting, abdominal pain, diarrhea, severe muscle and joint pain, muscular fibrillation and twitching, miosis and delirium, followed by coma and death from respiratory failure.

TREATMENT

1. Emetics followed by gastric lavage with 1:5000 potassium permanganate solution. Activated charcoal in water should be instilled through the lavage tube.
2. Oxygen therapy.
3. Calcium gluconate, 10 ml. of 10% solution, slowly intravenously.
4. Large amounts of fluids orally or intravenously.

49—234.   CURARE (Intocostrin, Metubine Iodide, d-Tubocurarine Chloride)

Acute toxic signs and symptoms may follow parenteral injection of any derivatives of curare as adjuncts to anesthesia or as muscle relaxants, and are characterized by prolonged apnea, bradycardia, vascular collapse and symptoms resulting from histamine release.

TREATMENT

1. Maintenance of a patent airway.
2. Positive pressure oxygen therapy by intratracheal catheter or face mask and rebreathing bag.
3. Neostigmine methylsulfate, 1 to 3 mg. intravenously, combined with 0.6 mg. to 1.2 mg. of atropine sulfate. Edrophonium, 10 mg. intravenously, repeated as necessary, may be helpful
4. Treatment of hypotension may be necessary.

49—235.   CYANIDES

SIGNS AND SYMPTOMS.   Victims of acute cyanide poisoning are usually either dead or in deep coma when first seen by a physician. Occasionally, recognition of the known exposure and the odor of bitter almonds on the breath may give time for administration of pure oxygen under pressure, followed by hydrogen peroxide and 5% sodium thiosulfate solution by mouth. If this therapy can be given while vital signs are still present, there is some − but very slight − chance of recovery. Following these measures, the routine treatment outlined below should be begun and continued in the ambulance en route to the hospital.

ROUTINE TREATMENT

1. Amyl nitrite inhalations for 15 to 20 seconds of every minute, alternating with oxygen therapy under positive pressure, while a 3% solution of sodium nitrite is being prepared. A syringe containing 1:1000 epinephrine hydrochloride (Adrenalin) should be ready at all times to combat a sudden drop in blood pressure.

2. Discontinue the amyl nitrite inhalations and inject 10 ml. of the freshly prepared sodium nitrite solution slowly intravenously, followed by 50 ml. of a 25% aqueous solution of sodium thiosulfate given over a period of 10 to 15 minutes and repeated every 30 minutes until a total of not more than 12 gm. has been given.

3. Gastric lavage with a 1:5000 solution of potassium permanganate but only *after* steps 1 and 2 (above) have been done. Administration of activated charcoal is of no value in cyanide poisoning.

4. Caffeine sodiobenzoate, 0.5 gm. intravenously. Parenteral atropine sulfate, pentylenetetrazol (Metrazol) and strophanthin may be tried but are of questionable value. Geiger's formula (a 1% solution of methylene blue containing 1.8% sodium sulfate) is no longer used in the treatment of cyanide intoxication.

5. Hospitalization for observation and follow-up care, including transfusions (14−12), because of the danger of sudden relapse.

PROGNOSIS. If the patient is alive 1 hour after exposure, there is some chance of recovery, but sudden unexplained fatal relapses may occur 4 to 5 hours after apparent improvement.

49−236. CYCLOPROPANE See 49−70. *Anesthetics, Inhalation*

49−237. CYCRIMINE HYDROCHLORIDE (Pagitane)

Excessive doses of this anti-Parkinsonian drug have been reported as causing decreased body temperature, restless, convulsive movements and impaired speech and vision. Symptoms clear completely after treatment

TREATMENT

1. Gastric lavage followed by activated charcoal in water by mouth or through the lavage tube if the medication has been taken within 2 hours.

2. Saline cathartics.

3. Intravenous fluids.

4. Sedation as required.

49−238. CYSTISINE

Chewing or eating the seeds, flowers or roots of common plants containing this toxic alkaloid results in gastrointestinal irritation, dyspnea, vertigo, myalgia, delirium and hallucinations. Death may occur from respiratory failure.

TREATMENT

1. Gastric lavage followed by activated charcoal by mouth or through the lavage tube.

2. Emptying the bowel by saline cathartics and enemas.

3. Intravenous administration of 5% dextrose in saline and other supportive measures as indicated.

49−239. DAPHNE (Wild Pepper, Dwarf Bay) See 49−906

49 – 240. DATURA STRAMONIUM (Devil's Apple, Jamestown Weed, Jimson-weed, Stinkweed, Thorn Apple)

Drinking a decoction or chewing the roots, leaves or seeds of this common annual plant results in a toxic picture caused by the alkaloids hyoscyamine and hyoscine, characterized initially by dryness of the mouth, fever, flushed skin, mydriasis and diplopia. Later symptoms are muscle weakness, confusion, delirium and loss of memory. Circulatory collapse and coma may develop.

A similar toxic picture has been reported from eating tomatoes grown on plants grafted to *Datura stramonium* roots.

TREATMENT
See **49 – 104.** *Atropine.*

49 – 241. DD COMPOUNDS (Chlorinated Propylene-propanes)

All of the chlorinated hydrocarbons are used full strength as fumigants. They are toxic by ingestion, by absorption through the intact skin and by inhalation but fortunately have a garlic-like odor which is offensive and repellent, even to small children. All may cause blistering of the skin on contact, eye and upper respiratory tract irritation, substernal pain, dyspnea, cyanosis, gastroenteritis and pulmonary edema (**51**) from inhalation of the fumes. Gastric pain, acute diarrhea and pulmonary edema (**51**) develop rapidly after ingestion.

TREATMENT
If on the skin
1. Remove contaminated clothing and wash the skin thoroughly with mild soap and water.
2. Treat blisters as second degree chemical burns (**25 – 9**).
If inhaled
1. Remove from exposure.
2. Start artificial respiration (**11 – 1**) at once, followed as soon as possible by oxygen inhalations under positive pressure using a face mask or endotracheal catheter and rebreathing bag.
3. Inject theophylline ethylenediamine (aminophylline) *slowly* intravenously if bronchospasm is present.
4. Give sedative cough mixtures – codeine preparations are particularly effective.
5. Treat pulmonary edema (**51**).
6. Hospitalize for at least 24 hours for observation after apparent recovery – delayed relapses often occur.
If ingested
1. Administer nonoily demulcents.
2. Empty the stomach immediately by gastric lavage with large amounts of water, leaving activated charcoal in water in the stomach. A saline cathartic should be given.
3. Control gastrointestinal pain with narcotics as needed.
4. Support the respiration with oxygen therapy, preferably under positive pressure.
5. Hospitalize for supportive and symptomatic care.

49 – 242. DDD (Tetrachlorodiphenylethane)

For toxicity and treatment, see **49 – 243.** *DDT.*

49 – 243. DDT (Dichlorodiphenyltrichlorethane, Chlorophenothane)

Used extensively as an insecticide, DDT has undoubtedly often been credited with the production of serious conditions – especially pulmonary edema (**51**) – caused in fact by the solvents used in the insect sprays, usually petroleum derivatives (**49—585**). However, if inhaled in strong concentrations, or if ingested, DDT has a definite toxic action which usually comes on 2 to 4 hours after exposure and is characterized by vomiting from gastric irritation, apprehension, acute depression, incoordination, giddiness, paresthesias of the face and lips, muscular tremors, convulsions (both tonic and clonic), dyspnea and cyanosis followed by respiratory failure. Death may occur from sudden ventricular fibrillation (**26—23**).

TREATMENT

1. Demulcents by mouth, followed by gastric lavage with large amounts of water, then by activated charcoal in water by mouth or through the lavage tube.

2. Magnesium sulfate (Epsom salts) 30 gm. by mouth.

3. Oxygen therapy under positive pressure by face mask or intranasal catheter and rebreathing bag (**11—2**) if signs of respiratory distress are present.

4. Caffeine sodiobenzoate, 0.5 gm. intramuscularly or intravenously.

5. Calcium gluconate, 10 ml. of a 10% solution intravenously, repeated as necessary.

6. Phenobarbital sodium, 0.06 to 0.2 gm. intravenously for control of convulsions.

7. Hospitalization for at least 24 hours under close observation because of the tendency toward relapse.

Chronic exposure to DDT has been reported as causing blurred speech, loss of coordination and other neurologic signs and symptoms.

49—244. DELPHINIUM (Larkspur)

The roots and seeds contain several toxic alkaloids. Ingestion may result in burning and dryness of the mucous membranes of the mouth and throat with stiffness of the facial muscles, nausea, vomiting, loss of urinary and rectal sphincter control, extreme hypotension and respiratory depression.

TREATMENT

1. Gastric lavage with large quantities of warm water followed by activated charcoal in water orally or via the lavage tube.

2. Emptying of the bowel by saline cathartics and enemas.

3. Supportive and symptomatic care.

49—245. DEMEROL (Meperidine, Isonipecaine, Dolantin, Dolosal, Pethidine, Endolat)

This commonly used synthetic narcotic is similar in action and addictive tendencies to the narcotic opium derivatives, although it is a weaker anodyne (**7—2**) and less powerful respiratory depressant. See **2—4.** *Addiction;* **7.** *Narcotics;* **49—495.** *Morphine.*

49—246. DEMETON (Systox) See **49—546.** *Organic Phosphates*

49—247. DEODORANTS AND DEODORIZERS

Preparations used to neutralize body odor usually contain 3 ingredients in varying proportions.

Antiperspirants—Usually aluminum salts (**49—50**) or zinc salts (**49—854**). Iron salts (**49—399**) and silver salts (**49—688**) are used occasionally but may cause discoloration. Zirconium salts have been reported as causing skin granulomas. The most commonly used anions are chlorides, hydroxychlorides, phenolsulfonates and sulfates.

Deodorants—usually halogenated salicylanides, hexachlorophene, QAC (**49—637**) and thiuram disulfide.

Perfumes—often with essential oil bases (**49–543**).

Deodorizers used in the home may contain formaldehyde (**49–340**), essential oils (**49–543**), *p*-dichlorobenzene (**49–258**), naphthalene (**49–510**) or isopropyl alcohol (**49–403**). Although most deodorant and deodorizer preparations contain only small amounts of toxic materials, ingestion of more than a minute quantity calls for emptying the stomach by emetics or gastric lavage followed by activated charcoal in water by mouth and a saline cathartic.

49–248. DEPILATORIES (Hair Removers)

These cosmetics usually contain a mixture of inert ingredients, with a small amount of barium sulfide, calcium sulfide, sodium sulfide or thallium. See **49–112.** *Barium Compounds;* **49–709.** *Sodium Sulfide;* **49–768.** *Thallium.*

49–249. DERRIS

Powdered derris root contains rotenone (**49–631.** *Pyrethrum*) and is used as a fish poison and insecticide. Exposure to the powder may cause severe dermatitis, which clears rapidly when exposure is terminated.

Ingestion of the fresh root has been reported as causing vomiting, collapse and congestive heart failure (**26–8**).

TREATMENT

1. Gastric lavage followed by activated charcoal by mouth or through the lavage tube.
2. Saline cathartics.
3. Circulatory support, preferably in a hospital.

49–250. DETERGENTS See **49–43.** *Alkyl Sodium Sulfates*

49–251. DEXTROAMPHETAMINE SULFATE See **49–64.** *Amphetamines*

49–252. DIALKYLPHOSPHATE

Although this substance is sometimes used medicinally in glaucoma and myasthenia gravis because of its anticholinesterase activity, its use as an insecticide causes most of the cases of acute poisoning. The signs and symptoms of toxicity and treatment are the same as outlined in **49–546.** *Organic Phosphates.*

49–253. DIAZOMETHANE

This dangerous gas is used in industry as a methylating agent. Inhalation can cause choking, dyspnea and severe chest pain followed by pulmonary edema (**51**) and severe shock (**53**).

TREATMENT

1. Removal from exposure.
2. Treatment of shock (**53–7**).
3. Oxygen under positive pressure by face mask and rebreathing bag.
4. Treatment of pulmonary edema (**51**).

49–254. DIBENAMINE HYDROCHLORIDE

Use of this drug in the treatment of hypertension may be associated with gastrointestinal irritation, mental confusion and hypotension. Symptoms subside slowly when the drug is discontinued.

49 — 255. 1,2-DIBROMOETHANE (Ethylene Bromide)

This substance is used as a grain fumigant and in fire extinguishers. On the skin it causes reddening and blisters; inhalation of the fumes results in headache, weakness, excitement, prolonged vomiting and diarrhea which is very resistant to treatment. Heavy concentrations may cause death from cardiac failure.

TREATMENT
1. Removal from exposure.
2. Oxygen by face mask and rebreathing bag.
3. Treatment of diarrhea, dehydration and shock (53 — 7).

49 — 256. DIBUCAINE HYDROCHLORIDE (Nupercaine, Percaine)

Nupercaine is less effective and also less toxic than cocaine. See 49 — 72. *Anesthetics, Local.*

49 — 257. DICHAPELATUM TOXICARIUM (Rat's Bane)

Ingestion of the seeds of this South American and African plant has resulted in a peculiar, often fatal, syndrome called "broke back," characterized by intense gastrointestinal irritation, incoordination and paralysis, areflexia and extreme hyperesthesia.

TREATMENT
1. Removal of the toxic substance by gastric lavage, saline cathartics, and enemas.
2. Sedation.
3. Symptomatic and supportive therapy.

49 — 258. DICHLOROBENZENE

Both the ortho isomer (used as a wood preservative) and the para isomer (used in mothproofing sprays) are toxic when inhaled or ingested. Signs and symptoms of toxicity and treatment are approximately the same as for naphthalene (49 — 510).

49 — 259. DICHLORODIETHYLETHER

Fumes from this insecticide, soil fumigant and solvent irritate the eyes and upper respiratory tract. A severe persistent cough with a peculiar glassy sputum is characteristic. Sensitization may occur. Eosinophilia is common.

TREATMENT
1. Removal from exposure.
2. Inhalation of a 5% sodium bicarbonate spray.
3. Symptomatic therapy.

49 — 260. DICHLOROETHANE

This liquid is used as a solvent for fats, gums, rubber and resins.

TOXIC SIGNS AND SYMPTOMS may be caused by inhalation or ingestion and consist of nausea, vomiting, diarrhea, somnolence, weakness and respiratory and circulatory collapse.

TREATMENT
1. If inhaled, immediate removal from the area contaminated with fumes to the fresh air. If ingested, emptying of the stomach by emetics and/or gastric lavage followed by saline cathartics.
2. Oxygen therapy under positive pressure.

3. Caffeine sodiobenzoate, 0.5 gm. intramuscularly. Treatment of shock (**53–7**) may be necessary.

4. Hospitalization in severe cases because of the tendency toward delayed liver and kidney damage.

49 – 261. DICHLOROHYDRIN

Inhalation of fumes causes symptoms in workers in the nitrocellulose and lacquer industries. The toxic manifestations range from nausea, vomiting and vertigo to somnolence, delirium and death.

TREATMENT

1. Removal from exposure.
2. Oxygen inhalations.
3. Symptomatic and supportive care.

By ingestion, the toxicity of dichlorohydrin is even greater; dysphagia, vomiting and severe gastric pain may be followed by conjunctival, scleral and gastric hemorrhage and coma. Toxic hepatitis, nephritis, hemolytic anemia and pulmonary edema (**51**) may develop.

TREATMENT

1. Gastric lavage followed by activated charcoal in water through the lavage tube.
2. Control of severe pain by small doses of meperidine (Demerol) or morphine.
3. Hospitalization for observation and supportive care because of the possibility of delayed appearance of pulmonary edema (**51**) or hepatic and renal pathology.

49 – 262. DICHLOROPHENE

Used as a mild antiseptic in antiperspirants, deodorants, tooth powders and toilet waters, dichlorophene may cause contact dermatitis, glossitis, stomatitis and cheilitis. Symptoms clear slowly when use of the offending preparation is stopped.

49 – 263. 2,4-DICHLOROPHENOXYACETIC ACID (2-4-D)

This acid, used in the preparation of herbicides utilized principally in the control of broad-leafed weeds, is a potentially dangerous substance. Peripheral neuropathy following exposure to the diethylamine salt during manufacture has been reported.

TREATMENT

1. Immediate gastric lavage unless there are signs of impending convulsions. If so, short-acting anticonvulsant drugs should be given cautiously.
2. Support of the circulatory system. Continuous ECG monitoring is advisable. Epinephrine (adrenalin) may precipitate ventricular fibrillation and should not be used.
3. Oral administration of quinidine sulfate to combat extreme muscle weakness and to prevent development of ventricular fibrillation (**26–23**).

49 – 264. DICODID (Eucodal)

Dicodid is used medicinally as a sedative and analgesic and gives toxic reactions similar to morphine. Addiction (**2–4**) has been reported. For treatment, see **49–495.** *Morphine.*

49 – 265. DICUMAROL (Dicoumarin, Melitoxin)

Because this anticoagulant causes bleeding which persists for some time after discontinuance of therapeutic use, emergency care may be required for some or all of the toxic effects — especially hemorrhage — listed below. 4-Hydroxycoumarin (**49–833.** *Warfarin*) — used as a rodenticide only — is even more toxic, especially to children.

SIGNS AND SYMPTOMS.   Generalized ecchymoses, purpura, hematuria, hemorrhage from the nose, gums or gastrointestinal tract, menorrhagia and extreme weakness from secondary anemia.

TREATMENT
1. Stop the anticoagulant. If a large amount has been ingested, empty the stomach immediately by gastric lavage followed by activated charcoal through the lavage tube.
2. Transfer for hospitalization for vitamin K therapy (42 — 34), fluid replacement (6) and transfusions (14 — 13).

49 — 266.   DIEFFENBACHIA SEGUINE (Dumb Cane)

Chewing the leaves of this common decorative house plant results in immediate burning of the lips and mouth with difficulty in talking and swallowing and, occasionally, difficulty in breathing. Swelling of the parts with which the juice comes in contact is immediate and intense. If the juice or pulp is swallowed, severe corrosion of the esophagus and stomach may occur. Systemic effects are due to oxalate poisoning (49 — 552) and include bradycardia, hypotension, vomiting, gastric cramping and acute respiratory distress.

For treatment, see 49 — 552. *Oxalic Acid.*

49 — 267.   DIELDRIN (Compound 497, Octalox)

Dieldrin is a chlorinated hydrocarbon insecticide and pesticide used when long-continued action is desirable, usually in combination with kerosene (49 — 408) and xylene (49 — 844), both of which may complicate the toxic picture. Central nervous system symptoms may be caused by absorption through the intact skin, by inhalation or by ingestion.

SIGNS AND SYMPTOMS of toxicity (delayed for 1 to 10 hours after ingestion) consist of severe headache, vertigo, nausea, vomiting, muscular twitching, tremors and respiratory failure. Severe epileptiform convulsions may be the first evidence of poisoning.

TREATMENT
1. Removal of contaminated clothing; thorough washing of the skin with soap and water. *The attendant must wear gloves.*
2. Prevention or control of convulsions by large doses of rapid-acting barbiturates.
3. Gastric lavage with large amounts of warm water if ingested. Activated charcoal in water should be left in the stomach.
4. Administration of oxygen under positive pressure by face mask or endotracheal catheter and rebreathing bag.
5. Immediate hospitalization with supportive treatment for at least 1 week after the last convulsion. Recovery is usually slow but complete.

49 — 268.   DIETHYLAMINE (Acetylarsen)

Therapeutic use of this antiluetic drug may result in gingival and gastrointestinal bleeding, encephalopathy and agranulocytosis.

TREATMENT
See 49 — 96. *Arsphenamine.*

49 — 269.   DIETHYL-BETACHLORETHYLAMINE

Fumes of this compound cause severe ophthalmic and respiratory irritation increasing in intensity for 10 to 12 hours after exposure. Delayed pulmonary edema (51) may occur.

For treatment, see mustard gas [under *War Gases* (49 — 832)].

49 – 270.   DIETHYLENE GLYCOL (Diethylene Ether)

Used in industry as a solvent, lubricant and hygroscopic agent, this liquid if ingested may have serious immediate and delayed effects, including ataxia, nausea, vomiting, abdominal cramping, heartburn, generalized weakness, myalgia (especially of the lumbar muscles), severe kidney damage, convulsions, coma and death from respiratory failure.

TREATMENT

1. Immediate emptying of the stomach by emetics or gastric lavage followed by activated charcoal in water orally or through the lavage tube.

2. Administration of oxygen under positive pressure by face mask or intranasal catheter and rebreathing bag if respiratory depression is acute.

3. Intravenous infusion of 1000 ml. of normal salt solution.

4. Hospitalization because of the tendency of diethylene glycol to cause delayed and severe kidney damage.

49 – 271.   DIETHYLSTILBESTROL

Therapeutic doses, or overdosage, of this estrogenic agent may cause extreme lassitude, nausea, vomiting and abdominal pain, followed by bloody diarrhea and temporary psychoses (50 – 1).

TREATMENT

1. Discontinue administration of the estrogen.

2. Administer sedation as needed.

49 – 272.   DIGITALIS

For mild toxic signs and symptoms following therapeutic use in cardiac patients, see 26 – 9.

Ingestion or injection of large amounts of digitalis preparations by accident or with suicidal intent results in headache, vomiting, drowsiness, slow pulse, bigeminal rhythm, visual disturbances (amblyopia, blurring, diplopia, bizarre color vision changes) and characteristic extreme ECG changes (26 – 9).

TREATMENT

1. Stop digitalis.

2. Apply external heat.

3. Start continuous electrocardiographic monitoring.

4. If seen early, before toxic symptoms are marked, empty the stomach by emetics or gastric lavage with 500 ml. of 1:5000 potassium permanganate solution, strong tea or a 1% solution of tannic acid.

5. Intravenous administration of potassium unless ECGs show definite A.V. block without atrial tachycardia. Potassium chloride (40 mEq. in 5% dextrose in water) may be given over a period of 1 hour. For children, the dose should be 5 to 10 mEq. dissolved in 100 ml. of 5% dextrose in water.

6. Atropine sulfate, 0.5 to 1.0 mg. subcutaneously or intravenously.

7. Inhalations of oxygen under positive pressure by face mask and rebreathing bag.

8. Sedation by cautious use of rapid-acting barbiturates.

9. If the patient's condition is degenerating, give 100 mg. of diphenylhydantoin (Dilantin) slowly intravenously, with frequent blood pressure and ECG monitoring. Diphenylhydantoin (Dilantin) can be continued as necessary intravenously or orally until the digitalis is excreted.

10. All of the above agents may cause hypotension; therefore, a pressor agent such as metaraminol bitartrate (Aramine) should be ready for immediate injection.

49 — 273. DIHYDROCODEINONE (Dicodid, Eucodal) See **49 — 264.** *Dicodid*

49 — 274. DIHYDROMORPHINONE (Hydromorphone) **HYDROCHLORIDE** See **49 — 277.** *Dilaudid*

49 — 275. DILAN

This insecticide is similar in action and toxicity to DDT (**49 — 243**).

49 — 276. DILANTIN (Sodium Diphenylhydantoinate)

Usual doses or overdosage of this drug, used for prevention of epileptic attacks and in the treatment of digitalis toxicity (**49 — 272**), may cause apprehension, tension, tremulousness, dizziness, ataxia, nausea, vomiting, blurring of vision, diplopia, generalized lymphadenopathy and hepatosplenomegaly.
TREATMENT
1. Discontinue therapeutic use, or decrease the size of the dose of the drug.
2. Impress on the patient or his family the need for further medical treatment. The patient should be made to understand that stopping the drug may cause an increase in the number and severity of convulsive seizures.

49 — 277. DILAUDID (Hydromorphone Hydrochloride)

The signs and symptoms of acute toxicity, addictive tendencies (**2 — 4**) and treatment of this powerful narcotic (formerly known as dihydromorphinone hydrochloride) are approximately the same as those for morphine (**49 — 495**), for which it may be substituted under certain emergency conditions (**7 — 2**). Naloxone hydrochloride (Narcan) is an effective antagonist.

49 — 278. DIMENHYDRINATE (Dramamine)

Usual doses prescribed for motion sickness may cause drowsiness, nausea, vomiting and paresthesias. Deaths have been reported from ingestion of large amounts, with preliminary hyperexcitability and convulsions.
TREATMENT
1. Gastric lavage followed by activated charcoal in water through the lavage tube.
2. Sedation with rapid-acting barbiturates if hyperactive.
3. Saline cathartics and enemas.
4. Supportive therapy.

49 — 279. DIMERCAPROL See **49 — 109.** *BAL*

49 — 280. DIMETHYLKETONE See **49 — 17.** *Acetone*

49 — 281. DIMETAN

Dimetan is a chlorinated hydrocarbon aphicide which is not absorbed through the skin. Ingestion may cause a toxic picture similar to that caused by DDT (**49 — 243**).

49 – 282.   DIMETHYLPHTHALATE

Ingestion of this insect repellant may cause an immediate burning sensation of the mucous membranes of the mouth, throat and pharynx and delayed coma coming on 1 to 2 hours after ingestion.

TREATMENT

1. Demulcents by mouth.

2. Emptying of the stomach by emetics and/or gastric lavage followed by activated charcoal in water orally or through the lavage tube.

3. Dextrose, 5% in saline, 500 ml. intravenously.

4. Caffeine sodiobenzoate, 0.5 gm. intramuscularly or intravenously.

49 – 283.   DINITROBENZENE

Evidence of acute toxicity may come on suddenly or may develop following several weeks of exposure in industry. Toxic symptoms may be precipitated by prolonged exposure to sunlight or by overindulgence in alcoholic beverages. The toxic picture consists of a bitter almond-like taste in the mouth, headache, vertigo, fatigue, dyspnea, nausea, vomiting with severe gastric pain and a peculiar cyanosis, ranging from pale yellow to a grayish black. Jaundice may be present. Marked blood picture changes may be a late development.

TREATMENT

1. Gastric lavage with normal salt solution followed by activated charcoal in water orally.

2. Saline cathartics.

3. Dextrose, 5% in saline, 500 to 1000 ml. intravenously.

4. Oxygen therapy under positive pressure.

5. Methylene blue (1% solution in 1.8% sodium sulfate solution), 50 ml. intravenously for cyanosis.

6. Hospitalization because of the tendency toward late development of serious heart, liver and blood damage.

49 – 284.   DINITROCRESOL

For symptoms and signs and treatment of toxic effects of this fungicide and pesticide, see **49 – 285.** *Dinitrophenol.*

49 – 285.   DINITROPHENOL (Capsine, Elgetol, Sinox)

Prescription or sale of this substance for use as a weight reducing medication is prohibited by law. It is used extensively in the explosives industry and as a fungicide, insecticide, miticide and herbicide.

SIGNS AND SYMPTOMS following inhalation or ingestion consist of temperature elevation, profuse perspiration, extreme thirst, fatigue, flushing of the skin followed by development of a yellow color, rapid deep breathing, restlessness, acute anxiety and sometimes convulsions and coma followed by death from respiratory failure.

TREATMENT

1. Gastric lavage with large amounts of 1:5000 potassium permanganate or 5% sodium bicarbonate solution, followed by activated charcoal in water by mouth via the lavage tube.

2. Reduction of temperature by cold packs, cold water enemas, alcohol rubs or other available means.

3. Dextrose, 5% in saline, 1000 ml. intravenously.

4. Oxygen under positive pressure by face mask and rebreathing bag.

5. Caffeine sodiobenzoate, 0.5 gm. intramuscularly or intravenously.

49 – 286.   DINITROTOLUENE

This drug may cause arthralgia, dyspnea, cyanosis, severe headache, dizziness, nystagmus and severe chest pain, usually in persons handling the material. Ingestion of alcohol in any form accentuates the toxic picture.

TREATMENT

See **49 – 283.** *Dinitrobenzene.*

49 – 287.   DIODRAST (Iodopyracet)

Diodrast is used in intravenous pyelography. Mild allergic reactions are relatively common; rarely, death may occur from acute hypersensitivity (**21**). All patients should be tested for sensitivity before injection of the contrast medium.

49 – 288.   DIOXANE

Low concentrations of this commercial solvent cause acute mucous membrane irritation of the respiratory tract, including the lungs. Inhalation of high concentrations results in dyspnea, nonreactive pupils, lung congestion, decreased reflexes and serious liver and kidney pathology.

TREATMENT

1. Removal from exposure.
2. Oxygen inhalations under positive pressure.
3. Hospitalization for supportive care.

49 – 289.   DIPHENHYDRAMINE (Benadryl, Amidryl) See **49 – 80.** *Antihistaminic Drugs*

49 – 290.   DIPHENYLHYDANTOID SODIUM See **49 – 276.** *Dilantin*

49 – 291.   DISULFIRAM See **49 – 77.** *Antabuse*

49 – 292.   DITHIOCARBAMATES (Blightox, Blistex, Blue Mold Dust, Corozate, D-14, Dithane, Ferbam, Maneb, Nabam, Zeneb, Zerlate, Ziram)

These substances, usually in an oily base, are used as insecticides. For toxic signs and symptoms see **49 – 77.** *Antabuse;* **49 – 848.** *Zerlate.*

49 – 293.   DJENKOL BEANS

These beans are used as a food by natives of Java and Sumatra and, as a rule, are well tolerated; however, occasionally they may cause acute and very uncomfortable effects, even in persons accustomed to them for years. There is a musty odor to the breath, severe bladder and inguinal pain, milky urine with a very offensive odor, hematuria, anuria and intense colic, with flatulence, vomiting and diarrhea.

TREATMENT

1. Large amounts of fluids by mouth.
2. Sodium bicarbonate, 2 to 4 gm. orally 3 to 4 times a day.
3. Morphine sulfate in small doses subcutaneously for severe pain.

PROGNOSIS.   Fatalities are rare. Complete recovery in 3 to 4 days is the usual course.

49 – 294. DOG PARSLEY See 49 – 910

49 – 295. DORIDEN See 49 – 352. *Glutethimide*

49 – 296. DULCAMARA (Bittersweet, Woody Nightshade)

The berries of this common North American and European plant contain a very toxic glucoside, solanine. For signs and symptoms of toxicity and treatment, see **49 – 712.** *Solanine.*

49 – 297. DYES

Aniline dyes. See **49 – 74.**

Azo dyes. The most commonly used azo dyes are alizarine blue S, brilliant vital red, Chicago blue, chlorazol fast pink, indigo carmine, Pyridium (a commonly used urinary antiseptic which may cause methemoglobinemia if given in large doses), scarlet red and toluidine blue. All the members of this group have approximately the same toxicity as scarlet red (**49 – 672**) and require the same treatment.

Benzidine dyes have been used extensively as trypanocides. The most commonly used members of this group are diamidinostilbene, pentamidine, trypan blue and trypan red. All are toxic if large amounts are ingested and all have a cumulative toxic action if therapeutic doses are continued over a long period.

SIGNS AND SYMPTOMS. Fever, acute dermatitis (often generalized, may be exfoliative), acute or chronic kidney irritation and occasional agranulocytosis.

TREATMENT. Withdrawal of the drug, although symptoms may persist for as long as 6 weeks afterward. Ingestion of large amounts requires immediate emptying of the stomach by emetics and/or gastric lavage followed by vigorous catharsis.

Coal tar dyes

This general heading includes all dyes derived from benzene (**49 – 119**) and includes all the headings listed in this section.

Flavins (acridine dyes) are derived from a coal tar base and, before the development of sulfa drugs and antibiotics, were frequently used in 1:1000 to 1:10,000 solutions to check surface infection. The two most common preparations are acriflavine and proflavine. Neither is toxic if applied to raw surfaces or ingested. Industrial exposure has been reported as causing acute conjunctivitis, lacrimation and acute dermatitis.

Gentian violet (methylrosaniline chloride) is a triphenylamine dye. Large amounts of gentian violet, as well as the other common triphenyl dyes (brilliant green, acid fuchsin and basic fuchsin) can be ingested without danger to life, although in some persons nausea, vomiting and diarrhea may occur.

TREATMENT

1. Removal of large amounts from the stomach by emetics and/or gastric lavage followed by activated charcoal in water by mouth or through the lavage tube.

2. Administration of magnesium sulfate (Epsom salts) by mouth to clear the lower gastrointestinal tract.

3. Assurance of the patient or family that the color of the skin, sclerae and mucous membranes will slowly return to normal.

Hair dyes. See **49 – 357.**

Methylene blue (tetramethylthionine chloride) is a coal tar dye which is often used medicinally (and usually ineffectively) for its supposed parasiticidal, antiseptic and analgesic action. It has a very low toxicity. A 1% solution in 1.8% sodium sulfate solution (Geiger's formula) is used intravenously in the treatment of acute methemoglobinemia from nitrite (**49 – 528**), acetanilid (**49 – 13**) and sulfanilamide poisoning (**49 – 731**) because of its ability to decrease the methemoglobin and to increase the oxygen-carrying capacity of the red blood corpuscles.

Ingestion of large amounts of methylene blue may cause gastrointestinal and bladder irritation, depression of the parasympathetic receptive system similar to that caused by atropine (**49-104**) and temperature elevation by central action.

TREATMENT

1. Emptying of the stomach as soon as possible by emetics and/or gastric lavage with 1:5000 potassium permanganate solution.

2. Administration of oxygen by mask and rebreathing bag if respiratory depression is present.

3. Injection of pilocarpine hydrochloride, 10 mg. subcutaneously every ½ hour or until the mouth becomes moist.

4. Sedation by barbiturates.

5. Hospitalization for observation if a large amount has been ingested. Transfusion (**14-13**) may be indicated for hemolysis and/or methemoglobinemia.

Phthalein dyes

Eosin (tetrabromofluorescein) is harmless if ingested, even in large amounts. Use of lipsticks containing eosin may cause acute dermatitis or gastrointestinal symptoms in certain sensitive individuals.

Fluorescein sodium (Uranine) is used locally in a 1 or 2% solution to demonstrate defects in the conjunctiva and cornea. The eye should be anesthetized with a few drops of ½% tetracaine (Pontocaine) before testing, and all fluorescein removed after examination by thorough irrigation with saline.

Fluorescein in a 20% solution can be given orally and intravenously for diagnosis of intraocular disease and for determination of renal function. If large, potentially dangerous amounts have been ingested, emptying of the stomach by emetics or gastric lavage may be indicated to prevent the characteristic yellowish discoloration of the sclerae and skin, which may be very disturbing to the patient. No other treatment is necessary.

Phenolphthalein. See **49-591.**

Phenoltetrachlorphthalein and phenolsulfonphthalein, used in liver function tests, are harmless. Tetrabromphenolphthalein, used in gallbladder visualizations, is usually nontoxic, although a few serious allergic reactions have been reported.

Shoe dyes. Ingestion may cause severe toxic reactions, as may absorption through the skin from recently dyed shoes. See **49-74,** *Aniline Dyes;* **49-529,** *Nitrobenzene.*

Triphenyl dyes (acid fuchsin, basic fuchsin, brilliant green, gentian violet) are relatively nontoxic.

49-298. EMETINE

This alkaloid occurs in ipecac and is used medicinally in the treatment of amebic dysentery and, in small doses, as an emetic and expectorant. It may cause nausea, vomiting, difficulty in swallowing, a sensation of tightness in the chest, acute stomach pain, intestinal cramping, diarrhea, cardiac depression and collapse.

TREATMENT

1. Absolute rest, with symptomatic and supportive therapy.

2. Stimulation with analeptic drugs, especially caffeine sodiobenzoate and amphetamine sulfate (Benzedrine) parenterally.

49-299. ENDRIN

This is an insecticide similar in action to but more toxic than *Dieldrin* (**49-267**).

49-300. EPHEDRINE (Racephedrine, l-sedrine)

Excessive use of nose drops or nasal sprays containing ephedrine may cause transient symptoms which clear rapidly when the medication is discontinued. Ingestion may cause extreme nervousness with tonic and clonic convulsions, cold clammy skin, mydriasis and dysphagia.

TREATMENT

1. Emptying of the stomach, preferably by emetics, but if necessary by gastric lavage.

2. Control of extreme nervousness and convulsions by sedation with barbiturates or paraldehyde.

PROGNOSIS. Complete recovery usually occurs even after ingestion of large amounts, although a few fatalities have been reported.

49—301. EPILEPSY "CURES"

These proprietary compounds usually contain barbiturates (49—111), bromides (49—144) or sodium diphenylhydantoinate [Dilantin (49—276)].

49—302. EPINEPHRINE (Adrenalin)

In certain hypersensitive persons, even minimal therapeutic doses may produce great discomfort from tenseness, restlessness, acute anxiety, tremors, dizziness, respiratory distress and palpitation. These symptoms are usually more uncomfortable than serious and in most instances can be cleared up rapidly by sedation with barbiturates. Severe, sometimes fatal, reactions from inadvertent, ill-advised or excessive intravenous injections of epinephrine hydrochloride have been reported. Persons with hyperthyroidism, cardiovascular disease and angina pectoris are notoriously susceptible. Aggravation of preexistent psychomotor symptoms and activation of psychoses (50—1) may take place. When epinephrine is given intravenously, its action is so rapid that no emergency measures are of any benefit. Severe reactions, almost always caused by the accidental injection of a large dose or by ingestion, are characterized by:

1. Cerebrovascular accidents (59—2).
2. Acute pulmonary edema (51).
3. Cardiac dilatation.
4. Ventricular fibrillation (26—23).

TREATMENT

1. Limitation of absorption by application of a tourniquet to an extremity proximal to the site of injection if the error in the amount injected is realized in time.

2. If ingested, emptying of the stomach *at once* by gastric lavage.

3. Sedation with paraldehyde or barbiturates, preferably given parenterally.

4. Oxygen inhalations by face mask and rebreathing bag.

5. Treatment of pulmonary edema (51).

6. Hospitalization for observation after acute symptoms have been controlled.

PROGNOSIS. Good if the patient survives the first half hour. No permanent ill effects are to be anticipated.

49—303. EPN See 49—546. *Organic Phosphates*

49—304. EPOXY RESINS

Used as concrete adhesives, these substances may cause severe contact dermatitis. The catalysts or hardeners used with epoxy compounds may cause erythema, pruritus, periorbital and facial edema and, apparently, permanent hypersensitivity. Inhalation of the fumes may result in severe and persistent bronchospasm.

49—305. EQUANIL See 49—448. *Meprobamate*

49—306. ERGOT (Spurred Rye)

Contamination of flour with this fungus may cause acute toxic symptoms, as may ingestion or injection of medicinal preparations.

SIGNS AND SYMPTOMS OF ERGOTISM. Extreme pallor of the face, with cyanosis of the extremities; small, weak rapid pulse; visual, auditory and sensory disturbances; hallucinations and myocardial infarction. Frequent use of large doses—especially as an abortifacient—results in a tabes-like clinical picture. Gangrene, especially of the fingertips and toes, may develop.

TREATMENT

1. Induction of vomiting followed by gastric lavage with 500 ml. of 1:5000 potassium permanganate solution if ingested.
2. Papaverine hydrochloride, 0.03 gm. subcutaneously.
3. Application of external heat.
4. Forced respiration of oxygen by face mask and rebreathing bag.
5. Hospitalization for observation. Gangrene of the extremities may occur.

49—307. ERGOTAMINE (Gynergen) See 49—306. Ergot

49—308. ERYTHRITYL TETRANITRATE

This is used commercially in the explosives industry and medicinally in the treatment of hypertension. Its toxic signs, symptoms and treatment are similar to those outlined in 49—528. Nitrites.

49—309. ESERINE See 49—603. Physostigmine

49—310. ETHANOL See 49—315. Ethyl Alcohol

49—311. ETHCHLORVYNOL (Placidyl)

SIGNS AND SYMPTOMS OF OVERDOSAGE

1. Characteristic aromatic odor on the breath.
2. Deep coma—often prolonged.
3. Respiratory depression; apnea.
4. Hypotension; bradycardia.
5. Complications include cardiac arrest (26—7) and pulmonary edema (51).

TREATMENT

1. Emptying the stomach as soon as possible by emetics and/or lavage.
2. Activated charcoal by mouth or via the lavage tube.
3. Support of cardiac and respiratory function, with frequent monitoring of blood gases.
4. Forced diuresis.
5. Peritoneal dialysis (14—9) or hemodialysis in severe cases.

49—312. ETHER See 49—70. Anesthetics, Inhalation

49—313. ETHIDE (Dichloronitroethane)

Inhalation of fumes or ingestion of this grain fumigant may cause severe toxic symptoms. The treatment is similar to that outlined in 49—553. Oxides of Nitrogen.

49 — 314. ETHINE See **49 — 24.** *Acetylene*

49 — 315. ETHYL ALCOHOL (See also **2 — 1.** *Addiction;* **15 — 1.** *Alcohol Intoxication Tests;* **29 — 13.** *Coma;* **34 — 1.** *Alcoholism;* **34 — 3.** *Delirium Tremens;* **46 — 8.** *Alcoholic Neuritis*)

Ethyl alcohol and isopropyl alcohol (**49 — 403**) vary in some side effects but give practically identical pictures following ingestion. Both are commonly used in rubbing alcohol compounds, and ethyl alcohol is the active agent in intoxicating beverages and the vehicle in many medicinal preparations. The denaturing substances commonly used to make rubbing compounds nonpotable give unpleasant symptoms but, as a rule, are harmless in themselves.

The amounts of ethyl and isopropyl alcohol necessary to produce acute toxic symptoms vary markedly, not only in different individuals but also in the same individuals at different times, depending on several modifying factors (**15 — 1**). Barbiturates, meprobamate, chlorpromazine and other commonly used tranquilizing drugs may potentiate the toxicity of alcohol to a dangerous degree.

Treatment of Acute Alcoholism

1. Obtain a blood specimen for alcohol level determinations (**15 — 1**) and for blood sugar level.

2. If the last ingestion of alcohol was within 2 hours, lavage with a large volume of water or 3 to 5% sodium bicarbonate solution, taking precautions against aspiration of vomitus or lavage fluid, leaving activated charcoal in water in the stomach. A saline cathartic should be given. Apomorphine hydrochloride should not be used as an emetic.

3. Apply external heat.

4. Support the respiration by expired air and mechanical means (**11 — 1**), with administration of oxygen as required. Circulatory support should be given by strong coffee orally or rectally, or by caffeine sodiobenzoate intramuscularly, repeated as necessary.

5. Treat stomach and bowel complaints symptomatically.

6. Give isotonic sodium chloride solution or 1/6 molar sodium lactate solution intravenously for dehydration and acidosis.

7. Combat hypoglycemia by intravenous glucose.

8. In the moribund patient, hemodialysis may be lifesaving.

9. Hospitalization under strict supervision and control for supportive care and evaluation and treatment of neurologic and psychiatric aspects. Parenteral multivitamin preparations probably are of little value.

49 — 316. ETHYL CHLORIDE See **49 — 70.** *Anesthetics, Inhalation*

49 — 317. ETHYLENE See **49 — 70.** *Anesthetics, Inhalation*

49 — 318. ETHYLENE CHLORHYDRIN

Used in the chemical and textile industries, this liquid gives acute toxic symptoms by absorption through the skin, inhalation of fumes and ingestion. The toxic picture is characterized by mucous membrane irritation (especially of eyes and nose), visual disturbances, dizziness, incoordination and paresthesias. Severe thirst, soft weak pulse and extreme hypotension develop, followed in severe cases by shock (**53**) and coma. Death is usually caused by brain congestion or pulmonary edema (**51**).

Treatment

1. If splashed on skin, thorough washing after removal of contaminated clothing.

2. If ingested, gastric lavage followed by activated charcoal in water.

3. Oxygen under positive pressure by face mask or endotracheal catheter.

4. Treatment of shock (53—7) and pulmonary edema (51).

PROGNOSIS. Very poor in severe cases. Because of the possibility of ventricular fibrillation, use of epinephrine is contraindicated.

49—319. ETHYLENEDIAMINE TETRAACETIC ACID (EDTA, Calsol, Sequestrene, Versene)

This chelating agent in therapeutic dosage may cause internal hemorrhage and symptoms of kidney irritation. Symptoms clear rapidly when use of the drug is discontinued.

49—320. ETHYLENE GLYCOL (Diethylene Glycol, Antifreeze, Prestone)

This toxic liquid is commonly used in automobile "permanent" antifreeze mixtures; hence, is often available for ingestion by children. Toxic effects are due to breaking down of these liquids to oxalic acid (49—552). The appropriate measures outlined below should be carried out if ingestion is even suspected; do not wait for symptoms to develop.

SIGNS AND SYMPTOMS of toxicity (usually delayed 1 to 2 hours after ingestion) consist of temporary exhilaration followed by development of progressively deepening coma, rapid weak pulse, acute respiratory distress, muscular paralysis and loss of reflexes. A positive Babinski sign may be present. If anuria and uremia develop, the condition is generally fatal.

TREATMENT

1. Induction of vomiting.

2. Gastric lavage with large amounts of a 1:5000 potassium permanganate solution followed by activated charcoal in water through the lavage tube.

3. Administration of oxygen under positive pressure by face mask and rebreathing bag.

4. Intravenous calcium gluconate to form insoluble calcium oxalate.

5. Injection of caffeine sodiobenzoate, 0.5 gm. intramuscularly. Treatment for shock (53—7) may be necessary.

6. Hospitalization for symptomatic care.

49—321. ETHYLENE OXIDE

Used as a food and textile fumigant, ethylene oxide fumes cause a peculiar sweetish taste in the mouth, vomiting, severe cough and vertigo. Bradycardia and extrasystoles are common, as is intense abdominal pain.

TREATMENT

1. Removal from exposure.

2. Oxygen inhalations.

3. Control of abdominal pain by small doses of morphine sulfate.

4. Symptomatic care as required.

49—322. ETHYL GASOLINE

The symptoms and treatment following ingestion are the same as for gasoline (49—349). Tetraethyl lead apparently is relatively nontoxic in the concentrations commonly found in ethyl gasoline, although persons concerned with its manufacture or those who experience prolonged cutaneous contact may develop the clinical picture of acute or chronic lead poisoning (49—420) from absorption through the intact skin.

49 – 323.   **ETHYLMORPHINE HYDROCHLORIDE** (Dionin)

Dionin is occasionally used therapeutically as an analgesic, antispasmodic and sedative. Sensitivity reactions (**21**) following local application are common. Use as a rectal suppository in a child has caused death.

49 – 324.   **EUCAINE** See **49 – 72.** *Anesthetics, Local*

49 – 325.   **EUCALYPTOL** (See also **49 – 543.** *Oil, Essential*)

Oil of eucalyptus (50% eucalyptol) is an ingredient of many widely used household remedies, especially counterirritant salves and lotions. Ingestion of even small amounts may have serious effects.

SIGNS AND SYMPTOMS of toxicity are nausea, vomiting, abdominal pain, diarrhea, miosis, dizziness, mental confusion, dysuria, hematuria, convulsions in children, dyspnea, cyanosis and circulatory collapse, followed by coma. Late development of pulmonary edema (**51**) and severe pneumonitis (**52 – 15**) may occur.

TREATMENT

1. If the patient is conscious and cooperative, have him swallow 60 to 120 ml. of liquid petrolatum. This is all that is necessary if the amount ingested is known to be small.

2. Empty the stomach by emetics and/or gastric lavage if a large amount has been swallowed, using all precautions to prevent aspiration.

3. Start oxygen inhalations by face mask.

4. Administer saline cathartics.

5. Hospitalize if a large amount has been ingested or if marked circulatory or respiratory depression has been present.

49 – 326.   **EUCODAL** (See also **49 – 264.** *Dicodid;* **49 – 495.** *Morphine*)

Addiction (**2 – 3**) has been described. Naloxone (Narcan) is an effective antagonist – dosage 0.4 mg. intramuscularly or intravenously, repeated as necessary.

49 – 327.   **EUDERMOL** (Nicotine Salicylate) See **49 – 523.** *Nicotine*

49 – 328.   **EUONYMIN**

Euonymin is a digitalis-like substance found in the fruit of many varieties of bushes and trees (arrowwood, bitter ash, burning bush, strawberry tree).

Ingestion may result in vomiting, watery diarrhea, hallucinations and somnolence deepening to coma.

TREATMENT

1. Emetics followed by gastric lavage, leaving a suspension of activated charcoal in the stomach.

2. Saline cathartics.

3. Supportive measures as required.

49 – 329.   **EUPATORIUM URTICAEFOLIUM** (Deerwort, Poolwort, Pool Root, Squaw Root, Rayless Goldenrod, Richweed, White Sanicle, White Snakeroot)

These plants are indigenous to the eastern and western parts of the United States and contain a toxic unsaturated alcohol, tremetol. For toxic picture and treatment, see **49 – 795.** *Tremetol.*

49–330. FAVA BEANS

Favism, characterized by chills, fever, nausea, vomiting, jaundice, red-brown or black urine, gastrointestinal bleeding and hemoglobinemia may be caused by ingestion of green or incompletely cooked broad (Windsor) beans or horse beans, or by inhalation of the pollen or by dust from grinding. Different individuals show wide variations in susceptibility; in addition, the same individuals may vary in susceptibility at different times.

TREATMENT

Immediate hospitalization for supportive therapy and blood transfusions.

49–331. FENFLURAMINE HYDROCHLORIDE (Pondimin)

Overdosage of this recently developed anorectic drug may cause agitation or drowsiness, confusion, fever, abdominal pain and hyperventilation.

TREATMENT

1. Emetics or gastric lavage.
2. Activated charcoal in water by mouth or through the gastric lavage tube.
3. Diuresis with acidification of the urine.
4. Circulatory support, preferably with cardiac monitoring.

49–332. FERRIC AND FERROUS SALTS See 49–399. *Iron Salts*

49–333. FINGERNAIL POLISH See 49–17. *Acetone;* 49–74. *Aniline Dyes*

49–344. FIRE EXTINGUISHERS

Toxic ingredients depend on the type.
1. Dry type—magnesium stearate, tricalcium phosphate.
2. Foam type—aluminum sulfate (49–50), methyl bromide (49–476).
3. Gas type—compressed carbon dioxide gas (49–170).
4. Liquid type—carbon tetrachloride (49–173), dichloromethane, chlorobromethane and trichlorethylene (49–800).
For treatment, see the specific toxic constituents.

49–335. FIREWORKS

Many acutely toxic substances may be present in the fuel, binders, oxidizers and coloring agents of fireworks. In some instances, mild transient toxic signs and symptoms may be caused by inhalation of fumes. Among commonly used toxic constituents are:

Antimony salts (49–81)	Mercury (49–455)
Arsenates (49–90)	Nitrates (49–525)
Barium salts (49–112)	Perchlorates (49–187. *Chlorates*)
Chlorates (49–187)	Phosphorus (49–602)
Copper salts (49–223)	Strontium salts
Lead salts (49–420)	Thiocyanates (49–774)

Ingestion of some types of fireworks by children may be fatal if the stomach is not emptied at once and careful symptomatic follow-up care administered.

49 – 336. FLUORIDES (See also **49 – 337.** *Fluoroacetates;* **49 – 338.** *Fluoro-silicates;* **49 – 378.** *Hydrofluoric acid*)

Sodium, barium and zinc fluorides are often the active toxic ingredients in ant, insect, roach and rodent poisons. Ingestion (especially by children) and inhalation of the dust during manufacture and use have caused many cases of acute and serious poisoning.

SIGNS AND SYMPTOMS of acute fluoride poisoning consist of nausea, vomiting, severe abdominal pain, burning, cramps, bluish gray cyanosis, muscular tremors, myalgia (especially of the calf muscles) and convulsions. Death usually occurs in 2 to 4 hours; the prognosis is good if the patient survives for 24 hours.

TREATMENT
1. If inhaled, removal from exposure followed by oxygen inhalations under positive pressure.
2. If ingested, immediate gastric lavage (even if evidence of corrosion is present) with large amounts of 1% calcium chloride or lime water. Follow with large amounts of milk or aluminum gel by mouth.
3. Oxygen inhalations under positive pressure.
4. Prevention of chilling.
5. Treatment of shock (**53 – 7**).
6. Maintain mild diuresis and correct dehydration.
7. Calcium gluconate, 10 ml. of 10% solution intravenously for severe myalgia; repeated in 30 minutes and every 4 to 6 hours until recovery is complete.
8. Hospitalization because of the danger of serious liver and kidney damage.

49 – 337. FLUOROACETATES

These compounds, used as rodenticides, are toxic in a different manner from other fluoride derivatives, apparently because of blocking of cellular energy production resulting in the slow development of convulsions.

SIGNS AND SYMPTOMS. Acute apprehension, anxiety, nausea, vomiting, aberrations of special senses [especially auditory, visual (nystagmus) and mental (hallucinations)], paresthesias (usually facial) and muscle twitching. Epileptiform convulsions are often followed by development of cardiac abnormalities [pulsus alternans, ectopic beats, ventricular tachycardia (**26 – 24**) and fibrillation (**26 – 23**)].

TREATMENT
1. Immediate emptying of the stomach by emetics and gastric lavage if fluoroacetic poisoning is even suspected. Activated charcoal in water should be left in the stomach.
2. Control of convulsions by rapidly acting barbiturates intravenously.
3. Administration of oxygen under positive pressure by face mask and rebreathing bag.
4. Glyceryl monoacetate (Monacetin), 0.5 ml. per kilogram of body weight, intra-muscularly, repeated in $\frac{1}{2}$ hour if necessary.
5. Hospitalization for close observation, ECG monitoring and symptomatic care.

49 – 338. FLUOROSILICATES (Silicofluorides)

These salts have approximately the same toxicity and require the same treatment as fluorides (**49 – 336**).

49 – 339. FOOD POISONING

Botulism (**49 – 141**). Evidence of toxicity from botulism usually does not develop until 18 to 36 hours after eating improperly processed canned foods; in some instances, the time lapse is much longer. The toxic picture is caused by an exotoxin produced under anaerobic conditions by *Clostridium botulinum.* The prognosis depends upon the amount of toxin ingested in relation to body weight. For treatment, see **49 – 141.**

Bacterial. From enterotoxins in food produced by the growth of staphylococci or by the organisms themselves (*Salmonella, Streptococcus*).

SIGNS AND SYMPTOMS of toxicity from staphylococcic enterotoxins develop in 2 to 6 hours after ingestion; from streptococcic contamination, in 2 to 12 hours. Both are characterized by vertigo, weakness, general malaise, salivation, nausea, vomiting, gastric pain, tenesmus, diarrhea, muscular cramps and shock – usually transient but may be severe and resistant to treatment (**53 – 7**).

TREATMENT

1. Empty the stomach at once by emetics or gastric lavage followed by activated charcoal.

2. Control severe pain by morphine sulfate subcutaneously, intramuscularly or intravenously, depending on the severity. Pentazocine lactate (Talwin), 15 to 30 mg. intramuscularly or intravenously, often is effective.

3. Give 30 ml. of castor oil, or 0.2 gm. of calomel (mercurous chloride) by mouth.

4. Decrease tenesmus and diarrhea by 1 gm. of bismuth subcarbonate or 7.5 gm. of kaolin by mouth. Camphorated tincture of opium (paregoric), 4 to 8 ml., may be given orally after each loose bowel movement.

5. Hospitalize if severe shock (**53**) or dehydration is present; usually it is not necessary.

Chemical. Ingestion of acid foods stored in containers lined with antimony (**49 – 81**), cadmium (**49 – 156**), lead (**49 – 420**) or zinc (**49 – 850**) may result in nausea, vomiting and diarrhea lasting 2 or 3 days if not treated. Eating unwashed fruit and vegetables which have been sprayed with preparations containing the metal salts may give the same picture. Food preservatives and sugar and salt substitutes may give toxic signs and symptoms. (See **49 – 528.** *Nitrites;* **49 – 658.** *Saccharin.*)

TREATMENT

1. Emetics followed by gastric lavage if profuse vomiting has not occurred. Activated charcoal in water should be given by mouth.

2. Saline cathartics.

3. Atropine sulfate, 0.5 mg. subcutaneously.

4. Bismuth subcarbonate by mouth.

5. Specific treatment as outlined under the offending metal.

Radioactive contamination. See **63 – 4** and **63 – 5.** *Wartime Emergencies.*

Rare causes of food poisoning. Poisoning from ingestion of certain plants and animal foods may be due to contaminants or to naturally occurring poisons contained in the foods. Among the foods or food contaminants which have been reported as giving toxic symptoms – usually from nonbacterial poisons – are the following:

Abalone. See *Mytilotoxism* (below); **49 – 504.** *Mussel Poisoning.*

Aconite. The roots of this plant, also called Friar's cowl, monkshood and mousebane, may be mistaken for edible horseradish. See **49 – 222.** *Coniine.*

Agrostemma githago (corn campion, corn cockle, corn rose). See **49 – 31.**

Amanita muscaria. This variety of mushroom is very toxic. Toxic symptoms develop in from a few minutes to 3 hours after ingestion. See **49 – 502.** *Mushroom Poisoning;* **49 – 500.** *Muscarine.*

Amanita pantherina. See **49 – 502.** *Mushroom Poisoning.*

Amanita phalloides. Delayed, severe, often terminal, toxic symptoms (6 to 24 hours) are characteristic of poisoning from this variety of poisonous mushroom. See **49 – 502.** *Mushroom Poisoning.*

Amanita verna. This variety of poisonous mushroom is responsible for many cases of acute toxicity in Europe. See **49 – 502.** *Mushroom Poisoning.*

Amberjack. See *Fish poisoning* (below).

Asari. See *Venerupin* (below).

Balloon fish. See *Fish poisoning* (below).

Barracuda. See *Fish poisoning* (below); **49 — 113.** For baracuda bites, see **24 — 2.**

Black ulna. See *Fish poisoning* (below).

Blaasoportoby. See *Fish poisoning* (below); **49 — 766.** *Tetraodontiae.*

Blood (Polish Kiszra) sausage. See *Sausage cyanosis* (below).

Blowfish. See *Fish poisoning* (below); **49 — 766.** *Tetraodontiae.*

Botete. See *Fish poisoning* (below); **49 — 766.** *Tetraodontiae.*

Bread poisoning. See *Senecio* (below); **49 — 680.** *Senecio.*

Bream. See *Haff disease* (below).

Broad beans. See **49 — 330.** *Fava Beans.*

Cadmium. See **49 — 156.** *Cadmium and Its Salts.*

Chlorinated hydrocarbon pesticides. Contamination of bulk cereal foods has resulted in several series of severe poisoning. Endrin (**49 — 299**) has been the most common offender.

Ciguatera. This is a gastrointestinal and neurotic disorder caused by ingestion of certain fish, which differs from all other types of fish poisoning because of its cholinesterase-inhibiting action. The toxic effects are similar to those described for organic phosphates (**49 — 546**). Treatment is symptomatic except that 2-PAM (Protopam chlorides) seems to have a neutralizing effect.

Clams. See *Mytilotoxism* (below).

Claviceps purpurea. Ergot fungus as a contaminant of cereal grains (especially rye) can cause acute circulatory symptoms followed by evidence of central nervous system damage. For treatment, see **49 — 306.** *Ergot.*

Coprinus atramentarius. This variety of edible mushroom, called "inky caps," gives toxic symptoms only in the presence of alcohol. For toxic picture and treatment, see **49 — 77.** *Antabuse.*

Corn campion. See **49 — 31.** *Agrostemma Githago.*

Corn cockle. See **49 — 31.** *Agrostemma Githago.*

Corn rose. See **49 — 31.** *Agrostemma Githago.*

Deathfish. See *Fish poisoning* (below); **49 — 766.** *Tetraodontiae.*

Dog parsley. The leaves may be mistaken for edible parsley. See **49 — 910.**

Eel. See *Fish poisoning* (below); *Haff disease* (below); **49 — 355.** *Gymnothorax Flavimarginatus.*

Ergot. See *Claviceps purpurea* (above); **49 — 306.**

Fava beans. See **49 — 330.**

Favism. See **49 — 330.** *Fava Beans.*

Fish poisoning (ichthyosarcotism) is widespread and is usually classified in 3 groups depending on the geographic area in which the fish are found.

Caribbean Type (amberjack, great barracuda, cavallas, groupers, sierra and fish of related species). Usually not fatal.

Pacific Type (barracuda, black ulna, eels, red snapper, sea bass, trigger fish). Mortality about 5%.

Japanese (Tetraodon) Type (balloon fish, globe fish, puffers). This type is limited to the waters bordering Japan. The mortality is about 70%. For toxic effects and treatment, see **49 — 766.** *Tetraodontiae.*

Fugu. See *Fish poisoning* (above); **49 — 766.** *Tetraodontiae.*

Fungicides. These preparations are sprayed on grain fields and may give toxic effects when the cereal is used as food. A large series of cases of acquired porphyria (**43 — 22**) in Turkey was caused by fungus control with hexachlorobenzene.

Galerina venenata. See **49 — 347.**

Globe fish. See *Fish poisoning* (above).

Groupers. See *Fish poisoning* (above).

Gymnothorax flavimarginatus. See **49 — 355.**

Haff disease. Eating bream, burbot, eels, perch and roach has resulted in an unusual type of food poisoning in countries bordering on the North Sea. The etiology of Haff disease is unknown, but it is characterized by agonizing pain in muscles of the back and extremities coming on about 18 hours after eating the fish. The condition clears spontaneously after 36 to 48 hours. The only treatment required is relief of the severe muscle pain.

Helvella (lorchel, morel, false morel). See **49—361; 49—502.** *Mushroom Poisoning.*

Honey. If bees collect the honey from certain plants it may be very toxic. See **49—374.**

Ichthyosarcotism See *Fish poisoning* (above).

Jatropha curcas. See **49—405.** *Jatropha Nut Oil.*

Jugfish. See *Fish poisoning* (above); **49—766.** *Tetraodontiae.*

Kiszka. See *Sausage cyanosis* (below).

Lathyrism. The exact etiology of this type of food poisoning, occurring in India, southern Europe and other tropical countries during times of famine, is not known; although ingestion of the seeds of *Lathyrus sativa L.* (Vetchling, green vetch) is suspect. It occurs mainly in middle-aged persons and is characterized by spastic paralysis, paresthesias, hyperreflexia and patellar and Achilles clonus. Symptomatic treatment is all that can be given.

Lead. Food poisoning from lead is usually due to ingestion of unwashed fruits or vegetables which have been sprayed with lead-containing insecticides. See **49—420.** *Lead Salts.*

Lolium tremulentum. See **49—430.**

Maki-maki. See *Fish poisoning* (above); **49—766.** *Tetraodontiae.*

Milk sickness. See **49—795.** *Trometol.*

Metals. Arsenic (**49—90**) and lead (**49—419**) may be present on unwashed vegetables and fruits. Antimony (**49—81**), cadmium (**49—156**), tin (**49—786**) and zinc (**49—850**) poisoning may be acquired by eating foods stored in containers lined with these metals. For treatment, see *Chemical poisoning* (above).

Mushrooms. See **49—502.** *Mushroom Poisoning, Amanita muscaria, Amanita pantherina, Amanita phalloides* and *Amanita verna* (above) and *Coprinus atramentarius* (above).

Mussels. See **49—504.** *Mussel Poisoning; Mytilotoxism* (below).

Mytilotoxism. (See also **49—504.** *Mussel Poisoning.*) On the Pacific Coast of North America, abalones, clams, mussels and oysters during certain months of the year (usually June to October) feed on dinoflagellates which contain a toxic substance which is not destroyed by cooking. Ingestion of the shellfish may cause nausea, vomiting, abdominal cramps, muscle weakness, peripheral paralysis and death from respiratory failure. Symptoms of toxicity appear within ½ hour of ingestion. The mortality is extremely high.

TREATMENT

1. Immediate emptying of the stomach by any available means (**49—3**). Vomiting must be initiated by tickling the throat, gargling with soapsuds or swallowing mustard and water as soon as the *possibility* of ingestion of toxic shellfish is known or even suspected. These measures should be followed by oral administration of syrup of ipecac (15 ml. in water) or subcutaneous injection of 5 mg. of apomorphine hydrochloride. This in turn should be followed by thorough gastric lavage, leaving activated charcoal in water in the stomach.

2. Administration of a saline cathartic.

3. Control of pain by small doses of meperidine (Demerol).

4. Oxygen under positive pressure by face mask and rebreathing bag.

5. Treatment of shock (**53—7**).

6. Fluid replacement to overcome dehydration and acid-base imbalance (**6**).

7. Hospitalization for several days after apparent improvement. Relapses are common.

PROGNOSIS. Good if the toxic material is completely removed from the stomach within ½ hour; poor if the clinical picture of mytilotoxism is full-fledged.

Organic phosphate pesticides. Contamination of bulk flour and sugar has resulted in several series of organic phosphate poisoning cases with many fatalities. For mode of action and treatment, see **49–546.** *Organic Phosphates.*

Oysters. See *Mytilotoxism* (above); **49–504.** *Mussel Poisoning.*

Panmyelotoxicosis. This disease is well known in Russia and is caused by ingestion of toxic substances elaborated by a fungus growing on cereal grains, especially millet. Toxic effects begin with burning in the mouth and throat followed in a few days by acute gastrointestinal symptoms lasting about a week. Four to 8 weeks later, purpura, anemia and thrombocytopenia may develop. Death is usually caused by severe sepsis and bronchopneumonia. Treatment has to be symptomatic and supportive.

Parathion. See **49–546.** *Organic Phosphates.*

Perch. See *Haff disease* (above).

Phalloidine. See **49–502.** *Mushroom Poisoning; Amanita phalloides* (above).

Phytolacca decandra. See **49–604.**

Potato. Sprouting or unripened potatoes contain a toxic amount of solanine (**49–712**).

Puffer. See *Fish poisoning* (above); **49–766.** *Tetraodontiae.*

Red Snapper. See *Fish poisoning* (above).

Rhubarb. See **49–651; 49–552.** *Oxalic Acid.*

Roach. See *Fish poisoning* (above).

Sausage cyanosis. Use of large amounts of nitrate–nitrite to preserve the blood-red color of Polish blood sausage has caused acute toxic effects due to methemoglobinemia. For treatment, see **49–528.** *Nitrites.*

Sea bass. See *Fish poisoning* (above).

Senecio. Native to South Africa, the seeds of several varieties of this plant as a contaminant of cereal grains have caused many cases of "bread poisoning," a high percentage of which have been fatal. Fatalities are usually the result of irreversible liver damage. For treatment, see **49–680.**

Shellfish. See *Mytilotoxism* (above); **49–504.** *Mussel Poisoning.*

Sierra. See *Fish poisoning* (above).

Solanine. See *Potato poisoning* (above); **49–712.**

Tin. See **49–786.**

Tetraodon. See *Fish poisoning* (above); **49–766.** *Tetraodontiae.*

Toadfish. See *Fish poisoning* (above); **49–766.** *Tetraodontiae.*

Tomato. Several series of cases have been reported, especially from the Middle West area of the United States, in which acute toxic symptoms have developed from eating tomatoes picked from plants grafted on *Datura stramonium* (jimsonweed, stinkweed) roots (**49–240**). The toxic picture and treatment are similar to that outlined under *Atropine* (**49–104**).

Tremetol. See **49–795.**

Trigger fish. See *Fish poisoning* (above).

Venerupin. Limited to Japan, this type of food poisoning follows ingestion of asari and oysters. Acute gastrointestinal symptoms develop in 24 to 36 hours, with evidence of liver damage and increase in blood coagulation time. The mortaility is about 30%.

TREATMENT

1. Emptying the stomach as soon as possible by emetics and gastric lavage followed by activated charcoal in water by mouth or via the lavage tube.

2. Saline cathartics.

3. Supportive and symptomatic care.

Vitamin A. Poisoning from excessive intake of Vitamin A is limited to Arctic regions where animal organs (especially of the polar bear, bearded seal, fox and husky dog) are used as food. Discontinuance of the food and symptomatic care is the only treatment required.

Windsor bean. See *Fava beans* (above).

Zinc. Storage of food in galvanized containers may cause symptoms of zinc poisoning. For treatment, see *Chemical poisoning* (above); **49–850.** *Zinc Chloride.*

49-340. FORMALDEHYDE

A solution of this pungent gas is the active ingredient in many commonly used household antiseptics, deodorizers and fumigants. It is also used to wrinkle-proof clothing. Inhalation of fumes or ingestion of solutions of the gas (**49-341**) may cause an acute toxic picture. The breath has a characteristic odor. If inhaled, acute irritation of the eyes, nose and upper respiratory tract, bronchospasm and/or laryngeal edema may occur. If ingested there is soreness of the mouth and throat with difficulty in swallowing. Nausea, vomiting, hematemesis, severe abdominal pain, diarrhea (often bloody), severe shock, convulsions, coma and death from respiratory failure is the chain of events in terminal cases.

TREATMENT

1. Have the patient swallow aromatic spirits of ammonia, 8 ml. in water. Follow with demulcents such as raw eggs and milk.

2. Induce vomiting by emetics, followed by gastric lavage with 0.2% ammonia in water. Activated charcoal in water should be left in the stomach.

3. Inject morphine sulfate subcutaneously for severe pain if respiratory depression is not acute.

4. Combat dyspnea by oxygen under positive pressure.

5. Begin treatment of shock (**53-7**) as soon as possible.

6. Hospitalize if convulsions have occurred or respiratory depression or severe shock (**53**) has developed.

49-341. FORMALIN

Formalin is an aqueous solution containing 40% formaldehyde and small amounts of ethyl and/or methyl alcohol. For treatment of poisoning, see **49-340**. *Formaldehyde.*

49-342. FORMIC ACID

Used in the chemical and leather industries, the fumes of formic acid cause acute inflammation of the eyes, nose and throat. Ingestion causes acute stomatitis, glossitis, esophagitis and gastritis with delayed serious kidney damage.

TREATMENT

1. Gastric lavage.

2. Instillation of ammonium chloride solution to which a small amount of sodium bicarbonate has been added.

3. Close observation of kidney function.

49-343. FOWLER'S SOLUTION See **49-90**. *Arsenic*

49-344. FREONS

These chlorinated-fluorinated hydrocarbons are used in refrigerators and as the propelling agents in aerosol containers. Inhalation of fumes may cause respiratory tract irritation from the freezing effect and mental confusion from the narcotizing effect. Another danger lies in contact of the containers with fire in the home. At high temperatures, freons break down into chlorine (**49-190**), fluorine, hydrogen fluoride (**49-336.** *Fluorides*) and phosgene (**49-599**)—all volatile gases which are dangerous in even low concentrations.

49-345. FURNITURE POLISH

Ingestion of these preparations by children is common and may cause severe illness and even death due to the toxic effects of the chief ingredient, mineral seal oil, a hydrocarbon distillate. These effects are similar to but more severe than gasoline (**49—349**) and kerosene (**49—408**). All children who have ingested furniture polish should be hospitalized for at least 24 hours because of the possibility of delayed development of severe pulmonary involvement.

49—346. GADOLINIUM CHLORIDE

This by-product of the uranium industry has caused cardiovascular collapse in laboratory animals, but no cases of human toxicity have been reported.

49—347. GALERINA VENENATA

Ingestion of this North American fungus has been reported as causing acute gastro-intestinal symptoms coming on after about 10 hours, followed by hypotension, convulsions and pulmonary edema (**51**).
TREATMENT
1. Gastric lavage, followed by activated charcoal in water through the lavage tube.
2. Saline cathartics.
3. Hospitalization for administration of intravenous fluids and because of the danger of delayed pulmonary edema (**51**).

49—348. GAMMEXANE (Gamma Benzene Hexachloride) See 49—120.
Benzene Hexachloride

49—349. GASOLINE

Its wide use as a motor fuel and as a cleansing agent makes gasoline one of the main present-day causes of poisoning. Toxic signs and symptoms may follow contact with the skin over large areas of the body, inhalation of fumes or ingestion. Repeated voluntary inhalation of gasoline fumes has been reported. See **49—358**. *Hallucinogens.*
Skin contact. Repeated or prolonged washing of the skin with gasoline results in removal of the protective fat layer, with subsequent lowering of resistance to infection. Exposure of large areas of skin to gasoline may cause severe toxic symptoms from absorption similar to those given below for inhalation of high concentrations. Acute symptoms from skin absorption are sometimes encountered following automobile accidents in which the clothing has been saturated with gasoline.
TREATMENT
1. Remove all contaminated clothing at once.
2. Wash the skin thoroughly with copious amounts of soap and water.
3. Give symptomatic therapy as outlined under inhalation of high concentration (below).
Inhalation. Low or medium concentrations of gasoline fumes cause flushing of the skin, staggering gait, confusion, incoherence and disorientation—a clinical picture which may be mistaken for acute alcohol intoxication.
TREATMENT
1. Removal from exposure.
2. Fresh air or inhalations of oxygen.
PROGNOSIS.   Complete recovery in a short time.
High concentrations may cause muscular twitching, tonic and clonic convulsions, dilated nonreactive pupils, delirium followed by sudden loss of consciousness and death from ventricular fibrillation (**26—23**) or complete respiratory arrest.
TREATMENT
1. Removal from exposure.

2. Oxygen inhalations under positive pressure by face mask and rebreathing bag.

3. Caffeine sodiobenzoate, 0.5 gm. intramuscularly, for circulatory failure. *Do not* give epinephrine hydrochloride (Adrenalin) because of the danger of inducing ventricular fibrillation.

4. Hospitalization as soon as possible. The acute stage may be followed in 2 to 3 hours by peripheral and retrobulbar neuritis, epileptiform seizures, paresthesias and pneumonitis.

PROGNOSIS. Fair if the patient survives the initial exposure. Permanent mental changes as well as serious kidney damage may develop.

Ingestion. Swallowing gasoline causes a burning sensation in the mouth and throat, nausea, vomiting and diarrhea, followed by extreme restlessness, with muscular twitching and incoordination. Aspiration of fumes when gasoline is swallowed may result in a severe chemical pneumonitis.

TREATMENT

1. No attempt should be made to induce vomiting. The mouth should be rinsed thoroughly and large quantities of milk given in mild cases, as when a mouthful of gasoline results from siphoning from one motor vehicle tank to another.

2. If a large quantity has been swallowed, gastric lavage with 120 ml. of olive oil followed by warm water should be done as soon as possible. Care should be taken to prevent aspiration, especially during withdrawal of the lavage tube.

3. Administration of a saline cathartic.

4. Caffeine sodiobenzoate, 0.5 gm. intramuscularly – repeated as necessary.

5. Oxygen inhalations under positive pressure, preferably by face mask and rebreathing bag.

6. Hospitalization for symptomatic and supportive care to minimize the chance of development of respiratory tract, kidney or brain damage. Antibiotics seem to have little value in preventing chemical pneumonitis.

49 – 350. GELSEMIUM (Yellow Jasmine)

Used medicinally in some localities as an antineuralgic and antispasmodic, gelsemium contains a toxic alkaloid (gelsemine).

SIGNS AND SYMPTOMS. Great weakness, unsteady gait, vertigo, headache, aphasia, paralysis of the tongue with inability to swallow, lowered body temperature and a pale clammy skin, which later becomes olive green, then flushed and cyanotic. The pupils are dilated and nonreactive. Ptosis of the eyelids is often present.

TREATMENT

1. Induction of vomiting by emetics, followed if necessary by gastric lavage with 1:5000 potassium permanganate solution. Activated charcoal in water should be left in the stomach.

2. Local heat.

3. Caffeine sodiobenzoate, 0.5 gm. intramuscularly – repeated as necessary.

4. Insurance of an open airway by positioning, suction, traction on the tongue, support of the angles of the jaw or insertion of a nasopharyngeal catheter or airway.

5. Oxygen therapy under positive pressure.

6. In severe cases, hospitalization is indicated. Tracheostomy (**14 – 12**) may be necessary.

49 – 351. GLUTAMIC ACID

Under the trade names of Accent, Lawry's Seasoned Salt, and others, the sodium salt of glutamic acid is used as a food flavoring. Allergic reactions characterized by abdominal discomfort, acute distention, eructations and epigastric fullness have been reported. All disappear when the offending preparation is discontinued.

49 – 352. GLUTETHIMIDE (Doriden)

Overdosage of this nonbarbiturate sedative results in dryness of the mucous membranes, fever, flushing of the skin, mydriasis, nystagmus, ataxia and coma.

TREATMENT

1. Gastric lavage, leaving 30 ml. of castor oil in the stomach.
2. Oxygen under positive pressure by face mask or endotracheal tube and rebreathing bag.
3. Administration of vasopressors if hypotension is present.
4. Limitation of fluids.
5. Hospitalization for possible peritoneal dialysis using a lipid-containing dialysate. This, however, should only be used as an adjunct to other therapy.

49 – 353. GOLD SALTS

Gold salts used medicinally in the treatment of arthritis and lupus erythematosus are extremely toxic. These salts are:

Gold sodium thiosulfate (Sanochrysine)
Sodium aurothiomalate (Myochrysine)
Aurothioglucose (Solganal)
Aurothioglycolanilide (Lauron)

Apparently there is great variation in personal tolerance of these drugs, not only in different individuals but also in the same person at different times.

SIGNS AND SYMPTOMS. Fever, characteristic facial puffiness, various skin disorders, intense pruritus, nausea, vomiting, abdominal pain and diarrhea. Polyneuritis affecting almost exclusively the motor nerves, liver and kidney damage and blood changes may occur.

TREATMENT

1. Stop administration of the offending drug.
2. Give sedatives, anodynes and narcotics as needed for pain.
3. Hospitalize at once for heavy metal poisoning therapy. See **49 – 90.** *Arsenic.*

PROGNOSIS. Good unless agranulocytosis has developed, then a mortality of about 30%.

49 – 354. GUAIACOL

Toxic signs, symptoms and treatment are similar to those listed under *Phenol* (**49 – 590**).

49 – 355. GYMNOTHORAX FLAVIMARGINATUS

Indigenous to Hawaii, the Philippines and South Africa, this edible eel for as yet undetermined reasons has been responsible for many cases of acute poisoning. Toxic symptoms, which consist of numbness of the lips, impaired speech, progressive paralysis and convulsions, usually last for several days and are followed by complete recovery without residual ill effects.

TREATMENT

1. Emetics or gastric lavage after control of convulsions by rapid-acting barbiturates. Activated charcoal in water should be left in the stomach.
2. Saline cathartics.
3. Intravenous fluids.
4. Supportive and symptomatic therapy.

49—356.   GYNERGEN See **49—306.** *Ergot*

49—357.   HAIR DYES AND SPRAYS

Many of the preparations used to color, curl, straighten or set hair contain ethyl alcohol (**49—315**), isopropyl alcohol (**49—403**), higher alcohols (**49—33**), borates (**49—138**), cadmium salts (**49—156**), caustic hydroxides (**49—39.** *Alkalies*), copper salts (**49—223**), dichromates (**49—207.** *Chromates*) and ether (**49—312**). These various substances may cause systemic poisoning through absorption from the scalp and surrounding skin or by ingestion, in addition to localized damage to the hair and scalp.

Among the more complex constituents which may give toxic reactions are:

Aminodiphenylamines	Henna
Aminonisole	Nitrodiamino compounds
Chloroaminophenols	Phenetols
Chlorodiamines	Polyvinylpyrrolidones
Diaminophenols	Pyrogallol

TREATMENT

In mild cases the only treatment required is to stop use of the preparation. More severe cases may require symptomatic treatment as outlined in **49—634.** *Pyrogallol.*

49—358.   HALLUCINOGENS

Plants containing small amounts of psychotomimetic (sometimes called "consciousness-expanding") drugs have been used for many years as a means of escape from reality in Asia and the Orient [e.g., hashish or marihuana (**49—441**)] and in religious rites in southwestern United States and Mexico where sliced peyote nuts [*Mescal* (**49—460**)] and certain varieties of mushrooms containing psilocybin (**49—502**) are chewed by participants. A synthetic derivative of lysergic acid, the diethylamide (LSD), has a similar but more powerful effect. Illegal sale and use of LSD has become common during the last few years. The toxic effects (hallucinations, increased perception, personality dissociation, etc.) last for from 6 to 8 hours to 2 to 3 weeks. Whether or not LSD causes permanent ill-effects has not as yet been finally and conclusively determined, due in part to laws in some areas which impose strict limitations on experimental studies. It is possible that some of the reported unpredictable ill-effects may be due to impurities resulting from improper synthesizing. True addiction to nonnarcotic hallucinogens does not occur.

In addition to the drugs and plants mentioned above, the following are some of the many substances which have been reported as having hallucinatory effects:

Acetanilid (**49—13**).

Alkyl mercury compounds (**49—42**).

Amantadine hydrochloride (Symmetrel). This is a recently developed chemical virostat used orally in prevention of influenza. Large doses have a definite hallucinatory effect.

Amyl nitrite (**49—69**).

Arsenic trioxide (**49—90.** *Arsenic*).

Arsine (**49—94**).

Asthma remedies (**49—103**).

Atropine (**49—104**).

Banana peel scrapings. The dried inner pulp of banana peels has been reported as having some hallucinatory effect. This, however, is very questionable.

Barbiturates (**49—111**).

Belladonna and its alkaloids (**49—116**).

Bromides (**49—144**).

Caffeine (**49 – 157**).
Camphor (**49 – 163**).
Carbon monoxide (**49 – 172**).
Carbon tetrachloride (**49 – 173**).
Colchicine (**49 – 220**).
Cortisone (**49 – 227**).
Dilantin (**49 – 276**).
DMT (dimethyltryptamine) is a hallucinogen which occurs naturally in certain plants. It can be synthesized very easily. Its action can be obtained only by intramuscular or intravenous injection and is more rapid but less prolonged than LSD.
Epinephrine hydrochloride (Adrenalin) solutions which have turned brown from age or exposure to light.
Ergot (**49 – 306**).
Euonymin (**49 – 328**).
Freons (**49 – 344**).
Gasoline fumes (**49 – 349**).
Hydrogen sulfide (**49 – 380**).
Hyoscyamus (**49 – 383**).
Insulin (**29 – 3.** *Hypoglycemia*).
Meperidine – large doses (**49 – 245.** *Demerol*).
Mercury fumes ("Mad Hatters' Syndrome").
Methamphetamine (**49 – 468.** *Methedrine*).
Model airplane glue and cement (**49 – 610**).
Morning glory seeds. Decoctions of the seeds have been used for their alleged hallucinatory effects. The active ingredient is closely related to LSD.
Morphine (**49 – 495**).
Muscarine (**49 – 500**).
Nitrous oxide (**49 – 70.** *Anesthetics, Inhalation;* **49 – 553.** *Oxides of Nitrogen*).
Nutmeg (**49 – 506.** *Myristicin*).
Oxygen – high concentrations (**49 – 555**).
Paradichlorobenzene (**49 – 567**).
Prophenpyridamine (**49 – 628**).
Quinine (**49 – 642**).
Saccharin (**49 – 658**).
Salicylic acid (**49 – 664.** *Salicylates*).
Scopolamine (**49 – 676**).
STP is a more powerful hallucinogen than LSD and is chemically related to amphetamine (**49 – 64**) and mescaline (**49 – 460.** *Mescal*).
Tetraethyl lead (**49 – 322.** *Ethyl Gasoline;* **49 – 349.** *Gasoline;* **49 – 761**).
Thallium (**49 – 768**).
Thiocyanates (**49 – 774**).
Trinitrotoluene (**49 – 809**).
Tripelennamine hydrochloride (**49 – 812**).
Yage. This plant has been used for centuries by Central American witch doctors to promote hallucinations. Its action is similar to LSD and mescaline (**49 – 460.** *Mescal*).
The table on pages 443 and 444 includes most of the mind-modifying substances usually encountered in drug abuse patients. (Modified from special edition, *Medical Economics*, April 20, 1970.)

TREATMENT

1. Close observation under controlled circumstances with a sympathetic and physically able attendant present at all times. Relapses may occur as long as several weeks after the original exposure.

NAME OF DRUG	SHORT-TERM EFFECTS	HOW TO SPOT ABUSER
Hallucinogens		
DMT	Exhilaration, excitation. Extremely potent when taken intravenously, producing a "blast." Smoking effects are milder.	Same symptoms as LSD.
LSD	Distortion and intensification of sensory perceptions, especially visual hallucinations. Suggestibility.	Dilation of pupils. Exhilaration. Rambling speech, talk of "hearing" or "tasting" colors and "seeing" sounds.
Marijuana and hashish (**49 – 441**)	Euphoria, heightened sensory awareness, time/space distortions, increased appetite or lessening of inhibitions. Transient loss of memory, and paranoia.	Euphoria with no physical signs of intoxication, tendency to talk excessively or giggle without provocation, odor of burnt leaves or hemp on breath or clothes, reddened eyes.
Mescaline (**49 – 460**)	Same general effects as LSD. High-dose symptoms similar to those after high dose of amphetamine. Acute episode may be mistaken for acute schizophrenia.	Same symptoms as LSD.
Psilocybin	Initial reactions of nausea, muscular relaxation, headaches, followed by visual and auditory hallucinations.	Same symptoms as LSD.
Depressants		
Barbiturates (**49 – 111**)	Sedation, relaxation. Relief from anxiety and mental stress. Resultant impaired memory, defective judgment, incoordination.	Drunken behavior with no smell of alcohol. Drowsiness, slowed reflexes, pulse, and respiration. Often not diagnosed until onset of acute withdrawal symptoms.

NAME OF DRUG	SHORT-TERM EFFECTS	HOW TO SPOT ABUSER
Depressants (Continued)		
Codeine (**49 – 219**)	Euphoria obtained only with large amounts, which may also cause excitement and restlessness. Used to "tide over" addict between "fixes" of his usual drug.	Very little evidence of general effect unless taken intravenously.
Heroin (**49 – 366**)	Rush of euphoria when injected intravenously, but requiring constantly increasing dosage. Drowsiness. Constipation, urinary retention.	Pinpoint pupils (less contraction in seasoned addicts), slow pulse and respiration, needle marks, "nodding."
Methadone (**49 – 464**)	Analgesia, euphoria. A synthetic narcotic, taken by abusers for its own sake, it is also given to opiate addicts for blockage of craving for and euphoria from their usual drug. Also blocks sickness otherwise produced by withdrawal from opiates.	Heroin-like symptoms.
Morphine (**49 – 495**)	Similar to heroin except lacking its characteristic euphoric rush.	Same symptoms as heroin.
Plastic or cement glue, cleaning fluids, aerosols, etc. (**49 – 610**)	Hazy euphoria. Impaired perceptions, coordination, and judgment. Irritation of mucous membranes, slurred speech. Initial excitation is followed by depression, stupor.	See short-term effects.
Stimulants		
Amphetamines (**49 – 64**)	Feeling of energy and excitation. Loss of appetite. Insomnia. Feeling of increased initiative. Euphoric rush when injected.	Extreme restlessness or nervousness. Tremor. Dryness of mouth. Tachycardia. Excessive sweating. Needle marks when injected.
Cocaine (**49 – 218**)	Flashing, intense euphoria, pleasurable hallucinations. Feeling of great mental and muscular strength.	Garrulity, restlessness, excitement. Hyperactivity of reflexes. Rapid pulse and irregular respiration.

2. Symptomatic and supportive therapy based on the hallucinogen used. Diazepam (Valium) in appropriate doses is a safe sedative. Chlorpromazine hydrochloride (Thorazine) should not be used in the treatment of unidentified hallucinogens. If STP is a component, fatalities may occur.

3. Psychiatric evaluation and treatment as needed.

49–359. HEADACHE REMEDIES

These proprietary compounds generally contain acetanilid (49–13) combined with caffeine (49–157), bromides (49–144) and salicylates (49–664).

49–360. HELLEBOREIN

This is one of several glucosides found in the roots and seeds of plants of the *Helleborus* family. Ingestion of even small amounts results in rapid development of nausea, vomiting, abdominal pain, diarrhea, headache, vertigo, tinnitus, dilation of the pupils, photophobia, visual disturbances and myalgia, especially of the calves. More serious cases develop delirium, convulsions, coma and death from respiratory collapse.

TREATMENT

1. Emetics followed by gastric lavage with large amounts of water. Activated charcoal in water should be left in the stomach.

2. Artificial respiration by expired air or mechanical methods (11–1), followed by administration of air or oxygen under positive pressure by face mask if respiratory depression is acute.

3. Administration of 10% calcium gluconate intravenously for acute myalgia.

4. Hospitalization for close observation for at least 24 hours after apparent complete recovery.

49–361. HELVELLA (False Morel, Lorchel, Morel)

Generally considered to be edible, these mushrooms occasionally cause severe toxic symptoms coming on from 6 to 8 hours after ingestion. For signs and symptoms of toxicity and treatment, see 49–502. *Mushroom Poisoning*.

49–362. HEMLOCK See 49–222. *Coniine*

49–363. HEPARIN

Purpura, ecchymosis and hematuria from the use of this anticoagulant may be severe enough to require immediate therapy for shock (53–7). Plasma volume expanders should be given for temporary support, and the patient hospitalized at once for thorough investigation and possible blood transfusions. (See also 42–34. *Hemorrhage After Anticoagulant Therapy;* 49–265. *Dicumarol*.)

49–364. HEPTACHLOR

Heptachlor is a complex insecticide which by inhalation, skin absorption or ingestion can give a toxic picture similar to that produced by chlordane (49–188). In addition, severe and permanent liver damage may occur.

49 – 365. HERACLEUM LANATUM (Cow Cabbage, Cow Parsnip, Hayweed, Masterwort)

The sap of this perennial meadow plant, indigenous to the northern section of the United States, on contact with the skin causes photosensitization and acute eczematous eruptions, which heal with permanent pigmentation.

49 – 366. HEROIN (Diacetylmorphine) (See also **2 – 4.** *Addiction*)

This powerful narcotic is more toxic and addictive than any of the other opiates. Prescription or administration of heroin is forbidden in the United States and many other countries, but because of its potency it is common in the illegitimate narcotic market, often adulterated with substances which in themselves may be toxic.

SIGNS AND SYMPTOMS of heroin overdosage [usually following intravenous ("mainline") injection].

1. Marked respiratory depression (apnea or 3 to 4 gasping respirations per minute).
2. Cyanotic, clammy pallor.
3. Pinpoint pupils (may be dilated if anoxia is extreme).
4. Weak pulse, but may be strong and full if extreme hypoxia is present. Arrhythmias and cardiac cessation may occur.
5. Evidence of pulmonary edema.
6. Areflexia, deep coma and death.

TREATMENT

1. Establish and maintain an adequate airway.
2. Start artificial ventilation by expired air or mechanical methods (**11 – 1**).
3. Begin external cardiac compression (**11 – 2**) if the heartbeat is very weak or absent. Monitor cardiac status by ECGs.
4. Inject naloxone hydrochloride (Narcan) intravenously, 0.01 mg. per kilogram of body weight. As much as 1.2 mg. can be given intravenously to an adult, repeated as often as necessary to obtain the desired affect. Naloxone is preferred to Lorfan and Nalline because it has no respiratory or cardiovascular depressant effects.
5. Inject 3 to 5 ml. of doxapram hydrochloride (Dopram) as a respiratory stimulant.
6. Give intravenous glucose and electrolytes.
7. Treat metabolic acidosis with intravenous sodium bicarbonate.
8. Treat pulmonary edema (**51**).

WITHDRAWAL SYMPTOMS from heroin are very uncomfortable but rarely life-threatening. Beginning about 10 to 12 hours after the last injection, reaching maximum intensity in about 36 hours and subsiding on about the fifth day, they are characterized by frequent exaggerated yawning and gaping, nausea, vomiting, abdominal cramping and diarrhea, hypersalivation, excessive tearing, photophobia, intense myalgia, jitteriness and insomnia.

TREATMENT

For pain and myalgia: Propoxyphene hydrochloride (Darvon), 130 mg. every 4 to 6 hours.

For gastrointestinal symptoms: Belladonna preparations or dicyclomine hydrochloride (Bentyl) every 4 hours.

For nervousness and sleeplessness: Phenobarbital, 30 mg., or diazepam (Valium), 5 to 10 mg. four times a day; chloral hydrate, 2.5 gm. at bedtime.

49 – 367. HETP (Hexaethyltetraphosphate, Bladan) See **49 – 546.** *Organic Phosphates*

49-368. HEXAMETHONIUM BROMIDE (Vegolysin)

Overtreatment of hypertension with this potent autonomic blocking agent can result in rapid fall in blood pressure, with vertigo, blurred vision, mydriasis, acute glaucoma and loss of vision. Urinary retention and paralytic ileus may occur, with terminal shock from cardiovascular collapse.

TREATMENT

1. Gradual decrease — not complete withdrawal — of the drug.
2. Treatment of shock (53-7).
3. Symptomatic and supportive therapy (49-4).

49-369. HEXAMETHYLENETETRAMINE (Methenamine, Urotropin)

In acid urine, this drug slowly releases formaldehyde. Excessively large doses may give mild toxic symptoms. See **49-340.** *Formaldehyde.*

49-370. HEXYLRESORCINOL

Use of high concentrations or large doses by mouth may give a picture suggestive of mild phenol poisoning. The treatment is the same as outlined in **49-590.** *Phenol.*

49-371. HIPPOMANE MANCINELLA (Mancellier, Manzinello)

Growing along the seashore of Florida, the Caribbean islands and Central America, this small tree exudes a latex which on contact gives a multiplicity of acute toxic eye symptoms — vesicles, bullae, conjunctivitis, photophobia and corneal ulcers. Ingestion of the fruit causes vomiting, violent gastric pain and bloody diarrhea which may be followed by cardiovascular collapse.

TREATMENT

1. Removal of the latex from the skin by thorough washing with soap and water.
2. Removal from the eyes by irrigation with large amounts of water.
3. Gastric lavage followed by activated charcoal in water and saline cathartics if ingested.
4 Supportive and symptomatic care (49-4).

49-372. HISTAMINE

Medical use of excessive amounts may cause severe, sometimes fatal, shock. For treatment, see 53-7.

49-373. HOMATROPINE

Therapeutic use in ophthalmology may cause a slow pulse, dysphagia, vertigo, weakness, excitement and collapse, as well as the expected mydriasis. Complete recovery in a short period is the rule. No special treatment is required.

Overdosage has been reported as causing excitement, confusion and coma, with very slow respiration, rapid pulse and hypotension.

TREATMENT

1. Stop the medication.
2. If ingested, empty the stomach by immediate gastric lavage, leaving activated charcoal in water in the stomach.
3. Give supportive treatment as required.

49 – 374.   HONEY

Nectar collected by bees from certain flowering plants may yield toxic honey. Among these plants are aconite (**49 – 27**), azalea (**49 – 867**), foxglove (**49 – 272.** *Digitalis*), gelsemium (**49 – 350**), laurel (**49 – 944**), oleander (**49 – 544**) and rhododendron (**49 – 988**).

49 – 375.   HORSERADISH See **49 – 222.** *Coniine*

49 – 376.   HYDROCHLORIC ACID See **49 – 26.** *Acids*

49 – 377.   HYDROCYANIC ACID (Prussic Acid) See **49 – 235.** *Cyanides*

49 – 378.   HYDROFLUORIC ACID

This extremely corrosive solution (hydrogen fluoride, 47% in water) is used in etching and engraving. It may cause severe toxic symptoms by contact with the skin or nails, contact with the eyes, inhalation of fumes and ingestion.

Skin contact. Even small amounts of hydrofluoric acid on the skin or nails will cause severe damage. The onset is insidious; after the acid is removed, the skin or nails will appear to be normal for about 1 hour. Erythema, followed by vesication and tissue destruction, then develops rapidly, resulting in a nonhealing ulcer that sometimes extends to the bone. Fingernails and nail beds may be completely destroyed.

TREATMENT

1. Immediate washing with water for 1 to 2 hours, followed by soaking for one hour in 70% alcohol and ice.

2. After lengthy washing and soaking, application of a paste made from equal parts of magnesium oxide and magnesium sulfate (Epsom salts).

3. Injection of calcium gluconate (10% solution) into, under and around the affected area. Nails should be partially cut away and the nail bed injected as above. Small ulcers should be excised en bloc and the base injected with 10% calcium gluconate. Following injection, the areas should be painted with Berwick's or other triple dye solution and treated as an open wound or third degree chemical burn.

Contact with the eyes may cause serious and permanent damage.

TREATMENT

1. Immediate washing with large amounts of water.

2. Instillation of 1% tetracaine hydrochloride (Pontocaine) to control pain, followed by 1% atropine sulfate to dilate the pupil.

3. Application of an eye patch.

4. Immediate referral for ophthalmologic care.

Inhalation of fumes

TREATMENT

1. Removal from exposure.

2. Inhalation of 1% calcium chloride solution sprayed into the respiratory tract with an atomizer.

3. Hospitalization if marked irritation of the respiratory tract is present.

Ingestion

TREATMENT

See **49 – 336.** *Fluorides.*

49 – 379.   HYDROGEN SELENIDE

Low concentrations of this colorless industrial gas may cause severe throat irritation (cough, hoarseness, dysphagia), rhinitis, anosmia, urticaria, extreme hypotension, dyspnea and cyanosis, followed by pulmonary edema (**51**).

TREATMENT
1. Removal from exposure.
2. Oxygen by face mask and rebreathing bag.
3. Antihistaminics if urticaria is marked.
4. Support of the circulation by plasma volume expanders intravenously.
5. Treatment of pulmonary edema (**51**).

49 – 380. HYDROGEN SULFIDE

Toxic symptoms from this foul smelling ("rotten egg") gas, formed by putrefaction of sulfur-containing material, are common among petroleum and sewer workers.

Low concentrations are irritant only and may cause acute conjunctivitis, photophobia and seeing of colored rings around bright lights, rhinitis with decrease or loss of the sense of smell, tracheitis, bronchitis, pneumonia (**52 – 14**) and pulmonary edema (**51**).
TREATMENT
1. Removal from exposure.
2. Instillation of olive oil into the eyes for conjunctivitis.
3. Oxygen therapy under positive pressure.

High concentrations are very depressant and may cause nausea, vomiting, progressively increasing somnolence, amnesia, transient unconsciousness coming on especially after exertion, dysphagia, rapid pulse, low blood pressure and eye signs (strabismus, diplopia, exophthalmos, fixed nonreactive pupils). Delirium and hallucinations may be followed by convulsions and death from respiratory failure. Extremely high concentrations are rapidly fatal.
TREATMENT
1. Removal from exposure. Complete rest.
2. Prolonged artificial ventilation (**11 – 1**) – preferably oxygen inhalations under positive pressure by mask or endotracheal catheter. Treatment of pulmonary edema (**51**) may be required.
3. Caffeine sodiobenzoate, 0.5 gm. intramuscularly. In severe cases intravenous administration of 4 ml. of 0.2% levarterenol bitartrate (Levophed) in 1000 ml. of 5% dextrose in saline may be necessary for circulatory support. Metaraminol bitartrate (Aramine), 50 to 100 mg., may be added to the dextrose solution in place of Levophed.
4. Atropine sulfate, 0.6 mg. subcutaneously.
5. In severe cases, use amyl nitrite therapy as outlined in **49 – 235. Cyanides.** Hospitalization for prevention or treatment of delayed sequelae (pneumonia, pulmonary edema, cardiac dilation, severe gastrointestinal symptoms and peripheral polyneuritis) is indicated. If evidence of pulmonary infection develops, antibiotic therapy should be instituted at once.

49 – 381. HYDROQUINONE

Most of the cases of acute poisoning from hydroquinone arise from its use as a photographic developer.
SIGNS AND SYMPTOMS. These include dizziness, ringing in the ears, rapid respiration, profuse sweating, nausea, vomiting, restlessness, muscular twitching, cyanosis (probably due to methemoglobinemia) and collapse.
TREATMENT
1. Emetics; if unsuccessful, gastric lavage with 1:5000 potassium permanganate solution followed by activated charcoal in water by mouth.
2. Oxygen under positive pressure by face mask and rebreathing bag if cyanosis is extreme.
3. Saline cathartics.
4. Hospitalization for thorough study because of the relatively frequent late development of severe hemolytic anemia.

49 – 382.   HYOSCINE See **49 – 104.** *Atropine Sulfate;* **49 – 676.** *Scopolamine*

49 – 383.   HYOSCYAMUS (Henbane)

If the foliage or stalks of this flowering garden plant are chewed, severe toxic symptoms similar to those from atropine (**49 – 104**) may develop. For the toxic picture and treatment, see **49 – 104.** *Atropine Sulfate.*

49 – 384.   HYPOCHLORITES (Chlorinated Lime, Clorox, Bleaching Powder, Labarraque's Solution, Dakin's Solution, Emergency Water Sterilizers)

Concentrated solutions have severe caustic alkali actions (**49 – 39**); dilute solutions cause only mild gastrointestinal symptoms. Although the antiseptic and bleaching actions depend on the chlorine content, this is too low to give toxic symptoms and can be disregarded in treatment.

TREATMENT

1. Immediate oral administration of demulcents (olive oil, crushed bananas, starch, egg albumin).

2. Emptying of the stomach by cautious gastric lavage (unless there is evidence of severe corrosion or perforation). Tap water or 1% sodium thiosulfate solution should be used for lavage fluid. Activated charcoal in water should be left in the stomach. Sodium bicarbonate and acidic antidotes are contraindicated.

3. Hospitalization if evidence of severe mucous membrane erosion is present.

4. Opiates for control of pain, as well as therapy for shock (**53 – 7**), may be necessary. Emergency tracheostomy (**14 – 12**) may be indicated. Strictures of the esophagus may occur and require prolonged treatment.

49 – 385.   IMPERIAL GREEN (Copper Acetoarsenite) See **49 – 90.** *Arsenic*

49 – 386.   INDELIBLE INKS, PENCILS AND STAINS See **40 – 7.** *Puncture Wounds of the Hand;* **49 – 74.** *Aniline Dyes*

49 – 387.   INDIGO

Ingestion of small amounts of natural or synthetic indigo may cause retching, vomiting, abdominal pain, diarrhea, fever, muscle twitching and renal colic.

TREATMENT

1. Emetics or gastric lavage with 1:5000 potassium permanganate solution. Activated charcoal in water should be left in the stomach.

2. Intravenous infusion of 500 to 1000 ml. of 5% dextrose in saline.

3. Calcium gluconate (10% solution) intravenously.

PROGNOSIS.   Complete recovery in 1 to 2 days.

49 – 388.   INK See **49 – 74.** *Aniline Dyes*

Marking inks may contain silver salts (**49 – 688**).

49 – 389.   INK ERADICATORS See **49 – 384.** *Hypochlorites;* **49 – 552.** *Oxalic Acid*

49 – 390.   INSULIN See **29 – 3.** *Diabetes Mellitus*

49 – 391.   IODATES

Intravenous use of solutions of sodium and potassium iodate in the treatment of sepsis at one time was common and accounted for a considerable number of fatalities. Iodates are no longer used for this purpose. No recent cases of iodate toxicity have been reported.

49 – 392.   IODIDES

Iodides are relatively nontoxic, but excessive doses or prolonged use of therapeutic doses can cause iodism (see **49 – 393.** *Iodine*), as well as enlargement of the salivary glands, which may be mistaken for mumps (**30 – 17**).

49 – 393.   IODINE

Local application causes mahogany-brown discoloration of the skin, with marked erythema and desquamation, vesication and corrosion of mucous membranes.

Exposure to fumes results in sparkling before the eyes, conjunctivitis, lacrimation, severe cough, headache, somnolence and swelling of the parotid glands (see **49 – 392.** *Iodides*).

Ingestion results in a characteristic metallic iodine taste, with severe pain and burning in the esophagus and stomach, often associated with brownish discoloration of the mucous membranes of the mouth and throat, nausea, vomiting (blue color of vomitus if the patient has been given starch), and extreme thirst. Convulsions may occur if large amounts have been swallowed.

TREATMENT

1. Give large amounts of starch solution by mouth.
2. Unless there is evidence of extensive mucous membrane corrosion, empty the stomach by gastric lavage with 1% sodium thiosulfate solution; repeat until the returned fluid no longer shows any blue color.
3. Control convulsions by rapidly acting barbiturates. Opiates may be necessary for severe pain.
4. Correct dehydration and acid-base imbalances by fluid and electrolyte replacement (**6**).
5. Apply external heat.
6. Inject caffeine sodiobenzoate, 0.5 gm. intramuscularly, for circulatory collapse. Severe shock requiring energetic management (**53 – 7**) may develop.

49 – 394.   IODOFORM

Absorption from wounds packed with iodoform gauze, or ingestion, may cause nausea, vomiting, rapid pulse, acute excitement and convulsions.

TREATMENT

1. Removal of packing (or emptying of the stomach by lavage if ingested).
2. Control of excitement and convulsions by rapidly acting barbiturates.

49 – 395.   IODOPYRACET See **49 – 287.** *Diodrast*

49 – 396.   IPECAC

Syrup of ipecac orally is an excellent emetic, with a wide margin of safety; however, deaths have occurred when the fluidextract (14 times as toxic as the syrup) has been administered by error in place of the syrup. In addition to its emetic action, ipecac is an efficient sedative. If satisfactory emptying of the stomach does not occur after 2 doses of syrup of ipecac, gastric lavage (**14 − 4**) should be done at once. Excessive vomiting can be controlled by chlorpromazine (Thorazine) parenterally. Treatment of shock (**53 − 7**) frequently is necessary. Continuous ECG monitoring is advisable because of the cardiotoxic effects of ipecac − bradycardia, atrial fibrillation, tachycardia and cardiac arrest.

49 − 397. IPRONIAZID (Marsalid)

Large doses used in the treatment of tuberculosis may cause vertigo, muscle twitching, hyperreflexia, difficulties in micturition, hepatitis and psychoses (**50 − 1**). All symptoms clear slowly when the drug is discontinued.

49 − 398. IRON OXIDE See 49 − 399. *Iron Salts;* 49 − 461. *Metal Fumes*

49 − 399. IRON SALTS

Since the common salts of iron oxidize rapidly on exposure to air to form basic ferric sulfate, acute poisoning from this source may occasionally be encountered. The majority of the cases of acute toxicity, however, result from ingestion by children of candy-coated ferrous sulfate tablets, with a mortality rate of about 30%.

SIGNS AND SYMPTOMS. A metallic taste in the mouth, vomiting of bluish green material, rapid weak pulse, hypotension, blackish diarrhea, often persistent enough to cause acute dehydration, and severe shock (**53**), especially in children.

TREATMENT

1. Administration of demulcents (raw eggs, starch solution, milk) by mouth, followed by gastric lavage with weak sodium bicarbonate solution, 5% mono- or disodium phosphate in water, or large amounts of tap water. Five to 10 gm. of deferoxamine (Desferal) should be left in the stomach.

2. Oxygen therapy under positive pressure.

3. Bismuth subcarbonate, 0.2 gm. orally every 4 hours as a demulcent.

4. Glucose (5% in saline) intravenously to combat dehydration.

5. Sodium bicarbonate intravenously if metabolic acidosis is present.

6. Treatment of shock (**53 − 7**), which may not appear for 12 hours. Whole blood transfusions may be required.

7. Immediate hospitalization for fluid replacement (**6**) and, in severe cases, continuation of therapy with deferoxamine (Desferal). The usual dose is 1 gm. given intravenously at a rate not to exceed 1.5 mg. per kilogram of body weight per hour. A specimen of gastric washing and a blood specimen taken before starting deferoxamine therapy should be obtained and sent to the laboratory for iron level determinations. Peritoneal dialysis and hemodialysis are of little, if any, value. Dimercaprol (BAL) therapy is ineffective. Antibiotics are indicated if there are any signs of infection.

49 − 400. ISODRIN

This complex substance is a powerful rodenticide. See **49 − 267.** *Dieldrin.*

49 − 401. ISOLAN See 49 − 546. *Organic Phosphates*

49 − 402. ISONIAZID

Large doses of this drug used in the treatment of tuberculosis may be toxic, especially in children.

SIGNS AND SYMPTOMS.   Nausea, vomiting, cyanosis of the extremities, generalized convulsions and coma.

TREATMENT

1. Emetics or gastric lavage followed by activated charcoal by mouth or through the lavage tube.
2. Oxygen therapy under positive pressure.
3. Plasma volume expanders and 5% dextrose in saline intravenously.
4. Barbiturates intramuscularly for control of convulsions.
5. Pyridoxine hydrochloride (vitamin B_6) therapy.

49–403. ISOPROPYL ALCOHOL (Avantine, Dimethylcarbinol)

Isopropyl alcohol has many uses—as a rubbing compound (usually with a denaturant to make it unpotable), as a solvent for waxes and resins, in the production of safety glass, paints, and varnishes, and in the manufacture of perfumes and cosmetics.

SIGNS AND SYMPTOMS (usually following ingestion but may be caused by inhalation of concentrated fumes) are dizziness, muscular weakness and incoordination (no exhilaration as with ethyl alcohol), severe headache, slow pulse with low blood pressure, acute gastrointestinal irritation with bloody vomitus and diarrhea, anuria and uremia.

TREATMENT

See **49–315.** *Ethyl Alcohol.*

49–404. ISUPREL HYDROCHLORIDE (Aleudrine, Aludrine, Isonorin, Norisodrine)

Used as an inhalant in asthmatic and allergic conditions, Isuprel in certain individuals can cause tachycardia, palpitation, precordial pain and irregularities in blood pressure. Large doses may cause dizziness and mental confusion.

All symptoms clear when use of the drug is discontinued.

49–405. JATROPHA NUT OIL

The nuts of this tropical South American and Asiatic shrub (Barbados nut tree, physic nut tree, purging nut tree) contain an oil known as Turkey red oil and "Hell" oil, which is a powerful purgative. It is used in the manufacture of soap. As an adulterant of olive oil, it has been responsible for several series of acute poisonings. Symptoms of toxicity and treatment are similar to those outlined in **49–232.** *Croton Oil.*

49–406. JEQUIRITY BEANS ("Crab Eyes")

The beans of the plant *Abrus precatorius,* indigenous to Florida and the Caribbean islands, especially Haiti, and some South Pacific Islands, are bright red with a small black spot and are very attractive—and dangerous—to tourists and children. For toxic effects of ingestion of the soft, easily chewed young beans, see **49–7.** *Abrus precatorius.*

When the beans mature and develop a hard shell, they become even more dangerous. They are used as ornamental beads on rosaries, as strands of beads on blouses and purses, as the eyes of native dolls and as decorations on "voodoo swizzle sticks." The drier they become, the more dust escapes from the hilum. If this powder is ingested, or enters the tissues through a break in the skin, it causes serious, often fatal, effects from abrin poisoning.

TREATMENT

See **49–7.** *Abrus precatorius L.*

49–407. JUTE

Processing of jute fibers in the manufacture of bags, mats and rope may cause severe allergic reactions—asthma, bronchitis, bronchospasm, laryngitis and tracheitis.

TREATMENT

1. Removal from exposure.
2. Management as outlined in **21.** *Allergic Reactions.*

49–408. KEROSENE (Coal Oil)

This common petroleum distillate has a wide use as a household fuel, solvent and cleanser and also as the inert ingredient in many types of household and garden sprays. Although often considered as being of low toxicity, the exact opposite is true; the mortality is close to 10% following ingestion, probably owing in great part to aspiration during ingestion, vomiting and gastric lavage. Inhalation of the fumes may cause transient excitement, headache, hallucinations and delirium, but these signs and symptoms clear rapidly when the concentration of the fumes is lowered by adequate ventilation. It is after these transient and uncomfortable symptoms clear up that the serious pathologic conditions (pneumonitis, pneumonia) become apparent.

SIGNS AND SYMPTOMS from ingestion are gastrointestinal irritation, circulatory disturbances, severe depression, coma, convulsions and pulmonary symptoms, especially aspiration pneumonia.

TREATMENT

1. *Do not* give emetics.
2. Unless a very large amount has been ingested do not wash the stomach—the risk of aspiration is very great.
3. Give large amounts of water or 3% sodium bicarbonate solution by mouth, followed by 30 to 60 ml. of vegetable (olive) oil. *Do not* substitute mineral oil.
4. Give a saline cathartic followed by a cleansing enema.
5. Oxygen under positive pressure by face mask and rebreathing bag.
6. Caffeine sodiobenzoate intramuscularly. [Dosage according to age (**4**). Do not administer to children under 6 years of age.]
7. Hospitalization as soon as possible. Prophylactic antibiotic therapy to guard against the possible results of aspiration should be considered. Administration of epinephrine (Adrenalin) hydrochloride, ethyl alcohol, and mineral oil should be avoided.

49–409. KETOBEMIDONE

The hydrochloride is a powerful narcotic which is extremely habit-forming. For signs and symptoms of toxicity and treatment, see **49–495.** *Morphine.*

49–410. KNOCKOUT DROPS See **49–184.** *Chloral Hydrate*

49–411. LACTIC ACID

Ingestion may cause severe burning of the mouth, pharynx, esophagus and stomach, nausea and vomiting, bloody emesis, rapid, weak pulse, cold perspiration, dyspnea, cyanosis and death from dehydration and exhaustion secondary to acute gastroenteritis.

TREATMENT

1. Gastric lavage with large quantities of lime water followed by activated charcoal in water given through the lavage tube.

2. Large amounts of fluid by mouth or intravenously.
3. Hospitalization after lavage and administration of fluids for symptomatic and supportive care.

49—412. LARKSPUR See 49—908. *Delphinium*

49—413. LAUDANUM (Tincture of Opium) See 49—495. *Morphine*

49—414. LAUREL OIL

Allergic skin reactions are common in hat makers who use laurel oil for "fattening" felts. Termination of exposure results in slow disappearance of symptoms.

49—415. LAURON See 49—353. *Gold Salts*

49—416. LEAD ACETATE See 49—420. *Lead Salts.*

49—417. LEAD ARSENATE AND ARSENITE

Both these substances, commonly used as insecticides, may cause toxic symptoms through inhalation. See 49—420. *Lead Salts.*

49—418. LEAD CHROMATE (Chrome Yellow)

Extremely toxic. See 49—420. *Lead Salts.*

49—419. LEAD OXIDE See 49—420. *Lead Salts;* 49—461. *Metal Fumes*

49—420. LEAD SALTS

In addition to exposure in industry, signs and symptoms of toxicity (plumbism) may occur, especially in children, from ingestion of flakes of old-fashioned paints and from use of improperly glazed china and other ceramics. Toxic symptoms also may be caused by inhalation of dust and fumes and by absorption through the skin. Several series of cases from illicitly distilled ("bootleg") whisky have been reported.

SIGNS AND SYMPTOMS of acute plumbism consist of a sweetish metallic taste, with dryness of the throat and extreme thirst, dizziness and severe cramping abdominal pain, with either constipation or bloody diarrhea. Severe arthralgia may occur, with paresthesias, convulsions and coma. There is often evidence of severe liver and kidney damage.

TREATMENT
1. Gastric lavage with 1% sodium sulfate solution.
2. Magnesium sulfate (Epsom salts), 30 gm. by mouth.
3. Application of external heat.
4. Control of abdominal pain and cramping in adults by morphine sulfate subcutaneously. Children should be given appropriate oral doses (4) of camphorated tincture of opium (paregoric). Calcium gluconate, 10 ml. of 10% solution intravenously, may help to control pain and colic.
5. Control of convulsions by intramuscular or intravenous injection of rapidly acting barbiturates, chloral hydrate orally or rectally, or paraldehyde intramuscularly.

6. Intravenous isotonic saline solution for control of dehydration and shock.

7. Hospitalization for deleading by ethylenediamine tetraacetate (EDTA) and sodium citrate. Dimercaprol (BAL) therapy is ineffective in lead poisoning.

49—421. LEMON GRASS OIL

This is a volatile (essential) oil (**49—543**) which not only is toxic if ingested but also causes a dermatitis similar to poison oak (**54—11**) on contact with the skin.

49—422. LETHANE

Lethane is used as a contact insecticide and may give acute toxic signs and symptoms if ingested. See **49—774**. *Thiocyanates (Organic derivatives).*

49—423. LEVOPROPOXYPHENE

This recently introduced antitussive drug may, in large doses, cause nausea, urticaria, dizziness, drowsiness, coma and cardiac arrest. Recovery usually follows gastric lavage and supportive therapy.

49—424. LIGUSTRUM VULGARE (Common Privet) See 49—970. *Privet*

49—425. LIME

Quicklime (unslaked lime, calcium oxide) is a powerful caustic which liberates heat when exposed to moisture. It may cause serious damage if ingested or allowed to come in contact with any portion of the eyes. By mouth the signs, symptoms and treatment are approximately the same as for any strongly caustic alkali (**49—39**). In the eyes it may cause hyperemia, edema and corneal ulceration, sometimes with resultant permanent opacities and loss of vision.

TREATMENT

Treatment of eye involvement consists of immediate prolonged washing with large amounts of water, followed by application of an eye patch (Figure 17) and referral to an ophthalmologist at the earliest possible opportunity.

Slaked lime is harmless.

49—426. LINDANE See 49—120. *Benzene Hexachloride*

49—427. LIPSTICKS See 49—228. *Cosmetics*

In general, the more "kiss-proof," the more the chance of toxic reactions—usually of the allergic or contact dermatitis type—which clear rapidly when use of the particular cosmetic is discontinued.

49—428. LITHIUM CHLORIDE

This is one of the substances which in minute amounts may cause acute toxic signs and symptoms in certain individuals. Apparently, the tolerance of different persons varies tremendously. Since in addition to its commercial use in fireworks and in soldering aluminum, it is a constituent of some mineral waters and sodium chloride substitutes, and is used medicinally in the treatment of certain mental conditions, familiarity with its toxic effects is important.

SIGNS AND SYMPTOMS. Tinnitus, vertigo, blurred vision, sleeplessness, generalized weakness, tremors of the extremities, often associated with muscular twitching, bizarre shifting disturbances in sensation, acute dysphagia, mental confusion, coma and (occasionally) death.

TREATMENT

Hospitalization for thorough investigation and possible extensive intravenous therapy, especially 1/6 molar lactic acid solution, is indicated in all cases when the history and findings suggest lithium poisoning. Marked hypersensibility to stimuli should be controlled by intravenous barbiturates or intramuscular paraldehyde before transfer.

PROGNOSIS. Guarded because of the marked variation in reactions and responses to therapy.

49−429. LOBELIA

Ingestion of leaves and seeds of this common plant causes serious symptoms due to a toxic alkaloid, lobeline. The characteristic picture consists of throat dryness, vomiting, abdominal pain, diarrhea, anxiety, muscular twitching and somnolence. In fatal cases severe convulsions precede death.

TREATMENT

1. Gastric lavage followed by activated charcoal in water by mouth or through the lavage tube.
2. Saline cathartics.
3. Intravenous fluids to combat dehydration.
4. Control of convulsions by rapidly acting barbiturates.
5. Symptomatic and supportive care.

49−430. LOLIUM TEMULENTUM (Darnel, Ivray, Poison rye-grass, Tares)

This widespread weed, as a contaminant of cereal grains and of their derivatives − especially linseed oil − has given rise to numerous cases of poisoning characterized by somnolence, vertigo, staggering and trembling. Eye signs are common, with blurred vision (often greenish) and dilated pupils. Severe cases show the symptoms of severe shock (53).

TREATMENT

1. Gastric lavage if ingestion has taken place within a few hours; otherwise saline cathartics.
2. Treatment of shock (53−7).
3. Symptomatic and supportive care.

49−431. LOMOTIL

Containing diphenoxylate hydrochloride and atropine sulfate, the first effects of overdosage with this popular diarrhea remedy are from atropine (49−104). Later, symptoms resembling those of morphine (49−495) develop, often complicated by hyperthermia.

TREATMENT

1. Immediate establishment of an adequate airway with respiratory assistance as needed.
2. Gastric lavage, even if many hours have elapsed since ingestion of Lomotil tablets.
3. Intravenous fluids to combat dehydration.
4. Administration of a morphine antagonist, preferably naloxone hydrochloride (Narcan), 0.01 mg./kg. of body weight intravenously, repeated as necessary.

49—432. LYE (Lixivium)

Lye originally was made by leaching wood ashes, but the term is now used for several of the strong alkalies, especially sodium and potassium hydroxide and carbonate. All act as severe caustics on direct contact with exposed parts of the body, and all may cause severe, often fatal, damage if ingested. Because lye is available in many households (washing powders, drain pipe cleaners, oven cleaners, paint removers, etc.), contact with the eyes or skin or ingestion by accident or with suicidal intent is relatively common.

In the eyes lye may cause severe conjunctivitis, chemosis, ulceration and loss of vision. It is more dangerous than most acids.

TREATMENT

1. Wash with large amounts of cold water immediately.
2. Apply an eye patch (Figure 17).
3. Refer to an ophthalmologist immediately.

On the skin lye may cause deep chemical burns with sloughing and loss of tissues.

TREATMENT

1. Wash with large amounts of cold water followed by a 10% solution of acetic acid (diluted vinegar will do).
2. Apply a sterile petrolatum gauze dressing.
3. Control severe pain by codeine sulfate or morphine sulfate subcutaneously, or pentazocine lactate (Talwin) intramuscularly.

If ingested, lye may cause whitish discoloration of mucous membranes of the mouth and throat (later becoming brownish); severe burning pain in the mouth, esophagus and stomach; bloody vomitus; rapid respiration with feeble pulse; collapse; coma and death. If it occurs within a few hours, death is usually due to hemorrhage and hypovolemic shock (**53**) or to edema of the glottis; later deaths are caused by lung lesions, pericarditis or peritonitis.

TREATMENT

1. Give demulcents by mouth at once—egg white, milk or olive oil.
2. Neutralize with diluted fruit juices, vinegar or 5% acetic acid by mouth. Give olive oil frequently in small doses.
3. Apply external heat.
4. *Do not* give emetics or attempt gastric lavage because of the danger of perforation.
5. Give small doses of narcotics as necessary for pain.
6. Treat shock by electrolyte solutions, plasma and whole blood intravenously.
7. Perform a tracheostomy (**14—12**) if edema of the glottis is severe enough to embarrass respiration.
8. After control of pain and shock, measures to determine whether or not severe esophageal damage has occurred (fluoroscopic examination during a barium swallow, esophagoscopy, etc.) should be undertaken.
9. If there is evidence of esophageal damage, prompt corticosteroid therapy should be instituted, together with broad spectrum antibiotics.
10. Prolonged hospitalization for supportive care, special liquid and soft diet, and possible esophageal bougienage.

49—433. LYSERGIC ACID DIETHYLAMIDE (LSD) See **49—358.** *Hallucinogens*

49—434. MAGNESIUM

Metallic magnesium is used in the manufacture of light metal alloys; grinding may cause fine, sharp fragments which perforate the skin and cause marked swelling and crepitus from formation of hydrogen bubbles.

TREATMENT. Surgical excision and primary closure.

Inhalation of finely ground metallic magnesium may cause metal fume fever (**49 — 461**).

49 — 435. MAGNESIUM OXIDE See **49 — 461.** *Metal Fumes*

49 — 436. MAGNESIUM SULFATE (Epsom Salts)

Especially in persons with impaired renal function, ingestion of excessive amounts, absorption through the rectum or intravenous injection may result in vomiting with acute gastric pain, dilation of the pupils, cyanosis, generalized weakness, and collapse from respiratory and cardiac failure.

TREATMENT

1. Artificial respiration by expired air and mechanical methods (**11 — 1**), especially oxygen under positive pressure by face mask or endotracheal catheter and rebreathing bag.
2. Calcium gluconate, 10 ml. of 10% solution intravenously, repeated as necessary.
3. Treatment of hypotension.
4. Administration of large amounts of fluids by mouth and intravenously.

49 — 437. MALATHION

This is one of the few organic phosphate insecticides approved for household use. In spite of its relatively low toxicity, treatment may be necessary if exposure has been excessive. See **49 — 546.** *Organic Phosphates.*

49 — 438. MALE FERN See **49 — 100.** *Aspidium*

49 — 439. MANGANESE

Although metal fume fever (**49 — 461**) may be caused by inhalation of finely ground magnesium, more serious toxic symptoms may follow inhalation of manganese dust by workers in the steel and battery industries and among ore handlers.

SIGNS AND SYMPTOMS are usually low grade and chronic, but severe acute muscular cramps (especially in the calves), uncontrollable laughter, slurred speech and staggering gait may require emergency therapy. Both the chronic and acute pictures can easily be mistaken for drug addiction (**2**).

TREATMENT

Hospitalization for thorough investigation is indicated if the history or symptoms suggest manganese poisoning. The incidence of a subsequent peculiarly virulent type of pneumonia is relatively high.

49 — 440. MANGANESE OXIDE See **49 — 461.** *Metal Fumes*

49 — 441. MARIHUANA (Bhang, *Cannabis sativa,* Hashish, Indian hemp, "Pot") (See also **49 — 358.** *Hallucinogens*)

SIGNS AND SYMPTOMS of marihuana intoxication are the same for ingestion or smoking and consist basically of inebriation, motor excitement, restlessness, euphoria and gaiety (sometimes anxiety) coming on about 1 hour after smoking or ingestion. Extreme thirst may be present as may wide dilation of the pupils with sluggish reaction to light. Aphrodisiac effects are much less marked than usually believed. Vertigo and transient collapse may occur.

TREATMENT
1. Symptomatic only—spontaneous recovery in a short time always occurs.
2. Psychiatric reference to determine the underlying causative factors. Contrary to wide publicity, no causal relationship to criminal offenses, sexual or otherwise, has ever been established. True addiction does not occur.

49 — 442. MATCHES

Most present-day matches contain phosphorus trisulfide or sesquisulfide which are almost inert chemically and therefore relatively nontoxic. "Safety matches" have no toxic ingredients in harmful amounts in the heads (the phosphorus compound is on the friction surface on the box or book); therefore, children who suck or eat the heads need no treatment except disciplining. Ingestion of large numbers of the heads of "strike anywhere" matches requires treatment, because many brands contain potassium chlorate and antimony sulfide in addition to a phosphorus compound. Old-fashioned "sulfur matches" contain yellow phosphorus and are dangerous; ingestion of 16 of these matches has been reported as fatal to an adult.
For toxic signs, symptoms and treatment, see **49 — 602.** *Phosphorus.*

49 — 443. MECAMYLAMINE (Inversine)

Used in treatment of hypertension because of its ganglion-blocking effect, mecamylamine may cause constipation and paralytic ileus, muscular weakness, palpitation, anginal pain, acute depressions and bladder atony.
TREATMENT
1. Gradual decreasing of the dose—*not* abrupt discontinuance, which may result in extreme hypertensive rebound.
2. Symptomatic and supportive care.

49 — 444. MECHOLYL (Methacholine)

Mecholyl is sometimes used in the treatment of urinary retention and cardiac arrhythmias. Therapeutic doses, as well as overdosage, may cause nausea and vomiting, generalized weakness, precipitation of asthmatic attacks in susceptible persons and momentary heart block.
TREATMENT
Atropine sulfate slowly intravenously in adequate doses (up to 2 mg.).

49 — 445. MELIA AZEDARACH (Bead Tree, Chinaberry, White Cedar)

The pulpy fruit (and to a lesser extent the leaves and bark) of the Australian variety of this tree is considered to be acutely toxic, although the North American variety is usually classified as nontoxic. The toxic picture, after ingestion, consists of mental confusion, dizziness, syncope and stupor.
TREATMENT
1. Gastric lavage followed by activated charcoal in water through the lavage tube.
2. Saline cathartics.
3. Supportive and symptomatic care.

49 — 446. MENTHOL

Ingestion may cause nausea, vomiting, severe abdominal pain, dizziness, staggering gait, slow respiration, flushed face, sluggishness, sleepiness and, in large amounts in children, coma.

TREATMENT
1. Emetics or gastric lavage.
2. Magnesium sulfate (Epsom salts) as a saline cathartic.
PROGNOSIS.   Complete recovery within a few hours.

49—447. MEPERIDINE HYDROCHLORIDE See 49—245. *Demerol*

The narcotic affects of Demerol can be neutralized by naloxone (Narcan), 0.01 mg. per kilogram of body weight intravenously, repeated as necessary.

49—448. MEPROBAMATE (Equanil, Miltown)

Usual doses may cause drowsiness or excitement, generalized diplopia, muscle weakness, acute hypersensitivity reactions, stomach pain, abdominal cramping and diarrhea.
TREATMENT
1. Withdrawal or reduction of dosage of the drug.
2. Treatment of hypersensitivity reactions (21).
Excessive doses (over 5 gm.) may cause shallow respiration with cyanosis, muscular weakness, loss of reflexes, hypotension and acute mental depression.
TREATMENT
1. Artificial respiration (expired air, or mechanical, after clearing the airway).
2. Emptying of the stomach by emetics or gastric lavage if meprobamate has been ingested in large amounts.
3. Support of the circulation and control of hypotension by caffeine sodiobenzoate or ephedrine sulfate intravenously. Severe cases may require slow intravenous injection of 4 ml. of a 0.2% solution of levarterenol bitartrate (Levophed) or 50 to 100 mg. of metaraminol bitartrate (Aramine) in 1000 ml. of 5% dextrose in saline.
4. Hospitalization for observation and supportive therapy. Hemodialysis may be helpful in extremely severe cases.
Sudden discontinuance can cause acute serious withdrawal symptoms, often magnified by the fact that many habitual users of tranquilizing drugs have prepsychotic tendencies. These symptoms consist of severe headache, persistent insomnia, excessive salivation and epileptiform convulsions. Activation of psychotic tendencies, especially acute depression states which may be presuicidal, has been reported.
TREATMENT
1. Mild cases need only symptomatic care with close supervision and observation at home.
2. Severe cases require hospitalization for symptomatic care and psychiatric evaluation and control.

49—449. MERBROMIN (Mercurochrome) See 49—456. *Mercury Antiseptics*

49—450. MERCAPTANS

Mercaptans are released during the process of petroleum refining. Inhalation of high concentrations of the fumes may cause fever, dyspnea, cyanosis, convulsions and coma.
TREATMENT
1. Removal from exposure.
2. Air or oxygen by face mask and rebreathing bag.
3. Hospitalization for observation for at least 24 hours; delayed pulmonary edema (51) may occur.

49—451. MERCOCREOSOL (Mercresin) See **49—456.** *Mercury Antiseptics*

49—452. MERCURIC CHLORIDE See **49—128.** *Bichloride of Mercury*

49—453. MERCUROCHROME (Merbromin) See **49—456.** *Mercury Antiseptics*

49—454. MERCUROUS CHLORIDE See **49—160.** *Calomel*

49—455. MERCURY

All forms of mercury are toxic if absorbed. This includes metallic mercury, mercurous chloride (calomel), corrosive sublimate, mercurial dyes and mercuric diuretic drugs. About 100 occupations offer definite industrial hazards, usually through inhalation of fumes or dust containing mercury. Fatalities in the home have occurred from fumes from gas heaters and radiators painted with "aluminum" paint. Mercury salts may cause toxic effects by absorption through the intact skin, open wounds, lungs and gastrointestinal tract.

Toxic Signs and Symptoms in industry are generally chronic and may be unrecognized until an acute picture develops or is superimposed. For signs, symptoms and treatment of acute toxicity, see **49—128.** *Bichloride of Mercury.*

49—456. MERCURY ANTISEPTICS

A wide variety of commercial compounds intended to utilize the antiseptic action of mercury are available. The most common are mercocresol (Mercresin), merbromin (Mercurochrome) and thimerosal (Merthiolate). All are relatively nontoxic.

Treatment (if a large amount has been ingested):
1. Empty the stomach by emetics and gastric lavage.
2. Give saline cathartics by mouth.

49—457. MERCURY DIURETICS

The effective irritant diuretic action of certain mercury compounds has led to the medical use of mersalyl (salyrgan), mercurophylline (Mercuzanthin) and many others. All may cause acute toxic signs and symptoms if given too frequently or in excessive doses.

Allergic reactions are characterized by chills, fever, urticaria and, occasionally, bronchospasm and laryngeal edema. For treatment see **21.** *Allergic Reactions.*

Immediate toxicity. Acute symptoms may come on during intravenous injection of the therapeutic dose to which the patient is accustomed. These symptoms consist of apprehension, substernal pain, dyspnea, cyanosis, bradycardia, hypotension, mental confusion, delirium and collapse, probably due to ventricular fibrillation (**26—23**).

Treatment
1. Stop the medication at once.
2. Limit absorption and extension if possible by application of a tourniquet and of ice packs.
3. Administer oxygen therapy by mask and rebreathing bag.
4. Give caffeine sodiobenzoate, 0.5 gm. intramuscularly for circulatory support, repeated as necessary.
5. Hospitalize for observation and symptomatic and supportive care.

Prognosis. Good unless the initial onset has been overwhelming.

Deferred toxicity. Coming on from 1 to 3 hours after injection, this type is characterized by chills and fever, dyspnea, cyanosis, asthmatic symptoms, pulmonary edema and evidence of sodium deficiency.

TREATMENT

1. Oxygen under positive pressure by face mask or endotracheal catheter and rebreathing bag.

2. Epinephrine hydrochloride (Adrenalin) (1:1000 solution) subcutaneously in small doses, repeated as necessary for asthmatic symptoms.

3. Administration of sodium if laboratory tests show depletion.

4. Hospitalization for observation because of the possibility of development of pulmonary edema (**51**).

49—458. MERCURY OXYCYANIDE

Local use as an antiseptic agent can cause severe mucous membrane erosion. If absorbed through mucous membranes or ingested, nausea, vomiting, abdominal pain and collapse may occur. Terminal cases usually die from cyanide poisoning resulting from the action of the gastric hydrochloric acid on the oxycyanide radical.

TREATMENT

See **49—235**. *Cyanides;* **49—128**. *Biochloride of Mercury.*

49—459. MERTHIOLATE (Thimerosal) See **49—456**. *Mercury Antiseptics*

49—460. MESCAL (Peyote)

Intoxication from ingestion of this substance, derived from a certain type of cactus, is sometimes encountered, especially in Mexicans, Indians and Negroes. Also see **49—358**. *Hallucinogens.*

SIGNS AND SYMPTOMS. A rapid fall in blood pressure and hallucinations similar to schizophrenia.

TREATMENT

Symptomatic only. Complete recovery without permanent ill effects occurs in 6 to 8 hours.

49—461. METAL FUMES

Inhalation of high concentrations of freshly formed metallic oxide fumes from smelting, brazing, galvanizing and welding may give rise to a type of poisoning known variously as metal fume fever, brass chills, metal ague, foundry workers' ague, zinc chills, spelter shakes or Monday morning fever. The clinical picture, treatment and prognosis are completely different from those for the toxic symptoms caused by ingestion of the different metals. The following metallic oxides may cause the condition:

Antimony (**49—81**)	Lead (**49—420**)
Beryllium (**49—126**)	Magnesium (**49—434**)
Cadmium (**49—156**)	Manganese (**49—439**)
Cobalt (**49—217**)	Nickel (**49—521**)
Copper (**49—223**)	Zinc (most common) (**49—852**)

SIGNS AND SYMPTOMS (usually coming on from 1 to 3 hours after exposure) consist of profuse perspiration, a peculiar metallic taste in the mouth, dryness of the throat, cough, tightness in the chest, nausea, vomiting, severe general malaise, exhaustion and an elevated temperature [rarely above 39°C. (102.2°F)].

TREATMENT

1. Absolute bed rest.

2. Codeine sulfate and acetylsalicylic acid (aspirin) by mouth every 4 hours.

3. Dextrose, 5% in saline, 500 to 1000 ml. intravenously.
PROGNOSIS.   Complete recovery from the acute phase in 1 to 2 days. Never fatal.

49 – 462. METALDEHYDE (Metafuel)

This toxic substance is a constituent of many snail baits. In the form of compressed
tablets it is used as fuel for small heaters.
SIGNS AND SYMPTOMS (usually a 1 to 3 hour time lag after ingestion before onset).
Salivation, nausea, vomiting, severe abdominal pain, flushed face, high temperature,
muscle twitching and incoordination and coma, sometimes fatal in 5 to 8 hours.
TREATMENT
1. Emetics, followed if necessary by gastric lavage.
2. Magnesium sulfate (Epsom salts), 30 ml. by mouth.
3. Application of external heat.
4. Caffeine sodiobenzoate, 0.5 gm. intramuscularly.
5. Hospitalization for prevention and treatment of liver and kidney damage.

49 – 463. METAPHEN See 49 – 456. *Mercury Antiseptics*

49 – 464. METHADONE (Dextrolevomethadone Hydrochloride, Adanon, Amidon, Butalgin, Diaminon, Dolophen, Hoeschst 10820, Miadone, Polamidon)

Methadone is a potent and long-acting, cumulative synthetic narcotic which has
strong addictive tendencies (2 – 3). The recent increase in treatment of heroin and
morphine addiction with oral methadone, often on an ambulatory basis, has resulted in
a considerable series of acute methadone poisoning, especially in children who are
attracted by the bright orange clover leaf shaped tablets and by methadone-containing
fruit juices. The usual maintenance dose does not cause any ill-effects in a narcotic
addict but can cause extreme respiratory depression in non-addicts.
TREATMENT
1. Empty the stomach immediately by gastric lavage followed by activated charcoal
through the lavage tube. Precautions to prevent aspiration should be taken.
2. Start expired air or mechanical respiration (11 – 1).
3. Give naloxone hydrochloride (Narcan) intravenously, 0.01 mg. per kilogram of
body weight, repeated if necessary in 5 minutes and again in 10 minutes. Naloxone is
the narcotic antagonist of choice because it has no significant respiratory depressant
effect.
4. Maintain adequate hydration by slow intravenous injection of glucose-saline solution (2 parts 5% glucose to 1 part saline), watching carefully for signs of fluid
overload.
5. Hospitalize under close observation until all signs of methadone affect have
cleared – usually about 2 days. Since naloxone hydrochloride (Narcan) has a short
antagonist action (2 to 3 hours) and the respiratory depressant affects of methadone
last for as long as 48 hours, repeated injections of naloxone are necessary to prevent
recurring coma, which may be terminal.
6. Analeptic drugs, hemodialysis and peritoneal dialysis are of no value.

49 – 465. METHANOL See 49 – 475. *Methyl Alcohol*

49 – 466. METHANTHELINE BROMIDE (Banthine)

Ordinary doses may cause acute skin reactions, even exfoliative dermatitis, and an
increase in intraocular tension. Overdosage may cause extreme weakness, loss of
sphincter control, mental confusion and stupor.

TREATMENT
1. Discontinuance of the medication.
2. Symptomatic and supportive care. Full recovery usually occurs.

49–467.   METHAPYRILENE HYDROCHLORIDE (Pyridine HCl, Histadyl HCl, Semikon HCl, Tenalin HCl, etc.)

Usual therapeutic doses of this antihistaminic drug may cause transient nausea, vomiting, headache and nervous tension. Large doses taken by accident or with suicidal intent have caused tetanic jerking, clonic convulsions, cyanosis, pulmonary edema, anuria and death.

TREATMENT
1. Gastric lavage followed by activated charcoal by mouth or through the lavage tube.
2. Saline cathartics.
3. Rapid-acting barbiturates for control of convulsions.
4. Treatment of pulmonary edema (51).

49–468.   METHEDRINE (Methamphetamine Hydrochloride, Desoxyephedrine HCl, Amphedroxyn, Desoxyn, Estimulex, Isophen, Syndrox, etc.)
See 49–64. *Amphetamines;* 49–715. *"Speed-balls"*

49–469.   METHENAMINE (Hexamethylenetetramine, Urotropin)

Toxic signs and symptoms are due to slow decomposition of methenamine into formaldehyde and are characterized by severe diarrhea, pain in the kidney and bladder, painful urination and albumin and blood in the urine.

TREATMENT
1. Emetics and/or gastric lavage followed by activated charcoal in water by mouth or through the lavage tube.
2. Codeine sulfate, morphine sulfate or pentazocine lactate (Talwin) parenterally for control of severe pain.
3. Large amounts of fluid by mouth and/or intravenously.
PROGNOSIS.   Complete recovery without residual ill effects

49–470.   METHIMAZOLE (Marcozole, Tapazole)

Skin rash and other allergic manifestations (21), arthralgia, gastrointestinal irritation, toxic hepatitis and neuropathy with footdrop may occur when methimazole is used in the treatment of hyperthyroidism. Loss of the sense of taste has been reported, as have serious reactive blood changes (Leukopenia, granulocytopenia and agranulocytosis).

TREATMENT
1. Discontinuance of therapeutic use.
2. Symptomatic care (49–4).

49–471.   METHOPHENOBARBITAL (Mephobarbital) See 49–111.
Barbiturates

49–472.   METHORPHINAN HYDROBROMIDE (Dromoran)

Overdosage with this synthetic narcotic gives toxic signs and symptoms similar to but less serious than morphine sulfate (49–495). Response to intravenous administration of the physiologic antagonist, naloxone hydrochloride (Narcan), may be slow, with frequent injections of naloxone required at short intervals.

49 – 473. METHOXYCHLOR

This insecticide is slightly less toxic than DDT, although signs and symptoms of toxicity are more prolonged. Muscular twitching, tremors and acute depression may require symptomatic care. No fatal cases of poisoning from methoxychlor have been reported. For treatment, see **49 – 243.** *DDT.*

49 – 474. METHYL ACETATE

Through inhalation of fumes or by ingestion, this solvent for nitrocellulose, resins and oils may give toxic signs and symptoms similar to methyl alcohol (**49 – 475**).

49 – 475. METHYL ALCOHOL (Methanol, Methyl Hydrate, Carbinol, Wood Alcohol, Wood Spirit, Wood Naphtha, Columbia Spirit, Colonial Spirit)

Widespread use of this toxic liquid as a solvent in industry, in antifreeze mixtures, in the chemical industry and as a fuel makes accidental ingestion fairly common. In addition, many serious cases have been caused by ingestion, by accident or intent, of methyl alcohol in place of ethyl alcohol. There is a wide variation in susceptibility of different individuals, but as little as 60 ml. has been fatal. Inhalation of the fumes also may give an acute toxic picture.

Mild cases are characterized by severe headaches, aching pain in the extremities, nausea, vomiting, gastric pain, dilated sluggish pupils and visual disturbances with temporary (sometimes permanent) blindness. Slow and labored respiration usually is present, often with dyspnea and cyanosis. If marked dyspnea or extreme metabolic acidosis is present, the prognosis is unfavorable.

Severe cases show all the signs and symptoms of mild cases but in greater degree. In addition, there is usually increased reflex hyperexcitability, with trismus, opisthotonos and convulsions, hypotension with a weak rapid pulse and hallucinations – sometimes mania. Acute visual disturbances and eye signs usually become acute 18 to 24 hours after ingestion. These consist of dilated fixed pupils, sometimes responsive to convergence tests but rarely to light, sensitivity of the eyeballs to pressure, painful eye motion, ptosis of the lids and retrobulbar neuritis with partial or complete permanent loss of vision. Acute peripheral neuritis is common.

TREATMENT

1. Gastric lavage with 4% sodium bicarbonate solution followed by activated charcoal in water by mouth or through the lavage tube.

2. Magnesium sulfate (Epsom salts) by mouth or through the lavage tube.

3. Control of severe pain by opiates as needed.

4. Oxygen by face mask and rebreathing bag for dyspnea and cyanosis.

5. Prevention and treatment of metabolic acidosis by intravenous sodium bicarbonate, 1 to 2 mEq. per kilogram of body weight, repeated every 4 hours as necessary.

6. Ethyl alcohol (50% in water, or whiskey, 30 ml. every 3 to 4 hours orally, until acidosis is corrected – continued as necessary for 2 to 3 days.

7. In severe cases hemodialysis may be sight- and lifesaving.

PROGNOSIS. Poor; the mortality rate is high even if relatively small amounts of methyl alcohol have been ingested. Death may be due to respiratory or cardiac failure or to severe kidney damage. If recovery occurs, it is a prolonged process. Residual eye, kidney and heart damage is common.

49 — 476.   METHYL BROMIDE

Acute toxic signs and symptoms from this dangerous volatile liquid (used in fire extinguishers, as a refrigerant and as an insecticide) do not develop for from 4 to 12 hours after inhalation of the fumes. On the skin, methyl bromide causes itching, prickling and blistering, followed by a sensation of cold and the development of the systemic toxic picture after 4 to 6 hours.

SIGNS AND SYMPTOMS. Transient blurred and double vision (sometimes followed by temporary blindness), nausea, vomiting, abdominal pain, sleepiness, loss of memory, profound weakness and slurred speech. Muscular twitching may be present, with incoordination and temporary paralysis. Mental confusion, psychoses, mania and epileptiform convulsions may develop. Pulmonary edema (**51**) or circulatory and/or respiratory collapse may be terminal.

TREATMENT

1. Remove from exposure. Undress the victim and wash contaminated areas of the body with soap and water.

2. If seen during the latent (asymptomatic) period give dimercaprol (BAL), 2.5 mg. per kilogram of body weight every 4 hours for 6 injections.

3. Clear the airway and begin expired air respiration (**11 — 1**) immediately. Substitute administration of oxygen under positive pressure by face mask and rebreathing bag as soon as possible.

4. Administer rapid-acting barbiturates for control of acute excitement or convulsions, preferably intravenously. Preliminary restraint may be required. Oversedation should be avoided.

5. Give caffeine sodiobenzoate, 0.5 gm. intramuscularly or intravenously. Levarterenol bitartrate (Levophed) or metaraminol bitartrate (Aramine) in 1000 ml. of 5% dextrose in saline intravenously may be necessary if circulatory collapse is profound.

6. Hospitalize for observation for at least 48 hours, even if the toxic picture is relatively mild, because of the tendency toward late development of pulmonary edema (**51**). Although severe metabolic acidosis rarely occurs, the cautious administration of alkalies is usually in order. Unlike methyl alcohol blindness (**49 — 475**), the impairment of vision from methyl bromide intoxication is temporary and clears spontaneously.

49 — 477.   METHYL CELLOSOLVE

Used in the leather industry, as a solvent and in stains, paints, enamels, nail polishes and varnishes, the fumes of methyl cellosolve may cause burning of the eyes, severe headache and signs and symptoms of encephalopathy. Severe reactive blood changes also occur.

TREATMENT

1. Stop exposure.

2. Give intravenous fluids.

3. Hospitalization for symptomatic and supportive care and whole blood transfusions.

49 — 478.   METHYL CHLORIDE

This toxic gas is used in refrigeration systems and in the chemical industry. For signs and symptoms of toxicity and treatment, see **49 — 476.** *Methyl Bromide.*

49 — 479.   METHYLENE BLUE See **49 — 297.** *Dyes*

49 – 480. METHYLENE DICHLORIDE

Fumes of this common solvent cause intense eye and mucous membrane irritation with central nervous system depression and pulmonary edema (**51**) if high concentrations have been inhaled.

TREATMENT
1. Removal from exposure.
2. Oxygen under positive pressure by face mask and rebreathing bag.
3. Supportive therapy, especially for pulmonary edema (**51**).

49 – 481. METHYLETHYLKETONE

This is an industrial solvent that on brief contact can cause extreme thickening of the fingernails, with permanent destruction of the nail beds.

TREATMENT is symptomatic only.

49 – 482. METHYL FORMATE

Widely used as a solvent in industry, methyl formate may cause severe toxic effects through absorption from the respiratory tract or by ingestion.

SIGNS AND SYMPTOMS. A feeling of suffocation and constriction of the chest, acute dyspnea and visual disturbances (amblyopia and nystagmus).

TREATMENT
As outlined under **49 – 475.** *Methyl Alcohol.*

49 – 483. METHYL IODIDE

Inhalation of small amounts of the fumes results in acute intoxication with dizziness, sleepiness, irritability and diarrhea. Higher concentrations cause marked nervous system involvement (slurred speech, amblyopia, nystagmus, acute excitement and delirium).

TREATMENT
1. Removal from exposure.
2. Oxygen under positive pressure.
3. Hospitalization for observation since signs of central nervous system involvement may not appear until apparent recovery from acute toxic effects.

49 – 484. METHYLPARAFYNOL (Dormison)

Overdosage with this hypnotic drug has resulted in slow pulse, rapid respiration, hypotension, coma and acute psychosis. For treatment, *see* **49 – 111.** *Barbiturates.* Post-therapy ataxia and apathy often persist for several weeks.

49 – 485. METHYLROSANILINE CHLORIDE (Methyl violet)

Methyl violet is used as an antiseptic and in the leads of indelible pencils. Skin contact may cause acute eczematous and acneform eruptions; contact with the lips may cause cheilitis and gingivitis, with a systemic picture of headache, malaise, vomiting, general weakness and low-grade kidney and liver damage.

Imbedded fragments of indelible pencil leads require immediate excision (**40 – 7.** *Puncture Wounds of the Hand*).

49—486. METHYL SALICYLATE (Oil of Sweet Birch, Teaberry Oil, Oil of Wintergreen)

This pleasant-smelling liquid is used as an aromatic flavoring extract, as a rubefacient in rubbing liniments and ointments, and as an antirheumatic and antiseptic agent. Because of its attractive smell and taste, it is frequently ingested by infants and children, with a very high mortality (about 55%). Absorption through the intact skin also can cause an acute toxic picture. Methyl salicylate is from 10 to 20 times as toxic as acetylsalicylic acid but is much more slowly absorbed from the gastrointestinal tract.

SIGNS AND SYMPTOMS. Odor of wintergreen or acetone on the breath, labored rapid "panting dog" respiration, cyanosis, sleepiness, profuse perspiration, nausea, persistent vomiting, dehydration, thirst, disturbances in sight and hearing, convulsions and coma. Circulatory and respiratory depression may be terminal.

TREATMENT
See **49—664**. *Salicylates.*
PROGNOSIS. Fair in adults; poor in infants and children, especially if hyperpnea is present. Nephritis, toxic hepatitis and acidosis are frequent sequelae.

49—487. METHYSERGIDE MALEATE

This congener of ergonovine is used for prevention of migraine attacks. Its toxic effects are similar to those caused by ergot (**49—306**), plus acute apprehension, excitement, nightmares, hallucinations and precipitation of psychotic states (**50—1**).

TREATMENT
1. Discontinuance of the drug.
2. Sedation as required.
3. Therapy as given under **49—306**. *Ergot.*

49—488. METRAZOL (Cardiazol, Pentylenetetrazol)

Although it is probably the safest of the potent analeptics, in hypersensitive individuals use of pentylenetetrazol (Metrazol) in therapeutic doses may result in brief but extremely violent convulsions and in auricular fibrillation. No treatment is indicated except protection against injury (fractures, dislocations, tongue biting, etc.), until the convulsion ceases. The auricular fibrillation is transient and not dangerous.

49—489. MEXICAN JUMPING BEANS

Diarrhea of varying degrees of intensity, probably caused by surface contaminants, may make a child who eats several of these peculiarly acting beans very uncomfortable and the parents very apprehensive. However, larvae in the beans which cause the "jumping" are harmless. Administration of a saline cathartic and reassurance of the parents are generally all that is required.

49—490. "MICKEY FINN"

Two formulas are occasionally (and illegally) added to alcoholic beverages in some disreputable cocktail lounges and bars to get rid of obstreperous or offensive customers:
Drops: 1 to 2 ml. of croton oil.
Powders; A mixture of powdered jalap and milk sugar.
Both are effective, although in different ways, and, in certain instances, dangerous.

Neither should be confused with "knockout drops," which contain chloral hydrate
(**49—184**) and which usually are administered with a more sinister purpose.

SIGNS AND SYMPTOMS.   An acute burning sensation in the mouth, nausea, violent
vomiting associated with tenesmus, severe abdominal pain, violent diarrhea, cold
clammy skin, weak pulse, hypotension and collapse. Death from respiratory and/or
circulatory failure may occur if an extremely large dose has been given.

TREATMENT

1. Give demulcents (white of eggs, flour, etc.) by mouth as soon as possible.

2. Empty the stomach (if vomiting has not been profuse) by emetics or lavage. Activated charcoal in water should be given orally or through the lavage tube.

3. Institute artificial respiration by expired air or mechanical means (**11—1**) if respiratory depression is severe.

4. Give large amounts of black coffee or strong tea by mouth, or inject caffeine
sodiobenzoate, 0.5 gm. intramuscularly. In extreme cases, support the circulation by
intravenous ephedrine sulfate, levarterenol bitartrate (Levophed) or metaraminol
bitartrate (Aramine).

5. Hospitalize if respiratory or circulatory depression is profound. Sudden collapse
may occur several hours after apparent control of acute signs and symptoms of toxicity.

49—491.   MILTOWN See **49—448.** *Meprobamate*

49—492.   MIPAFOX (Phosphorodiamedic Fluoride)

Used as an insecticide, Mipafox has a toxic effect similar to, but less severe than,
parathion. For symptoms and treatment, see **49—546.** *Organic Phosphates.*

49—493.   MONOCHLOROBENZENE See **49—194.** *Chlorobenzene*

49—494.   MONOSODIUM L-GLUTAMATE (MSG)

Used to enhance the flavor of Chinese food, this substance may cause paresthesias
and a sense of facial pressure, chest pain and (occasionally) severe headache. The
amounts necessary to produce symptoms vary markedly in different individuals, and
in the same same individuals at different times.

These symptoms, although often extremely uncomfortable, are self-limiting and
require no treatment.

49—495.   MORPHINE (See also **2—4.** *Addiction;* **7.** *Narcotics in Emergency Cases;* **29—13.** *Coma—Poisons*)

Acute morphinism may follow ingestion, subcutaneous, intramuscular or intravenous
injection, or (occasionally) absorption of morphine through mucous membranes. If
subcutaneous or intramuscular injections are given to a patient whose circulatory system is extemely depressed (for instance, in severe shock), overwhelmingly cumulative—even lethal—toxic effects may occur when the circulation improves.

SIGNS AND SYMPTOMS.   Pinpoint nonreactive pupils (during terminal asphyxia the
pupils may dilate), subnormal temperature, gradually slowing respiration with slowly
increasing cyanosis and increasing somnolence deepening into coma. Convulsions are
common in children, rare in adults. Collapse from respiratory failure is the final stage.

TREATMENT

1. If seen during the pre-coma stage keep the patient awake and moving if possible.
Muscular activity such as walking is beneficial in mild cases but can be detrimental if

respiratory depression is acute. Strong black coffee by mouth, or caffeine sodiobenzoate, 0.5 gm. intramuscularly or intravenously, may be helpful.

2. If ingested within the past few hours, lavage with 1:5000 potassium permanganate solution or a weak iodine solution (1 ml. of tincture of iodine to 1 liter of water), taking care to avoid aspiration. Attempts at induction of vomiting by emetics are usually unsuccessful and are often dangerous.

3. If only a short time has elapsed after subcutaneous or intramuscular injection into an extremity, apply a tourniquet proximal to the injection site—tight enough to shut off the venous return but not tight enough to interfere with the arterial pulse. An icebag may delay absorption.

4. Combat hypoxemia and cyanosis by expired air methods (11–1) followed by administration of oxygen under positive pressure by face mask or endotracheal catheter and rebreathing bag.

5. Inject naloxone hydrochloride (Narcan) intravenously, 0.01 mg. per kilogram of body weight, repeated in 5 minutes and again in 10 minutes. If marked improvement in the patient's condition does not occur, look for another cause, or causes, for coma (29). If the patient is an addict who is suffering from overdosage, naloxone may bring on acute withdrawal symptoms requiring immediate treatment as outlined in 49–366. *Heroin.*

6. Apply external heat by warm blankets, a bed warmer or cast dryer. Hot water bags should not be used unless other means of applying heat are not available.

7. Correct dehydration and electrolyte imbalance (6), avoiding overhydration. Diuretics are of no value.

8. Treat hypotension.

9. Hospitalize for symptomatic and supportive therapy after control of acute symptoms. Antibiotic therapy for prevention of pneumonia should be considered.

PROGNOSIS. If the patient can be kept alive for 6 to 8 hours, he will usually make a complete recovery, although remissions sometimes occur from reabsorption from the gastrointestinal tract.

Chronic morphinism with withdrawal symptoms (see also 2–4. *Addiction*).

This serious condition is a true emergency. Since many states and countries consider prescribing opiates of any type for an addict a crime, except in extreme emergency or as a lifesaving measure, symptomatic supportive therapy and sedation through barbiturates, paraldehyde and/or phenothiazines is indicated until the patient can be transferred for treatment to a properly accredited institution. A generally recognized exception to this rule is that if the patient has been booked and is in police custody, narcotics may be administered for control of acute withdrawal symptoms. Also, it is becoming increasingly recognized in many parts of the world that persons who seek relief from addiction or from withdrawal symptoms should be treated as patients and not as criminals.

For methadone treatment of morphine addiction and its complications, see 49–464.

49 – 496. MOTHER OF PEARL

Although the osteitis caused by inhalation of mother of pearl dust is usually chronic, flareups may be acute. These flareups consist of sudden acute arthralgia and myalgia, with low-grade fever. Symptomatic treatment usually gives relief.

49 – 497. MOTH REPELLENTS

These may be of several strengths. For slightly toxic repellents, see 49–567. *Paradichlorobenzene;* for moderately toxic kinds, 49–163. *Camphor;* and for extremely toxic types, 49–510. *Naphthalene.*

49 — 498. MOVELLAN (Hydroxystrichnic Acid Hydrochloride)

Therapeutic use as a tonic or use as an abortifacient has resulted in symptoms resembling mild strychnine poisoning.

For toxic picture and treatment, see **49 — 729.** *Strychnine.*

49 — 499. MUCUNA PRURIENS (Cowhage, Cow-itch, Elephant's Scratchwort, Stinging Bean)

The seed pods of this Central American plant contain a proteolytic enzyme which causes transient extremely severe itching, pain and edema of the skin on contact. Symptoms subside rapidly when exposure is terminated.

49 — 500. MUSCARINE

This toxic substance occurs in certain varieties of poisonous mushrooms ("fly mushrooms") and toadstools (**49 — 502**), but not in most fungi.

SIGNS AND SYMPTOMS after ingestion. Rapid onset and course with acute symptoms lasting only 1 to 3 hours. Death from cardiac arrest (**26 — 7**) or complete collapse may occur in a few hours. In nonfatal cases, complete recovery usually occurs in 1 to 2 days. The toxic signs and symptoms are due to parasympathetic stimulation characterized by lacrimation, salivation, miosis, sweating, dyspnea, abdominal pain, vomiting, diarrhea and intense excitement, followed by circulatory and respiratory depression.

TREATMENT

1. Induction of vomiting.

2. Gastric lavage with 1:5000 potassium permanganate solution followed by activated charcoal in water.

3. Subcutaneous or intravenous injection of atropine sulfate, the physiologic antagonist of muscarine. Doses up to 1 mg. may be necessary; repeated until the muscarine effect has been neutralized.

4. Administration of magnesium sulfate (Epsom salts), 30 mg. by mouth.

5. Symptomatic and supportive care.

49 — 501. MUSCLE RELAXANT DRUGS (See also 49 — 234. *Curare*)

The toxic effects of average doses of drugs commonly used for muscle relaxation are uncomfortable but rarely serious. Among these drugs are:

Carisoprodol (Soma, Rela)   Orphenadrine citrate (Norflex)
Chlormethazanone (Trancopal)   Phenyramidol hydrochloride (Analexin)
Chlorzoxazone (Paraflex)   Styramate (Sinaxar)
Methocarbamol (Robaxin)

SIGNS AND SYMPTOMS of toxicity consist of drowsiness, apathy, anorexia, nausea (rarely vomiting), headache, dizziness and dryness of the mouth and throat.

All disappear slowly when the drug is discontinued.

49 — 502. MUSHROOM POISONING

Rapid poisoning. Acute toxic signs and symptoms developing from a few minutes to 3 hours after ingestion and occasionally causing death are usually due to the muscarine contained in *Amanita muscaria* and *Amanita pantherina*. Considerable variation in the degree of toxicity in different localities has been noted; for example, in Switzerland *A. muscaria* ("fly agaric") is considered to be very dangerous, while in Alaska it is eaten by Eskimos as a source of pleasurable intoxication. For treatment, see **49 — 500.** *Muscarine.*

Delayed poisoning. Toxic signs and symptoms coming on 6 to 24 hours after ingestion are almost invariably due to *A. phalloides* and allied forms in the United States and to *A. verna* in Europe. These varieties of bulb agarics account for about 90% of all fatalities from mushroom poisoning; ingestion of the "amanita toxins" has a mortality rate of 50%. A less frequent offender is the Helvella (false morel) (**49—361**), which may cause acute toxic signs and symptoms coming on from 6 to 8 hours after ingestion.

Identification. Members of the amanita family are responsible for practically all cases of serious mushroom poisoning; hence, one simple rule may be lifesaving: *never eat a mushroom that has two swellings on the stalk!* These 2 enlargements—the annulus just below the gills, and the volva at or slightly beneath ground level—are characteristic of the deadly amanita family only; other mushrooms may have 1, but no other important variety has both. An even simpler rule: *Never eat uncultivated mushrooms!*

SIGNS AND SYMPTOMS (after a latent period of 6 hours or more). Sudden severe abdominal pain, nausea, bloody vomitus, diarrhea with blood and mucus, extreme thirst, dehydration and rapidly developing weakness. Apparent marked improvement, usually lasting a few hours may occur, followed by sudden development of acute cyanosis with coldness of the skin of the extremities and collapse of the circulatory system and progressive central nervous system involvement. Death usually occurs 48 to 72 hours after ingestion.

TREATMENT

1. Induction of vomiting by whatever means are necessary, including apomorphine subcutaneously. This is essential so that fragments of the ingested mushroom can be recovered for identification. Vomiting, even if profuse, should be followed by lavage with 1:5000 potassium permanganate solution. Activated charcoal in water should be left in the stomach.

2. Administration of morphine sulfate subcutaneously or intravenously for severe pain and apprehension. Codeine sulfate or meperidine hydrochloride (Demerol) may be of value in less severe cases.

3. Intravenous injection of 500 to 1000 ml. of 10% dextrose in saline to combat dehydration.

4. Emptying of the bowel by magnesium sulfate (Epsom salts).

5. Hospitalization as soon as possible even if apparent improvement has been noted. In severe cases, peritoneal dialysis and hemodialysis may assist in the removal of amanita toxins.

Hallucinogenic effects. Psilocybin, an unsaturated indole, is the active toxic agent in certain varieties of mushrooms used in religious rites in Mexico because of their peculiar ability to produce hallucinations (**49—358**). Recovery in 8 to 10 hours after ingestion is to be expected. No specific treatment is required.

49—503. MUSHROOM "MIASMA"

In certain localities crews engaged in dumping compote and cleaning the bins used in growing mushrooms have developed dryness of the nose and throat lasting about 8 hours, nausea and restlessness, with a burning sensation in the nose and throat. These symptoms are followed after 24 hours by fever, rapid pulse, dry cough, dermatitis (usually involving the nose, the area below the eyes and the scrotum), fever, sweating, chills and chest pain lasting until about the 8th day after exposure. Gradual abatement of signs and symptoms occurs in about 2 weeks. The cause is not known. Symptomatic treatment only is required. No fatalities have been reported.

49—504. MUSSEL POISONING [See also **49—339**. *Rare causes of food poisoning (Mytilotoxism)*]

Poisonous heat-stable alkaloids are present in certain seafoods during certain months. Mussels, clams, oysters or abalone may be affected.

...

SIGNS AND SYMPTOMS. Acute progressive respiratory paralysis coming on without warning generally causes the patient to be brought for emergency care. The diagnosis depends wholly upon the history—usually several members of the same family or party are affected.

TREATMENT

1. Apomorphine hydrochloride, 4 to 5 mg. subcutaneously, as an emetic. The original dose should not be repeated; if apomorphine does not cause vomiting, it may produce extreme respiratory depression requiring intravenous naloxone hydrochloride (Narcan), 0.01 mg. per kilogram of body weight, repeated as necessary.

2. Magnesium sulfate (Epsom salts) as a purgative.

3. Long-continued administration of oxygen under positive pressure by face mask or endotracheal catheter and rebreathing bag. Recovery from respiratory depression with establishment of normal breathing may occur after several hours.

4. Hospitalization for observation and supportive care for at least 24 hours. Relapses are common.

49−505. MUSTARD GAS See 49−832. *War Gases (Vesicants)*

49−506. MYRISTICIN

Myristicin is the active ingredient of oil of nutmeg and nutmeg flower oil. Ingestion of these substances or of 2 or 3 ground nutmegs may cause a rapid pulse, clammy skin, tremors, acute excitement, hallucinations and unconsciousness.

TREATMENT

1. Gastric lavage followed by a saline cathartic.

2. Symptomatic and supportive therapy (49−4).

49−507. NAIL POLISH See 49−74. *Aniline Dyes;* 49−340. *Formaldehyde;* 49−477. *Methyl Cellosolve*

49−508. NAIL POLISH REMOVERS See 49−17. *Acetone*

49−509. NAPHTHA See 49−119. *Benzene and Its Derivatives*

Do not confuse with Naphthol (49−511).

49−510. NAPHTHALENE (Naphthalin, Tar Camphor)

This is the most toxic of the insect repellants commonly found in moth balls. It is also a constituent of some brands of deodorant cakes. Toxic signs and symptoms may be caused in children by contact with clothes that have been stored in mothballs as well as by ingestion.

SIGNS AND SYMPTOMS FOLLOWING INGESTION. Characteristic odor on the breath, nausea, vomiting, gastroenteritis and profound depression, with development after 3 to 7 days of symptoms due to hemolysis.

TREATMENT

1. Give demulcents such as egg white or gelatin. Fatty substances (including milk) should be avoided.

2. Induce vomiting by warm water, ipecac or other emetics. Follow with activated charcoal in water by mouth.

3. Place the patient at absolute rest with application of external heat.

4. Force fluids by mouth or give 500 to 1000 ml. normal salt solution intravenously.

5. Give caffeine sodiobenzoate, 0.5 gm. intramuscularly, for circulatory support.
6. Hospitalize severe cases; deferred hemolysis may require repeated transfusions. Acute renal failure may occur. Peritoneal dialysis may be beneficial.

49—511. NAPHTHOL

Both the alpha and beta isomers of naphthol may give severe toxic signs and symptoms after ingestion as well as after absorption through the intact skin.
SIGNS AND SYMPTOMS.   Nausea, vomiting, convulsions, coma, severe liver, kidney and spleen damage, jaundice, albuminuria and anemia.
TREATMENT
1. If ingested, gastric lavage with 1:5000 potassium permanganate solution.
2. Hospitalization of all cases for observation because of the possibility of serious liver, kidney and spleen damage.

49—512. NAPHTHYLAMINE

The beta isomer of naphthylamine may cause fever and severe bladder irritation after ingestion or inhalation of fumes.
TREATMENT
1. If inhaled, oxygen therapy by face mask and rebreathing bag using positive pressure.
2. If ingested, emetics or gastric lavage with 1:5000 potassium permanganate solution followed by activated charcoal in water orally or through the lavage tube.
3. Referral to a urologist if persistent hematuria or acute dysuria is present.

49—513. NARCISSUS (Daffodil)

Ingestion of the bulbs of these European and North American spring-flowering plants may cause violent vomiting with delayed development of tetanic convulsions.
TREATMENT
1. Emptying the stomach by emetics or gastric lavage, followed by activated charcoal by mouth and a saline cathartic.
2. Control of convulsions by rapid-acting barbiturates.
3. Symptomatic and supportive care. Complete recovery is the rule.

49—514. NARCYLENE See 49—24. *Acetylene*

49—515. NEOARSPHENAMINE (Neosalvarsan) See 49—96. *Arsphenamine*

49—516. NEOCINCHOPHEN See 49—212. *Cinchophen*

49—517. NEOMYCIN (Myfradin) See 49—78. *Antibiotics*

49—518. NEOSTIGMINE BROMIDE (Prostigmin)

Overdosage—especially in the treatment of myasthenia gravis (46—7)—may cause difficult respiration, giddiness, anxiety and muscular twitching.
TREATMENT
1. Administration of the physiologic antagonist, atropine sulfate, in effective doses.
2. Supportive and symptomatic care (49—4).

49 — 519. NERVE GASES See **49 — 546.** *Organic Phosphates;* **49 — 832.** *War Gases*

49 — 520. NIACIN See **49 — 524.** *Nicotinic Acid*

49 — 521. NICKEL (See also **49 — 522.** *Nickel Carbonyl*)

Acute dermatitis, gingivitis and stomatitis may be caused by dust and fumes of nickel and its salts. Removal from contact and symptomatic treatment usually result in rapid recovery.

49 — 522. NICKEL CARBONYL

Inhalation of the fumes of this industrial liquid may result in acute poisoning. More than 1 part of fumes to a million parts of air may cause severe, even fatal, toxic effects characterized by nausea, vomiting, dizziness and severe cephalgia.

TREATMENT

Removal of the patient to fresh air usually results in apparent recovery, but observation for 2 to 3 days is absolutely necessary. Delayed toxic signs and symptoms (latent period of 12 to 30 hours) may develop, with thoracic pain, a feeling of constriction in the chest, severe cough, slow pulse, rapid respirations, dyspnea, cyanosis and convulsions. Enlargement of the liver may be present after even short exposure.

1. Removal from exposure.
2. Oxygen inhalations under positive pressure.
3. Caffeine sodiobenzoate, 0.5 gm. intramuscularly.
4. Calcium gluconate, 10 ml. of 10% solution intravenously, very slowly.
5. Dimercaprol (BAL) intramuscularly, 2.5 mg. per kilogram of body weight every 4 hours for 2 days.
6. Hospitalization for observation and treatment because of the possibility of delayed development of severe brain, lung and liver damage.

PROGNOSIS. Good in most cases. If convulsions or cyanosis is present, the chances of bronchopneumonia are much increased.

49 — 523. NICOTINE (See also **49 — 210.** *Cigarettes and Cigars;* **49 — 790.** *Tobacco*)

Nicotine poisoning is characterized by depression; muscular weakness; prostration; pupils first contracted, then dilated; nausea; vomiting; profuse diarrhea; dyspnea; tachycardia and muscular tremors, followed by convulsions.

TREATMENT

1. Gastric lavage at once with 1:5000 potassium permanganate solution. Speed is essential because nicotine is absorbed very rapidly. Activated charcoal in water should be given by mouth or through the lavage tube.
2. Caffeine sodiobenzoate, 0.5 gm. intramuscularly or intravenously.
3. Application of heat.
4. Control of convulsions by small doses of rapid-acting barbiturates.
5. Artificial respiration and oxygen therapy started as soon as possible and continued until dyspnea has cleared.

49 — 524. NICOTINIC ACID (Niacin)

Used as a preservative in foods and as a medication, nicotinic acid may give toxic signs and symptoms in both therapeutic and excessive doses.

SIGNS AND SYMPTOMS are characterized by a sensation of heat starting in the face and spreading to arms and hands, then to the body, especially the perianal region; flushing of the face; generalized itching and vague, nonlocalized abdominal discomfort.

Although the effects are uncomfortable, complete recovery in 1 to 1½ hours always takes place.

49 – 525. NITRATES

Nitrates are used for many purposes in industry, especially in the processing and pickling of meat products. Contamination of well water with organic matter may cause sufficient concentration of nitrates to give toxic signs and symptoms. Fatalities have been reported from inhalation of silage gases. Potassium nitrate is a constituent of many asthma remedies (40 – 103).

Small doses may cause methemoglobinemia and resultant cyanosis. Breaking down of nitrates to nitrites by bacterial action in the intestine is the causative factor. For signs and symptoms of nitrite toxicitity, see 49 – 528. *Nitrites.*

Large doses may cause nausea and vomiting, with tenesmus, bloody diarrhea and generalized weakness, cardiac irregularities, dysuria and hematuria, convulsions and collapse – sometimes death.

TREATMENT

See 49 – 528. *Nitrites.*

49 – 526. NITRIC ACID See 49 – 26. *Acids*

49 – 527. NITRIC OXIDE (NO) See 49 – 553. *Oxides of Nitrogen*

49 – 528. NITRITES (See also 49 – 525. *Nitrates*)

Poisoning from nitrites may occur through inhalation or through ingestion.

SIGNS AND SYMPTOMS of nitrite poisoning consist of flushing of the face, dyspnea, cyanosis, a slow, weak and irregular pulse and sudden collapse with extreme hypotension.

TREATMENT

1. Gastric lavage with 1:5000 potassium permanganate solution if ingested. Activated charcoal in water should be left in the stomach.

2. Oxygen inhalations for dyspnea and cyanosis.

3. Treatment of shock (53 – 7).

4. Methylene blue, 1% solution in 1.8% sodium sulfate solution, 50 ml. (1 to 2 mg. per kilogram of body weight) intravenously.

5. Hospitalization in severe cases or if methylene blue solution has been given. Transfusions with whole blood or plasma expanders may be necessary. Epinephrine hydrochloride (Adrenalin) and other vasoconstrictor drugs are contraindicated.

49 – 529. NITROBENZENE (Oil of Almond, Oil of Mirbane)

Nitrobenzene is a common ingredient in shoe polishes and dyes, often in combination with aniline dyes (49 – 74). Ingestion may cause tinnitus, vertigo, incoordination, nausea, vomiting, dyspnea, cyanosis, convulsions and coma.

TREATMENT

1. Gastric lavage with normal salt solution followed by activated charcoal in water orally or through the lavage tube.

2. Oxygen inhalations.

3. Dextrose, 5% in saline, 500 to 1000 ml. intravenously.
4. Methylene blue, 1% solution in 1.8% sodium sulfate solution, 50 ml. intravenously, for cyanosis.
5. Saline cathartics.
6. Hospitalization for symptomatic and supportive therapy because of the tendency toward delayed development of cardiac, hepatic and renal damage.

49—530. NITROCHLOROBENZENE

Ingestion may cause rapid onset of staggering gait, pallor or cyanosis from the formation of methemoglobinemia, dyspnea, excitement and hallucinations.

Inhalation may cause a similar picture except that the toxic effects usually are less severe and do not become apparent for 1 to 2 hours.

TREATMENT
See **49—529.** *Nitrobenzene.*

49—531. NITROFURAZONE (Furacin, Vabrocid)

Used as a bacteriostatic agent, nitrofurazone on surface application may cause maculopapular and vesicular rashes and occasionally exfoliative dermatitis. Symptoms clear slowly when topical use is discontinued.

49—532. NITROGEN

Short exposure to high concentrations of nitrogen causes dizziness and dyspnea; prolonged exposure may result in unconsciousness and respiratory arrest.

TREATMENT
1. Removal from exposure.
2. Expired air ventilation (**11—1**) followed by oxygen under positive pressure by face mask and rebreathing bag.
3. Supportive and symptomatic care.

49—533. NITROGEN DIOXIDE (NO$_2$) See **49—553.** *Oxides of Nitrogen*

49—534. NITROGEN MUSTARD (Dichloren, Mustine, Mustargen)

Industrial exposure has resulted in acute skin reactions, liver damage and bone marrow depression. Overdosage in the treatment of Hodgkin's disease and lymphosarcoma may result in severe psychoses, leukemia, thrombocytopenia and bone marrow abnormalities.

TREATMENT
1. Discontinuance of industrial exposure or therapeutic use.
2. Symptomatic care—usually long term.

49—535. NITROGEN TETROXIDE (N$_2$O$_4$) See **49—553.** *Oxides of Nitrogen*

49—536. NITROGLYCERIN See **49—528.** *Nitrites*

49—537. NITROPRUSSIDE

Accidental or suicidal ingestion may result in pallor, mydriasis and respiratory paralysis.

TREATMENT
1. Gastric lavage followed by activated charcoal in water by mouth on through the lavage tube.
2. Saline cathartics.
3. Respiratory support.

49 – 538.   NITROUS OXIDE (N₂O) See **49 – 70.** *Anesthetics, Inhalation*

49 – 539.   NOVOCAIN (Procaine) See **49 – 72.** *Anesthetics, Local*

49 – 540.   NUX VOMICA See **49 – 729.** *Strychnine*

49 – 541   NYLON

Certain individuals develop transient skin erythema, hyperhydrosis and whitened erythematous patches on the soles of the feet from contact with nylon.

49 – 542.   OBESITY "CURES" See **49 – 64.** *Amphetamines;* **49 – 111.**
Barbiturates; **49 – 272.** *Digitalis;* **49 – 771.** *Thiazide Diuretics;*
49 – 785. *Thyroid*

49 – 543.   OILS

Of Absinthe. See **49 – 8.** *Absinthe.*
Of Almond (Artificial). See **49 – 529.** *Nitrobenzene.*
Of Apiol. See **49 – 811.** *Triorthocresyl Phosphate.*
Of Argemone. See **49 – 87.**
Banana. See **49 – 66.** *Amyl Acetate.*
Beechnut. See **49 – 114.**
Of Betula. See **49 – 486.** *Methyl Salicylate.*
Of Bitter Almond. See **49 – 65.** *Amygdalin;* **49 – 235.** *Cyanides.*
Of Cajeput. See *Oil, Essential* (below); **49 – 213.** *Cineol.*
Camphorated. See **49 – 163.** *Camphor.*
Cashew Nut. See **49 – 176. 54 – 16.** *Urushiols.*
Castor. See **49 – 177.**
Of Cedar. See **49 – 180.** *Cedar Oil.*
China. See **49 – 584.** *Peru Balsam.*
Chinawood. See **49 – 814.** *Tung Oil and Nuts.*
Coal. See **49 – 408.** *Kerosene.*
Croton. See **49 – 232.**
Diesel. See **49 – 408.** *Kerosene.*
Essential
    Oils of absinthe, apiol, cajeput, cedar, eucalyptus, menthol, nutmeg, pennyroyal, rue, savin and tansy are complex mixtures of alcohols, esters, ketones and hydrocarbons. Ingestion of very small amounts (less than 30 ml.) may be fatal. The signs and symptoms of toxicity are similar to those under Eucalyptol (**49 – 325**) and Turpentine (**49 – 815**). Treatment follows the same lines.
Of Eucalyptus. See **49 – 325.** *Eucalyptol.*
Fuel. See **49 – 408.** *Kerosene.*
Of Gautheria. See **49 – 486.** *Methyl Salicylate.*
Gingilli. See **49 – 681.** *Sesame Oil.*

"Hell." See **49—405.** *Jatropha Nut Oil.*

Jatropha Nut. See **49—405.**

Kerosene. See **49—408.**

Laurel. See **49—414.**

Lemon Grass. See **49—421.**

Linseed, Contamination of. See **49—430.** *Lolium Temulentum.*

Lubricating

In general, the toxicity of lubricating oils varies inversely with their viscosities. Treatment following ingestion of lighter grades should follow that outlined for *Kerosene* (**49—408**); for heavier grades, all that is required is gastric lavage and administration of saline cathartics.

Macassar. See **49—660.** *Safrole.*

Mineral

Habitual use may cause fibrosis of the lung or pneumonia. The section of the lung involved depends on the user's position in bed after his nightly dose.

Of Mirbane. See **49—529.** *Nitrobenzene.*

Of Nutmeg. See **49—506.** *Myristicin.*

Nutmeg Flower. See **49—506.** *Myristicin.*

Olive, Adulteration of. See **49—405.** *Jatropha Nut Oil.*

Pear. See **49—66.** *Amyl Acetate.*

Of Pennyroyal. See **49—959.** *Pennyroyal.*

Of Peppermint. See **49—446.** *Menthol.*

Pine. See **49—608.**

Prickly Poppy. See **49—87.** *Argemone Oil.*

Of Rosemary. See **49—654.**

Of Rue. See *Oil, Essential* (above).

Of Saffron. See **49—659.**

Of Sage. See **49—661.**

Of Sassafras. See **49—660.** *Safrole.*

Of Savin. See *Oil, Essential* (above).

Sesame. See **49—681.**

Of Sweet Birch. See **49—486.** *Methyl Salicylate.*

Of Tansy. See **49—741.** *Tanacetum Vulgare.*

Teaberry. See **49—486.** *Methyl Salicylate.*

Terpene. See **49—754.** *Terpineol.*

Tung. See **49—814.** *Tung Oil and Nuts.*

Turkey Red. See **49—405.** *Jatropha Nut Oil.*

Turpentine. See **49—815.**

Of Vitriol (Sulfuric Acid). See **49—26.** *Acids.*

Volatile. See *Oil, Essential* (above).

Of Wintergreen. See **49—486.** *Methyl Salicylate.*

Wormseed. See **49—182.** *Chenopodium.*

49—544. OLEANDER

Chewing the leaves, flowers or bark of this common ornamental shrub may result in fatal poisoning. Cases have been reported from eating food roasted while spitted on oleander sticks. There is usually a time lag of 2 to 5 hours before the onset of nausea, vomiting, severe abdominal pain, localized cyanosis of the ears, lips and fingertips and cold perspiration. The respiration becomes shallow and weak and the temperature subnormal; hypotension develops. Pinpoint nonreactive pupils and increasing sleepiness are followed by coma and collapse, with death from acute respiratory paralysis.

TREATMENT

1. Gastric lavage with 1:5000 potassium permanganate solution followed by activated charcoal in water or through the lavage tube.

2. Magnesium sulfate (Epsom salts) by mouth.

3. Oxygen inhalations under positive pressure by face mask or catheter and rebreathing bag.

4. Caffeine sodiobenzoate, 0.5 gm. intramuscularly or intravenously.

5. Dextrose, 5% in saline, 500 to 1000 ml. intravenously. If hypotension is extreme, levarterenol bitartrate (Levophed) or metaraminol bitartrate (Aramine) should be added to the dextrose in saline and given slowly until a satisfactory blood pressure level is obtained.

6. Hospitalization for supportive care.

49—545. OPIUM [Laudanum (Tincture of Opium); Paregoric (Camphorated Tincture of Opium)] (See also 2—4. *Addiction, 7. Narcotics; 49—495. Morphine*)

The milky exudate of the unripe capsules of certain varieties of poppy (Papaver Somniterum and Papaver Album DeC) contains a complex mixture of toxic alkaloids, the most important of which is morphine (**49—495**). Opium eating and smoking, common in the Orient, give similar pictures to injection of morphine, although withdrawal symptoms may be more severe and more resistant to treatment.

TREATMENT
See **49—495**. *Morphine.*

49—546. ORGANIC PHOSPHATES (See also **49—832**. *War Gases*)

Originally developed for wartime use, organic phosphate esters are now used as insecticides and pesticides by spraying and dusting, often by airplane. Accidental contamination of bulk cereal foods has been responsible for fatalities. The clinical picture may be confused with asthma (**52—1**), encephalitis (**48—24, 62—1; 62—5**), food poisoning [especially botulism (**49—141**) and mushroom poisoning (**49—502**)], pilocarpine intoxication (**49—607**) and heat exhaustion (**57—3**).

Common compounds

Azodrin	Fenthion (Baytex)
Bidrin	Gruthion
Chlorthion	Malathion
Ciodrin	Metacide
Co-ral	OMPA
Delnay	Parathion
Demeton (Systox)	Paroxon
Dialkylphosphate	Phosdrin
Diazinon	Phosphamidon
Dibrom	Ronnel (Korlan)
Dicapthon	Sulfotepp
Dimethoate	TEPP (Bladex, Tetrin)
Dipterix (Trichlorfon)	Thimet
Di-Syston	Trithion
EPN	

All of these compounds are available under numerous trade names. Each must bear a label stating the name and amount of each toxic constituent.

Mode of action. In all of these compounds the organic phosphorus-containing portion of the molecule is strongly cholinesterase-inhibiting; hence, the accumulation of acetylcholine in the body may result in stimulation of the entire parasympathetic nervous system [muscarine effect (**49—500**) and nicotine effect (**49—523**)]. Acquired sensitivity to or tolerance for these compounds has not been reported, and skin lesions do not occur. There is marked variation in the toxicity of the various compounds and in the amounts required to cause toxic effects in different individuals.

Entrance into the body may be through the intact skin, by inhalation or by ingestion.

Incidence of poisoning. Anyone who comes in contact with dust-spraying or dusting apparatus or plants or vegetables to which organic phosphate preparations have been applied within 30 days may develop toxic signs and symptoms. Poisoning has occurred in:

Agricultural, greenhouse and nursery workers; formulators, packagers and distributors.

Crop dusters (pilots, flagmen and mechanics; persons servicing equipment used in application).

Occupants of houses in or near treated areas, especially to the leeward; children playing in or near treated areas.

Persons handling contaminated clothing (housewives, laundry workers, etc.).

Travelers passing the fields during application; casual trespassers.

Beekeepers.

Time of onset of toxic effects varies from 15 minutes to 24 hours – most commonly within $1/2$ hour of exposure or while in bed at night. Exposure may not take place until a workman changes his contaminated clothing at the end of the day's work. If an individual gives a history of exposure within 24 hours to any of the organic phosphate (phosphate ester) pesticides and presents, even mildly, any of the signs and symptoms listed below (especially severe headache, fixed contracted pupils and rapid respiration), treatment should be begun at once. Laboratory tests are of no value as an emergency measure, but a specimen of vomitus or of material obtained on gastric lavage should be saved for later analysis.

SIGNS AND SYMPTOMS OF ORGANIC PHOSPHATE (PHOSPHATE ESTER) POISONING. Premonitory indications are headache, fatigue, giddiness, nausea, salivation, lacrimation and excessive perspiration. Acute toxic signs and symptoms ($1/2$ to 1 hour after the premonitory stage) are dim vision, fixed miosis, dizziness, fainting, severe headache, rapid difficult breathing, vomiting (with or without diarrhea) and increasing cyanosis. Severe poisoning is indicated by sphincter incontinence, muscular twitching, tonic convulsions, respiratory failure, pulmonary edema (**51**), total collapse and death.

TREATMENT

1. Respiratory support by insurance of a patent airway, removal of secretions by suction and administration of oxygen under positive pressure. Tracheostomy may be necessary. Pulmonary edema may occur and require therapy (**51**).

2. Decontamination. All clothing should be removed and the skin, hair and nails washed thoroughly with soap and water. The eyes should be irrigated for 5 to 10 minutes with normal saline or water. *Attendants must wear rubber gloves and protective clothing.*

3. Atropine sulfate parenterally in large doses. Mild cases usually require 1 to 2 mg. intravenously or intramuscularly, repeated whenever symptoms reappear. Patients with severe cases should be given 2 to 4 mg. intravenously every 5 to 10 minutes until signs of atropinization appear and then every 30 to 60 minutes until the toxic effects of the organic phosphate subside – often many hours. Dosages for children should be adjusted by age or weight (**4**). Poisoned persons commonly receive too little, practically never too much, atropine.

4. 2-PAM (Protopam chloride). Although this drug is a specific chemical antidote for organic phosphates, it should be used as an adjunct to, not as a substitute for, large doses of atropine. In mild cases, 0.5 gm. should be given slowly intravenously. Severe cases require 1 gm. intravenously, followed in 30 minutes by 0.5 gm. [dosage by age or weight in children (**4**)].

5. If the material has been ingested and there has not been profuse vomiting, institute gastric lavage with warm water only, followed by activated charcoal and a saline cathartic.

6. Hospitalization as soon as possible if seen during the prodromal or premonitory

stage but not until an adequate dose of atropine (No. 3, above) has been administered. Since onset of acute toxic symptoms may be terminal if proper symptomatic and supportive treatment is not given at once, the patient should, if possible, be accompanied during transportation to an emergency hospital by a physician, registered nurse or other trained attendant. Close observation in the hospital for at least 48 hours after the disappearance of acute symptoms, or after the last injection of atropine sulfate or 2-PAM, is essential.

Do not give

1. Natural or synthetic narcotics of any type.
2. Apomorphine hydrochloride or ipecac as an emetic.
3. Barbiturates or phenothiazines. If sedation is necessary, chloral hydrate rectally or paraldehyde intramuscularly in the smallest effective doses should be used. Need for extreme sedation indicates that atropinization is not adequate.
4. Calcium gluconate, aminophylline, theophylline or chlorotheophylline.
5. Large amounts of fluids intravenously.
6. Atropine or 2-PAM for first aid or prophylactic use – either drug may mask prodromal symptoms or give a false sense of security and thus prevent prompt medical treatment.

PROGNOSIS. Poor, unless the condition is recognized and given proper emergency treatment at once. Good, if proper immediate treatment is given – complete recovery without residual ill effects usually occurs even after severe exposure. After plasma and red cell cholinesterase are normal, the patient can usually be allowed to return to his regular work with the warning that any exposure to organic phosphates should be avoided for several months.

49 – 547. ORRIS (White Flag)

The powdered rhizomes of certain varieties of iris, used in adhesive plaster, cosmetics and tooth powders, contain substances which may cause skin reactions, rhinitis and acute asthmatic symptoms which clear rapidly when exposure is terminated.

49 – 548. ORTHODICHLOROBENZENE

For treatment of toxic effects of this wood preservative, See **49 – 510.** *Naphthalene.*

49 – 549. OSMIUM TRIOXIDE (Osmic Acid)

Contact of osmium preparations with the skin causes intense dermatitis with black discoloration. Inhalation of the fumes results in acute eye, nose and throat irritation, bronchitis and pneumonia and, occasionally, hematuria and other evidences of kidney damage.

TREATMENT

1. Removal from the skin by thorough washing.
2. Removal from exposure to fumes, followed by oxygen inhalations.
3. Close observation because of the danger of delayed development of pneumonia and nephritis.

49 – 550. OUABAIN

The toxic effects of this rarely used digitalis-like alkaloid are much greater and less predictable than the more frequently used digitalis preparations. See **49 – 272.** *Digitalis.*

49–551. OXALATES See **49–552.** *Oxalic Acid;* **49–617.** *Potassium Oxalate*

49–552. OXALIC ACID

This acid is the active agent in many household bleaching and cleansing preparations and in some ink eradicators. It also occurs in the leaves and blades (not the stalks) or rhubarb plants (**49–651**), and in the leaves of a common household plant, dieffenbachia (**49–266**). *Treatment of oxalic acid ingestion does not follow the outline given under acids* (**49–26**).

SIGNS AND SYMPTOMS. Burning of the mouth, throat and esophagus; dysphagia; rapid weak pulse; cold clammy skin; bloody vomitus caused by erosion of the gastric mucosa and violent diarrhea and subsequent acute dehydration.

TREATMENT

1. Have the patient swallow large amounts of calcium lactate, lime water (0.15% calcium hydroxide solution), chalk (or plaster off the wall if necessary), egg white, liquid petrolatum or olive oil. *Do not* include vomiting or pass a stomach tube if concentrated oxalic acid has been swallowed and there is any evidence of mucosal erosion. In mild cases, cautious gastric lavage with a large amount of lime water may be done. *Do not* give the usual alkalies used to neutralize strong acids; they form salts with oxalic acid which may be more corrosive than the acid itself.

2. Inject 10 to 20 ml. of calcium gluconate (10% solution) slowly intravenously; repeated as necessary to prevent hypocalcemic tetany.

3. Apply external heat. Force fluids by mouth to promote diuresis.

4. Support the circulation by cautious intravenous injection of isotonic saline solution. Caffeine sodiobenzoate, 0.5 gm. intramuscularly, or ephedrine sulfate, metaraminol bitartrate (Aramine) or levarterenol bitartrate (Levophed) intravenously may be necessary if circulatory collapse is extreme.

5. Control severe pain by morphine sulfate subcutaneously.

6. Hospitalize as soon as the patient's condition will allow. Acute edema of the glottis may require tracheostomy (**14–12**) before transfer. Esophageal strictures may occur, as may serious renal damage.

49–553. OXIDES OF NITROGEN

All of these substances are volatile and all can cause acute toxic symptoms following inhalation of relatively small amounts.

Exposure to toxic concentrations may occur in commercial production of explosives, nitrocellulose and photographic and x-ray films, photoengraving, metal etching and pickling, welding and oxyacetylene operations, use of the carbon arc and in silo cleaning. Decomposition of nitrates in silage may result in a fatal concentration of nitrogen oxides.

Modes of toxic action

Anesthetic action. See **49–70.** *Anesthetics, Inhalation.* This is unimportant in industry since nitrous oxide is never present in high enough concentration to cause anesthetic symptoms.

Nitrite action resulting from breaking down of NO, NO_2 and N_2O_4 in the lungs. See **49–528.** *Nitrites.*

Local irritative and corrosive action in the lungs due to NO_2 and N_2O_4.

Clinical types of toxic reactions

Shock type. Immediate death from asphyxia may occur. There is generally no time for treatment of any kind.

Irritant gas type. This type is characterized by an immediate burning sensation in the mouth and throat, with violent nonproductive cough. A latent period of up to 24 hours may follow, with secondary development of severe, frequently fatal, pulmonary edema (**51**). If the patient survives the initial acute symptoms, pneumonia or pulmonary fibrosis is a frequent complication.

Reversible type. This type is characterized by mild respiratory irritation, with nausea, vomiting, vertigo, severe dyspnea, cyanosis and syncope. These persons generally recover spontaneously and completely.

Combined type. Various combinations of the types outlined above.

TREATMENT

1. Immediate termination of exposure. The patient should be instructed to breathe deeply and rapidly.

2. In any case where a history of possible exposure is obtained, the patient should be at complete rest and comfortably warm. Immediate transfer to a hospital by ambulance should be arranged with symptomatic treatment (cleansing and insurance of the patency of the airway, administration of air or oxygen under pressure, supportive measures, etc.) continued during transfer.

3. Morphine sulfate intramuscularly in small doses to alleviate dyspnea and anxiety.

4. Removal of frothy, foamy exudate from the respiratory tract by suctioning, postural drainage and sodium bicarbonate–sodium chloride aerosols.

5. Treatment of extreme venous congestion by rotating tourniquets.

6. Penicillin and broad spectrum antibiotics if there is evidence of respiratory infection.

49 — 554. OXOPHENARSINE HYDROCHLORIDE (Mapharsen) See 49 — 96. *Arsphenamine and Neoarsphenamine*

49 — 555. OXYGEN (See also 49 — 653. *Rocket Fuels*)

In addition to retrolental fibroplasia in premature infants, high concentrations of oxygen can cause pulmonary hyaline membrane disease to develop shortly after birth in full-term infants. In adults, prolonged administration of concentrations of 60% or more can cause severe cough and acute chest pain associated with decreased vital capacity. In persons with chronic pulmonary disease, oxygen may cause a decrease in respiration by "washing out" of carbon dioxide.

Inhalation of oxygen at high pressures may cause severe poisoning in flyers and in professional and sport divers (**23 — 5**).

SIGNS AND SYMPTOMS.   Restlessness; nervousness; extreme hilarity; impaired cerebration, judgment and sensation and muscle fibrillation and spasm, followed by severe convulsions.

TREATMENT

1. Rescue.

2. Artificial respiration (**11 — 1**) *at once* by expired air or mechanical methods if cyanosis is present.

3. Immediate transfer to a pressure chamber for recompression if the patient has become unconscious while diving with any type of gas-filled apparatus (**23 — 5**). Artificial respiration must be continued en route.

49 — 556. OXYQUINOLINE DERIVATIVES

Overdosage of these amebicides may result in acute symptoms which are practically never fatal provided proper treatment is obtained.

SIGNS AND SYMPTOMS.   Nausea, vomiting, upper abdominal pain (sometimes severe enough to be mistaken for an acute surgical condition) and hepatitis (with or without jaundice).

TREATMENT
1. Stop administration of the drug at once.
2. Give 5% dextrose in water, 500 to 1000 ml. intravenously.
3. Sedate by barbiturates as needed. Morphine sulfate may be given subcutaneously or slowly intravenously if the pain is severe.
4. Hospitalize severe cases.
5. Instruct the patient in use of a high carbohydrate diet.
6. Arrange for follow-up care if evidence of hepatitis is present.

49−557. OXYTETRACYCLINE (Terramycin) See 49−78. Antibiotics

49−558. OZONE

Consumable electrode welding has resulted in an increase in the number of cases of acute ozone poisoning. In addition, ozone-producing equipment, allegedly of therapeutic benefit, may give toxic concentrations of ozone (more than 0.1 part per million of air).

SIGNS AND SYMPTOMS. Headache, lethargy, generalized malaise, persistent (usually nonproductive) cough, and chest pain−sometimes severe enough to be mistaken for the pain caused by a myocardial or pulmonary infarct. There are usually only minimal clinical and x-ray findings in spite of the acute clinical picture.

TREATMENT
1. Remove from exposure.
2. Control restlessness and pain by administration of sedatives and anodynes orally. Severe cases may require subcutaneous injections of small doses of meperidine hydrochloride (Demerol) or morphine sulfate for relief of pain.
3. Give oxygen inhalations under positive pressure by face mask and rebreathing bag if dyspnea is acute or accompanied by cyanosis.
4. Keep under observation until acute symptoms have subsided. Delayed pulmonary edema (51) may occur.

49−559. PAINT See 49−90. Arsenic; 49−207. Chromates, Chromic Acid, Chromium Trioxide; 49−349. Gasoline; 49−408. Kerosene; 49−420. Lead Salts; 49−475. Methyl Alcohol; 49−477. Methyl Cellosolve; 49−787. Titanium Tetrachloride; 49−815. Turpentine

White lead (a basic carbonate) and red lead (the tetroxide) are the bases of many paints. Petroleum solvents give toxic signs and symptoms similar to gasoline and kerosene. Harmless titanium salts are the base of many modern inside house paints.

49−560. PAINT REMOVERS See 49−17. Acetone; 49−119. Benzene (Benzol) and Its Derivatives; 49−173. Carbon Tetrachloride; 49−260. Dichloroethane; 49−432. Lye; 49−475. Methyl Alcohol; 49−481. Methylethylketone; 49−815. Turpentine

49−561. PAMAQUINE NAPHTHOATE

Under the trade name of Plasmochin, this drug is used for specific antimalaria therapy. Excessive or prolonged dosage may cause dizziness, drowsiness, cyanosis and jaundice.

TREATMENT
1. Stop administration of the drug.

2. Give oxygen therapy under positive pressure for cyanosis.

3. Inject methylene blue, 50 ml. of a 1% solution in 1.8% sodium sulfate solution intravenously.

4. Hospitalize severe cases for symptomatic care. Permanent ill effects are rare.

49 — 562. PANTOPON

Containing about 50% morphine, Pantopon is a mixture of opium alkaloids which is used as an analgesic and narcotic.

TREATMENT

See **49 — 495.** *Morphine.*

49 — 563. PAPER PRODUCTS

Ornamental paper products, such as colored crepe, are often sucked or chewed by children. They are not toxic.

49 — 564. PARA-BROMOANILINE

Absorption through the intact skin may cause headache, dizziness, cyanosis and coma.

TREATMENT

1. Prolonged washing of the exposed part of the body with soap and water.

2. Treatment of systemic effects as outlined in **49 — 73.** *Aniline.*

49 — 565. PARACHLOROMETACRESOL (PCMC)

Although ordinary commercial concentrations do not cause skin irritation, ingestion gives a toxic picture similar to that from phenol (**49 — 590**).

49 — 566. PARACHLOROMETAXYLENOL (PCMX)

This complex insecticide can give an acute picture by penetration of the skin as well as by ingestion. For toxic signs, symptoms and treatment, see **49 — 590.** *Phenol.*

49 — 567. PARADICHLOROBENZENE (PDB)

This is the least toxic of the active agents used in moth repellent balls and flakes. Ingestion rarely causes acute toxicity, but prolonged exposure to fumes may be serious.

TREATMENT

See **49 — 510.** *Naphthalene.*

49 — 568. PARALDEHYDE

Although this effective sedative has a large margin of safety, some hypersensitive patients react unfavorably to even small doses. Paraldehyde solutions deteriorate rapidly in the presence of light, with formation of toxic products.

SIGNS AND SYMPTOMS.   Sudden onset of rapid pulse, accelerated respiration, cyanosis, coma and cardiac and respiratory failure.

TREATMENT

1. Gastric lavage with 1:5000 potassium permanganate followed by activated charcoal in water by mouth or through the lavage tube.

  2. Saline cathartics.
  3. Oxygen therapy by face mask and rebreathing bag for cyanosis.
  4. Caffeine sodiobenzoate, 0.5 gm. intramuscularly.
  5. Symptomatic and supportive care (**49 – 4**). Complete recovery usually occurs.

49 – 569.   PARASULFONEDICHLORAMIDOBENZOIC ACID (Halazone)

Combined with borates and sodium chloride, this complex substance is marketed in tablet form as a drinking water purifier and sterilizer. Accidental ingestion of a large number of tablets has been reported as causing a bizarre toxic picture with coma, tremors, convulsions, hyperreflexia, positive Babinski and amnesia lasting for several days.
TREATMENT
  1. Gastric lavage followed by activated charcoal in water and a saline cathartic.
  2. Control of convulsions by rapid-acting barbiturates.
  3. Close observation and symptomatic care. Recovery is usually slow but complete.

49 – 570.   PARATHION (Alkron, E605, Niran, Paraphos, Thiophos)

This compound is one of the most toxic of the organic phosphate insecticides. See **49 – 546.** *Organic Phosphates.*

49 – 571.   PAREGORIC (Camphorated Tincture of Opium) See **7.** *Narcotics;* **49 – 495.** *Morphine;* **49 – 812.** *Tripelennamine Hydrochloride ("Blue Velvet")*

49 – 572.   PARIS GREEN (Copper Acetoarsenate, Schweinfurth Green) See **49 – 90.** *Arsenic*

49 – 573.   PARTHENOCISSUS QUINQUEFOLIA (Virginia Creeper, American Woodbine, False Grape, Wild Wood Vine)

Although this North American climbing vine is usually considered to be nontoxic, chewing the leaves and eating the berries has caused violent vomiting, diarrhea, stupor and collapse.
TREATMENT
  1. Emetics or gastric lavage followed by activated charcoal in water orally or through the lavage tube.
  2. Sedatives.
  3. Supportive and symptomatic care.

49 – 574.   PCM See **49 – 565.** *Parachlorometacresol*

49 – 575.   PCMX See **49 – 566.** *Parachlorometaxylenol*

49 – 576.   PDB See **49 – 567.** *Paradichlorobenzene*

49 – 577.   PELLETIERINE (Punicine)

This toxic alkaloid is found in the bark (especially in the root bark) of the pomegranate tree. Ingestion of moderate amounts may cause mydriasis, partial blindness, severe headache, vertigo, vomiting, diarrhea and convulsions.

TREATMENT
1. Tincture of iodine, 1 ml. in 100 ml. (15 drops in ½ glass of water) by mouth.
2. Gastric lavage with large amounts of water followed by activated charcoal in water by mouth or through the lavage tube.
3. Aspirin for headache.
4. Rapid-acting barbiturates intravenously as necessary for control of convulsions.

49 – 578. PENICILLIN See 49 – 78. *Antibiotics*

49 – 579. PENNYROYAL (Squaw Mint) See 49 – 543. *Oil, Essential;* 49 – 972

49 – 580. PENTOTHAL SODIUM

This relatively safe and effective intravenous anesthetic may cause cardiac arrest (26 – 7) in certain hypersensitive persons or if administered improperly or carelessly. It should never be used in children under 12 years of age.
TREATMENT
1. Stop administration of the anesthetic at once.
2. In moderately severe cases, give respiratory and cardiac stimulants and oxygen under pressure. Complete recovery usually occurs.
3. In severe cases with cardiac arrest (26 – 7), institute external cardiac massage (11 – 2) immediately.

49 – 581. PENTYLENETETRAZOLE (Cardiazol, Metrazol) See 49 – 488. *Metrazol*

49 – 582. PERFUMES

The exact constituents of most perfumes are closely guarded professional secrets of the various manufacturers, but, basically, ambergris, volatile hydrocarbons, alcohols and natural or synthetic scents are used.
TREATMENT
If more than 4 ml. has been ingested, gastric lavage followed by activated charcoal in water and by symptomatic and supportive therapy is indicated.

49 – 583. PERTHANE (Q-137)

This insecticide is similar in action and toxicity to DDT, but without its ability to penetrate skin. For treatment, see 49 – 243. *DDT.*

49 – 584. PERU BALSAM (China Oil)

A mixture of resins and aromatic esters, balsam of Peru is used topically in the treatment of indolent ulcers and pediculosis. Absorption may cause a rapid pulse, convulsions and nephritis, with slow recovery when use is discontinued.

49 – 585. PETROLEUM DISTILLATES See 49 – 119. *Benzene (Benzol) and Its Derivatives;* 49 – 349. *Gasoline;* 49 – 408. *Kerosene;* 49 – 509. *Naphtha;* 49 – 723. *Stoddard Solvent*

49 – 586. PEYOTE See 49 – 460. *Mescal;* 49 – 358. *Hallucinogens*

49 – 587.   PHENACEMIDE (Phenurone)

This anticonvulsant drug may cause severe, even terminal, liver damage. Early signs of toxicity resemble infectious hepatitis (**62 – 8**). The hepatic damage is reversible if detected early.

TREATMENT
1. Discontinuance of the drug.
2. Blood transfusions.
3. Administration of crude liver extract.
4. Symptomatic and supportive care.

49 – 588.   PHENACETIN See **49 – 21**. *Acetphenetidin*

49 – 589.   PHENOBARBITAL (Barbenyl, Dormiral, Gardenal, Luminal, Somonal, etc.)

In some persons even small doses of this long-acting sedative may cause headache, dizziness, acute skin changes (including exfoliative dermatitis) and personality changes.

TREATMENT
See **49 – 111**. *Barbiturates.*

49 – 590.   PHENOL (Carbolic Acid)

Acute toxic signs and symptoms may occur from absorption through the skin, absorption through the mucous membrane of the rectum or vagina and ingestion by accident or with suicidal intent.

SIGNS AND SYMPTOMS following ingestion are acute and consist of the odor of phenol on the breath, burning in the mouth and throat, with whitish discoloration of the tongue and mucous membrane of the throat, nausea, vomiting, severe abdominal pain, slow weak pulse, faintness, hypotension and coma.

TREATMENT
1. Removal as soon as possible by washing the skin or eyes with large amounts of water, or by giving warm water enemas or douches. If ingested, the stomach should be washed with large quantities of warm water until the odor of phenol has disappeared. This should be followed by activated charcoal in water by mouth or through the lavage tube.
2. Olive or salad oil by mouth. Mineral oil should *not* be used. Alcohol increases absorption of phenol and is contraindicated.
3. Artificial respiration (**11 – 1**) and oxygen therapy as required.
4. Morphine sulfate or meperidine (Demerol) in small doses for control of pain.
5. Sodium bicarbonate intravenously for correction of metabolic acidosis.
6. Treatment of incipient or actual pulmonary edema (**51**).
7. Normal salt solution, 500 to 1000 ml. intravenously.
8. Application of external heat to prevent chilling.
9. Hospitalization as soon as possible for supportive therapy. Renal insufficiency may develop. Esophageal strictures are a rare complication.

49 – 591.   PHENOLPHTHALEIN

This cathartic is the active ingredient in several popular "candy laxatives." Although phenolphthalein is relatively nontoxic, large doses, especially in children, may cause severe enteritis and colitis lasting for 3 to 4 days. Aside from treatment of dehydration, no specific therapy is required.

49 – 592. PHENOTHIAZINES

Used in the treatment of gastrointestinal and psychiatric complaints, phenothiazines may cause characteristic side effects following average as well as excessive
doses.

Common preparations

Acetophenazine (Tindall)
Carphenazine (Proketazine)
Chlorpromazine (Thorazine)
Fluphenazine (Permitil)
Methoxypromazine (Tentene)
Perphenazine (Trilafon)

Prochlorperazine (Compazine)
Promazine (Sparine)
Thiopropazate (Dartal)
Thioridazine (Mellaril)
Trifluoperazine (Stelazine)
Triflupromazine (Vesprin)

Extrapyramidal reactions. Dyskinesia, dystonia, cervical muscle spasm, facial muscle
spasm (trismus, sardonic grin, etc.), lack of control of movements of the tongue,
bizarre involuntary movements of the extremities and embarrassment of respiration.

Parkinsonian symptoms. Drooling, tremor, rigidity, abnormal posture and gait, restlessness and profuse speech.

TREATMENT

1. Discontinue or decrease the dose of the medication.
2. Give diphenhydramine (Benadryl), 25 mg. intravenously, or 50 mg. intramuscularly; in milder cases, oral administration may be substituted.
3. Administer barbiturates for sedation.
4. Support respiration as needed.
5. If continuation of phenothiazine therapy is necessary, decrease the dosage and
give antiparkinsonian agents.

Hypotension and shock. For treatment, see **53 – 7.**

Jaundice, dermatitis and agranulocytosis. These may persist for lengthy periods after the
drug has been stopped.

Somnolence. This usually clears rapidly when the phenothiazine is discontinued.

49 – 593. PHENYLBUTAZONE (Butazolidin) and OXYPHENBUTAZONE (Tandearil)

Both of these drugs have important toxic side effects.

SIGNS AND SYMPTOMS. Acute gastrointestinal symptoms including activation of
healed ulcers, fluid retention, acute skin changes; sometimes severe exfoliative
dermatitis, stomatitis, sore throat and serious progressive blood changes which may
develop rapidly and which may be irreversible.

Prevention and early recognition of toxic reactions

1. Limitation of dosage to 300 mg. daily. A base-line complete blood count should be
established.
2. Discontinuance at the end of 1 week if no clinical improvement.
3. Hematologic examinations every week for the first 6 weeks of treatment; then
every 6 to 8 weeks for as long as therapy is continued.

TREATMENT

1. Stop administration at once.
2. Symptomatic care, local and general. Mild cases as a rule do well under home care;
severe cases require hospitalization for control of edema and fluid imbalance, transfusions, etc.

49 – 594. PHENYLENEDIAMINE

Used in eyelash dyes, this substance may give severe toxic reactions (**21**) in hypersensitive individuals.

LOCAL REACTIONS. Severe smarting and pain in the eyes, edema, lacrimation and acute conjunctivitis with photophobia and corneal ulcerations.

SYSTEMIC REACTIONS. Headache; sleepiness; bizarre paresthesias; nausea; epigastric pain; edema of the face, neck and glottis; asthmatic attacks (probably allergic) and severe liver damage.

TREATMENT

1. Immediate termination of exposure.
2. Administration of pilocarpine nitrate, 5 mg. by mouth, as a diaphoretic.
3. Injection of 0.3 to 1 mg. of 1:1000 epinephrine hydrochloride (Adrenalin) intramuscularly for asthmatic manifestations, repeated as necessary.
4. Hospitalization if facial and/or cervical edema is marked or if there are signs of liver damage. All cases should be checked by an ophthalmologist, since permanent eye damage may result if prompt treatment is not given.

49–595. PHENYLHYDRAZINE

Accidental ingestion or therapeutic use in the treatment of polycythemia vera may cause severe toxic manifestations.

SIGNS AND SYMPTOMS. Fatigue, headache, vertigo, edema of the eyelids and upper extremities, acute gastritis with or without diarrhea, cyanosis secondary to blood destruction and toxic hepatitis with severe anemia.

TREATMENT

1. Stop administration of the drug. Mild cases will recover completely in a short time.
2. Hospitalize severe cases immediately for blood transfusions and symptomatic and supportive therapy.

49–596. PHENYL SALICYLATE (Salol)

Mild toxicity is due to phenol (**49–590**), not to salicylates.

49–597. PHENOZUIN See **49–212**. *Cinchophen*

49–598. PHOSDRIN See **49–546**. *Organic Phosphates*

49–599. PHOSGENE (Carbonyl Chloride)

Although phosgene originally was used as a war gas (see **49–832**. *War Gases*), toxic signs and symptoms from respiratory tract irritation occur occasionally in the chemical industry.

SIGNS AND SYMPTOMS. A foul taste in the mouth, with a "scratchy" feeling in the throat. Anosmia develops after the first few whiffs, so that large amounts of the gas may be inhaled without knowledge of its presence. Dyspnea, severe cyanosis, bronchitis, emphysema, pulmonary edema (**51**), bronchospasm and acute cardiac failure may occur.

TREATMENT

1. Removal from exposure. Contaminated clothes should be removed.
2. Absolute rest; prevention of chilling.
3. Oxygen under positive pressure by face mask and rebreathing bag.
4. Caffeine sodiobenzoate, 0.5 gm. intramuscularly.
5. Epinephrine hydrochloride (Adrenalin), 0.5 ml. of 1:1000 solution subcutaneously for bronchospasm, repeated as necessary.
6. Hospitalization because of the danger of development of pulmonary edema (**51**) and acute cardiac failure even after apparent recovery.

49—600. PHOSPHINE (Phosphoretted Hydrogen)

Formed by the decomposition of phosphides in industrial processes, this foul-smelling gas in low concentrations may cause headache, dizziness, restlessness, tremors, general fatigue, burning substernal pain, nausea, vomiting and diarrhea. Bronchitis with fluorescent green sputum, acute dyspnea and pulmonary edema (**51**) may develop. Death is usually preceded by tonic convulsions which may occur suddenly after the patient has apparently completely recovered.

TREATMENT
1. Absolute rest after removal from exposure.
2. Oxygen inhalations under positive pressure by face mask and rebreathing bag.
3. Dextrose, 5% in saline, 500 to 1000 ml. intravenously, unless there is evidence of pulmonary edema (**51**).
4. Caffeine sodiobenzoate, 0.5 gm. intramuscularly.
5. Hospitalization even if the patient has apparently recovered because of the tendency of phosphine to cause serious delayed symptoms—especially pulmonary edema (**51**).

49—601. PHOSPHORIC ACID

For systemic effects, see **25—22**. *Phosphorus Burns;* **49—26**. *Acids;* **49—602**. *Phosphorus.*

Locally, phosphoric acid burns require special emergency therapy (**25—22**).

49—602. PHOSPHORUS (See also **25—22**. *Phosphorus Burns*)

Yellow and white phosphorus are extremely toxic; red phosphorus is insoluble and hence nontoxic. Acute poisoning may arise from ingestion of rat or roach poisons, certain types of fireworks, imported matches (especially from China and Japan) and old-fashioned "sulfur" matches. Severe, even terminal, effects have been caused by the ingestion of the heads of "strike anywhere" kitchen matches, or of the friction striking areas of "safety" book or box matches (**49—442**. *Matches*).

SIGNS AND SYMPTOMS of phosphorus poisoning after ingestion are a garlicky taste in the mouth and odor on the breath, a burning sensation in the mouth and throat, nausea, vomiting (the vomitus may be luminous in the dark), abdominal pain, slow weak pulse, faintness and collapse. Severe systemic damage may be evident 2 to 3 days after apparently complete recovery. Fatty enlargement of the liver, intense icterus, severe hemorrhage and serious blood dyscrasias may occur.

TREATMENT
1. Immediate gastric lavage with 60 ml. of 1% copper sulfate solution, followed by large amounts of 1:5000 potassium permanganate solution. The patient and attendants must be protected from contact with vomitus and gastric washings.
2. Administration of 100 ml. of liquid petrolatum by mouth or lavage tube. Digestible fats and oils should be avoided.
3. Application of external heat.
4. Treatment of severe shock. Corticosteroid therapy may be of value.
5. Control of convulsions by rapid-acting barbiturates.
6. Injection of 1000 ml. of 5% dextrose in saline intravenously.
7. Vitamin K_1 intravenously to combat hypoprothrombinemia. Fresh blood transfusions may be necessary.
8. Hospitalization for observation to ascertain possible liver and kidney damage.
For local and systemic effects of burns from phosphorus-containing bombs, rockets and flares in wartime. see **25—22**. *Phosphorus Burns.*

49–603. PHYSOSTIGMINE (Eserine)

This is a powerful parasympathetic stimulator which may cause bradycardia, intense salivation, miosis, twitching of skeletal muscles, coma and collapse.

TREATMENT

Administration of the physiologic antagonist, atropine sulfate, in large doses. Gastric lavage, followed by activated charcoal in water and administration of analeptics may be indicated if large amounts have been ingested.

49–604. PHYTOLACCA DECANDRA L. (Ink Berry, Pokeweed) See 49–978. *Pokeweed.*

49–605. PICRIC ACID

Used industrially in the manufacture of explosives and dyes and medicinally (usually as the picrate) as an antiseptic ointment, picric acid may cause bright yellow discoloration of the skin, intense bitter taste, nausea, vomiting, abdominal pain, epigastric tenderness, bladder tenesmus and severe liver and kidney damage.

TREATMENT

1. Administration of emetics followed by gastric lavage with 5% sodium bicarbonate solution. A saline cathartic should be left in the stomach.
2. Administration of large amounts of fluid by mouth and/or intravenously (6).
3. Hospitalization if there is evidence of kidney damage.

49–606. PICROTOXIN

Picrotoxin is the toxic ingredient of the bright red berries of an East Indian plant, commonly known as "fish eggs." Medicinally it was formerly used as an analeptic, especially in barbiturate poisoning, but its use for this purpose is gradually becoming less prevalent.

SIGNS AND SYMPTOMS after ingestion: A burning sensation in the mouth, pallor, cold perspiration, nausea, vomiting and shallow respiration. After ½ to 3 hours, confusion, stupor, unconsciousness and clonic or tonic convulsions may occur, especially in children.

TREATMENT

1. If ingested, emetics followed by gastric lavage with 500 to 1000 ml. of 1:5000 potassium permanganate solution. Activated charcoal in water should be left in the stomach.
2. Control of convulsions by phenobarbital sodium, 0.1 to 0.2 gm. intravenously, or paraldehyde, 5 ml. intramuscularly.
3. Administration of saline cathartics.

PROGNOSIS. The mortality from ingestion is very low. Ill-advised injection of picrotoxin in the treatment of coma may cause uncontrollable convulsions and death.

49–607. PILOCARPINE

Toxic manifestations and treatment are approximately the same as given for *Physostigmine* (49–603).

49–608. PINE OIL

Ingestion of small amounts of this complex mixture of terpene alcohols may cause acute toxic effects, especially gastritis (sometimes hemorrhagic), decreased body temperature, central nervous system depression and respiratory failure. For treatment, see 49–754. *Terpineol;* 49–815. *Turpentine.*

49–609. PLASTER OF PARIS (Anhydrous Calcium Sulfate or Dihydrate)

Plaster of Paris has no intrinsic toxicity, but if swallowed may harden and cause obstruction requiring surgical relief. *Immediate* ingestion of large amounts of water, gelatin or glycerin will sometimes delay setting long enough to allow removal by gastric lavage.

49–610. PLASTIC CEMENTS AND GLUES (Model Airplane Cement)

Sniffing the fumes from model airplane adhesive materials has recently become common. Transient exhilaration, euphoria and increased tolerance to pain result— probably due to the solvents employed, often amyl acetate (49–66). Habitual glue-sniffing may result in intoxication and coma. Similar effects have been reported from sniffing paint thinner, lacquer and marking pencil fumes. Whether or not permanent organic brain or nervous system damage may result has not yet been determined.

TREATMENT.   Symptomatic and supportive.

49–611. PLASTICS

Ever-widening uses of plastic materials have focused attention on 3 main types of toxic reactions:

1. Irritation of the skin and mucous membranes during manufacture. This is often due to solvents, plasticizers and dyes and is rarely serious.
2. Polymer fume fever. The exact cause of this condition is unknown. The toxic picture and treatment are similar to metal fume fever (49–461).
3. Acute toxic signs and symptoms may be caused by decomposition products resulting from heating plastic materials used in industry and medical and surgical therapy, i.e., fluorocarbons such as Teflon. Under certain conditions, extremely toxic substances, including hydrocyanic acid (49–235. *Cyanides*), oxides of nitrogen (49–553) and tetrafluoroethylene, may result from exposure of plastics to intense heat.

49–612. PMA (Phenyl Mercuric Acetate)

This fungicide is more toxic than mercuric chloride. For treatment, see 49–128. *Bichloride of Mercury.*

49–613. POISON IVY, OAK, SUMACH See 54–11 and 54–16. *Urushiol Contact Dermatitis*

49–614. POLYMER FUME FEVER See 49–611. *Plastics*

49–615. POSTERIOR PITUITARY EXTRACTS

The most commonly used extracts are posterior pituitary (Pituitrin), oxytocin (Pitocin) and vasopressin (Pitressin). All are oxytocic agents and may cause nausea, vomiting, intestinal cramping, extreme facial pallor and cramping similar to menstrual cramps in women.

TREATMENT

No physiologic antagonist to posterior pituitary extracts is known; therefore, symptomatic treatment (oxygen inhalations, sedation by barbiturates and moderate doses of vasopressor drugs) is all that is indicated.

PROGNOSIS.   Complete and rapid disappearance of symptoms, provided the offending extract has been discontinued.

49 – 616. POTASSIUM CHLORATE

Many household toilet articles and medications (cough mixtures, gargles, mouth-washes and toothpastes) contain potassium chlorate. Ingestion of large amounts may cause nausea, vomiting, epigastric pain, dyspnea, cyanosis, acute delirium, anuria and jaundice.

TREATMENT

1. Egg white or other demulcents by mouth.
2. Application of external heat.
3. Gastric lavage with dilute salt solution, followed by activated charcoal.
4. Methylene blue, 50 ml. of a 1% solution in 1.8% sodium sulfate solution intravenously.
5. Oxygen inhalations under positive pressure by face mask or endotracheal catheter and rebreathing bag.
6. Caffeine sodiobenzoate, 0.5 gm. intramuscularly or intravenously.
7. Careful follow-up medical care; severe degenerative nephritis may be a delayed complication.

49 – 617. POTASSIUM OXALATE (See also 49 – 552. *Oxalic Acid*)

Potassium oxalate is the active constituent of many popular household cleansing and bleaching agents. Acute toxic, even fatal, effects may be caused by ingestion (accidental or with suicidal intent), by injection into the vagina or uterus in an attempt to produce an abortion or by inhalation of fumes or steam from cleansing or bleaching solutions.

SIGNS AND SYMPTOMS of oxalate toxicity consist of a burning sensation in the mouth and throat with difficulty in swallowing, edema of the glottis, nausea, vomiting, often bloody and associated with severe epigastric pain, weak pulse, low blood pressure, muscular fibrillation and twitching, exaggerated reflexes with patellar clonus, uremic convulsions, coma and death from circulatory collapse.

TREATMENT

Treatment is based on the formation of insoluble calcium oxalate. For details, see **49 – 552.** *Oxalic Acid.*

49 – 618. POTASSIUM PERMANGANATE

Crystals or solutions of potassium permanganate are common in many household medical cabinets and often are available to children. Ingestion of a few crystals usually does no harm, but larger amounts may be dangerous. Severe mucous membrane burns, even perforation and peritonitiis, have occurred following attempts at induction of an abortion by insertion of large amounts of the crystals into the vagina. Ingestion causes a film in the mouth or on other mucous membranes which may be violet or dark brown, stomatitis, nausea, vomiting, acute gastroenteritis with abdominal tenderness and shock from circulatory collapse (**53**), which may be severe and resistant to therapy.

TREATMENT

1. Local treatment of mucous membrane burns (**25 – 18**).
2. Administration of demulcents such as egg white.
3. Gastric lavage with large quantities of normal salt solution followed by activated charcoal in water and saline cathartics.
4. Control of pain by small doses of narcotics.
5. Treatment of shock (**53 – 7**).
6. Hospitalization if there is evidence of deep erosion or penetration of any mucous membrane.

PROGNOSIS. Good unless a concentrated solution (more than 3%) or a large amount of crystals have been swallowed, or perforation of a body cavity or viscus has occurred.

49—619. PREDNISOLONE (Delta-Cortef, Hydeltra, Meticortelone)

This synthetic steroid is used in the treatment of arthritis and may give a toxic picture similar to cortisone (**49—227**).

49—620. PREDNISONE (Deltasone, Deltra, Meticorton) See **49—227**. *Cortisone*

49—621. PRIMIDONE (Mysoline)

Used as an anti-epileptic drug, primidone in large doses may cause drowsiness, ataxia, vertigo and psychotic episodes. Toxic symptoms subside when use is stopped.

49—622. PRIMROSE (Primula)

Hypersensitivity to this common garden plant is common and is characterized by acute skin reactions and swelling, burning and itching of the fingertips. Symptoms clear slowly when contact is avoided.

49—623. PRIVINE (Naphazoline Hydrochloride)

Ingestion, as well as local use, of this powerful vasoconstrictor may result in disturbing and uncomfortable (but rarely dangerous) toxic effects.Many persons are hypersensitive to Privine and show extreme reactions after relatively small doses (**21.** *Allergic Reactions*).

SIGNS AND SYMPTOMS.   Severe headache, acute anxiety and excitement, cold perspiration and cyanosis, especially of lips and fingertips, followed by respiratory failure.

TREATMENT

1. If ingested, syrup of ipecac by mouth or gastric lavage followed by activated charcoal in water by mouth or through the lavage tube.
2. Oxygen inhalations under positive pressure by face mask and rebreathing bag.
3. Caffeine sodiobenzoate, 0.5 gm. intramuscularly or intravenously.
4. Barbiturates intramuscularly for control of excitement or anxiety.

PROGNOSIS.   Complete recovery after 1 to 2 hours.

49—624. PROCAINAMIDE HYDROCHLORIDE (Pronestyl)

In hypersensitive persons or in large doses, Pronestyl may produce bradycardia and cardiac arrest (**26—7**), sometimes preceded by extreme hypotension. Sore throat, fever, dysphagia and bone marrow depression have also been reported.

TREATMENT

1. Discontinue therapeutic use at once.
2. Treat cardiac arrest (**26—7**).
3. Give symptomatic and supportive therapy as required.

49—625. PROCAINE HYDROCHLORIDE (Novocain) See **49—72**. *Anesthetics, Local*

49—626. PROLAN

Readily absorbable through the intact skin, this chlorinated hydrocarbon insecticide gives a toxic picture similar to chlordane (**49—188**).

49 — 627.   PROPANONE See **49 — 17.** *Acetone*

49 — 628.   PROPHENPYRIDAMINE (Trimeton)

Overdosage of this complex drug used in the treatment of allergic conditions may cause facial flushing, mydriasis, muscle stiffness, dizziness, ataxia, confusion, delirium and hallucinations.

TREATMENT

1. Gastric lavage followed by activated charcoal in water by mouth or through the lavage tube.
2. Rapid-acting sedatives.
3. Large amounts of fluids to increase excretion through the kidneys.

49 — 629.   PROPOXYPHENE (Darvon)

Either convulsions or coma may result from an overdose of this popular analgesic agent. Both may be preceded by deep respiratory depression, cardiac arrhythmias and signs and symptoms of cerebral and pulmonary edema.

TREATMENT

1. Gastric lavage followed by activated charcoal in water by mouth or through the lavage tube.
2. Assisted respiration by expired air or mechanical methods (**11 — 1**).
3. Continuous ECG monitoring with symptomatic treatment depending upon the findings (right conduction abnormalities, bigeminy, lengthening of the QRS complex with ST wave modifications).
4. Control of convulsive seizures by rapid-acting barbiturates.
5. Naloxone hydrochloride (Narcan) 0.01 mg. per kilogram of body weight intravenously, repeated as necessary.
6. Injection of sodium bicarbonate intravenously to prevent development of metabolic acidosis.
7. Treatment of pulmonary edema (**51**), which must be differentiated from aspiration pneumonitis.

49 — 630.   PYRAMIDON (Aminopyrine)

This is a dangerous drug because of its tendency to produce malignant granulopenia and irreversible neurologic changes. It is a constituent of some proprietary medicines. For treatment, see **49 — 12.** *Acetanilid.*

49 — 631.   PYRETHRUM (Persian Insect Powder)

Many household and garden insecticides contain this relatively nontoxic compound, often combined with other more toxic insecticides, especially DDT (**49 — 243**). Pyrethrum sprays often have a kerosene (**49 — 408**) or xylene base.

SIGNS AND SYMPTOMS after inhalation or ingestion of large amounts consist of nausea, vomiting, acute gastrointestinal pain followed by diarrhea and a burning and stinging sensation around the anus.

TREATMENT

Treatment is symptomatic only unless pyrethrum is combined with more dangerous insecticides or suspended in harmful vehicles (distillate, kerosene, xylene, etc.). Pyrethrum alone rarely causes dangerous toxic effects.

49-632. PYRIDINE

Used commercially as a solvent and medicinally as an antiseptic and antispasmodic, pyridine may cause acute but transient toxic reactions following inhalation of the fumes or ingestion.

SIGNS AND SYMPTOMS.   Headache, restlessness, insomnia, vertigo, muscular incoordination, disturbances in hearing and severe peripheral neuritis.

TREATMENT

1. If inhaled, air or oxygen inhalations under positive pressure by face mask and rebreathing bag.

2. If ingested, emetics or gastric lavage with 1:5000 potassium permanganate solution followed by activated charcoal in water by mouth or through the lavage tube.

3. Control of restlessness by rapid-acting barbiturates.

4. Intravenous administration of 5% dextrose in normal saline.

49-633. PYROCATHECHOL (Catechol)

This substance has, in general, the same actions as phenol but is more toxic, especially in its tendency to cause convulsions. For treatment, see 49-590. Phenol.

49-634. PYROGALLOL (Pyrogallic Acid)

Pyrogallol is used commercially in hair dyes and proprietary ringworm "cures." Severe toxic signs and symptoms similar to those caused by phenol (49-590) may occur from absorption through the intact skin as well as by ingestion. In addition, renal damage, methemoglobinemia and red blood cell destruction similar to the effects of aniline (49-73) have been noted after prolonged use. Toxicity is usually manifested by the sudden onset of collapse, convulsions and albuminuria due to severe toxic nephritis. This characteristically sudden onset may occur after use of a preparation containing pyrogallol for a long period without apparent previous ill effects. Dyspnea, cyanosis and acute respiratory depression may occur.

TREATMENT

1. Apomorphine hydrochloride hypodermically if the substance has been ingested by an adult; oral emetics if ingested by a child. Activated charcoal in water should be left in the stomach. Any secondary respiratory depressant effect of apomorphine can be neutralized by intravenous naloxone hydrochloride (Narcan), 0.01 mg. per kilogram of body weight, repreated as necessary.

2. Caffeine sodiobenzoate, 0.5 gm. intramuscularly or intravenously.

3. Oxygen inhalations for dyspnea and cyanosis.

4. Purgation with magnesium sulfate (Epsom salts).

5. Hospitalization because of the characteristic severe blood and kidney damage.

49-635. PYROLAN

This is a phosphate ester pesticide, similar in action and toxicity to parathion. For treatment, see 49-546. Organic Phosphates.

49-636. Q-137 See 49-583. Perthane

49-637. QUATERNARY AMMONIUM SALTS (QAC)

In 0.01 to 1% concentrations, many complex combinations of quaternary ammonium salts are used as antiseptics, deodorants and fungicides. Lauryl benzyl dimethyl ammonium chloride is used commonly in medicine under the U.S.P. name of benzalkonium chloride and the proprietary name of Zephiran.

Ingestion of large amounts of concentrated solutions, or absorption from a mucous membrane-lined cavity such as the vagina, may cause severe toxic effects. A few fatalities coming on 1 to 2 hours after ingestion have been reported.

SIGNS AND SYMPTOMS.   A severe burning sensation in the mouth, throat and stomach if a concentrated solution has been ingested; restlessness; apprehension; dyspnea; cyanosis; generalized muscle weakness and death from respiratory failure, sometimes preceded by convulsions.

TREATMENT

1. Removal from the skin by thorough washing with soap and water.

2. Large amounts of demulcents (egg white, milk, soapsuds) by mouth, followed by a slurry of activated charcoal in water and a saline cathartic. If concentrated QAC solutions have been swallowed, avoid emetics and gastric lavage.

3. Rapidly acting barbiturates for control of convulsions.

4. Oxygen under positive pressure by face mask or endotracheal catheter and rebreathing bag.

5. Treatment of hypotension and circulatory shock (**53**).

6. Hospitalization for supportive therapy if extreme muscle weakness or convulsions have been present. Curare antagonists such as neostigmine (**49 – 518**) and edrophonium (Tensilon) are ineffective.

49 – 638. QUICKLIME

Quicklime is unslaked lime, a powerful and dangerous caustic alkali. For treatment, see **49 – 39.** *Alkalies;* **49 – 425.** *Lime.*

49 – 639. QUICKSILVER See **49 – 455.** *Mercury*

49 – 640. QUINACRINE (Atabrine)

Effective therapeutic doses used in the treatment of malaria may cause severe toxic effects, as may overdosage. Individual tolerance varies markedly. Signs and symptoms of toxicity following excessive doses are similar to those given in **49 – 201.** *Chloroquine Phosphate.*

49 – 641. QUINIDINE

Quinidine is used in the treatment of auricular fibrillation and other cardiac arrhythmias (**26**). Overdosage (or therapeutic doses in hypersensitive persons) may produce cardiac abnormalities, including extrasystoles, paroxysmal tachycardia, heart block (**26 – 10**), ventricular fibrillation (**26 – 23**) and cardiac arrest (**26 – 7**). In addition, respiratory paralysis and pulmonary infarction may occur.

For treatment, see **49 – 642.** *Quinine.* Cardiac irregularities are less likely to occur if the patient is digitalized; they usually subside rapidly when quinidine therapy is discontinued.

49 – 642. QUININE

The most important alkaloid of cinchona bark, quinine is used in the treatment of malaria (**30 – 14**), as a tonic and as a hair dressing and is an ingredient of many common proprietary preparations. Allergic hypersensitivity reactions (**21**) are common.

Acute quinine poisoning is characterized by nausea, vomiting, abdominal pain, diarrhea, generalized edema and hypotension. The patient may have decreased vision and hearing, severe headache, tinnitus and auditory hallucinations. Jaundice and evidence of renal damage may develop. Fatalities are the result of excessive dosage and are due to respiratory arrest.

TREATMENT

1. Gastric lavage with 1:5000 potassium permanganate solution or 1% tannic acid solution followed by activated charcoal in water by mouth or through the lavage tube.
2. Administration of saline cathartics.
3. Control of excitement by rapid-acting barbiturates.
4. Oxygen inhalations if cyanosis is present.
5. Intravenous injection of a 1 M solution of sodium lactate (30 to 50 mg.), repeated every 2 to 3 hours to prevent and control metabolic acidosis.
6. Constant ECG monitoring because of the danger of cardiac arrest (26-7).
7. Hospitalization for close observation, and symptomatic and supportive care. The clinical picture of acute quinine poisoning may resemble that of acute malaria (30-14), the disease for which the drug is often prescribed.

49-643. QUINOPHEN See 49-212. Cinchophen

49-644. RANUNCULUS SCLERATUS (Buttercup, Crowfoot)

Chewing or swallowing flowers or leaves of this common flowering meadow plant results in acute salivation, peeling of the surface of the tongue, loss of taste and colicky gastric pain. All symptoms are of short duration and leave no permanent ill-effects.

49-645. RAT KILLERS (Rodenticides) See 49-90. Arsenic; 49-112. Barium Compounds; 49-235. Cyanides; 49-336. Fluorides; 49-647. Red Squill; 49-699. Sodium Fluoroacetate; 49-729. Strychnine; 49-768. Thallium; 49-833. Warfarin, 49-853. Zinc Phosphide

49-646. RAUWOLFIA ALKALOIDS (Reserpine, Serpasil)

Rauwolfia and its alkaloids in therapeutic doses may cause nasal congestion and epistaxis, acute gastrointestinal symptoms, flare-ups of healed ulcers, acute colitis simulating an acute surgical abdomen, acute mental depression and parkinsonism.

TREATMENT

Decrease in dosage or stopping administration of the drug usually results in spontaneous and complete clearing of symptoms. In severe cases, treatment is as follows:

1. Even if several hours have passed since ingestion, gastric lavage with large amounts of water, followed by activated charcoal via the lavage tube and a saline cathartic.
2. Maintenance of a normal body temperature by blankets or other means.
3. Conservative therapy if coma and hypotension are present. Analeptic and vasopressor drugs should be avoided, as should rapid intravenous infusions.
4. Give small doses of atropine for control of parasympathomimetic side effects.
5. Local antacid therapy for gastric pain.
6. Antiparkinsonian drugs for control of stiffness and tremors.
7. Frequent ECG monitoring regarding cardiac abnormalities. Rapid digitalization may be beneficial.

49–647.   RED SQUILL

Ingestion of even small amounts of this commonly used rat poison causes a toxic picture similar to that caused by digitalis (**49–272**).

49–648.   REFRIGERATING AGENTS See **49–59**. *Ammonia;* **49–476.** *Methyl Bromide;* **49–478.** *Methyl Chloride;* **49–736.** *Sulfur Dioxide;* **49–826.** *Vinyl Chloride*

49–649.   RESORCINOL

Similar in many respects to phenol in its toxicity, resorcinol may give acute signs and symptoms from skin absorption as well as from ingestion. The toxic picture is generally not as severe as that caused by phenol, although the tendency toward convulsions is greater.

Hexylresorcinol (**49–370**) is slightly less toxic than resorcinol.

For treatment, see **49–590**. *Phenol.*

49–650.   RHODOTYPOS KERRIOIDES (Jet Bead Tree)

A native of Japan, this flowering tree produces drupes called "jet beads." Ingestion by children of 2 or 3 of these attractive drupes has caused dilated pupils, tonic-clonic convulsions and glucosuria—all transient.

49–651.   RHUBARB

Ingestion of large amounts of rhubarb greens (leaves or blades) may be dangerous. For signs and symptoms of toxicity and treatment, see **49–552**. *Oxalic Acid.*

49–652.   ROACH PASTE See **49–90**. *Arsenic;* **49–336**. *Fluorides*

49–653.   ROCKET FUELS

None of the chemical substances now in use as rocket propellants are new; their properties and toxicities have been well known to chemists, laboratory workers and toxicologists for many years. What is new is the utilization of their peculiar physical and chemical properties in rocketry. Elaborate methods of protection from toxic effects of persons working with tremendous amounts of these dangerous substances have been put in effect, so far successfully. Protection of the general public from transportation accidents, wind-blown fumes, explosions, etc., so far has been effective.

The list on page 503 contains some of the chemicals in use at the present time, with a notation regarding toxicity or other dangerous characteristics.

49–654.   ROSEMARY

Oil of rosemary is used medicinally as a rubefacient but is extremely toxic if ingested.

SIGNS AND SYMPTOMS.   Nausea, vomiting, severe gastric pain, rapid weak pulse, hyperactive reflexes, pulmonary edema (**51**), marked albuminuria, collapse and coma.

TREATMENT

1. Gastric lavage with 1:5000 potassium permanganate solution followed by activated charcoal in water through the lavage tube.

2. Caffeine sodiobenzoate, 0.5 gm. intramuscularly or intravenously.

CHEMICAL	CHARACTERISTICS AND TOXICITY
Ammonia	Fumes acutely toxic (**49 – 59**).
Anhydrous hydrazine	Explosive; fumes toxic.
Aniline	Acutely toxic (**49 – 73**).
Boron derivatives	Flammable; fumes acutely toxic; all exposed personnel required to wear special masks and protective clothing.
Chlorine trifluoride	Reacts violently; toxic effects of both chlorine (**49 – 191**) and fluorides (**49 – 336**).
Decaborane	See *Boron derivatives* (above). In addition, borates break into flame on contact with the atmosphere; therefore, special containers are necessary for transportation. Boron fires cannot be controlled by the usual methods.
Diborane	See *Decaborane* (above).
Ethyl nitrate	Will explode when exposed to slight shock or temperature variations; fumes acutely toxic.
Fluorine (liquid)	Will ignite spontaneously in the presence of another chemical (hypergolic); fumes toxic.
Fuming nitric acid	Hypergolic; fumes toxic (**49 – 553**); severe burns on contact.
Hydrazine	See *Anhydrous hydrazine* (above).
Hydrogen (liquid)	Explosive. Exposure to air may result in severe burns before the presence of a fire is recognized, since hydrogen burns with a completely nonluminous flame.
Hydrogen peroxide (90%)	Explosive; causes severe burns on contact; fumes toxic.
Isocyanates	Toxic; see **49 – 235**. *Cyanides.*
LOX	See *Oxygen (liquid)*, below.
Mixed amines	Ignite spontaneously on contact with nitric acid (hypergolic).
Nitrogen tetraoxide	Must be kept absolutely dry; in presence of moisture forms nitric acid. See **49 – 553**. *Oxides of Nitrogen.*
Nitroglycerin	Extremely sensitive to percussion; see **49 – 528**. *Nitrites.*
Oxygen (liquid)	Acutely flammable; reacts violently with hydrocarbons and other combustible materials.
Pentaborane	See *Decaborane* (above).
Perchlorates	Break down into hydrochloric acid and corrosive substances.
UDMH (unsymmetrical dimethylhydrazine)	Highly explosive, flammable; fumes toxic. Based on experimental evidence, injection of pyridoxine hydrochloride, 25 mg. per kilogram of body weight, has been recommended.

3. Treatment of shock (**53 – 7**).

4. Hospitalization if treatment of pulmonary edema (**51**) is or has been required or if evidence of renal irritation is present.

49 – 655.   ROTENONE See **49 – 249**. *Derris;* **49 – 631**. *Pyrethrum*

Rotenone is widely used as an insecticide, often in combination with DDT (**49 – 243**) and pyrethrum (**49 – 631**), because it has a low toxicity for plants and animals. No human fatalities have been reported. For treatment see **49 – 631**. *Pyrethrum.*

49—656. RUBBING ALCOHOL See 49—315. *Ethyl Alcohol;* 49—403. *Isopropyl Alcohol*

The substances used to make rubbing alcohol unpotable cause nausea and vomiting but are otherwise harmless even if ingested in large quantities. Contrary to common belief, rubbing alcohol never contains methanol (49—475).

49—657. RUMEX ACETOSA L. (Sorrel)

In some localities sorrel is sometimes used as a salad green. Ingestion of large amounts gives a toxic picture similar to rhubarb (49—651), due to the oxalate content. See 49—552. *Oxalic Acid.*

49—658. SACCHARIN (Garantose, Glucide, Saccharinol, Sycose)

Commonly used as a sugar substitute in diabetic or reducing diets, this benzoic acid derivative may give toxic reactions in hypersensitive persons or if excessively large doses are ingested.

SIGNS AND SYMPTOMS. Loss of appetite, nausea, vomiting, gastric cramps and pain, diarrhea, acute myalgia with muscular fibrillation and twitching, delirium and hallucinations (especially auditory).

TREATMENT
1. Emptying of the stomach by emetics or gastric lavage.
2. Oral administration of saline cathartics.
3. Intravenous injection of 10 ml. of a 10% solution of calcium gluconate, repeated as necessary for control of muscle pain.
4. Hospitalization if large amounts have been ingested.

49—659. SAFFRON

Although oil of saffron is occasionally used as a flavoring and coloring agent, most of the cases of acute toxicity which have been reported have been caused by drinking strong teas or concentrated decoctions in attempts to induce abortions.

SIGNS AND SYMPTOMS of saffron poisoning consist of vomiting of blood-tinged material, severe gastric pain, bloody diarrhea, rapid weak pulse, hypotension, hematuria, convulsions and coma.

TREATMENT
1. Gastric lavage with a 1:5000 solution of potassium permanganate followed by activated charcoal by mouth or via the lavage tube.
2. Caffeine sodiobenzoate, 0.5 gm. intramuscularly, repeated as necessary for circulatory support.
3. Copious fluids intravenously and orally.
4. Hospitalization for symptomatic and supportive therapy if bleeding from the gastrointestinal or urinary tracts is excessive or persistent.

PROGNOSIS. Good, although irritative symptoms referable to the stomach, intestines and kidneys may persist for several weeks.

49—660. SAFROLE

Safrole, the active ingredient in oil of sassafras and Macassar oil, is extremely toxic. Ingestion of a few milliliters has caused vomiting, hallucinations, vascular collapse and coma. Local application of oil of sassafras to the scalp has caused vertigo, stupor, aphasia and circulatory collapse.

TREATMENT
1. Gastric lavage followed by activated charcoal in water orally or via the lavage tube.
2. Saline cathartics.
3. Symptomatic care. Psychic disturbances (**50—1**) may persist for weeks after other symptoms have cleared.

49—661. SAGE

Oil of sage if ingested in small amounts may cause marked dyspnea, weak rapid pulse, lowered blood pressure, shock (**53**) and epileptiform convulsions.
TREATMENT
1. Gastric lavage with large amounts of water followed by activated charcoal in water by mouth or through the lavage tube.
2. Administration of a saline cathartic.
3. Treatment of shock (**53—7**).
4. Oxygen inhalations under positive pressure.
5. Rapid-acting barbiturates intramuscularly or intravenously for control of convulsions.
6. Hospitalization for observation and supportive and symptomatic care.

49—662. SALICYLAMIDE

Use of salicylamide as an antirheumatic agent has resulted in a high incidence of toxic reactions characterized by drowsiness, heartburn, anorexia and diarrhea. Gingival and petechial bleeding and thrombocytopenia have been reported.
TREATMENT
1. Discontinuation of the drug.
2. Supportive therapy. Blood transfusions may be required.

49—663. SALICYLANILIDE (Ansadol, Shirlan)

Used for mildew control and as a fungicide, salicylanilide can cause both aniline and salicylate poisoning by inhalation or by ingestion. For treatment, see **49—73.** *Aniline;* **49—664.** *Salicylates.*

49—664. SALICYLATES (See also **49—101.** *Aspirin;* **49—486.** *Methyl Salicylate*)

Salicylic acid and all of the soluble salicylates may cause severe toxic signs and symptoms, grouped under the heading of "salicylism," by skin absorption as well as by ingestion. The widespread use of oil of wintergreen (**49—486.** *Methyl Salicylate*) and candy-coated "baby aspirin" tablets makes therapeutic and accidental poisoning relatively common in children; the highest mortality is in the 1 to 4 age group. Any dosage over 65 mg. per year of age every 4 hours will produce acute toxic signs and symptoms in a child under 8 years old in a short time; if renal function is impaired even smaller doses may be dangerous. The minimal lethal dose of acetylsalicylic acid (aspirin) is usually considered to lie between 0.3 and 0.4 gm. per kilogram of body weight. Peak serum salicylate levels are usually reached about 2 hours after ingestion and may be roughly estimated by the following equation:

$$\frac{\text{Amount ingested in milligrams}}{\text{Total body water (70\% of body wt. in grams)}} \times 100 = \begin{array}{l}\text{Mg. of salicylate per}\\\text{100 ml. of serum}\end{array}$$

For peak serum salicylate levels after a single dose, see Figure 29. For qualitative test for salicylates, see **15—6.** *Salicylate Ingestion Test.*

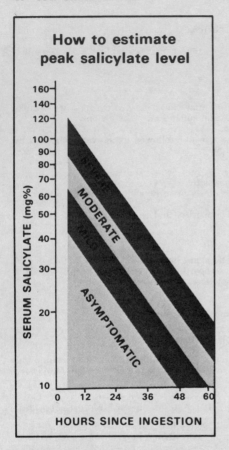

Figure 29. Hours after a single aspirin overdose it is possible to estimate peak salicylate level and severity of intoxication by using this nomogram. (From Done, A. K., Pediatrics, 26:800, 1960.)

The clinical picture of salicylate intoxication consists of faintness, tinnitus, loss of hearing, disturbed vision, nausea, vomiting, gastrointestinal hemorrhage and dehydration. There may be an acetone odor on the breath (for methyl salicylate only). Salicylism and diabetes (**29–3**) may give practically the same clinical picture. Rapid hyperpneic ("panting dog") respiration is common in children. Cyanosis is usually present. Edema of the larynx may be serious. Convulsions (especially in children), delirium, coma and hemorrhage secondary to hypoprothrombinemia may occur. Ingestion of massive doses causes death through irreversible respiratory collapse.

TREATMENT

Therapy for salicylate overdosage should be monitored by frequent tests of serum salicylate level and acid-base and electrolyte studies. The pH of the blood should be kept at about 7.0.

If the peak serum salicylate level [2 to 4 hours after ingestion for aspirin (**49–101**);

much longer for oil of wintergreen (**49−486**)] is below 40 mg.%; little, if any, treatment is required−spontaneous recovery will take place.

From 40 to 70 mg.%: Mild symptoms require emptying the stomach and supportive care. Hospitalization usually is not needed, although the patient should be kept under close observation for several hours.

From 70 to 100 mg.%: Moderate toxic symptoms are to be expected. The patient should be hospitalized for supportive and definitive care.

From 100 to 140 mg.%: Severe, critical symptoms (hyperventilation, acute dehydration, severe metabolic acidosis, convulsions, coma) require treatment as outlined below.

Above 140 mg.%: Very severe, often fatal.

Treatment of Severe Salicylate Intoxication

1. Immediate emptying of the stomach by emetics or gastric lavage with 3% sodium bicarbonate solution, followed by activated charcoal in water orally or through the lavage tube.

2. Large amounts of fluids intravenously and orally to increase renal excretion. Expansion of plasma volume can be obtained by intravenous isotonic solutions (lactated Ringer's or isotonic sodium bicarbonate, 20 mg. per kilogram of body weight) repeated in one hour if necessary.

3. Sodium bicarbonate solution intravenously to combat metabolic acidosis and to alkalinize the urine.

4. Potassium chloride intravenously in large doses. As much as 40 mEq. of KCl per liter of intravenous fluids may be required to make up the extreme potassium deficit.

5. If oliguria persists, give a 20% solution of mannitol (1 gm. per kilogram of body weight) intravenously−rate, 1 ml. per minute−to increase renal clearance.

6. Control of hyperpyrexia by cooling blankets or other means.

7. If forced alkaline diuresis as outlined above has not resulted in definite clinical improvement, peritoneal dialysis should be done and repeated 2 to 3 times if necessary. The dialysis fluid should consist of 5% human albumin in an electrolyte solution (Albumisol), to which 5 mEq. per liter of potassium has been added. If equipment is available, hemodialysis is very effective.

8. All patients requiring hospitalization should receive parenteral Vitamin K therapy.

49−665. SALT (See also 49−696. *Sodium Chloride*)

Several series of accidental severe poisoning in nursery infants have been reported. Severe toxic symptoms have followed the use of a strong solution of table salt as a household emetic.

49−666. SALTPETER (Potassium Nitrate)

Potassium nitrate is used in the manufacture of gunpowder and fireworks, as a fertilizer, in the chemical industry and as a constituent of some proprietary asthma remedies (**49−103**). Use as a food preservative and medicinally for suppression of sexual excitement is no longer common. Chile saltpeter is sodium nitrate.

For treatment of toxic effects, see **49−525.** *Nitrates.*

49−667. SAMARIUM CHLORIDE

This is a by-product of the uranium industry. Like gadolinium chloride (**49−346**), it is toxic to laboratory animals, but there have been no reports of human toxicity.

49−668. SANOCHRYSINE (Gold Sodium Thiosulfate) See 49−353. *Gold Salts*

49-669. SANTONIN (Wormseed) See **49-182.** *Chenopodium*

49-670. SAPONIN

Saponin occurs in many common plants and has the ability to produce foam with water. Ingestion of the seeds may result in acute toxic symptoms. For the toxic picture, see **49-31.** *Agrostemma Githago.*

49-671. SAPROL

Toxic effects are due to 40% cresols. For signs and symptoms of toxicity, see **49-590.** *Phenol.*

49-672. SCARLET RED (Aminoazotoluene)

In ointment form, scarlet red is used medicinally to promote epithelization. Its attractive color may result in ingestion by children, producing a toxic picture similar to that resulting from absorption from wound surfaces.

SIGNS AND SYMPTOMS.   Nausea, vomiting, abdominal pain, diarrhea, fever, general malaise and hypotension.

TREATMENT
1. Discontinue at once if used locally.
2. If ingested, gastric lavage with 1:5000 potassium permanganate solution followed by activated charcoal in water by mouth or through the lavage tube.
3. Saline cathartics.
4. Administration of copious fluids, especially if diarrhea is marked.

49-673. SCHEELE'S GREEN (Copper Arsenite) See **49-90.** *Arsenic;* **49-91.** *Arsenic Color Pigments*

49-674. SCHRADAN See **49-546.** *Organic Phosphates*

49-675. SCHWEINFURT GREEN See **49-90.** *Arsenic;* **49-91.** *Arsenic Color Pigments*

49-676. SCOPOLAMINE

An alkaloid occurring naturally in Datura stramonii and Hyoscyamus niger, scopolamine on ingestion gives a toxic picture resembling that of atropine sulfate. For treatment, see **49-104.** *Atropine Sulfate.*

49-677. SCORPION VENOM See **56-11.** *Scorpion Stings;* **61.** *Venoms*

49-678. SEDORMID

Ingestion of large amounts of this sedative and hypnotic drug has caused somnolence, stupor and pulmonary edema (**51**) as well as thrombocytopenia with diffuse hemorrhages. Symptoms clear under supportive care when administration of the drug is stopped.

49 – 679. SELENIUM AND ITS SALTS

This nonmetallic element is dangerous only if vaporized; however, its salts are acutely toxic by inhalation of dust or fumes, skin absorption or ingestion. The treatment is the same as given for arsenic (**49 – 90**) except that BAL is ineffective and should *not* be used.

49 – 680. SENECIO

Several varieties of this South African plant as a contaminant of cereal grains have caused numerous cases of food poisoning, with many fatalities.

Senecio glicifolius and burchelli seeds cause bloody vomiting, epigastric pain, enlargement of the liver with ascites, pleural effusion and collapse. The mortality rate from this type of poisoning is very high.

Senecio vulgaris (groundsel) seeds cause "bread poisoning" characterized by nausea, vomiting, epigastric pain, bloody diarrhea and evidence of acute liver damage. The presence of ascites makes the prognosis very poor.

Senecio canicida. The toxic principles of this variety are contained in the roots and resemble picrotoxin (**49 – 606**).

TREATMENT
1. Gastric lavage followed by activated charcoal by mouth or through the lavage tube.
2. Saline cathartics.
3. Intravenous fluids to combat dehydration.
4. Symptomatic and supportive therapy.

49 – 681. SESAME OIL (Benne, Teel, Gingilli Oil)

Large doses of this complex mixture of glycerides produce extreme catharsis. Acute dehydration may require oral or intravenous fluid replacement.

49 – 682. SHEEP DIP See 49 – 90. *Arsenic;* 49 – 590. *Phenol*

49 – 683. SHELLAC

White shellac contains rosin; other colors contain arsenic trisulfide. All varieties are dissolved in ethyl or methyl alcohol to which various aliphatic hydrocarbons and ketones in small amounts have been added. For treatment, see **49 – 90**. *Arsenic;* **49 – 475**. *Methyl Alcohol.*

49 – 684. SHOE CLEANERS

Usually shoe cleaners contain a small amount of trisodium phosphate with isopropyl alcohol (**49 – 403**).

49 – 685. SHOE DYES AND POLISHES See 49 – 74. *Aniline Dyes;* 49 – 403. *Isopropyl Alcohol;* 49 – 529. *Nitrobenzene*

49 – 686. SILICOFLUORIDES See 49 – 336. *Fluorides;* 49 – 338. *Fluorosilicates*

49 – 687. SILVER POLISH See 49 – 235. *Cyanides*

49−688. SILVER SALTS AND COMPOUNDS

Silver acetate and nitrate are available in many households and are acutely toxic if ingested. Silver nitrate caustic pencils may be broken up and eaten by children. Less than 2 gm. is generally harmless; larger amounts may cause burning of the throat and epigastrium, black vomitus, violent abdominal pain and convulsions, and coma which may be terminal.

TREATMENT

1. Sodium chloride, 15 gm., well diluted, by mouth.

2. Gastric lavage with large amounts of warm water followed by activated charcoal in water by mouth.

3. Codeine sulfate or morphine sulfate for pain.

4. Magnesium sulfate (Epsom salts) by mouth as a purgative.

5. Hospitalization for symptomatic and supportive therapy if more than 2 gm. has been swallowed or if convulsions or coma has been present.

PROGNOSIS.   Good with small amounts. Ingestion of 2 to 10 mg. of silver nitrate may be fatal; over 10 gm. almost always causes death.

49−689. SLAKED LIME See 49−425. *Lime*

49−690. SNAIL BAITS See 49−462. *Metaldehyde*

Some older proprietary products may contain arsenic (**49−90**).

49−691. SNAKE VENOM See 24−19. *Snake Bites;* **61.** *Venoms*

49−692. SNUFF See 49−523. *Nicotine*

49−693. SOAPS AND DETERGENTS

White, unperfumed household soaps are harmless even if ingested in large quantities; addition of antiseptics, disinfectants, deodorants, coloring or perfume may cause nausea, vomiting and mild gastrointestinal irritation but no serious symptoms. Some laundry soaps contain enough caustic alkalies to cause severe mucous membrane damage and require treatment as outlined in **49−39.** *Alkalies,* together with fluid replacement if vomiting has been prolonged.

Detergents are divided into 3 classes, depending on the purpose for which they are intended.

Class 1. Light-duty, high sudsing: For dishes, baby clothes, etc.—these are slightly toxic.

Class 2. All-purpose, high sudsing: For laundry and general use—moderately toxic.

Class 3. Washday, low sudsing: Made for use in automatic washers—relatively high toxicity. Deaths from ingestion have been reported.

TREATMENT FOR CLASSES 1 AND 2

1. Immediate dilution with large amounts of water, milk, olive oil or other demulcents.

2. Induction of vomiting if large amounts have been swallowed and vomiting has not already occurred. After the stomach has been emptied, activated charcoal in water should be given by mouth.

3. Calcium gluconate, 10 ml. of 10% solution intravenously, to prevent development of hypocalcemia.

TREATMENT FOR CLASS 3

1. Dilution; administration of demulcents and absorbents, especially activated charcoal.

2. Gastric lavage (if mucous membrane erosion is not extreme), followed by a saline cathartic.

3. Control of pain. Small doses of a narcotic may be required.

4. Administration of air or oxygen by face mask and rebreathing bag.

5. Tracheostomy (**14 – 12**) for laryngeal edema.

6. Recognition and treatment of pulmonary edema (**51**).

7. Hospitalization for prolonged observation, supportive and symptomatic treatment. Permanent strictures of the esophagus may occur.

49 – 694. SODIUM ARSENATE AND ARSENITE

These contain about 50 and 75% arsenic (**49 – 90**), respectively and, because they are very soluble, are extremely toxic. See **49 – 90**. *Arsenic.*

49 – 695. SODIUM AUROTHIOMALATE See **49 – 353**. *Gold Salts*

49 – 696. SODIUM CHLORIDE (Salt)

Common table salt in excess can cause severe toxic effects in infants and small children, characterized by nausea, vomiting, excitement, hypertonicity, extensor spasticity, convulsions and eventual coma. *Table salt and water should never be used as an emetic.*

TREATMENT

1. Control of hypertonicity and convulsions by sedatives.

2. Prevention of dehydration and potassium depletion (**6.** *Fluid Replacement*).

3. Removal of salt by repeated peritoneal dialyses (**14 – 9**), using 5% dextrose in water as the dialysate, may be necessary in severe cases.

49 – 697. SODIUM CYANIDE

Inhalation or ingestion of even minute amounts may be fatal. See **49 – 235**. *Cyanides*

49 – 698. SODIUM FLUORIDE See **49 – 336**. *Fluorides*

49 – 699. SODIUM FLUOROACETATE (See also **49 – 337**. *Fluoroacetates*)

Sodium fluoroacetate is a tremendously toxic substance which occurs naturally in a South African plant (*Dichapetalum cymosum*), which has caused many fatalities. The synthetic commercial preparation (Compound 1080) is used as a rodenticide. Accidental ingestion of a few crystals has caused tingling around the mouth and nose, severe vomiting, blurred vision from loss of focusing ability, epileptiform convulsions, stupor and coma.

TREATMENT

1. Gastric lavage with sodium bicarbonate solution, leaving magnesium sulfate solution in the stomach.

2. Control of convulsions by rapid-acting barbiturates intravenously.

3. Calcium gluconate (5%) or dextrose (5%) in saline intravenously.

4. Hospitalization for supportive therapy and close observation for several days. Delayed hypertension and cardiac dilatation may occur.

49 – 700. SODIUM FLUOROSILICATE See **49 – 338**. *Fluorosilicates*

49 – 701. SODIUM HYDROXIDE (Caustic Soda) See **49 – 39.** *Alkalies*

49 – 702. SODIUM MONOFLUOROACETATE (Compound 1080) See **49 – 699.** *Sodium Fluoroacetate*

49 – 703. SODIUM NITRITE See **49 – 528.** *Nitrites*

49 – 704. SODIUM OXALATE See **49 – 552.** *Oxalic Acid*

49 – 705. SODIUM PENTOTHAL See **49 – 580.** *Pentothal Sodium*

49 – 706. SODIUM PERBORATE See **49 – 138.** *Borates, Boric Acid and Boron*

49 – 707. SODIUM RHODANATE (Sodium Thiocyanate) See **49 – 774.** *Thiocyanates*

49 – 708. SODIUM SELENATE See **49 – 679.** *Selenium and Its Salts*

49 – 709. SODIUM SULFIDE

Usually mixed with barium sulfide or thallium salts, sodium sulfide is the main active agent in many depilatories (hair removers). Toxic effects following ingestion are due partly to local corrosive action on the mucous membranes and partly to the formation of hydrogen sulfide, and consist of a foul breath from the odor of hydrogen sulfide, a burning sensation in the mouth, throat and stomach, rapid onset of pulmonary irritation and edema (**51**). Convulsions and coma followed by death from respiratory paralysis may occur.

TREATMENT

1. Immediate cautious emptying of stomach by lavage unless evidence of severe corrosion is present. Activated charcoal in water should be left in the stomach and followed by a saline cathartic.

2. Oxygen inhalations under positive pressure by face mask or endotracheal catheter and rebreathing bag, continued as long as there is any evidence of heart action.

3. Control of convulsions by rapid-acting barbiturates.

4. Hospitalization for observation for at least 24 hours after control of the acute signs and symptoms. Pulmonary edema (**51**) may be a late complication.

49 – 710. SODIUM SULFOCYANATES See **49 – 774.** *Thiocyanates*

49 – 711. SOIL FUMIGANTS See **49 – 241.** *DD Compounds;* **49 – 821.** *Vapam*

49 – 712. SOLANINE

A mixture of very toxic glucosides, including solanine, is present in several species of plants. Among these are:

Bittersweet (**49 – 872**). The toxic alkaloid occurs in the leaves, berries and seeds. Green berries contain large amounts of solanine; ripe berries, very little.

Jerusalem cherry. The fruit contains a large amount of solanine and is extremely poisonous.

Nightshade (49—967). The green, unripened berries and the leaves of several varieties of this plant are toxic; the ripe berries are relatively nontoxic.

Potato. In the sprouts, leaves, berries and seeds.

Tomato. In the leaves and stems.

SIGNS AND SYMPTOMS.   Poisoning is usually delayed for 1 to 3 hours after ingestion; symptoms consist of a cold clammy skin, nausea, vomiting, multiple soft stools, mental confusion, delirium, muscular twitching, mydriasis and acute respiratory and cardiac depression.

TREATMENT

1. Emetics or gastric lavage with potassium permanganate (1:5000 solution) followed by activated charcoal in water orally or through the lavage tube.

2. Administration of saline cathartics.

3. Sedation by parenteral administration of rapid-acting barbiturates if muscular twitching is extreme.

4. Respiratory and cardiovascular support as required.

5. Observation for at least 6 hours after ingestion because of the tendency of solanine to cause delayed toxic effects.

49—713. SOMINEX

This proprietary preparation, extensively advertised as a safe somnifacient, has caused numerous cases of acute toxicity due to its scopolamine content. See 49—104. *Atropine;* 49—676. *Scopolamine.*

49—714. SOMNIFENE

This is a potent sedative and hypnotic. For toxic signs, symptoms and treatment, see 49—111. *Barbiturates.*

49—715. "SPEED-BALLS"

Two well-known preparations have recently been substituted by ingeniously minded individuals—often narcotic addicts—for the more difficult to obtain drugs heroin, morphine and meperidine. These are:

Percodan. A proprietary preparation containing dihydrocodeinone, homatropine, acetylsalicylic acid, acetophenetidin and caffeine in a nonsterile tablet for oral use.

Methamphetamine Hydrochloride (Methedrine). Usually 15 or 30 mg. sterile solution in ampules, suitable for intravenous injection.

One Percodan tablet is usually dissolved in 1 ampule of Methedrine to produce a "speed-ball" which is injected intravenously with an effect similar to powerful opiates (see 49—495. *Morphine*) but of much shorter duration.

Since the Percodan tablets are not sterile, habitual "speed-ball" users may show evidence of multiple abscesses in different stages of healing at the sites of injections.

49—716. SPIDER VENOM See 24—20. *Spider Bites;* 61. *Venoms*

49—717. SPIRITS OF NITRE See 49—528. *Nitrites*

49—718. SQUILL (Sea Onion)

White squill is used medicinally as a diuretic and cardiac agent; red squill is used as a rat poison. The toxicity and treatment are practically the same as outlined in 49—272. *Digitalis.*

49 – 719. SQUIRREL POISONS

These preparations usually contain sodium fluoroacetate (**49 – 699**), thallium (**49 – 768**) or strychnine (**49 – 729**).

49 – 720. STANNIC AND STANNOUS SALTS See **49 – 786**. *Tin*

49 – 721. STILBESTROL See **49 – 271**. *Diethylstilbestrol*

49 – 722. STINGRAY (Stingaree) VENOM See **56 – 13**. *Stings;* **61**. *Venoms*

49 – 723. STODDARD SOLVENT

This is a petroleum distillate which has about the same toxicity as kerosene. For treatment, see **49 – 408**. *Kerosene.*

49 – 724. STRAMONIUM

Stramonium is found in common plants (jimsonweed, stinkweed, thorn apple, etc.) in many localities. The toxicity and treatment are similar to that outlined for *Atropine Sulfate* (**49 – 104**). It has a mild hallucinogenic effect (**49 – 358**). Stramonium poisoning has been reported following ingestion by immature persons of Asthamaclor, a stramonium-belladonna mixture.

49 – 725. STREPTOKINASE-STREPTODORNASE (Varidase)

Allergic reactions to this mixture of proteolytic enzymes have been reported. These include chills, restlessness, apprehension, profuse perspiration, chest pain, dyspnea and anaphylactic shock. For treatment, see **21**. *Allergic Reactions.*

49 – 726. STREPTOMYCIN See **49 – 78**. *Antibiotics*

49 – 727. STROBANE See **49 – 794**. *Toxaphene*

49 – 728. STROPHANTHIN See **49 – 272**. *Digitalis*

49 – 729. STRYCHNINE

Strychnine is an alkaloid contained in the seeds of the nux vomica plant. It is a powerful poison which formerly had wide use medicinally as a tonic and respiratory stimulant and commercially as a rodenticide. A household hazard for children is often present in patent medicines (usually laxatives and tonics) which may contain appreciable quantities. Strychnine acts by increasing the reflex excitement of the spinal cord and the medullary center. The toxic picture can be confused with acute tetanus (**30 – 31**) and is characterized by dyspnea, cyanosis, a feeling of suffocation, profuse perspiration, opisthotonos and tetanic convulsions. No matter how acute the poisoning, the patient is always fully conscious.

TREATMENT

1. Absolute rest in a quiet room to prevent initiation of tetanic convulsions by external stimuli.

2. Activated charcoal in water by mouth. Unless the patient is seen within a few minutes of ingestion do not give emetics or attempt gastric lavage.

3. Pentobarbital sodium intravenously for control of convulsions, repeated as necessary.

4. Ether (very light inhalations), to relax the tightness of the diaphragm and allow efficient respiration.

5. Assistance with ventilation by mechanical methods (**11 – 1**) if necessary.

6. Hospitalization for close observation and symptomatic treatment. Relapses after several hours are common.

7. *Do not use:*

Emetics of any type. Choking, strangling and aspiration of vomitus may result.

Gastric lavage, unless within 10 minutes of ingestion (see No. 2, above). If the stomach is washed, 1:5000 potassium permanganate or 2% tannic acid solution should be used. If not seen within a few minutes, attempts to empty the stomach should be postponed until reflex irritibility and convulsions have been completely controlled.

Caffeine. It increases the strychnine effect.

Bromides. Their action is too slow to be beneficial.

Opiates or synthetic narcotics. They react synergistically with strychnine and may cause acute respiratory depression.

Cathartics, purgatives and diuretics. They are of no value.

PROGNOSIS.   Good if the patient can be kept alive for 5 to 6 hours.

49 – 730. SULFOBROMOPHTHALEIN SODIUM (Bromsulphalein)

Hypersensitivity reactions to this substance used in liver function tests occasionally occur. They are characterized by acute anxiety, severe squeezing chest pain, dyspnea and vomiting. For treatment, see **21 – 5.** *Less Serious Allergic Reactions.*

49 – 731. SULFONAMIDES

The sulfonamides currently in common use include:

Acetyl sulfamethoxypyridazine
    (Kynex Acetyl)
Para-nitrosulfathiozole
    (Nisulfazole)
Phthalylsulfathiazole
    (Sulfathalidine)
Salicylazosulfapyridine
    (Azulfidine)
Sodium sulfacetamide
    (Sodium Sulamid)
Succinylsulfathiazole
    (Sulfasuxidine)
Sulfacetamide
    (Sulamid)
Sulfachlorpyridazine
    (Sonilyn)
Sulfadiazine

Sulfadimethoxine
    (Madribon)
Sulfaethiodole (Sul-Spansim)
Sulfamerazine
Sulfamethizole
    (Thiosulfil)
Sulfamethoxazole
    (Gantanol)
Sulfamethoxypyridazine
    (Kypex, Midicel)
Sulfisomidine
    (Elkosin)
Sulfisoxazole
    (Gantrisin)

All may give acute toxic reactions following overdosage or accidental ingestion of large amounts. Some persons may demonstrate hypersensitivity to small doses. Toxic manifestations of greater or lesser degree occur in about 50% of adults and 20% of children. Although the symptoms may be alarming, few fatalities have been reported.

Minor toxic effects consist of fever, usually accompanied by skin rashes suggestive of measles, pruritus, cyanosis, gastrointestinal irritation, precordial and abdominal pain, acidosis, central nervous system disturbances, confusion, restlessness, headache, vertigo, nausea, vomiting, depression (or elation) and lassitude.

TREATMENT

1. Temporary decrease or discontinuance of the drug.
2. Administration of oxygen by face mask and rebreathing bag.
3. Referral of the patient if possible back to the physician who prescribed the medication. A brief summary of the signs, symptoms and treatment should be sent with the patient.

Dangerous toxic effects are characterized by:

Skin Rashes. Generalized serious exfoliative dermatitis may occur, sometimes associated with hepatitis.

Jaundice. The acute hemolysis apparently has no relationship to the level of sulfonamides in the blood. There is usually an associated hemoglobinuria.

Toxic nephrosis.

Acute hemolytic anemia with hemoglobinuria, severe leukopenia and agranulocytosis.

Crystalluria.

Renal calculi with resultant suppression of kidney function.

TREATMENT

1. Stop the administration of the medication at once.
2. Give emetics or lavage if large amounts have been ingested. Activated charcoal should be left in the stomach.
3. Give copious amounts of fluids by mouth and intravenously.
4. Hospitalize for determination of the blood sulfonamide level and for symptomatic and supportive treatment.

49 – 732. SULFONMETHANE (Sulfonal)

Large doses, or prolonged use, of Sulfonal may cause skin eruptions, gastrointestinal irritation, vomiting with an acetone odor, staggering gait, motor weakness and paralysis of the bladder. Since Sulfonal is excreted slowly, cumulative effects may be serious. The presence of coproporphyrinuria makes the prognosis poor.

TREATMENT

1. Gastric lavage followed by activated charcoal in water by mouth or through the lavage tube.
2. Saline cathartics.
3. Fluids by mouth and intravenously.
4. Prolonged hospitalization for symptomatic and supportive care because of slow elimination of the drug.

49 – 733. SULFOTEPP (Tetraethyl Pyrophosphate) See 49 – 546. *Organic Phosphates*

49 – 734. SULFUR

Sulfur has a relatively low toxicity. Toxic signs and symptoms may develop after ingestion of large amounts which break down in the large intestine to hydrogen sulfide (**49 – 380**).

49 – 735. SULFUR CHLORIDE

Sulfur chloride is a commonly used insecticide which in the presence of moisture breaks down into hydrochloric acid and sulfur dioxide. For treatment, see **49 – 26.** *Acids;* **49 – 736.** *Sulfur Dioxide.*

49 – 736. SULFUR DIOXIDE

Sulfur dioxide is used as an insecticide and as a food preservative. It is one of the toxic components of the "smog" common in highly industrialized areas. Even moderate concentrations cause irritation of the upper respiratory tract (choking, coughing, sneezing, dyspnea, cyanosis) and pulmonary edema (**51**). Acidosis (**43 – 1**) may develop. Convulsions and reflex respiratory arrest may be terminal.

TREATMENT

1. Removal at once from exposure to fumes.

2. Insurance of a clear airway.

3. Immediate oxygen inhalations under positive pressure, preferably by face mask and rebreathing bag.

4. Application of external heat.

5. Intravenous injection of 500 to 1000 ml. of normal salt solution.

6. Control of bronchospasm by subcutaneous injection of 0.3 to 0.5 ml. of 1:1000 solution of epinephrine hydrochloride (Adrenalin), repeated as necessary.

7. Treatment of acidosis (**43 – 1**).

49 – 737. SULFURIC ACID (Oil of Vitriol) See 49 – 26. *Acids*

49 – 738. SULFURYL CHLORIDE

Inhalation of the fumes of this solvent, used in the chemical and rubber industries, causes severe mucous membrane and skin irritation with conjunctivitis, palpebral edema, rhinitis, tracheitis, bronchitis and pneumonitis.

TREATMENT

1. Removal from exposure.

2. Inhalation of a 5% sodium bicarbonate solution mist.

49 – 739. SUN TAN CREAMS AND LOTIONS

These cosmetic preparations are used as "sun screens" to absorb ultraviolet rays and to prevent sunburn and usually contain Dicumarol and amyl salicylate. Toxic effects from skin absorption usually do not develop except in allergic individuals. If ingested, severe toxic effects may develop due to the Dicumarol (**49 – 265**) and the salicylate (**49 – 664**) content.

49 – 740. TALC (French Chalk)

Talc (magnesium silicate) is harmless unless large amounts are aspirated, but some popular brands of talcum powder contain a considerable amount of boric acid (**49 – 138**) and zinc stearate (**49 – 854**).

49 – 741. TANACETUM VULGARE (Tansy)

The stems and leaves of this perennial plant contain a mixture of toxic terpenes and volatile oils. "Therapeutic" doses given as abortifacients and anthelminthics have been fatal.

TREATMENT

1. Gastric lavage followed by activated charcoal by mouth or through the lavage tube.

2. Saline cathartics.

3. Symptomatic and supportive care.

49 – 742.   TANNIC ACID (Tannin)

By ingestion this powerful astringent will cause uncomfortable but never fatal signs and symptoms, including nausea, vomiting, gastritis and lower bowel disturbances.

In contrast, by injection it is a deadly poison and may cause severe convulsions, circulatory and/or respiratory collapse and death from hepatic necrosis.

49 – 743.   TAR

All types and derivatives of tar are toxic if ingested, because of their cresol content. For signs and symptoms of toxicity and treatment, see **49 – 590.** *Phenol.*

49 – 744.   TARTAR EMETIC (Antimony and Potassium Tartrate) See **49 – 81.** *Antimony*

49 – 745.   TARTARIC ACID

Although relatively nontoxic, large doses of tartaric acid may cause severe signs and symptoms. Fatalities have been reported.

SIGNS AND SYMPTOMS.   Nausea, vomiting, severe abdominal cramping, diarrhea and circulatory collapse.

TREATMENT

1. Emptying of the stomach as soon as possible by emetics or gastric lavage with large quantities of warm water followed by activated charcoal in water.

2. Administration of saline cathartics by mouth or through the lavage tube.

3. Large amounts of fluids by mouth and/or intravenously.

49 – 746.   TAXUS BACCATA L. (English Yew)

The leaves, stems and, to a lesser extent, the fruit of this ornamental evergreen tree contain toxic substances which, if ingested, cause vomiting, gastric and abdominal pain, pallor, dizziness and respiratory and cardiac embarrassment.

TREATMENT

1. Emetics or gastric lavage followed by activated charcoal in water by mouth or through the lavage tube.

2. Saline cathartics.

3. Supportive care.

49 – 747.   TCA (Trichloracetic Acid)

This is a powerful local caustic but has no systemic toxic actions. See **49 – 26.** *Acids.*

49 – 748.   TCE (Tetrachlorethane)

TCE is similar in action to but more dangerous than carbon tetrachloride. For treatment, see **49 – 173.** *Carbon Tetrachloride.*

49 – 749.   TDE (Tetrachlorodiphenylethane)

Used as an insecticide, TDE is much safer than most of the others used for the same purpose. Signs and symptoms of toxicity following inhalation or ingestion (general malaise, prostration and collapse) are usually relatively mild, with recovery in 2 to 4 days without residual ill effects. Treatment is similar to that outlined for DDT (**49–243**).

49–750. TEETHING POWDERS

These usually contain calomel (**49–160**) with talc (**49–740**) or chalk. Some brands contain small amounts of boric acid or borates (**49–138**) and bromides (**49–144**).

49–751. TEFLON See **49–611**. *Plastics*

Finely divided Teflon dust causes a condition similar to metal fume fever (**49–461**). Inhalation of fumes has been reported as causing pulmonary edema (**51**).

49–752. TELLURIUM

Most of the cases of toxicity from tellurium are caused by inhalation of the fumes of the oxide. A garlicky odor to the breath is characteristic, with gastric pain, fatigue and severe headache. Accidental ingestion of potassium tellurite has resulted in a similar picture followed by cyanosis, dyspnea, hepatic involvement and death.

TREATMENT

1. Removal from exposure to fumes followed by administration of oxygen under positive pressure.
1. Gastric lavage if ingested, leaving activated charcoal in water in the stomach.
3. Supportive and symptomatic care. BAL (**49–109**) is ineffective.

49–753. TEPP (Tetraethyl Pyrophosphate, TEP) See **49–546**. *Organic Phosphates*

49–754. TERPINEOL (Lilacin)

This toxic substance occurs in pine oil and because of its attractive lilac odor is a constituent of many perfumes and cosmetics. Ingestion of preparations containing terpineol in even small amounts may cause acute gastritis (sometimes hemorrhagic), general malaise, weakness, decreased body temperature, vertigo, excitement, drowsiness, convulsions and other signs of central nervous system disturbances and respiratory depression.

TREATMENT

See **49–815**. *Turpentine.*

49–755. TERPIN HYDRATE

This commonly used expectorant in large doses gives a toxic picture similar to that of turpentine. For signs and symptoms from overdosage and treatment, see **49–815**. *Turpentine.*

49–756. TETRACAINE HYDROCHLORIDE (Pontocaine) See **49–72**. *Anesthetics, Local*

49–757. TETRACHLORODIPHENYLETHANE (DDD)

This insecticide has the same action as but less toxicity than DDT (**49–243**).

49–758. TETRACHLOROETHYLENE See **49–173.** *Carbon Tetrachloride*

49–759. TETRACYCLINES See **49–78.** *Antibiotics*

49–760. TETRAETHYL DITHIOPYROPHOSPHATE (Sulfotepp) See **49–546.** *Organic Phosphates*

49–761. TETRAETHYL LEAD See **49–322.** *Ethyl Gasoline;* **49–349.** *Gasoline*

Used as an antiknock component of gasoline, tetraethyl lead may cause toxic symptoms by absorption through the intact skin or by inhalation of the fumes. Acute poisoning is characterized by sleeplessness, restlessness, mental confusion, hallucinations, delirium and maniacal outbursts. Later developments are tremors, fibrillary twitching, myoclonus and spasticity.

TREATMENT

1. Removal from exposure to fumes.
2. Removal of all clothing saturated with ethyl gasoline, followed by thorough washing with soap and water.
3. Sedation by rapid-acting barbiturates. Opiates, synthetic narcotics and chloral hydrate are ineffective in tetraethyl lead intoxication and should not be used.
4. Large amounts of fluid orally and intravenously.
5. Alkalinization of the urine.
6. Symptomatic and supportive care.

49–762. TETRAETHYLPYROPHOSPHATE (TEPP, Nifos, Tetrin) See **49–546.** *Organic Phosphates*

49–763. TETRAFLUOROETHYLENE See **49–611.** *Plastics*

49–764. TETRAHYDRONAPHTHALENE (Tetralin)

Inhalation of the fumes of this commercial solvent for fats, oils and waxes causes severe headache, acute conjunctivitis, nasotracheobronchitis and nephritic irritation, with grass-green urine.

TREATMENT

1. Removal from exposure.
2. Administration of oxygen under positive pressure by face mask and rebreathing bag.
3. Prescription of sedative cough mixtures.
4. Reference for follow-up care. The toxic nephritis usually clears in 7 to 10 days without permanent ill-effects.

49–765. TETRAMETHYLTHIURAM DISULFIDE See **49–779.** *Thiram*

49–766. TETRAODONTIAE (See also **49–339.** *Rare causes of food poisoning*)

The viscera, especially the ovaries, of this world-wide variety of edible fish contain a tremendously toxic substance, tetradotoxin, which is heat resistant and not destroyed by usual cooking methods, and which varies in amount in different species in different seasons. Local names for the fish vary in different countries—in Australia they are called toadfish, in Great Britain puffers, in the Hawaiian Islands death fish or maki-maki, in Japan fugus, in the Philippines botete, in South Africa blaasoportoby and in the United States blowfish, jugfish or puffers.

The clinical picture of poisoning from all types develops at any time up to 36 hours after ingestion and is characterized by facial tingling, numbness of the extremities, intense pruritus, vomiting, abdominal pain, arthralgia, myalgia, paralysis and prostration. Hypotension may reach shock levels.

TREATMENT

1. Absolute bed rest.

2. Emptying of the stomach as soon as possible by emetics followed by gastric lavage unless several hours have elapsed since ingestion. Whether or not the stomach is emptied, activated charcoal in water should be given by mouth.

3. Administration of oil base cathartics.

4. Morphine sulfate in small doses subcutaneously for severe pain and myalgia.

5. Intravenous fluids to combat shock (**53–7**) and dehydration, followed if necessary by whole blood transfusions.

49–767. TETRIN (TEPP, Nifos, Tetraethyl Pyrophosphate) See 49–546. *Organic Phosphates*

49–768. THALLIUM

With or without the sulfides of barium (**49–112**) and sodium, thallium acetate is used in depilatories (hair removers) in spite of the fact that it is only slightly less toxic than arsenic (**49–90**). Thallium sulfate is the active toxic ingredient in some brands of ant poisons (**49–75**) and rodenticides (**49–719.** *Squirrel Poisons*).

Toxic signs and symptoms usually develop 1 to 2 hours after ingestion, but may be delayed for as long as 36 hours if thallium has been administered medicinally.

SIGNS AND SYMPTOMS of thallium poisoning consist of nausea, vomiting, severe abdominal pain, bloody diarrhea, ulcerative stomatitis, bizarre paresthesias, ptosis, strabismus, mydriasis, facial palsies, superficial ecchymoses and petechiae, convulsions, delirium and delayed respiratory failure.

TREATMENT

1. Expired air respiration (**11–1**) followed if necessary by oxygen inhalations under positive pressure.

2. Application of external heat.

3. Gastric lavage with 1% sodium or potassium iodide (to form insoluble thallium iodide), followed by activated charcoal in water.

4. Control of convulsions by intravenous barbiturates or intramuscular paraldehyde.

5. Catharsis by castor oil or magnesium sulfate (Epsom salts).

6. Intravenous injection of 100 ml. of 5% dextrose in normal salt solution. Ephedrine sulfate, levarterenol bitartrate (Levophed) or metaraminol bitartrate (Aramine) to counteract circulatory collapse may be necessary.

7. Hospitalization for extensive, and sometimes prolonged, symptomatic and supportive treatment. Administration of BAL (**49–109**) may be beneficial. Permanent neurologic damage may occur.

49–769. THEOBROMINE

Occurring naturally in cacao beans and cola nuts, theobromine is used medicinally as a myocardial stimulant and diuretic. Large doses (2 to 5 gm.) may cause severe headaches, nausea, vomiting, gastric pain, diarrhea, acute excitement and tremors.

TREATMENT
1. Discontinue therapeutic use.
2. Supportive and symptomatic care.

49−770. THIAMINE HYDROCHLORIDE (Vitamin B₁ Hydrochloride)

Hypersensitivity reactions are common not only in patients receiving thiamine to correct B₁ deficiency but also in pharmaceutical workers. In addition to pruritus, urticaria, angioneurotic edema and respiratory distress, herpes zoster (**46−8.** *Neuritis*) may occur.
For treatment, see **21.** *Allergic Reactions.*

49−771. THIAZIDE DIURETICS

This group of drugs has practically replaced mercurial diuretics. Among available preparations are:
Benzydroflumethiazide (Benuron, Naturetin)
Benzthiazide (Aquatag, Exna)
Chlorothiazide (Diuril)
Cyclothiazide (Anhydron)
Flumethiazide (Ademol)
Hydrochlorothiazide (Esidrex, Hydrodiuril, Oretic)
Hydroflumethiazide (Saluron)
Methyclothiazide (Enduron)
Polythiazide (Renese)
Trichlormethiazide (Metahydrin, Naqua)
Usual therapeutic doses of any of these may cause many side effects, including aggravation of preexistent systemic conditions such as diabetes and gout and accentuation of the effects of drugs such as digitalis. Potassium depletion often requires replacement therapy. Other side effects are muscular weakness, gastroenteritis, pancreatitis, jaundice, hepatic cirrhosis, glomerulonephritis, photosensitization and (rarely) blood dyscrasias.
TREATMENT
1. Discontinuance of offending thiazide.
2. Symptomatic therapy is all that is required except in extreme cases requiring correction of potassium depletion (**6.** *Fluid Replacement*).

49−772. THIMET See 49−546. *Organic Phosphates*

49−773. THINNER INTOXICATION

Use of paint thinner as an intoxicating agent and hallucinogen has been reported among teenagers. Ordinary paint thinner made up of benzene, butyl acetate, butyl alcohol, ethyl acetate, ethyl alcohol and toluene is used to saturate a handkerchief which is held over the nose. Another method is to spray the thinner into the nose with an ordinary atomizer. All degrees of intoxication can be obtained.
TREATMENT
Treatment is similar to that outlined for acute alcoholic intoxication (**49−315**). See also **49−349.** *Gasoline* and **49−610.** *Plastic Glues and Cements.*

49−774. THIOCYANATES (Sulfocyanates, Rhodanates)

Inorganic salts (ammonium, potassium, sodium, etc.) present a completely different toxic picture from that given by the more complex organic (aliphatic) thiocyanates.

Average therapeutic doses in certain individuals may cause nausea, vomiting, acute gastric pain, diarrhea, acute depression, exhaustion, edema of the glottis or larynx and signs of hypothyroidism.

Larger doses (with a thiocyanate level above 12 mg. per 100 ml.) may cause high fever, angina, gastric hemorrhage, purpura, enlargement of the thyroid, hyperactive reflexes, muscular twitching, convulsions, hallucinations, motor paralysis of the lower extremities, toxic hepatitis, coma and collapse.

TREATMENT

1. Stop the medication at once.
2. Force fluids by mouth and intravenously.
3. Hospitalize as soon as possible for symptomatic and supportive care.

Organic (aliphatic) derivatives

These substances are used almost exclusively as contact insecticides, usually in kerosene or toluene bases. Not only does their toxicity differ from that of inorganic thiocyanates, but also the various members of the aliphatic group have different toxic characteristics.

Ethyl, isopropyl and methyl thiocyanates. Treat as outlined under **49—235.** *Cyanides.*

All other derivatives (Lauryl, Lethane, Thanite, etc.).

TREATMENT

1. Empty the stomach by lavage with large amounts of water, followed by lavage with at least 100 ml. of mineral oil, leaving a small amount of oil, together with 30 gm. of magnesium sulfate (Epsom salts), in the stomach.
2. Combat convulsions by intravenous injection of rapid-acting barbiturates.
3. Administer oxygen under positive pressure by face mask and rebreathing bag.
4. Give caffeine sodiobenzoate, 0.5 gm. intramuscularly or intravenously.
5. Hospitalize for continued supportive therpay and for evaluation and treatment of possible liver damage.

49—775. THIOGLYCOLLATES

These salts are the active ingredients of several "cold-wave" hair setting preparations. On the skin and scalp they may cause acute dermatitis with extreme edema and, occasionally, bleeding. If ingested they have a mild caustic action. Treatment consists of stopping use of the "cold wave" preparation.

49—776. THIONYL CHLORIDE

Skin contact may cause first and second degree burns. Inhalation of the fumes results in intense upper respiratory irritation.

TREATMENT

1. *Do not wash the skin with water;* instead, cleanse thoroughly with petroleum solvents.
2. Inhalations of 5% sodium bicarbonate mist.
3. Symptomatic and supportive therapy.

49—777. THIOPENTAL SODIUM See **49—580.** *Pentothal Sodium*

49—778. THIOURACIL

Used in the treatment of hyperthyroidism, thiouracil and its more modern prototype, propylthiouracil, may cause severe hypersensitivity reactions, parotitis and liver dysfunction. Exophthalmos from the primary disease may be increased. Blood dyscrasias occur frequently

TREATMENT
1. Discontinuance of use of the drug.
2. Supportive care, including pyridoxine, folic acid and crude liver extract.

49 — 779. THIRAM (Tetramethylthiuram Disulfide)

This substance is used extensively as a fungicide and in the rubber industry. It is the methyl analogue of disulfiram (Antabuse) and has approximately the same toxic action. For signs and symptoms of toxicity and treatment following ingestion of small amounts, see **49 — 77**. *Antabuse.* If large amounts have been ingested, gastric lavage with large amounts of water should be done. Ingestion of fats, oils and ethyl alcohol should be avoided for at least 1 week.

49 — 780. THOMAS SLAG

A by-product of the Thomas steel process, quadribasic calcium phosphate is used in a finely ground state as a fertilizer. Inhalation of the dust causes severe pneumonia, probably on an infectious, not a chemical, basis.
For treatment, see **52 — 15**. *Pneumonitis.*

49 — 781. THORIUM OXIDE

Insoluble thorium oxide is a by-product of the uranium industry. Inhalation of dust causes deposits of radioactive particles in the lungs and pulmonary lymph nodes, which are, for practical purposes, permanent.
No serious toxic effects from inhalation of thorium oxide particles have been reported as yet, although a preparation of thorium dioxide (Thorotrast) which was used by intravenous injection as a roentgenolographic contrast medium about 10 years ago has been related to several radiation-induced malignant tumors of the liver.

49 — 782. THORN APPLE (Jimsonweed)

These plants contain stramonium. The signs and symptoms of toxicity and treatment are the same as for atropine sulfate (**49 — 104**) and stramonium (**49 — 724**).

49 — 783. THUJA (Arbor Vitae, Yellow Cedar) See **49 — 864**. *Arbor Vitae*

49 — 784. THYMOL

Thymol has been used as an oral antiseptic and mouthwash, as a deodorant in dirty draining wounds and as a specific anti-hookworm agent.
SIGNS AND SYMPTOMS of thymol poisoning consist of a sensation of warmth in the stomach, followed by nausea, vomiting and severe epigastric pain. There may be dizziness, ataxia, acute excitement, subnormal temperature, rapid soft pulse, marked generalized weakness and collapse with cyanosis.
TREATMENT
1. Emetics or gastric lavage with 1:5000 potassium permanganate solution followed by activated charcoal in water by mouth or through the lavage tube. Oily substances and alcohol increase absorption and should be avoided.
2. Oxygen therapy if cyanosis is marked.
3. Magnesium sulfate (Epsom salts) by mouth for purgation.
4. Caffeine sodiobenzoate, 0.5 gm. intramuscularly.

5. Hospitalization if evidences of toxicity are still present after the treatment outlined above.

49−785. THYROID

Overdosage with thyroid or drugs of similar action [Sodium levothyroxine (Synthroid sodium), sodium liothyronine (Cytomel), thyroglobulin (Proloid)] may result in palpitation, excessive sweating, tremors, nervousness, fever, intolerance to heat, tachycardia, increased pulse pressure and diarrhea.

TREATMENT
1. Discontinuance or decrease in dosage of the offending drug.
2. Sedation as required.

49−786. TIN

Acute tin poisoning is rare but does occur occasionally following ingestion of canned foods. Usually 5 or 6 hours elapse before vomiting, chest pain, a metallic taste in the mouth and diarrhea develop. Symptoms are usually more uncomfortable than serious and subside after a few hours under symptomatic therapy.

49−787. TITANIUM TETRACHLORIDE

This substance is highly corrosive to soft tissues on contact and its fumes are extremely irritating if inhaled. Severe chemical bronchitis and pneumonia, followed by pulmonary edema (51), may be caused by inhalation of a high concentration of fumes. Titanium salts used in paints are harmless.

TREATMENT FOLLOWING INHALATION
1. Remove from exposure at once.
2. Give expired air respiration (11−1) at once, followed as soon as possible by oxygen inhalation under positive pressure.
3. Hospitalize for care of the irritated respiratory tract.

TREATMENT FOLLOWING SPLASHES ON SKIN OR IN EYES
Do not wash or irrigate. Addition of water causes production of extreme heat. Instead, wipe the affected parts (including the eyes) with a soft cloth until they are absolutely dry; wait several minutes and then irrigate with copious amounts of water. All eye cases should be referred to an ophthalmologist as soon as possible.

49−788. TNT See 49−809. Trinitrotoluene

49−789. TOADSTOOLS See 49−347. Galerina Venenata; 49−500. Muscarine; 49−502. Mushroom Poisoning

49−790. TOBACCO See also 49−210. Cigarettes and Cigars; 49−523. Nicotine)

Commercial tobacco contains 1 to 2½% nicotine. A cigarette contains about 25 mg. Except for the fact that tobacco causes vomiting, ingestion of 2 or 3 cigarettes could well be fatal to an adult unaccustomed to tobacco. Fatalities have been reported in small children from ingestion of ½ of 1 cigarette. Statistics indicate an increase in the incidence of bronchogenic carcinoma in habitual users of tobacco. For treatment of toxic effects, see 49−523. Nicotine.

49—791. TOLUENE (Toluol) See **49—119.** *Benzene (Benzol) and Its Derivatives*

49—792. TOLUIDINE

Toluidine is similar in action but more toxic than aniline and causes more renal damage. For treatment, see **49—73.** *Aniline.*

49—793. TOOTHPASTES AND POWDERS See **49—547.** *Orris;* **49—616.** *Potassium Chlorate*

49—794. TOXAPHENE (Compound 3956, Octochlorocamphene, Chlorinated Camphene)

Toxaphene is a moderately toxic insecticide and pesticide which is not destroyed by heat; therefore, cases of poisoning from eating cooked vegetables have been reported.

SIGNS AND SYMPTOMS from inhalation and ingestion are of about equal intensity. Toxaphene has only a slight irritant effect on the skin and mucous membranes, but inhalation or ingestion may cause dizziness, involuntary muscle tremors and epileptiform convulsions.

TREATMENT

1. If inhaled, symptomatic treatment only is indicated. Rapid recovery usually occurs. If on the skin, remove by prolonged washing with soap and water.

2. If ingested, emetics or gastric lavage, followed by activated charcoal in water orally or through the lavage tube. Any type of oil should be avoided.

3. Prevention and control of convulsions by rapid-acting barbiturates. The patient should be protected against strong external stimuli.

4. Saline cathartics.

49—795. TREMETOL

An unsaturated alcohol called tremetol occurs in many native uncultivated plants in many parts of the United States. It is the cause of "trembles" in cattle and of "milk sickness" in humans resulting from ingestion of milk of animals who have eaten the leaves or shoots. Plants which contain tremetol include the deerwort, rayless goldenrod, witchweed, squaw seed and white snakeroot.

Tremetol intoxication is manifested by the slow onset of toxic effects, beginning with weakness, fatigue, anorexia, subnormal temperature, acetone-like odor on the breath and constipation. Severe vomiting and abdominal pain may develop 24 to 36 hours after ingestion, followed by coma and collapse.

TREATMENT

1. Sodium bicarbonate by mouth in large amounts (as much as 10 gm.), followed by gastric lavage with large quantities of water.

2. Magnesium sulfate (Epsom salts), 30 gm. by mouth or through the lavage tube.

3. Dextrose, 5% in saline, 500 to 1000 ml. intravenously.

4. Hospitalization as soon as the patient's condition will allow. Supportive therapy over a lengthy period may be necessary.

PROGNOSIS. The mortality from tremetol poisoning is about 50%. If the patient survives the acute stage, it is usually many months before he regains full strength and endurance.

49—796. TRIALKYLTHIOPHOSPHATE (Parathion) See **49—546.** *Organic Phosphates*

49 – 797. TRIBROMOETHANOL (Avertin)

Sudden, unpredictable side effects (pallor, constricted pupils, hypotension, shallow respiration) may follow rectal administration of "safe" doses of this narcotic. Late development of bronchitis, pneumonia, toxic hepatitis, yellow atrophy of the liver, anuria and uremia may occur – sometimes 3 to 5 days after rectal medication.

TREATMENT

1. Prevention of further absorption by rectal lavage.
2. Hospitalization for close observation until the danger of delayed complications has passed.

49 – 798. TRICHLOROACETIC ACID (TCA) See 49 – 26. *Acids;* 49 – 747. TCA

49 – 799. TRICHLOROBENZENE

Used in termite control, trichlorobenzene fumes may cause mild irritation of the eyes, nose and throat. For treatment, see 49 – 510. *Naphthalene.*

49 – 800. TRICHLOROETHYLENE (Ethylene Trichloride, Trilene)

Used as a solvent for fats and greases in industry, trichloroethylene is rapidly replacing carbon tetrachloride because inhalation of its fumes does not cause hepatic and renal damage. It is also used medicinally as an anesthetic.

SIGNS AND SYMPTOMS FOLLOWING INGESTION. Severe burning in mouth, throat, esophagus and stomach; nausea; vomiting; acute excitement followed by depression; hyperactive reflexes; muscular tremors; in severe cases, repiratory and/or cardiac collapse with serious liver damage.

Following inhalation of excessive or narcotic concentrations, pallor, profuse perspiration, dyspnea, cyanosis, bradycardia, hypotension and unconsciousness may develop, with death from respiratory and/or cardiac failure.

TREATMENT

1. Following inhalation of concentrations not sufficient to cause immediate death from cardiorespiratory failure, recovery generally takes place as soon as exposure is stopped; in severe cases, oxygen therapy and analeptic drugs may be indicated. Analeptics, however, should be used with extreme caution because of their tendency to cause cardiac irregularities. For detailed treatment, see 49 – 70. *Anesthetics, Inhalation.*
2. If trichloroethylene has been ingested, the following measures are in order:
   a. Administration of demulcents by mouth.
   b. Emptying the stomach by emetics or gastric lavage. Activated charcoal in water should be left in the stomach.
   c. Purgation by magnesium sulfate (Epsom salts) solution, 30 ml. by mouth or through the lavage tube.
   d. Hospitalization for supportive care and observation for at least 48 hours.

49 – 801. TRICHLORONITROMETHANE (Chloropicrin) See 49 – 832. *War Gases*

49 – 802. 2,4,5-TRICHLOROPHENOXY ACETIC ACID (2-4-5-T)

Used as a weed and shrub killer, 2-4-5-T has toxic effects similar to 2-4-D (49 – 263).

49 – 803. TRICRESOL See 49 – 590. *Phenol*

49 – 804.   TRICYCLIC ANTIDEPRESSANTS [Amitriptyline Hydrochloride (Elavil), Desmethylimipramine Hydrochloride (Norpramin), Imipramine Hydrochloride (Tofranil), Nortriptyline Hydrochloride (Aventyl), Protriptyline (Vivactil)]

Overdosage of any of these drugs may cause extreme restlessness, twitching, hyperreflexia, hyperpyrexia and persistent tachycardia. Hallucinations may occur. Convulsions and cardiac arrythmias are rare complications.

TREATMENT

1. Gastric lavage with large amounts of water, repeated every hour until symptoms subside.

2. Respiratory assistance by expired air or mechanical methods (**11 – 1**).

3. Neutralization of atropine-like symptoms by physostigmine (**49 – 104**).

4. Frequent ECG monitoring with appropriate treatment. Various cardiac arrythmias and cardiac arrest may be late developments.

5. Convulsions are usually self-limiting but may require short-acting barbiturates or paraldehyde for control.

Therapeutic doses of tricyclic antidepressants given concomitantly with monamine oxidase (MAO) inhibitor drugs [isocarboxid (Marplan), nialamid (Niamid), phenelzine sulfate (Nardil), tranylcypromide (Parnate), etc.] can cause serious toxic symptoms, including hypotension (or hypertension), hyperpyrexia and convulsions. These symptoms clear rapidly under symptomatic care when use of MAO inhibitors and tricyclic antidepressant drugs at the same time is discontinued.

49 – 805.   TRIETHYLENE GLYCOL See **49 – 320.** *Ethylene Glycol*

49 – 806.   TRIIODOMETHANE See **49 – 394.** *Iodoform*

49 – 807.   TRIMET See **49 – 546.** *Organic Phosphates*

49 – 808.   TRINITROBENZENE

The signs and symptoms of toxicity and treatment are approximately the same as for dinitrobenzene (**49 – 283**).

49 – 809.   TRINITROTOLUENE (TNT)

Inhalation of the fumes and dust from TNT may cause a serious toxic picture, characterized by loss of appetite, nausea, vomiting, acute diarrhea, cyanosis of the fingertips, ears and lips, delirium, hallucinations, convulsions, hepatitis, jaundice and aplastic anemia.

TREATMENT

1. Immediate removal from exposure.

2. Oxygen therapy under positive pressure by face mask and rebreathing bag.

3. Sedation by rapidly acting barbiturates.

4. Intravenous administration of 500 to 1000 ml. of 5% dextrose in saline.

5. Hospitalization for symptomatic and supportive therapy.

49 – 810.   TRIONAL See **49 – 111.** *Barbiturates*

49 – 811. TRIORTHOCRESYL PHOSPHATE (o-Tricresyl Phosphate)

This substance is the toxic agent in so-called "jake poisoning," caused by drinking extract of ginger or ingestion of parsley extract (apiol).

SIGNS AND SYMPTOMS. Nausea, vomiting and gastrointestinal irritation lasting for 2 to 3 days. After an interval of 5 days to 3 weeks (usually about 10 days), footdrop and wristdrop may develop. Other muscle groups may be involved.

TREATMENT

1. Emptying of the stomach by emetics or gastric lavage if ingested within the past 24 hours. Activated charcoal in water should be left in the stomach.

2. Administration of saline cathartics by mouth.

3. Hospitalization for symptomatic and supportive care, including support of paralyzed parts in functional position.

PROGNOSIS. Poor – muscle weaknesses and paralysis may be permanent.

49 – 812. TRIPELENNAMINE HYDROCHLORIDE (Pyribenzamine Hydrochloride)

See **49 – 80.** *Antihistaminics* for signs and symptoms of toxicity following therapeutic or excessive doses.

"Blue velvet" is the name for a peculiarly vicious mixture of tripelennamine and paregoric used by opiate addicts as a substitute for morphine or heroin. Both of the ingredients can be obtained cheaply without a prescription in many localities. One ounce of paregoric is boiled to get rid of the camphor and other volatile ingredients and a 50 mg. tripelennamine oral tablet is crushed into the liquid. This mixture is then injected intravenously, giving a euphoric effect lasting 2 to 3 hours. Since the oral antihistaminic tablets contain talc, veins are rapidly occluded. Pulmonary hypertension, severe bacterial infections and hepatitis may occur. In addition to treatment for acute addiction to opiates (**49 – 495.** *Morphine*), symptomatic care of the serious complications resulting from intravenous injection of an irritative nonsterile substance often is necessary.

49 – 813. TTD (Disulfiram, Antabuse) See 49 – 77. *Antabuse;* **49 – 779.** *Thiram*

49 – 814. TUNG OIL (Chinawood Oil) AND NUTS

Tung oil is nontoxic, but ingestion of the Brazil-nut-like nuts may cause severe gastric pain with vomiting and profuse diarrhea, painful muscle cramping and complete prostration from shock and respiratory depression.

TREATMENT

1. Gastric lavage with 1:5000 potassium permanganate solution followed by activated charcoal in water by mouth or through the lavage tube.

2. Oxygen inhalations by face mask and rebreathing bag if dyspnea or cyanosis is severe.

3. Dextrose (5%) in salt solution, 1000 to 1500 ml. intravenously. If shock is severe, 4 ml. of 0.2% levarterenol bitartrate (Levophed) should be given slowly in the dextrose solution with the rate of injection controlled by frequent blood pressure checks. Metaraminol bitartrate (Aramine) may be used in place of Levophed.

4. Calcium gluconate, 10 ml. of 10% solution intravenously.

5. Magnesium sulfate (Epsom salts), 30 gm. by mouth.

PROGNOSIS. Complete recovery without residual ill effects.

49 – 815.   TURPENTINE (Gum Turpentine, Oil of Turpentine, Spirits of Turpentine)

Varying combinations of terpenes, especially o-pinene, are responsible for the toxicity of this common solvent and medication. Although ingestion is more common, inhalation of high concentrations of fumes as well as absorption through the skin can cause acute toxicity.

SIGNS AND SYMPTOMS.   Characteristic odor on the breath, a sensation of burning in the mouth, throat, esophagus and stomach, nausea, vomiting, diarrhea, severe abdominal pain, ataxia, delirium and acute excitement, often followed by convulsions and painful urination with a violet-like odor of the urine. Later, hematuria and albuminuria may be present. Death usually occurs from respiratory failure, often secondary to aspiration pneumonitis.

TREATMENT
1. Gastric lavage with warm water or weak sodium bicarbonate solution even after the lapse of many hours since ingestion. Prevention of aspiration is essential.
2. Oxygen therapy by face mask or endotracheal catheter using positive pressure.
3. Rapid-acting barbiturates intravenously for control of acute excitement and convulsions.
4. Magnesium sulfate (Epsom salts) solution by mouth.
5. Camphorated tincture of opium (paregoric) by mouth or codeine sulfate intramuscularly for colic.
6. Caffeine sodiobenzoate, 0.5 gm. intramuscularly or intravenously for circulatory support.
7. Application of external heat.
8. Large amounts of fluids intravenously and by mouth.
9. Hospitalization if large amounts have been ingested, if a lengthy period has elapsed since ingestion, if convulsions have developed or if there is evidence of aspiration of fumes or vomitus. Pulmonary edema (**51**) may be a late development.

49 – 816.   TWO-FOUR-D (2-4-D) See **49 – 263**. *2,4-Dichlorophenoxyacetic Acid*

49 – 817.   ULTRAMARINE (Lapis Lazuli)

This mineral decomposes in the presence of acid to hydrogen sulfide (**49 – 380**). It is used in the painting of fabrics and as a bluing agent. Ingestion causes a toxic picture similar to that of hydrogen sulfide (**49 – 380**).

49 – 818.   URANIUM SALTS

Inhalation of dust of the insoluble radioactive oxide results in accumulation in the lungs and pulmonary lymph nodes; it is slowly but never completely eliminated after termination of exposure.
To date, no cases of acute toxicity caused by uranium salts have been reported.

49 – 819.   VACCINIUM ULIGINOSUM L. (Bilberry, Whortleberry)

This berry-producing shrub, which grows in America, Asia and Europe, differs from true blueberry (*Vaccinium myrtillis L.*) in that its juice is colorless instead of purple. Ingestion of the berries has caused a feeling of inebriation, euphoria, headache, bradycardia, dyspnea and abberations of vision (white appears to be blue and green appears yellow).

TREATMENT
1. Emetics or gastric lavage followed by activated charcoal in water orally or through the lavage tube.
2. Symptomatic care. Complete recovery usually occurs in 3 to 5 hours.

49−820. VANADIUM

Vanadium poisoning is usually caused by the pentoxide and occurs in persons working around oil-burning furnaces and oil refineries, in the manufacture of vanadium steel and in the dyeing industry.

SIGNS AND SYMPTOMS.   Greenish-black discoloration of the tongue, dry nonproductive cough, severe headaches resistant to all therapy, disturbances in vision, hemoptysis, nervousness, psychic derangement and gastrointestinal and urinary disturbances, all persisting for 2 to 3 weeks

TREATMENT
1. Removal from exposure.
2. Intravenous fluids if dehydration is acute.
3. Sedative cough mixtures.
4. Ascorbic acid by mouth in large doses−up to 1 gm. per day.
5. Hospitalization because of the persistence of headaches, cough and uncomfortable gastrointestinal complaints.

PROGNOSIS.   Good in acute cases; chronic cases may show permanent renal damage.

49−821. VAPAM

This soil fumigant acts much like disulfiram (Antabuse) if ingested. For signs of toxicity and treatment, see **49−77.** *Antabuse.*

49−822. VARNISH AND VARNISH REMOVERS See **49−17.** *Acetone;* **49−39.** *Alkalies (Sodium Hydroxide);* **49−119.** *Benzene (Benzol) and Its Derivatives;* **49−173.** *Carbon Tetrachloride;* **49−315.** *Ethyl Alcohol;* **49−349.** *Gasoline;* **49−420.** *Lead Salts;* **49−475.** *Methyl Alcohol;* **49−478.** *Methyl Chloride;* **49−481.** *Methylethylketone;* **49−509.** *Naphtha;* **49−791.** *Toluene (Toluol);* **49−814.** *Tung Oil;* **49−815.** *Turpentine*

49−823. VENEZUELA (Coco de Mono) NUTS

Ingestion of these nuts has been reported as causing nausea, vomiting, chills, malaise and prostration followed in 7 to 10 days by complete loss of hair from the scalp and body.

TREATMENT
1. Emetics or gastric lavage followed by activated charcoal in water.
2. Saline cathartics.
3. Symptomatic care. No treatment seems to effect the loss of body hair, which grows back slowly. No fatalities have been reported.

49−824. VERATRINE (Cevadine)

Veratrine is a complicated mixture of alkaloids sometimes used in the treatment of pediculosis capitis and certain types of neuralgia. It (or an allied substance of similar action) is also found in the "death camas" (*Zygadenus*) plant (**49−857**) common in the grazing lands of the northwestern United States. Ingestion may cause burning in the mouth and stomach, salivation, nausea, vomiting, acute abdominal pain, diarrhea, acute anxiety, headache, vertigo, slow and feeble pulse, extreme hypotension, dilated pupils and muscular twitching. Respiratory and circulatory collapse may occur. In spite of the severity of the symptoms, most patients are conscious at all times.

TREATMENT

1. Gastric lavage with 1:5000 potassium permanganate solution followed by activated charcoal in water by mouth or through the lavage tube.

2. Magnesium sulfate (Epsom salts) solution by mouth or through the lavage tube.

3. Normal salt solution, 1000 ml. intravenously.

4. Caffeine sodiobenzoate, 0.5 gm. intramuscularly or intravenously, as a stimulant and diuretic. Ephedrine sulfate, levarterenal bitartrate (Levophed) or metaraminol bitartrate (Aramine) may be necessary for support of the circulation.

5. Oxygen therapy under positive pressure if respiratory depression is profound.

6. Hospitalization, since the toxic substances are excreted very slowly (probably through the kidneys) and a relapse may occur after apparent improvement.

PROGNOSIS.   Fair only, because of the profound respiratory and cardiac depression.

49 – 825. VERATRUM VIRIDE (Green Hellebore, White Hellebore) (See also 49 – 41. *Alkavervir*)

Acute toxic signs and symptoms may occur following ingestion of the roots, drinking of "herb teas," or through confusion with certain other tinctures used medicinally, expecially tincture of valeriana. The toxic action is due mainly to the alkaloid protoveratrine, which should not be confused with cevadine, the toxic agent in veratrine (**49 – 824**).

Although veratrum is a reliable cardiac depressant, medicinal use is now unusual. Most cases of poisoning occur from accidental ingestion of the powder, which is used as an insecticide. The toxic picture is characterized by burning in the throat and stomach, pain on swallowing, vomiting, diarrhea, bradycardia, hypotension, muscular cramping and convulsions, with or without loss of sphincter control.

TREATMENT

1. Administration of demulcents.

2. Gastric lavage with large quantities of warm water even though profuse vomiting has occurred. Activated charcoal in water should be left in the stomach.

3. Caffeine sodiobenzoate, 0.5 gm. intramuscularly for circulatory support.

4. Purgation with magnesium sulfate (Epsom salts) solution.

5. Calcium gluconate, 10 ml. of a 10% solution intravenously for muscle twitching and myalgia, repeated as necessary.

PROGNOSIS.   Most cases of veratrum viride poisoning recover in a short time because of its immediate violent emetic action.

49 – 826. VINYL CHLORIDE

Similar in action to but weaker than ethyl chloride (**49 – 70.** *Anesthetics, Inhalation*), this substance is used as a refrigerant and occasionally as an inhalation anesthetic. Its toxic effects are transient and require only symptomatic treatment.

49 – 827. VIOSTEROL (Vitamin D)

Although commonly and indiscriminately used medicinally in the treatment of many conditions (rickets, osteomalacia, arthritis, etc.), viosterol is a dangerous substance. Large doses (150,000 to 600,000 units per day) may result in serious, sometimes fatal, toxic reactions from hypercalcemia.

SIGNS AND SYMPTOMS. Nausea and vomiting associated with abdominal cramping and pain, with or without diarrhea. The abdominal pain may be severe enough to be mistaken for an acute surgical abdomen. Headache, general lassitude, dyspnea, neuralgia, myalgia and signs of urinary tract irritation (polyuria, nocturia, albuminuria) may be present, as may urticaria, asthma (52–1) and congestive heart failure (26–8).

TREATMENT

1. In mild cases, decrease in the dosage of vitamin D will result in complete recovery.

2. Severe cases may require:

Oxygen therapy for dyspnea.

Epinephrine hydrochloride (Adrenalin), 0.2 to 0.5 ml. subcutaneously, repeated as necessary for control of urticaria and asthma.

Codeine sulfate or morphine sulfate subcutaneously or pentazocine lactate (Talwin) intramuscularly if muscular pain is severe.

Hospitalization if signs and symptoms of severe hypercalcemia (43–12) are present, for correction of fluid-electrolyte imbalance (6. *Fluid Replacement*) and for corticosteroid therapy.

49–828. VITAMIN A

Acute hypervitaminosis A in infants causes vomiting and bulging of the fontanelles. In adults it is associated with nausea, vomiting, headache, mental irritability, sleepiness and localized peeling of the skin. Although excessive intake is the most common cause, hypervitaminosis A may be due to ingestion of food containing large amounts of the vitamin. See **49–339.** *Food Poisoning, Rare Causes.*

In acute cases signs and symptoms of toxicity subside rapidly when excessive intake of the vitamin is stopped; in chronic cases lengthy supportive and symptomatic care usually is required.

49–829. VITAMIN B See 49–770. *Thiamine Hydrochloride*

49–830. VITAMIN D See 49–827. *Viosterol*

49–831. VITAMIN K₁

Therapeutic doses may cause flushing, sweating and a sense of constriction of the chest. Acute sensitivity reactions (21) are fairly common. In certain susceptible persons usual therapeutic doses may result in hypotension, rapid irregular pulse, severe chest pain, cyanosis and coma.

Recovery occurs rapidly under symptomatic and supportive therapy after the drug has been discontinued.

49–832. WAR GASES

Lacrimators (brombenzylcyanide and chloroacetophenone).

SIGNS AND SYMPTOMS. Profuse lacrimation, smarting and burning of eyes, blurred vision and temporary blindness. The effects are panic-inducing but transient and usually not dangerous. See **49–192.** *Chloroacetophenone.*

TREATMENT

1. Irrigate the eyes thoroughly with 2% sodium bicarbonate solution.

2. Protect the eye with dark glasses. Do not bandage.

Pulmonary irritants (chlorine, chloropicrin, palite, phosgene). All of these gases produce symptoms with an insidious onset and are very dangerous.

Signs and Symptoms. Bronchospasm, dyspnea, pulmonary edema (**51**), intense cyanosis, nausea, vomiting, coma and collapse.

Treatment

1. Bed rest; prevention of chilling.

2. Insurance of an adequate airway.

3. Oxygen therapy under positive pressure by face mask and rebreathing bag. An endotracheal catheter may be necessary.

4. Epinephrine hydrochloride (Adrenalin), 0.5 to 1.0 ml. intramuscularly for bronchospasm.

Irritant smokes diphenylaminechlorarsine and diphenylchlorarsine).

Signs and Symptoms. Violent sneezing, nausea, vomiting, coughing, dyspnea and pulmonary edema (**51**). Dangerous only if very severe.

Treatment

1. Wash the nose and mouth with water or 2% sodium bicarbonate solution.

2. Prescribe absolute rest.

3. Give inhalations of oxygen, preferably under positive pressure.

Vesicants [mustard gas (dichloroethylsulfide) and lewisite (chlorvinyldichlorarsine)]

Signs and Symptoms. Itching, blistering, blurred vision, sneezing, blindness, collapse from severe shock (**53**) and delayed arsenic poisoning (**49 – 90**).

Treatment for Mustard Gas in the Eyes

1. Wash the eyes with large amounts of water or 2% sodium bicarbonate solution.

2. Instill tetracaine (Pontocaine) into the eyes to relieve pain.

Treatment for Mustard Gas on the Skin

1. Wash the contaminated areas with 2% sodium bicarbonate solution followed by soap and water.

2. Spot sponge with alcohol or gasoline; avoid spreading.

3. Rub in a paste of chlorinated lime or wipe with sodium hypochlorite solution.

Treatment for Lewisite on the Skin

1. Wipe with sodium hypochlorite solution and alcohol; then wash with soap and water.

2. Neutralize with BAL by local and systemic administration (**49 – 109**).

3. Treat the blisters as second degree burns (**25 – 2**).

4. Treat for collapse and shock (**53 – 7**).

49 – 833. WARFARIN [Compound 42, Coumachlor (Coumadin Sodium), Deathmore, Decon, Fumarin, Pival, Tomarin, Warficide]

This powerful anticoagulant is used in powder form as a rodenticide. It is toxic if ingested but is not absorbed through the skin. For signs and symptoms of toxicity and treatment, see **49 – 265**. *Dicumarol.*

49 – 834. WATER GLASS

Used as an egg preservative, as an adhesive, for fireproofing fabrics and as a detergent, water glass contains about 40% sodium silicate which has a definite caustic alkali effect (**49 – 39**) on the skin and mucous membranes. Ingestion causes a burning sensation in the mouth and throat, inability to swallow, vomiting and gastric pain.

Treatment

1. Thorough washing of the mouth with copious amounts of water.

2. Administration of demulcents.

3. Gastric lavage followed by activated charcoal in water by mouth or through the lavage tube. A saline cathartic should be given.

4. Symptomatic and supportive therapy.

49–835. WATER HEMLOCK (Musquash Root, Spotted Cowbane)

The roots of this plant are toxic if ingested. For signs, symptoms and treatment, see **49–209.** *Cicuta virosa.*

49–836. WATER PURIFIERS See 49–384. *Hypochlorites*

49–837. "WATERFRONT COCKTAILS"

For a small amount of money, persons who cannot afford the usual alcoholic beverages can obtain about 50 ml. of rubbing alcohol (**49–656**) and 100 ml. of white (nonethyl-containing) gasoline (**49–349**). This mixture, when ingested, results in acute intoxication, terminated in 2 to 3 hours by vomiting, triggered by the substances added to the alcohol to make it unpotable.

Treatment

Symptomatic and supportive, as outlined in **49–315.** *Ethyl Alcohol.*

49–838. WHITE HELLEBORE See 49–825. *Veratrum Viride*

49–839. WHITE VITRIOL See 49–855. *Zinc Sulfate*

49–840. WINTERGREEN OIL See 49–486. *Methyl Salicylate*

49–841. WOOD

In addition to skin reactions commonly caused by many different types of wood, several tropical woods used in cabinetmaking may give rise to acute toxic symptoms, apparently resulting from absorption of toxic substances through the intact skin or from inhalation of dust or fumes.

Signs and Symptoms. Swelling and stiffness of the hands and fingers associated with a heavy feeling in the arms, severe headaches, visual disturbances, dyspnea, rapid pulse, dysphagia and water diarrhea with dehydration.

Treatment

1. Removal from exposure.
2. Treatment of dyspnea by oxygen inhalations.
3. Administration of large amounts of fluids by mouth or intravenously.

Prognosis. Complete recovery is the rule, although some fatalities have been reported. Desensitization to certain tropical woods has been successful.

49–842. WOOD ALCOHOL (Methanol) See 49–475. *Methyl Alcohol*

49–843. WORMSEED See 49–182. *Chenopodium*

49–844. XYLENE (Xylol) See 49–119. *Benzene and Its Derivatives*

49–845. YATREN see 49–556. *Oxyquinoline Derivatives*

49–846. YELLOW CEDAR See 49–864. *Arbor Vitae*

49 — 847.   ZEPHIRAN (Benzalkonium Chloride)

The 1% aqueous or alcoholic solution of Zephiran has been used extensively for cold sterilization of surgical instruments and supplies. See **49 — 637.** *Quaternary Ammonium Salts.*

49 — 848.   ZERLATE (Zinc Dimethyldithiocarbamate)

Combined with an oily base, this substance is an effective insecticide. It also has toxic properties similar to those of disulfiram (Antabuse).
For signs and symptoms of toxicity and treatment, see **49 — 77.** *Antabuse.*

49 — 849.   ZINC ARSENATE AND ARSENITE

Arsenic, not zinc, is the toxic ingredient in these salts. For treatment, see **49 — 90.** *Arsenic.*

49 — 850.   ZINC CHLORIDE

Zinc chloride is used medicinally as an escharotic, astringent, deodorant and disinfectant and commercially in zinc plating and in alloys. Inhalation of fumes (common) and ingestion (rare) may cause acute toxic signs and symptoms; about 50% of ingestion cases are fatal. Inhalation cases generally recover, although there is a tendency toward delayed development of severe pneumonia.

Signs and Symptoms Following Inhalation of Fumes. Hoarseness, loss of voice, chest pain, rapid pulse and respiration, tracheobronchitis and sometimes severe and even fatal pneumonia.

Treatment

1. Removal from exposure.
2. Oxygen inhalations by face mask and rebreathing bag.
3. Immediate hospitalization. Antibiotic therapy to minimize the chances of development of a severe respiratory tract infection is indicated if hospitalization must be delayed.

Signs and Symptoms Following Ingestion.   Severe gastric and substernal pain, swollen lips, edema of the glottis, severe vomiting, bloody diarrhea, cold skin, low blood pressure, dyspnea and collapse with the picture of acute shock (**53**). Perforation of a viscus may occur.

Treatment

1. Gastric lavage with 1:5000 potassium permanganate solution.
2. Activated charcoal in water by mouth or through the lavage tube.
3. Oxygen inhalations by face mask and rebreathing bag.
4. Treatment of shock (**53 — 7**).
5. Immediate hospitalization. If acute edema of the glottis is present, tracheostomy (**14 — 12**) should be done before transfer.

49 — 851.   ZINC CYANIDE

This zinc salt is a powerful insecticide. For signs and symptoms of toxicity and treatment, see **49 — 235.** *Cyanides.*

49 – 852. ZINC OXIDE

Inhalation may cause metal fume fever (**49 – 461.** *Metal Fumes*). Ingestion causes toxic signs and symptoms from formation of zinc chloride in the stomach. The treatment is the same as outlined in **49 – 850.** *Zinc Chloride*.

49 – 853. ZINC PHOSPHIDE

Decomposition of this zinc salt by water and acids results in the formation of phosphine. If inhaled, the treatment given in **49 – 600.** *Phosphine* should be followed; if ingested, this treatment should be preceded by gastric lavage with 1:5000 potassium permanganate solution.

49 – 854. ZINC STEARATE

Inhalation of the fine dust from zinc stearate talcum powder by infants may result in pneumonia, with a mortality of over 20%. Hospitalization is indicated in all cases.

49 – 855. ZINC SULFATE (White Vitriol, Zinc Vitriol)

SIGNS AND SYMPTOMS FOLLOWING INGESTION. Violent vomiting with severe abdominal pain, bloody diarrhea and sudden collapse. Signs of severe kidney injury (albuminuria, acetonuria, glycosuria) may develop after apparent complete recovery.

TREATMENT
1. Gastric lavage with a 1:5000 solution of potassium permanganate, followed by activated charcoal in water by mouth.
2. Control of pain with opiates.
3. Hospitalization for observation for at least 48 hours because of the possibility of severe delayed kidney damage.

49 – 856. ZIRAM See **49 – 848.** *Zerlate*

49 – 857. ZYGADENUS VENENOSUS (Death Camas)

A native of northwestern America from British Columbia to northern California, this perennial plant contains a very toxic alkaloid, zygadenzine, which is similar in action to veratrine (**49 – 824**). The toxic principle is found in all parts of the plant and is not destroyed by drying.

For treatment, see **49 – 824.** *Veratrine (Cevadine)*.

For Your Personal Notes Regarding Poisons

For Your Personal Notes Regarding Poisons

For Your Personal Notes Regarding Poisons

For Your Personal Notes Regarding Poisons

POISONOUS CULTIVATED OR GARDEN PLANTS

The flowers, plants and shrubs listed in the following section are some of those which, planted for their decorative effect or growing as weeds in gardens, may cause toxic symptoms following ingestion. Most of the victims of plant poisoning are children between the ages of 4 and 10— usually motivated by curiosity, mimicry, practical jokes or the mistaken belief that anything that looks attractive is good to eat. The most frequently ingested plants are bittersweet (**49 — 872**), castor bean (**49 — 893**), dumb cane (**49 — 915**), lantana (**49 — 942**), mushrooms and toadstools (**49 — 502.** *Mushroom Poisoning*), deadly nightshade (**49 — 911**), pokeweed (**49 — 978**) and yew (**49 — 1017**).

49 — 858.   ACACIA

A toxic sap is exuded by those varieties which grow in Africa. See **49 — 9.**

49 — 859.   AKEE

After apparent recovery from acute gastrointestinal irritation from eating this saponin-containing fruit, convulsions, hypertension and coma may develop.

49 — 860.   ALFALFA See 49 — 36.

49 — 861.   ALOES

All species of aloes contain aloin (**49 — 47**), a strong gastrointestinal irritant. Treatment consists of gastric lavage, saline cathartics and sedation. Toxic effects are usually more uncomfortable than dangerous.

49 — 862.   AMERICAN NIGHTSHADE See 49 — 978. *Pokeweed*

49 — 863.   ANGEL'S TRUMPET

Toxic signs and symptoms from ingestion are due to depression of the parasympathetic mechanism and to stimulation of the central nervous system. For toxic effects and treatment, see **49 — 104.** *Atropine Sulfate.*

49 — 864.   ARBOR VITAE (Red Cedar, Thuja, Yellow Cedar)

The twigs and leaves may cause severe toxic symptoms if chewed. Decoctions of the young twigs have been used in attempts to induce abortions.

Signs and Symptoms.   Severe abdominal pain, diarrhea, frothing at the mouth, difficult respiration, pulmonary edema (**51**), tonic or clonic convulsions and circulatory failure.

Treatment
1. Emetics or gastric lavage.
2. Activated charcoal or other demulcents by mouth.
3. Oxygen therapy under positive pressure by face mask and rebreathing bag.
4. Caffeine sodiobenzoate, 0.5 gm. intramuscularly.

5. Treatment of pulmonary edema (**51**).

6. Hospitalization for close observation and symptomatic and supportive care because of the tendency of thuja to cause delayed genitourinary symptoms.

49 – 865.   ARNICA (Sororia, Cordifolia)

Ingestion of the flowers and roots of this plant may cause acute gastrointestinal symptoms and coma. For treatment, see **49 – 88.**

49 – 866.   AUTUMN CROCUS

Post-ingestion effects and treatment are similar to those outlined for colchicine (**49 – 220**).

49 – 867.   AZALEA

Andromedotoxin, the poisonous substance contained in these plants, is similar to aconite in many respects; in addition, it has a curare-like effect on voluntary muscles and a depressant action on the heart. See **49 – 27.** *Aconite;* **49 – 234.** *Curare.*

49 – 868.   BEAD TREE See **49 – 445.** *Melia Azedarach*

49 – 869.   BELLADONNA See **49 – 104.** *Atropine Sulfate*

49 – 870.   BILBERRY (Whortleberry) See **49 – 819.** *Vaccinum Oliginosum L.*

49 – 871.   BIRD OF PARADISE (Strelitzia)

Acute gastrointestinal irritation, vertigo and drowsiness may follow ingestion. After emptying the stomach, symptomatic treatment should be given.

49 – 872.   BITTERSWEET (Blue Nightshade, Climbing Nightshade, Woody Nightshade)

Ingestion of the green berries or leaves may cause acute signs and symptoms due to solanine and dulcamarin. The riper the berries, the less the toxicity. See **49 – 712.** *Solanine.*

49 – 873.   BLACK CHERRY See **49 – 895.** *Deadly Nightshade;* **49 – 712.** *Solanine*

49 – 874.   BLACK LAUREL

All parts of this shrub contain andromedotoxin (see **49 – 867.** *Azalea*).

49 – 875.   BLACK LOCUST

The bark and leaves of this shrub or tree contain a dangerous toxalbumin, phytotoxin. The signs and symptoms of toxicity and treatment are similar to those outlined in **49 – 893.** *Castor Bean.*

49–876. BLACK NIGHTSHADE

The leaves and green fruit contain solanine (**49–712**).

49–877. BLEEDING HEART (Dutchman's Breeches)

All parts contain a mixture of alkaloids which may cause respiratory distress, ataxia and convulsions. The treatment is symptomatic and supportive.

49–878. BLOODROOT

All parts of the plant contain a toxic substance (sanguinarine) which on ingestion causes nausea, vomiting, diarrhea and collapse. Treatment consists of emptying the stomach by emetics or gastric lavage, administration of activated charcoal in water and purgation by saline cathartics.

49–879. BLUEBERRY LEAVES

Blueberry leaves contain myrtillin, an antiglycemic agent which may cause severe and permanent liver damage
TREATMENT
1. Emetics and gastric lavage with 1:5000 solution of potassium permanganate followed by activated charcoal in water.
2. Saline cathartics.
3. Close observation for several weeks for possible liver damage.

49–880. BLUE LUPINE

The symptoms and treatment following ingestion of the flowers, leaves or stalks of this flowering plant are given in **49–222**. *Coniine.*

49–881. BLUE NIGHTSHADE (Bittersweet) See **49–872**. *Bittersweet;* 49–712. *Solanine*

49–882. BLUE WEED (Vipers bugloss)

The stems and leaves contain a toxic alkaloid, pyrrolizidine. Ingestion may cause a picture similar to acute toxic hepatitis.

49–883. BOXWOOD

Boxwood contains an alkaloid, buxine—a powerful intestinal irritant and central nervous system depressant. For treatment, see **49–40**. *Alkaloids.*

49–884. BRIONIA

Brionia is a strong irritant poison and may cause severe gastrointestinal irritation followed by severe shock.
TREATMENT
Treatment consists of gastric lavage, activated charcoal by mouth and supportive therapy.

49 — 885.   BROOM TOP (Scoporius)

This plant contains an alkaloid, sparteine, similar in action to coniine (**49 — 222**) and nicotine (**49 — 523**).

49 — 886.   BUCKEYE

The flowers, seeds and nuts contain toxic glycosides. Treatment consists of emptying the stomach by emetics or gastric lavage, with symptomatic and supportive measures.

49 — 887.   BUCKTHORN (Coyotillo, Tullidora, Wild Cherry)

Ingestion of the drupes of this shrub, indigenous to northern Mexico, Texas and New Mexico, causes gradual development of symmetrical polyneuropathy, starting in the legs and progressing to quadriplegia, respiratory involvement and bulbar paralysis. It can be distinguished from Guillain-Barré syndrome by the absence of spinal fluid abnormalities. If the patient survives the initial acute progressive stage, complete recovery without residual permanent disability usually takes place.

TREATMENT is symptomatic and supportive.

49 — 888.   BUTTERCUPS See **49 — 644.** *Ranunculus Scleratus*

49 — 889.   CALABAR BEAN See **49 — 603.** *Physostigmine (Eserine)*

49 — 890.   CALADIUM

The varicolored leaves and the roots contain calcium oxalate crystals, which can cause severe irritation of the tongue and mucous membranes. Treatment consists of emetics or gastric lavage followed by demulcents.

49 — 891.   CALLA LILIES

Ingestion causes severe irritation of the mouth and throat, with acute gastro-enteritis and ulceration. Large amounts may cause severe shock and death.

TREATMENT

Treatment consists of removal by mouthwashes, emetics and gastric lavage, followed by activated charcoal in water and a saline cathartic. Supportive measures may be necessary.

49 — 892.   CAMELLIA

The seeds contain a glucoside which acts like digitalis (**49 — 272**).

49 — 893.   CASTOR BEAN (Ricinus communis)

The large varicolored beans of this shrub are very attractive and dangerous to children since they contain a deadly poison, ricin. Ingestion of 4 or 5 seeds is usually fatal to a child; the mortality in recorded cases in all age groups is about 6%.

Evidences of castor bean poisoning usually do not come on for 1 to 3 days after ingestion and consist of severe headache, nausea, persistent vomiting, and acute gastro-enteritis, often with bloody diarrhea. Jaundice may be present. Convulsions may be followed by death in 6 to 10 days.

TREATMENT
1. Immediate emptying of the stomach followed by activated charcoal in water, even if ingestion is only suspected.
2. Hospitalization for observation for at least 3 days.
For toxic reactions during commercial processing of castor beans, see **49 – 177**.

49 – 894. CEDAR (Red) See **49 – 864**. *Arbor Vitae*

49 – 895. CHERRY

The bark, leaves and pits of certain cherry trees, especially the wild black cherry *(Prunus serotina)*, are toxic owing to the presence of amygdalin (**49 – 65**), which breaks down into hydrocyanic acid. See also **49 – 206**. *Chokecherry;* **49 – 918**. *Finger Cherry;* **49 – 1009**. *Wild Cherry.*

49 – 896. CHINABERRY See **49 – 445**. *Melia Azedarach*

49 – 897. CHRISTMAS PLANTS See **49 – 930**. *Holly;* **49 – 958**. *Mistletoe;* **49 – 979**. *Poinsettia.*

49 – 898. CHRISTMAS ROSE

The roots contain a toxic glucoside, helleborein. Ingestion of small amounts causes a severe intractable diarrhea but generally no other systemic effects. See **49 – 360**. *Helleborein.*

49 – 899. CLEMATIS

This gastrointestinal irritant gives a toxic picture similar to aloes (**49 – 861**).

49 – 900. CLIMBING NIGHTSHADE See **49 – 872**. *Bittersweet*

49 – 901. COLUMBINE

Like aloes (**49 – 861**) this climbing plant contains a substance in the stalks and leaves which, following ingestion of a small amount, causes intense gastrointestinal distress and sometimes a shock-like state.

49 – 902. CORN CAMPION (Corn Cockle, Corn Rose) See **49 – 31**. *Agrostemma Githago*

49 – 903. COW CABBAGE See **49 – 365**. *Heracleum lanatum*

49 – 904. COWSLIP See **49 – 161**. *Caltha palustris*

49 – 905. COYOTILLA See **49 – 887**. *Buckthorn*

49 — 906.   CROCUS

The stigmas contain saffron (49 — 659).

49 — 907.   CRYBABY TREE

Ingestion of the leaves, bark or shoots may cause a paralysis similar to that caused by curare (49 — 234).

49 — 908.   CYCLAMEN

The stalks and leaves contain a saponin which causes intense gastrointestinal symptoms without nausea or vomiting. Ingestion of large amounts may cause convulsions or coma. Gastric lavage followed by activated charcoal in water and saline cathartics and supportive therapy is indicated.

49 — 909.   DAFFODIL

The bulbs contain a substance which if ingested causes nausea, vomiting and diarrhea, which is uncomfortable but not dangerous. For treatment, see 49 — 926. *Grape Hyacinth.*

49 — 910.   DAPHNE (Dwarf Bay, Wild Pepper)

The attractive red berries and the bark of this shrub are sometimes ingested by children, with a fatality rate of about 20%. Contact of the juice with the skin may cause severe and even fatal symptoms, although recovery following this method of absorption usually occurs.

TREATMENT
1. Immediate gastric lavage with a 1:5000 solution of potassium permanganate, followed by activated charcoal by mouth or through the lavage tube.
2. Magnesium sulfate (Epsom salts) solution by mouth.
3. Caffeine sodiobenzoate, 0.5 gm. intramuscularly.
4. Large amounts of fluids by mouth and intravenously.
5. Hospitalization because of the danger of severe kidney damage.

49 — 911.   DEADLY NIGHTSHADE

The leaves and berries contain several toxic glucosides, especially solanine (49 — 712).

49 — 912.   DELPHINIUM (Larkspur)

SIGNS AND SYMPTOMS of toxicity after ingestion include burning and dryness of the mucous membranes of the mouth and throat, stiffness of the facial muscles, nausea, vomiting, loss of urinary and rectal sphincter control, extreme hypotension and respiratory depression.

TREATMENT
1. Gastric lavage with large quantities of warm water followed by activated charcoal.
2. Emptying of the bowel by enemas or saline cathartics.
3. Symptomatic and supportive therapy.

49—913.   DIEFFENBACHIA See **49—266.** *Dieffenbachia Sequine*

49—914.   DOG PARSLEY

Transient toxic signs and symptoms, very uncomfortable but never fatal, have followed accidental ingestion in place of edible parsley.

SIGNS AND SYMPTOMS are caused by irritation of the gastrointestinal tract and disappear rapidly.

TREATMENT

1. Emptying of the stomach by emetics or gastric lavage followed by activated charcoal.

2. Administration of saline cathartics.

49—915.   DUMB CANE See **49—266.** *Dieffenbachia Sequine*

49—916.   DWARF BAY See **49—910.** *Daphne*

49—917.   ELEPHANT'S EAR See **49—266.** *Dieffenbachia Sequine*

49—918.   FINGER CHERRY

The fruit of this Australian flowering shrub may cause sudden onset of complete and permanent blindness from optic nerve damage. If ingested, signs and symptoms of toxicity usually do not develop for 18 to 24 hours; hence, only symptomatic treatment can be given.

49—919.   FIRE BUSH See **49—984.** *Pyrocantha*

49—920.   FIRE THORN See **49—984.** *Pyrocantha*

49—921.   FOUR-O'CLOCK

The roots and seeds contain a mildly narcotic gastrointestinal irritant which causes immediate nausea and vomiting without permanent ill effects.

49—922.   FOXGLOVE See **49—272.** *Digitalis*

49—923.   FRIAR'S COWL See **49—27.** *Aconite*

49—924.   GELSEMIUM See **49—350.**

49—925.   GLORIOSA (Climbing Lily)

Ingestion of the roots, stalks or leaves of this climbing lily results in a toxic picture similar to that caused by colchicine (**49—220**).

49-926. GRAPE HYACINTH

Although this plant is a strong irritant, its action is mostly on the gastric mucosa; hence, vomiting with removal of the toxic substances usually results before much absorption has taken place. Treatment consists of gastric lavage followed by activated charcoal by mouth even if the patient has vomited.

49-927. HEATHER

Andromedotoxin is the active toxic agent in all varieties of heather. See **49-27.** *Aconite;* **49-234.** *Curare.*

49-928. HEDEOMA See **49-972.** *Pennyroyal*

49-929. HENBANE See **49-383.** *Hyoscyamus*

49-930. HOLLY (Ilex aquifolium)

Severe gastroenteritis with prolonged vomiting and diarrhea may follow ingestion of any portion of this plant. Eating 20 to 30 berries may be fatal to children.

TREATMENT
1. Immediate emptying of the stomach by emetics or gastric lavage.
2. Activated charcoal in water by mouth or through the lavage tube.
3. Correction of fluid and electrolyte depletion (**6**) if gastroenteritis has been severe and prolonged.

49-931. INDIAN TOBACCO (Lobelia inflata) See **49-946.** *Lobelia*—Do not confuse with wild tobacco (**49-1011**)

49-932. INKY CAPS (See also **49-502.** *Mushroom Poisoning*)

This variety of mushroom is considered by some authorities to be edible but in the presence of alcohol can give toxic effects similar to disulfiram [**49-77.** *Antabuse (Disulfiram)*].

49-933. IRIS

All members of this family contain solanine (**49-712**), mostly in the underground stems.

49-934. JACK-IN-THE-PULPIT

All parts contain calcium oxalate which may cause severe irritation of the mouth, tongue and upper gastrointestinal tract. Treatment consists of aluminum hydroxide by mouth as a demulcent.

49-935. JASMINE, YELLOW See **49-350.** *Gelsemium*

49—936. JET BEAD TREE See **49—650.** *Rhodotypos Kerrioides*

49—937. JET BERRY BUSH

The berries contain amygdalin (**49—65**).

49—938. JIMSONWEED

All parts contain alkaloids which act like atropine (**49—104.** *Atropine Sulfate;* **49—116.** *Belladonna Alkaloids*).

49—939. JONQUIL See **49—926.** *Grape Hyacinth*

49—940. KENTUCKY COFFEE TREE See **49—238.** *Cystisine*

49—941. LABURNUM (Golden Chain)

The flowers, leaves and shoots of this ornamental tree contain a toxic alkaloid, cystisine (**49—238**) similar in action to nicotine (**49—523**).

49—942. LANTANA (Red Sage, Wild Sage)

Fatalities have been reported from ingestion of the berries of this ornamental plant. Acute toxic symptoms resemble those from atropine. For treatment, see **49—104.** *Atropine Sulfate;* **49—116.** *Belladonna Alkaloids.*

49—943. LARKSPUR See **49—912.** *Delphinium*

49—944. LAUREL

All varieties of laurel contain andromedotoxin. See **49—27.** *Aconite;* **49—234.** *Curare.*

49—945. LILY OF THE VALLEY

The flowers, leaves, stalks and roots contain a glucoside, convallamarin, similar to digitalis (**49—272**) in action and toxicity.

49—946. LOBELIA (Indian Tobacco)

Plants of this species contain toxic alkaloids that act like nicotine (**49—523**).

49—947. LOCUST

The seeds of certain varieties of these common ornamental trees contain a toxic substance similar to that found in castor beans (**49—893**).

SIGNS AND SYMPTOMS are usually less severe than in castor bean poisoning and the mortality rate is lower. The treatment is the same.

49—948. LUPINE

All parts of this flowering plant contain lupinine, an alkaloid which causes respiratory and circulatory depression, paralysis and convulsions if ingested in even small amounts.

TREATMENT
1. Immediate emptying of the stomach by emetics or gastric lavage followed by activated charcoal by mouth.
2. Oxygen by face mask and rebreathing bag.
3. Support of the circulation by caffeine sodiobenzoate, ephedrine sulfate or, in severe cases, levarterenol bitartrate (Levophed) or metaraminol bitartrate (Aramine).
4. Control of convulsions by rapid-acting barbiturates.
5. Hospitalization as soon as possible for synptomatic and supportive care.

49—949. MAGNOLIA

The seeds of all of the numerous varieties of magnolias contain a substance similar in action and toxicity to picrotoxin (49—606).

49—950. MANGO

The skin and sap can cause severe dermatitis and gastrointestinal irritation. The treatment is symptomatic.

49—951. MANZINELLO (Manchineel) See 49—371. *Hippomane Mancinella*

49—952. MARIHUANA (Indian Hemp)

Marihuana plants growing in gardens, unless planted for illicit purposes, usually come from scattered birdseed. See 49—441.

49—953. MARSH MARIGOLD (Cowslip) See 49—161. *Caltha Palustris*

49—954. MAYAPPLE (Mandrake)

The leaves, roots and green fruit contain a powerful cathartic, podophyllin. The treatment is symptomatic and supportive.

49—955. MEADOW SAFFRON See 49—220. *Colchicine*

49—956. MILKWEED

Milkweed contains a resin which is highly irritant to the gastrointestinal tract. Treatment consists of emptying the stomach by emetics or gastric lavage followed by activated charcoal by mouth.

49—957. MIMOSA

This saponin-containing plant has toxic effects similar to those of cyclamen (49—908).

49-958. MISTLETOE

All parts, but especially the berries, contain a potent hypertensive adrenolytic substance, tyramine, which on ingestion may give severe toxic effects. Fatalities have been reported from use of a decoction of the berries as an abortifacient.

Signs and symptoms of toxicity consist of acute gastroenteritis with vomiting and diarrhea, hypertension, dyspnea, delirium, hallucinations and cardiovascular collapse.

TREATMENT

1. Induction of vomiting to remove larger particles.
2. Gastric lavage to remove smaller particles, followed by activated charcoal in water by mouth or through the lavage tube.
3. Treatment for shock and cardiovascular collapse (53-7).
4. Appropriate therapy for dehydration and electrolyte imbalance (6).

49-959. MOCK ORANGE See 49-859. *Akee*

49-960. MONKSHOOD

Aconite (49-27) is the toxic principle. It is found only in the root.

49-961. MOONSEED

Ingestion of the roots and fruit may cause acute gastrointestinal symptoms. The sharp-edged pits may cause mechanical intestinal injury.

49-962. MORNING GLORY

The seeds of this climbing plant have a mild hallucinatory effect (49-358).

49-963. MOUNTAIN LAUREL (Mountain Ivy, Ivy Bush)

This flowering shrub contains a toxic resinoid, andromedotoxin, in its twigs, leaves, flowers and pollen. Ingestion, or eating contaminated honey causes toxic symptoms resembling those caused by aconite (49-27) and curare (49-234).

49-964. MUSHROOMS See 49-502.

49-965. NARCISSUS (Daffodil, Jonquil)

The toxic action of these bulbs is similar to that given in 49-926. *Grape Hyacinth.*

49-966. NIGHT BLOOMING CEREUS

Night blooming cereus contains a toxic active principle with actions similar to digitalis (49-272).

49-967. NIGHTSHADE See 49-872. *Bittersweet;* 49-911. *Deadly Nightshade*

49—968. NUTMEG

The seeds contain myristicin, a substance which may cause elation, hallucinations, acute stomach distress, double vision, drowsiness, delirium and stupor. Treatment consists of mineral or castor oil by mouth followed by gastric lavage and demulcents.

49—969. OLEANDER See 49—544.

49—970. PANSY

The roots contain a mildly toxic alkaloid, violine. For treatment, see **49—40.** *Alkaloids.*

49—971. PAWPAW See 49—95. *Arsinima Triloba*

49—972. PENNYROYAL (Hedeoma, Squaw Mint)

The leaves and flowers of this plant contain substances which are powerful stimulants, carminatives and emmenagogues. Ingestion has been reported as causing symptoms of shock, confusion, delirium, twitching and respiratory depression.
TREATMENT
1. Empty the stomach by emetics or gastric lavage followed by activated charcoal by mouth.
2. Give a saline cathartic.
3. Increase diuresis by intravenous fluids.

49—973. PHILODENDRON

The leaves and stalks of this common household plant contain clusters of small needle-sharp crystals of calcium oxalate which may cause an acute inflammatory process in the mouth or throat; swelling of the throat may be severe enough to interfere with breathing. Systemic reactions to the oxalate are rare.

49—974. PHYSIC NUT TREE See 49—405. *Jatropha Nut Oil*

49—975. PHYTOLACCA See 49—978. *Pokeweed*

49—976. PIGEONBERRY See 49—978. *Pokeweed*

49—977. PINKS

The seeds are the only toxic part of the plant. Ingestion may cause intense gastrointestinal irritation—never fatal because of the emetic action. Treatment is symptomatic only.

49—978. POKEWEED (Inkberry, Phytolacca)

All parts of this common plant (especially the unripe berries) contain a saponin and resin which is an intense gastrointestinal irritant. Toxic effects (burning in the mouth, severe gastroenteritis, drowsiness, impaired vision and respiratory depression) develop about 2 hours after ingestion.

TREATMENT

1. Emetics or gastric lavage followed by activated charcoal in water by mouth.
2. Symptomatic and supportive therapy.

49–979. POINSETTIA

The sap from this plant can cause severe contact dermatitis and temporary blindness. Chewing the leaves results in irritation and swelling of oropharyngeal mucosa, gastroenteritis, vomiting, and diarrhea.

TREATMENT IF INGESTED

1. Induction of vomiting followed by activated charcoal by mouth.
2. Treatment of fluid and electrolyte depletion (6) if gastroenteritis has been prolonged or severe

49–980. POMEGRANATE

The bark and stems contain toxic alkaloids. See **49–577.** *Pelletierine.*

49–981. POPPIES

California poppies contain a mixture of alkaloids with a depressant action on heart muscle. Oriental poppies have a high content of opium alkaloids. For treatment, see **49–40.** *Alkaloids;* **49–495.** *Morphine*

49–982. POTATOES

Seeds, sprouts, leaves and berries contain toxic glucosides. See **49–712.** *Solanine.*

49–983. PRIVET

The leaves and berries of this hedge shrub have a toxic effect similar to those of aloes (**49–861**) and andromedotoxin. See **49–27.** *Aconite;* **49–234.** *Curare.*

49–984. PYROCANTHA (Fire Bush, Fire Thorn)

Ingestion of the berries causes a toxic picture similar to that caused by belladonna. See **49–104.** *Atropine Sulfate;* **49–116.** *Belladonna and Belladonna Alkaloids.*

49–985. RAGWORT

Ragwort, if ingested, causes severe liver damage without other toxic effects.

49–986. RAYLESS GOLDENROD See **49–329.** *Eupatorium Urticaefolium;* **49–795.** *Tremetol*

49–987. RED CEDAR See **49–864.** *Arbor Vitae*

49 – 988. RHODODENDRON

The foliage and shoots of the numerous flowering plants in this family contain andromedotoxin; the signs and symptoms of toxicity and treatment after ingestion are similar to those for aconite (**49 – 27**) and curare (**49 – 234**).

49 – 989. RHUBARB See **49 – 651**

49 – 990. SCOKE See **49 – 978**. *Pokeweed*

49 – 991. SCOTCH BROOM See **49 – 885**. *Broom Top*

49 – 992. SORREL See **49 – 657**. *Rumex Acetosa L.*

49 – 993. SPANISH BAYONET (Yucca)

Plants of this family contain toxic saponins, which on ingestion produce irritation of the gastrointestinal tract. See **49 – 908**. *Cyclamen.*

49 – 994. SPIDER LILY

The bulbs contain a toxic alkaloid (lycocine). Fatalities are rare because of its rapid irritant action on the stomach.

49 – 995. SPINDLE TREE See **49 – 328**. *Euonymin*

49 – 996. SQUAW MINT See **49 – 972**. *Pennyroyal*

49 – 997. SQUAW WEED See **49 – 795**. *Tremetol*

49 – 998. STAGGERBUSH

Staggerbush contains andromedotoxin, which may cause toxic effects that may be mistaken for acute alcoholic intoxication. The action is primarily a peripheral paralysis of the vagus and depression of the brain associated with a voluntary muscle effect similar to that from curare (**49 – 234**).

49 – 999. STAR ANISE

This plant belongs to the magnolia family. Ingestion of its seeds may result in toxic symptoms similar to those caused by picrotoxin (**49 – 606**).

49 – 1000. STAR OF BETHLEHEM (Snow drop)

Star of Bethlehem contains a toxic resin similar to that described under milkweed (**49 – 956**).

49—1001. SWEET PEAS

The stalks and stems of sweet peas contain active toxic alkaloids. Ingestion of large amounts has been known to cause cerebral motor paralysis and acute cardiac depression. The clinical syndrome from ingestion resembles that of curare (**49—234**) and is known as lathyrism (**49—339**. *Rare causes of food poisoning*).

TREATMENT

1. Tincture of iodine, 1 ml. in 100 ml. (15 drops in ½ glass of water), by mouth.
2. Gastric lavage followed by activated charcoal in water by mouth or through the lavage tube.
3. Symptomatic and supportive therapy.

49—1002. TULIPS

A toxic alkaloid, tulipine, contained in the bulbs may cause a severe reaction if ingested in even small amounts. The action and treatment are similar to colchicine (**49—220**).

49—1003. TULLIDORA See 49—887. *Buckthorn*

49—1004. VIOLETS

The rhizomes contain violine, a toxic alkaloid. See **49—40**. *Alkaloids*.

49—1005. VIRGINIA CREEPER See 49—573. *Parthenocissus Quinquefolia*

49—1006. WATER HEMLOCK See 49—209. *Cicuta Virosa*

49—1007. WHITE CEDAR See 49—445. *Melia Azedarach*

49—1008. WHITE FLAG See 49—547. *Orris*

49—1009. WILD CHERRY See 49—887. *Buckthorn*

49—1010. WILD PEPPER See 49—910. *Daphne*

49—1011. WILD TOBACCO

All parts of this plant contain nicotine (**49—523**).

49—1012. WILD TOMATO (Horse Nettle, Sand Briar)

The green fruit contain solanine (**49—712**).

49 – 1013.   WISTERIA

The pods if ingested cause severe gastrointestinal symptoms, sometimes followed by collapse. Treatment consists of emptying the stomach by emetics or gastric lavage followed by activated charcoal in water. Supportive therapy may be necessary.

49 – 1014.   WOODBINE See 49 – 573. *Parthenocissus Quinquefolia*

49 – 1015.   WOODY NIGHTSHADE (Bittersweet) See 49 – 712. *Solanine*

49 – 1016.   YELLOW CEDAR See 49 – 864. *Arbor Vitae*

49 – 1017.   YEW

The leaves, shoots and berries of the American, English, Irish and Japanese varieties contain a toxic alkaloid, taxine. For treatment, see 49 – 746. *Taxus Baccata L.*

For Your Personal Notes Regarding Poisons

For Your Personal Notes Regarding Poisons

50. PSYCHIATRIC EMERGENCIES

50 – 1. ORGANIC PSYCHOSES

Organic psychoses are caused by abnormalities in circulation, innervation, metabolism or nutrition, infection, injury, intoxication (alcohol, drugs, etc.) and neoplasms.

SIGNS AND SYMPTOMS vary, but, in general, consist of personality changes and progressive loss of brain function, especially of the higher centers. This functional impairment is manifested by loss of calculating ability and specialized knowledge, poor judgment and memory, faulty orientation, delirium, acute excitement states (**34**), confusion, anxiety, hallucinations, ataxia, tremors and slurred speech.

TREATMENT

1. Prevention of self-injury and injury to others by gentle physical restraint if necessary. If forcible restraint is required, sedation is indicated.

2. Sedation by one of the following drugs:

Sodium amobarbital (Amytal), 100 to 250 mg. intramuscularly or slowly intravenously.

Chloral hydrate orally (1 mg.), repeated if necessary at hourly intervals. Rectal administration is slow but effective.

Chlorpromazine hydrochloride (Thorazine, 50 to 100 mg. orally or intramuscularly.

Paraldehyde, 10 to 15 ml. orally, intramuscularly or rectally.

Prochlorperazine (Compazine), 10 to 15 mg. orally or intramuscularly.

Pentothal sodium intravenously, administered if possible by an anesthesiologist.

3. Hospitalization for treatment of the underlying cause.

50 – 2. PSYCHOGENIC PSYCHOSES (See also **34.** *Excitement States*)

Recognition of these conditions, so that early arrangements for psychiatric care can be made, is one of the chief responsibilities of the emergency physician.

Manic-depressive psychoses

Persons suffering from these conditions show marked changes in behavior and personality, with fluctuation between acute excitement and depression, and may demonstrate complete lack of comprehension of their condition.

Paranoia. Characterized by intense feelings of guilt and failure, these patients are potentially homicidal and suicidal (**13**).

Schizophrenia. Inability to distinguish between actual environment and a fantasy world is the chief distinguishing characteristic of an acute schizophrenic.

Suicidal tendencies. (See also **13**. *Suicide.*) Physical signs are suggestive only and consist of decrease in appetite, weight loss, insomnia, disturbances in bowel function, menstrual abnormalities and impotency. Abnormal activity, ranging from catatonia to mania, may be present. Psychologically, there may be deep depression, disorientation, disorganization, hallucinations and delusions.

TREATMENT

1. Tactful handling of the patient *with an able-bodied attendant present at all times.*

2. Sedation as needed, with avoidance if possible of physical restraint. If physical restraint is necessary, sedation is inadequate.

3. Arrangement for hospitalization for psychiatric evaluation and treatment either in a private hospital equipped for care of mentally disturbed patients or in an institution designated by local law enforcement authorities.

50 – 3. DELIRIUM TREMENS See 34 – 3

50 – 4. FAINTING (Vasodepressor Syncope) See **50 – 11**. *Differential Diagnosis;* **59 – 5**. *Syncope*

50 – 5. HYPERVENTILATION See 34 – 6.

50 – 6. HYSTERIA (See also **50 – 10**. *Unconsciousness, Episodic;* **50 – 11**. *Differential Diagnosis*)

Emotional or physical strain in certain individuals may cause bizarre hysterical symptoms severe enough to require emergency care.

Common manifestations of hysteria

Coma. See **50 – 10**. *Unconsciousness, Episodic;* **50 – 11**. *Differential Diagnosis.*

Globus. A subjective sensation of a lump in the throat, sometimes so severe that the patient is convinced that he is unable to swallow.

Hyperventilation. See **34 – 6**.

Paralysis. Transient, partial or complete, usually not corresponding to any motor nerve distribution.

Sensory abnormalities. Usually hypesthesias or paresthesias, often of stocking or glove distribution. Gag and corneal reflexes may be absent.

TREATMENT

1. Sedation by barbiturates, chlorpromazine hydrochloride (Thorazine) or reserpine (Serpasil).
2. Explanation of the condition in simple terms to the patient and responsible members of the family
3. Reference for psychiatric evaluation if the condition is severe, persistent or recurrent.

50 – 7. INSOMNIA

Persons who request emergency care for sleeplessness usually complain of difficulty in getting to sleep, inability to stay asleep long enough to become rested or inability to sleep soundly enough to become rested. Except in those instances where severe emotional trauma is a factor, most cases of insomnia are chronic and require emergency therapy only because previous medical and psychiatric care and lack of rest have resulted in complete exhaustion. After emphasizing to the patient or members of the family that only emergency treatment is being given, one of the following drugs may be administered:

DRUG	DOSE	METHOD
Chloral hydrate	0.6 to 2.0 gm.	Orally, diluted with water or milk.
Paraldehyde	2 to 8 ml. or 5 to 10 ml.	Orally, with fruit juice or cracked ice. Intramuscularly, deep in the glutei.
Flurazepam HCl	15 to 30 mg.	Orally

All patients should be advised to make arrangements for further care and told that treatment on an urgent emergency basis will not be repeated. Large quantities of barbiturates, bromides, "tranquilizers" or sedatives should not be prescribed for home use. Under no circumstances should opiates or synthetic narcotics be administered or prescribed.

50 – 8. MANIC-DEPRESSIVE PSYCHOSES

All medications should be in the possession of a responsible family member for dispensing.

50 – 8. MANIC-DEPRESSIVE PSYCHOSES See **50 – 2.** *Psychogenic Psychoses*

50 – 9. SCHIZOPHRENIA See **50 – 2.** *Psychogenic Psychoses*

50 – 10. UNCONSCIOUSNESS, EPISODIC See **50 – 11.** *Differential Diagnosis*

Common causes. Between 90 and 95% of the cases of transient and recurrent loss of consciousness are due to epilepsy (**31.** *Convulsive Seizures*), hysteria (**50 – 6**), hyperventilation (**34 – 6**) or vasodepressive syncope (**50 – 11.** *Differential Diagnosis;* **59 – 5.** *Syncope*).

Causes of episodic loss of consciousness (complete or partial):

1. Carotid sinus syncope. These attacks generally follow twisting the neck in a certain way or pressure (tight collar, etc.) over the junction of the external and internal carotid arteries at the level of the upper border of the thyroid cartilage. The diagnosis can be confirmed by applying pressure *over one side only* with the patient lying down. Atropine for intravenous administration should be at hand in a syringe. This test is not without danger and should not be done unless facilities for combating cardiac arrest (**11 – 2**) are immediately available.

2. Cardiac arrhythmias and standstill. See **26.** *Cardiac Emergencies;* **48 – 15.** *Cardiac Emergencies in Children.*

Complete heart block (Adams-Stokes syncope). See **26 – 10;** **48 – 15.** *Cardiac Emergencies in Children.*

Aortic stenosis.

Paroxysmal auricular tachycardia (**48 – 15.** *Cardiac Emergencies in Children*).

Ventricular fibrillation (**26 – 23**).

3. Intermittent cerebral ischemia (**59 – 8**).

4. Accidental or surreptitious intake of causative drugs. See **13.** *Suicide;* **49.** *Poisons.*

5. Orthostatic hypotension. Persons with this condition lose consciousness *in the upright position only.* No emergency treatment (except for injuries sustained in falls) is indicated

50 — 11. DIFFERENTIAL DIAGNOSIS OF EPISODIC UNCONSCIOUSNESS

Differential diagnosis between the four common causes of episodic loss of consciousness requires a careful history, especially in regard to previous episodes and onset of symptoms, and detailed examination. The most important points are summarized in the table on pages 572 and 573.

51. PULMONARY EDEMA

See also **26 — 8.** *Congestive Heart Failure.*

Acute pulmonary edema is a life-threatening emergency which requires prompt and effective treatment for control.

CAUSES.   Congestive heart failure (cardiac asthma, acute left or combined ventricular failure) is the most common cause. Pulmonary embolism may be a precipitating factor.

Acute poisoning from absorption, ingestion, injection or inhalation of many drugs, gases and other toxic substances. Among these are:

Aconite (**49 — 27**)
Acrolein (**49 — 29**)
Barbiturates (**49 — 111**)
Cadmium salts (**49 — 156**)
Carbon monoxide (**49 — 172**)
Chlorates (**49 — 187**)
Cyanides (**49 — 235**)
Dinitrophenol (**49 — 285**)
Epinephrine hydrochloride (**49 — 302**)
Ethylene (**49 — 70.** *Anesthetics, Inhalation*)

Hydrogen sulfide (**49 — 380**)
Iodine (**49 — 393**)
Kerosene (**49 — 408**)
Methyl bromide (**49 — 476**)
Morphine (**49 — 495**)
Phosgene (**49 — 599**)
Pyrogallol (**49 — 634**)
Salicylates (**49 — 664**)
Thallium (**49 — 768**)
Thuja (**49 — 864.** *Arbor Vitae*)

Barotrauma, including effects of high altitude (**23 — 6.** *Mountain Sickness*) and submersion (**23 — 5.** *Thoracic Squeeze*).

Acute trauma with massive thoracic concussion (**28 — 1** to **28 — 8.** *Chest Injuries*).

Interstitial pneumonia (**62 — 11**) — diffuse, due to acute viral infections [particularly *Varicella* (**30 — 36**)], and Eaton agent.

SIGNS AND SYMPTOMS.   Acute apprehension (sometimes apparent several hours before other signs and symptoms develop), a choking sensation, violent cough with frothy (sometimes blood-stained) sputum and gradually or rapidly developing dyspnea and cyanosis.

DIFFERENTIAL DIAGNOSIS OF EPISODIC UNCONSCIOUSNESS

	EPILEPSY (Grand Mal) (See **31**. *Convulsive Seizures*)	HYPERVENTILATION (See **34-6**. *Excitement States*)	HYSTERIA (See **50-6**)	VASODEPRESSOR SYNCOPE (Fainting) (See **59-5**)
Onset	Rapid; may be prodromal symptoms	Gradual – vertigo first	Slow or rapid, depending upon surrounding attention	Rapid, often preceded by stretching and yawning
Duration of symptoms	Usually 5 to 10 minutes; may be longer	Not over 2 to 5 minutes	Often prolonged	2 to 3 minutes
Type, results of fall	Sudden; may result in severe injury	Gradual and slow; generally no injury	Careful; practically never any injury	Sudden; may result in injury
Unconsciousness	Total; no response to stimuli	Usually partial, brief	Partial or complete; usually respond to painful stimuli	Complete but very brief
Time or place of onset	Anywhere, even when asleep	In the presence of any situation causing anxiety	In the presence of potential sympathizers	In the presence of real or imagined severe suffering
Muscular movements	Rhythmical and symmetrical	Spasmodic twitching	Inconstant, irregular and bizarre	None

Recovery	Slow; confused, partially disoriented for 10 to 30 minutes	Gradual but complete	Complete at once	Usually complete in a few moments
Skin	Cyanotic from apnea	Usually normal	Normal	Pallor and sweating
Pulse	Normal	Rapid	Normal	Usually slow
Blood pressure	Slightly elevated during episode	Lower than normal	Normal	Marked transient hypotension
Neurologic changes	None except loss of response to pain; occasionally positive Babinski sign	Signs of tetany (43–25)	Decreased corneal and gag reflexes; usually response to painful stimuli	None
Treatment	1. Prevention and treatment of injury 2. Gentle restraint 3. Sedation 4. Long-term care	1. Rebreathing (paper bag method) 2. Sedation by barbiturates 3. Investigation and treatment of cause	1. Sedation by barbiturates if necessary 2. Psychiatric care	1. Supine position 2. Aromatic spirits of ammonia inhalations 3. Treatment of injuries
Prognosis	Good for recovery from immediate attack	Complete recovery	Guarded; complete psychiatric evaluation indicated	Excellent for complete recovery

51. PULMONARY EDEMA

Dyspnea and cyanosis, though simple to recognize, may be complex in origin and due to 1 or more of the following factors:

CAUSE OF RESPIRATORY DISTRESS	EMERGENCY CORRECTION
1. Environment abnormality in gas content (e.g., low oxygen, high carbon dioxide).	Move to normal gas environment. Administer oxygen.
2. Partial mechanical ventilatory failure of muscles (diaphragm, intercostals, accessory muscles) or impaired elastic recoil of the lungs.	Ventilate (11 — 1. *Resuscitation*).
3. Airway obstruction, partial or complete.	Remove or bypass obstruction. See 11 — 1. *Resuscitation,* 14 — 12. *Tracheostomy,* 36 — 4. *Foreign Bodies in Respiratory Tract* and 52 — 1. *Acute Bronchospasm.*

4. Impairment of gas exchange between alveolar air and pulmonary capillary blood due to:
    Structural/functional changes of the alveolar wall.
    Abnormal segmental gas distribution and/or abnormal segmental pulmonary capillary blood flow to significant proportions of the alveoli.
	Improve ventilation and partial gas pressures (see treatment below).
	
	Refer for surgical evaluation of potentially correctable segmental lesions. Treat any specific infections or inflammatory processes.

5. Mechanical or electrical failure, partial or complete, of the cardiovascular pump function.	See treatment below. Also see 11. *Resuscitation,* 26 — 7. *Cardiac Arrest,* 26 — 8. *Congestive Heart Failure* and 53. *Shock.* Surgical evaluation for installation of a temporary pump mechanism may be of value.
6. Inadequate blood gas carrying mechanism due to insufficient hemoglobin or to abnormal alteration of hemoglobin [congenital or acquired (poisoning, e.g., carbon monoxide)]	Administration of oxygen by nasal tube to enhance hemoglobin and soluble oxygen content of blood. Transfusion of whole blood or packed blood cells. Removal from exposure to poisoning substance; give specific antidote if available. Consider transfusion or exchange transfusion; hyperbaric oxygen.
7. Impaired cellular metabolism due to enzymatic poisons, shock, metabolic disorders and acid — base or electrolyte disorders.	See: *Fluid Replacement* (6). *Metabolic Disorders* (43). *Poisons* (49). *Shock* (53).

page 574

TREATMENT

Treatment of acute pulmonary edema will vary dependent upon whether the primary cause is (1) cardiac in origin with pulmonary venous congestion or (2) due to acute development of interstitial fluid and functional impairment of alveolar wall exchange of oxygen and carbon dioxide (with possible secondary development of pulmonary venous congestion). It is also important to differentiate these primary causes of respiratory distress from patients with chronic obstructive lung disease with superimposed acute infections, in whom morphine and other narcotics as well as unsupervised oxygen administration may have a deleterious effect.

Differentiation by history and physical examination will usually suffice for initiation of immediate treatment, with chest x-rays, electrocardiograms, venous pressure determinations and arm-to-tongue circulation time to be obtained later. Arterial blood gas analysis may be essential in assisting in diagnosis in some cases as well as in evaluating efficiency of treatment. Since râles are not produced by ventilatory air with interstitial edema alone, auscultatory findings may reveal clear breath sounds even in the presence of roentgenologic evidence of gross diffuse pulmonary edema.

Any or all of the above signs and symptoms of pulmonary edema may develop rapidly or may not appear for as long as 18 hours after apparent complete recovery from acute poisoning.

TREATMENT FOR ACUTE PULMONARY VENOUS CONGESTION

1. Position of maximum comfort. Usually the patient prefers a semi-Fowler position or insists on sitting on the edge of the bed with his legs hanging down. An attendant must be present at all times.

2. Oxygen by mask or nasal catheter at 6 to 8 liters per minute.

3. Morphine sulfate, 10 to 15 mg. in 10 ml. of sterile water, given slowly intravenously until pain decreases, numbness around the mouth begins or respirations slow. Minimal doses only should be used in patients with kidney disease, chronic pulmonary pathology or hypothyroidism (**33−5.** *Hypothyroid Emergencies*). Opiates and synthetic narcotics are contraindicated in the presence of severe chronic pulmonary insufficiency; in this instance, pentazocine lactate (Talwin), 15 to 30 mg. intravenously may be given in place of morphine.

4. "Bloodless phlebotomy" by application of tourniquets serially to the most proximal portions of 3 or 4 extremities with periods of release of 1 tourniquet at a time for 15 minutes. These tourniquets

—rubber tubing or blood pressure cuffs—should be tight enough to obstruct venous return but not to cut off the arterial flow (arterial pulse should remain). The use of blood pressure cuffs adds greater precision to the procedure than rubber tubing. The cuffs generally should be inflated to 60 to 80 mm. of Hg pressure and kept above 60 mm. of Hg in the arms and approximately 30 to 40 mm. higher for the thighs. The tourniquets should be released 1 at a time at 15 minute intervals to avoid sudden overburdening of the pulmonary circulation; reapplication to a "free" extremity may be done as needed. On infrequent occasions, actual phlebotomy with removal of 250 to 500 ml. of venous blood may be an advisable and effective adjunct to the use of serial tourniquets, particularly in the presence of polycythemia.

5. Rapid diuresis by intravenous injection over a 5 minute period of sodium ethacrynate (Edecrin), 0.5 to 1 gm., in 50 ml. of 5% dextrose in water, or by furosemide (Lasix), 40 mg. orally, intramuscularly or intravenously.

6. Digitalization (for the previously undigitalized patient). Digoxin (usual digitalizing dose: 1.5 mg.) has the advantages of fairly rapid onset of maximal effect ($1\frac{1}{2}$ to 5 hours) and of maintenance therapy with the same preparation. Start with an intravenous dose of 1 mg. and supplement with further doses of 0.25 mg. to 0.5 mg. at 4 to 8 hour intervals until adequate digitalization is obtained. Start daily maintenance doses (0.25 to 0.75 mg.—range approximately 50% less in elderly persons) in 12 to 24 hours; initially, it may be preferable to give $\frac{1}{2}$ of the anticipated maintenance dose every 12 hours.

In more severe cases of pulmonary edema, deslanoside (Cedilanid-D)—average digitalizing dose 1.6 mg.—is preferred because of more rapid onset of maximum effect. Give 0.8 to 1.2 mg. of deslanoside (Cedilanid-D) intravenously followed by 0.2 to 0.4 mg. every 2 to 4 hours until the desired effect is obtained. Digoxin (see step 6) is usually utilized for maintenance therapy.

7. Intermittent positive pressure breathing (IPPB). Combined with an aerosol (absolute ethyl alcohol and water, 1:1 to 1:5 solution) to reduce surface tension, intermittent positive pressure breathing by face mask can be of great value. However, if breathing through the mask causes the patient to panic, or makes his condition worse, the procedure should be stopped.

8. Insertion of a cuffed endotracheal tube with positive pressure ventilation may be lifesaving if the patient is unconscious and cyanotic.

TREATMENT OF ACUTE PULMONARY EDEMA NOT PRIMARILY
DUE TO ACUTE PULMONARY VENOUS CONGESTION
1. Position of maximum comfort; complete rest.
2. Close observation for changes in condition.
3. Oxygen by mask or intranasal catheter (100% at 8 liters per minute). Acidosis must be corrected (**43−1**).
4. Removal from exposure to inciting toxic agents. [Variations in atmospheric pressure (**23.** *Barotrauma*), poisonous gases and dusts (**49.** *Poisons*), etc.]
5. Sedate with caution, preferably with agents that have a minimal depressant effect on the respiratory center (e.g., chloral hydrate, 0.5 to 1 gm. orally, or 1.5 to 2 gm. by rectal route, every 4 to 6 hours.
6. Bronchial dilatation by intermittent use of an aerosol of 0.2 to 0.5 ml. of 1:200 solution of isoproterenol hydrochloride (Isuprel) in 15 ml. of water if bronchial spasm is present, with close observation for cardiac arrhythmia; do not use in presence of rapid tachycardia (greater than 140 per minute).
7. Treatment of any specific bacterial infection (**30−41.** *Antimicrobial Drugs of Choice*).
8. Steroid therapy. Dexamethasone, 15 mg., or prednisone, 100 mg., in a single loading dose by oral or parenteral route, repeated in divided doses through the ensuing 24 hours, can produce dramatic improvement in severe life-threatening interstitial pulmonary edema and following aspiration of gastric contents.

52. RESPIRATORY TRACT CONDITIONS

A large number of persons who request emergency care have signs and symptoms referable to the respiratory tract which are more uncomfortable than serious. Some of the acute respiratory conditions which may warrant emergency care are listed below. See also *Causes of Respiratory Distress, Pulmonary Edema* (**51**).

52−1. ASTHMA (See also **48−6.** *Asthma in Children*).

Wheezing due to bronchospasm may be caused by allergic reactions (**21**), foreign bodies in the upper respiratory tract (**36−4**), infections, and left heart failure (**26.** *Cardiac Emergencies*).

Treatment of Acute Severe Bronchospasm
Hospitalize as soon as possible.
1. Elimination of foreign bodies (**36−4; 48−44.** *Localization Chart*) as causative factors by history and examination.
2. Hydration by intravenous infusion of 1000 ml. of 5% dextrose in 0.45% or 0.9% saline.
3. Correction of hypercapnea and acidosis by rapid intravenous administration of 25 to 100 ml. of sodium bicarbonate (44.6 mEq./50 ml.)
4. Bronchodilation by:
Epinephrine hydrochloride (Adrenalin), 0.25 to 0.5 ml. of 1:1000 solution subcutaneously, repeated in 15 to 20 minutes if bronchospasm has not decreased.
Aminophyllin (Theophylline ethylenediamine), 0.25 gm. in 10 ml. of sterile water, *slowly* intravenously; repeat in 15 to 20 minutes if bronchospasm has not decreased.
Usually tachycardia precludes use of intravenous isoproterenol hydrochloride (Isuprel); if no tachycardia is present, slow infusion of 1 to 2 mg. in 1000 ml. of 5% dextrose in water may be tried.
5. Oxygen under positive pressure using a face mask or intranasal catheter. Discontinue if breathing becomes more difficult; in chronic pulmonary disease, stimulation of the respiratory center by alveolar carbon dioxide may be what is keeping the patient alive — washing it out may be fatal.
6. Intermittent positive pressure breathing with aerosol: initially use 0.1 gm. of Aminophyllin and 1 ml. of 50% alcohol.
7. Sedation as required. The most effective sedative drugs in treatment of bronchospasm are the rapid acting barbiturates (e.g., amobarbital), chloral hydrate and chlorpromazine hydrochloride (Thorazine). Oversedation must be guarded against.
8. Steroids by intravenous route, 250 to 1000 mg. of hydrocortisone sodium succinate (Solu-Cortef) or 50 to 250 mg. of prednisolone (Meticortelone or Solu-Medrol).
9. Tracheostomy, deep sedation with intravenous amobarbital and diazepam (Valium), artificial ventilation using a cuffed tracheostomy tube and bronchial lavage with 30 to 60 ml. of ¼ to ½% lidocaine in normal saline gradually instilled over ½ hour and suctioning periodically, may be required in the most severe cases. Efforts at artificial ventilation may be impossible and self-defeating in the most severe cases until relief of smooth muscle spasm of the bronchi has occurred.

10. Determination of blood pH, pO_2 and pCO_2 are important in guiding therapy.

TREATMENT OF SLIGHT OR MODERATE ASTHMATIC ATTACKS

1. Hydration by:

Large amounts of fluids by mouth (**6**).

Dextrose 5% in 0.45% saline, 500 to 1000 ml. intravenously.

2. Bronchodilation by:

Ephedrine sulfate, 25 mg. orally every 4 hours.

Epinephrine hydrochloride (Adrenalin), 1:1000 solution by nebulizer, or, in severer cases, 0.25 to 0.5 ml. of 1:1000 solution subcutaneously every 20 minutes.

Aminophylline (Theophylline ethylenediamine) rectally or slowly intravenously.

Sedation by barbiturates or chlorpromazine hydrochloride (Thorazine) in the smallest possible effective doses.

Thinning of bronchial secretions by oral iodides.

3. Administration of oxygen by face mask and rebreathing bag.

4. Arrangement for detailed medical supervision on an ambulatory basis. The need for further care should be stressed most emphatically since many patients after relief from an acute attack will postpone medical care until another acute episode occurs.

Do Not

1. Administer opiates or synthetic narcotics in any form; any of these drugs may cause depression of the respiratory center, decrease of the cough reflex and, if repeated frequently, addiction.

2. Oversedate.

3. Allow use of stramonium fume inhalations.

4. Permit excessive use of tobacco. On the other hand, attempting to cure the tobacco habit is not a part of the emergency therapy of asthma.

5. Prescribe or administer corticosteroids of any type as emergency therapy until hospitalization or supervised ambulatory care is in effect.

6. Encourage the patient to cough forcibly to raise tenacious sputum.

7. Prescribe or administer antibiotics unless infection is a proved causative factor.

8. Recommend a climate change.

52 – 2. BRONCHITIS (See also 48 – 48. *Bronchitis in Children*)

TREATMENT

1. Penicillin tetracycline, 500 mg. by mouth; then 250 to 500 mg. every 6 hours.
2. Cough mixtures containing codeine sulfate or dihydrocodeinone bitartrate (Hycodan) and ammonium chloride.
3. Aerosol inhalations if tenacious mucus is present.
4. Bed rest with large amounts of fluids by mouth.

52 – 3. CORYZA (See also 48 – 48. *Laryngotracheobronchitis and Nasopharyngitis in Children; 62 – 3. Common Colds*)

No satisfactory treatment for "colds" except bed rest and copious fluids is known. The following measures may give symptomatic relief:

1. Sedative cough mixtures containing codeine sulfate or dihydrocodeinone (Hycodan) mixtures will usually relieve persistent coughs. Ammonium chloride is useful if tenacious mucus is present.
2. Codeine sulfate and acetylsalicylic acid (aspirin) by mouth every 4 to 6 hours.
3. Fluids in large amounts by mouth.
4. Phenylephrine hydrochloride (Neo-Synephrine) nose drops (0.25%). Naphazoline hydrochloride (Privine) should not be used or prescribed because of the relatively high percentage of allergic reactions (49 – 623).

52 – 4. CROUP See 48 – 19

52 – 5. DEAFNESS See 32 – 5

52 – 6. EPIGLOTTITIS

Acute swelling of the epiglottis is often overlooked as a cause for respiratory obstruction in children. Its development is very rapid and fatalities have been reported. Diagnosis is based on direct inspection of the swollen epiglottis. A single lateral inspiratory x-ray may show characteristic changes (ballooned hypopharynx, thickening of the epiglottis, widening of the aryepiglottic fold).

Treatment

1. Immediate tracheostomy (**14—12**) for impending, partial or frank signs of respiratory obstruction. Attempts at intubation should be avoided. Constant observation is required.

2. Treatment of the causative infection.

52—7.   HICCUPS (Singultus)

In infancy, this condition is often caused by overdistention of the stomach by food or swallowed air. Pressure over the upper abdomen ("burping") usually gives relief. A teaspoonful of weak sodium bicarbonate solution or lemon juice may be tried. In adults, hiccups may be idiopathic but also may occur with gastric distention, posterior myocardial infarction and uremia or during administration of general anesthesia.

Mild attacks can sometimes be controlled by 1 or more of a long list of "household cures." Among these are:

1. Pressing on or application of ice to the back of the neck.
2. Holding the breath as long as possible.
3. Swallowing finely cracked ice.
4. Pressing on the eyeballs (not too hard!).
5. Pulling on the tongue.
6. Cervical traction and manipulation.
7. Drinking a glass of water while holding a pencil crossways between the teeth.
8. Manipulation of single long hairs in the external auditory canal with a cotton applicator.

Severe attacks may yield to some of the following measures:

1. Rebreathing using a paper bag or face mask.
2. Inhalations of Carbogen or ether.
3. Gastric lavage.
4. Stimulation of the pharyngeal wall by insertion of a catheter. For maximum efficiency the tip of the catheter should be at the level of C_2–C_3.
5. Extreme sedation by chloral hydrate, paraldehyde or barbiturates.
6. Chlorpromazine hydrochloride (Thorazine), 25 to 50 mg. intramuscularly; repeated in 3 hours if necessary.
7. Hyoscine hydrobromide, 0.4 to 0.6 mg. subcutaneously.
8. Opiates, especially apomorphine hydrochloride, 5 mg. subcutaneously.

9. Amphetamine sulfate (Benzedrine), 10 to 20 mg. subcutaneously or slowly intravenously.

10. Adiphenine hydrochloride (Trasentine), 75 mg. subcutaneously (1 dose), or every 4 hours by mouth.

11. Breath-holding with the head acutely hyperextended.

12. Atropine sulfate, 1 mg. subcutaneously.

13. Calcium gluconate, 10 ml. of 10% solution intravenously.

Prolonged intractable cases require hospitalization for replacement fluids (**6**) and for treatment of extreme exhaustion which may be terminal.

52−8. HYPERVENTILATION See 34−6

52−9. LARYNGITIS

The emergency treatment is the same as outlined for *Bronchitis* (**52−2**).

52−10. MASTOIDITIS See 32−10

52−11. METAL FUME FEVER See 49−461

52−12. OTITIS MEDIA See 32−13

52−13. PLEURISY

TREATMENT

1. If possible, identify and give symptomatic treatment for the underlying pulmonary or cardiac conditions, with arrangements for follow-up care by an internist.

2. If pain is severe, limit respiratory excursion as much as possible by strapping or application of a binder. However, partial immobilization should be avoided as a routine measure; adequate aeration lessens the chance of development of intrapleural pathology.

3. Give acetylsalicylic acid (aspirin) and codeine sulfate by mouth as needed.

4. Hospitalize if the pain is severe or if there is evidence of fluid by clinical or x-ray examination.

52 – 14.   PNEUMONIA (See also **48 – 45.** *Pneumonia in Children;* **62 – 11.** *Interstitial Pneumonia*)

The patient's general condition should be the deciding factor in the management of cases of suspected or proved pneumonia. Many patients with extensive lung involvement can be treated satisfactorily at home by bed rest, antibiotics, sulfonamides, analgesics and good nursing care. Penicillin in adequate doses is often all that is necessary for control, but chlortetracycline (Aureomycin), oxytetracycline (Terramycin) and other antibiotics may be more effective if a mixed infection or a penicillin-resistant organism is present. Perform a gram stain and culture sputum secretions.

Severe pain on respiration, dyspnea and cyanosis, plus the physical findings of pneumonia, establish the diagnosis, but laboratory studies and x-rays may be necessary to determine the extent of involvement, causative organism and disposition of the case. Lobar pneumonia almost invariably, bronchopneumonia often and viral pneumonia rarely require hospitalization.

52 – 15.   PNEUMONITIS

Irritation of the alveolar spaces of the lungs may be caused by viral or bacterial infections, trauma to the chest (**28**), especially severe crushing injuries, and inhalation of toxic substances, e.g., gasoline (**49 – 349**) and kerosene (**49 – 408**).

TREATMENT

1. Limited activity; bed rest in severe cases.

2. Sedative cough mixtures.

3. Penicillin, 600,000 units intramuscularly, and/or chlortetracycline (Aureomycin) and oxytetracycline (Terramycin) in large doses by mouth depending on the sensitivity of the causative organism.

4. Hospitalization if the condition is extensive or severe, if it is associated with severe injury to the bony thorax or if other types of acute or chronic chest pathology are present.

52 – 16.   PNEUMOTHORAX (See also **28 – 4.** *Traumatic Pneumothorax;* **28 – 5.** *Tension Pneumothorax;* **48 – 46.** *Pneumothorax in Children*)

Spontaneous pneumothorax. Usually a benign process, spontaneous rupture of an air-containing vesicle or of an alveolus may result in the passage of air into the pleural cavity or mediastinum. X-rays are useful not only in establishing the diagnosis but also in disclosing underlying causative diseases. Symptomatic treatment is generally all that is required. Oxygen inhalations for cyanosis and dyspnea may be needed, followed by sedation and bed rest, preferably in a hospital, for a few days. Underlying disease processes should be recognized and arrangements made for proper care.

Tension pneumothorax. See **28 — 5; 48 — 46.** *Pneumothorax in Children.*

Traumatic pneumothorax. See **28 — 4; 48 — 46.** *Pneumothorax in Children.*

Therapeutic pneumothorax. Emergency care may be needed for bleeding following therapeutic injection of air.

TREATMENT

1. Sedation by intramuscular or intravenous barbiturates.
2. Slow (1 ml. per minute) intravenous injection of 1 ml. of Pituitrin, in 20 ml. of normal saline.
3. Hospitalization if bleeding is severe or persistent.

52 — 17. PULMONARY EMBOLISM See 59 — 4

52 — 18. PULMONARY HEMORRHAGE See 42 — 17. *Bleeding from the Lungs*

52 — 19. PULMONARY EDEMA See 51

52 — 20. RHINORRHEA

Drainage of spinal fluid, usually mixed with blood, from the nose indicates a basal fracture of the skull (**41 — 16**), whether or not x-rays show bony injury. See **41 — 17.** *Middle Fossa Fractures.*

52 — 21. SINUSITIS

TREATMENT

1. Penicillin, 600,000 units intramuscularly, or chlortetracycline (Aureomycin), 250 mg. by mouth, every 4 to 6 hours.
2. Phenylephrine hydrochloride (Neo-Synephrine) nose drops (0.25%) to shrink the engorged mucous membranes and promote drainage. Postural drainage may be effective.

3. Application of local heat.

4. Bed rest; copious fluids.

5. Acetylsalicylic acid (aspirin) and codeine sulfate by mouth for pain and headache.

6. Ultrasound therapy over the frontal and maxillary sinuses for 7 to 10 minutes daily may be of great value in promoting drainage.

7. Referral to an otolaryngologist for further treatment if symptoms persist.

52 – 22.   TONSILLITIS See **48 – 48** (*Tonsillitis*)

52 – 23.   VIRUS INFECTIONS See **62**

53.   SHOCK

53 – 1.   DEFINITION

Shock is "a rude unhinging of the machinery of life" (Samuel D. Gross, 1872) which is still incompletely understood, although it is recognized that its dramatic and various clinical pictures are based more on impairment of cellular function than on specific anatomic changes. It may be induced by injury, blood loss, fright, dehydration, cardiac inadequacy, hypersensitivity reactions, endotoxins from gram negative organisms, impairment of nervous function, blockage of blood flow in major vessels, impaired function of certain endocrine glands and many poisons. Any of these conditions may cause reduction of effective tissue perfusion to a level which is too low to sustain general cellular metabolism. This, in turn, further impairs tissue perfusion. Thus, shock begets shock.

53 – 2.   PHYSIOLOGIC EVALUATION OF SHOCK

An important contribution to the understanding of the pathophysiology of shock and of effects of treatment (including use of vasodilator and vasoconstrictor drugs) has been the recognition of the role of pre- and post-capillary vasoconstriction mechanism. If effective treatment is started in the earlier or ischemic stage, reversal of the process with improvement of tissue perfusion occurs more readily than if treatment is delayed until the stagnant phase has become established.

Peripheral arterial blood pressure measurements as single tests are not the most efficient means of determining the degree or severity of shock or of evaluating response to treatment, but rather represent one of the valuable methods for minute-by-minute monitoring of essential organ tissue perfusion and function outlined in Table 1 (page 587).

53-3. TYPES OF SHOCK

The following classification of the types of shock is not satisfactory in some ways, but it does furnish a basis for rapid evaluation and emergency therapy. A combination of the types listed below may be present in the same patient at a given time and may, by a common mode or interrelated action, cause disruption of tissue perfusion and cellular metabolism.

1. **Hypovolemic shock** is the result of gross loss of 1 or more of the following: blood, plasma, water, saline and electrolytes, either from the body or into a relatively inaccessible "third compartment" (peritoneal and pleural cavities, massive soft tissue effusion).

2. **Cardiogenic shock** results from electrical or mechanical failure of the heart and/or peripheral vascular collapse. Acute myocardial infarction, serious cardiac dysrhythmias and acute cor pulmonale — particularly from pulmonary embolus — are the most common causes.

3. **Septic shock** is caused by bacterial toxins or by endotoxins from gram-negative organisms.

53-4. SIGNS AND SYMPTOMS OF SHOCK

The clinical manifestations of shock will depend to a large extent upon the cause, magnitude and duration as well as upon the patient's prior general health. An individual showing the characteristic picture of shock is prostrated but usually conscious, restless and apprehensive, with moist cool clammy skin, circumoral pallor and sunken eyeballs ("Hippocratic facies"). Cyanosis may occur except when profound anemia is present. The pulse is rapid, feeble

TABLE 1. METHODS FOR RAPID CLINICAL MONITORING OF CELLULAR METABOLISM AND ORGAN PERFUSION

PARAMETER	PRIMARY ORGAN OR SYSTEM
Respiratory rate, tidal volume (estimated and measured), skin color, temperature, capillary blanching and filling	Pulmonary and ventilatory system. Peripheral cellular metabolism and perfusion
Pupillary size; sensorium	Central nervous system
Pulse and heart rate; stethoscope; oscilloscope with electrocardiograph (cardiac rate and rhythm; ventricular depolarization and repolarization)	Heart
Urinary output determined by indwelling bladder catheter	Kidney
Tilt test, jugular vein filling, capillary blanching test, venous and pulse pressure	Extracellular and intravascular fluid volume

Other periodic measurements (cardiac output, blood pH, expired air and arterial blood gas determinations and blood volume) may be necessary in some cases but are not as simple or immediately available as those listed above

and of small volume. Measured urine output is scanty or absent. The blood pressure becomes progressively (and sometimes rapidly) lower, with the systolic pressure usually falling more rapidly than the diastolic. Increasing acidosis (**43 — 1**) due to progressive hypoxemia of the tissues develops.

Duration of the acute shock state is a reliable index of prognosis — the longer the duration the worse the prognosis. Therefore, treatment of shock takes precedence over all other emergency measures except control of gross hemorrhage and insurance of adequate oxygenation. Any adult patient with a systolic blood pressure 40 to 50 mm. of mercury below his usual resting level, or below 80 to 90 mm. of mercury, should be checked thoroughly for other signs of shock (Table 3) and treatment should be instituted accordingly.

TABLE 2. COMMON PHYSICAL FINDINGS BY TYPE OF SHOCK

HYPOVOLEMIC	CARDIOGENIC	SEPTIC
Whole Blood Loss History of prior focal bleeding, blood dyscrasia or anticoagulant therapy (**49 — 79**) Acute trauma Observed gross bleeding Extreme pallor, including the conjunctivae and palmar creases Palpation, percussion and needle aspiration of large blood masses	Signs and symptoms of myocardial infarction (**26 — 12**) or congestive heart failure (**26 — 8**) ——————————— Serious arrhythmias and abnormal rates (increased or decreased) Gallop rhythm and murmurs Poor heart tones Cardiac enlargement	Feverishness Malaise Symptoms of genitourinary disease or disorder or prior treatment and instrumentation thereof ——————————— Toxic appearance Fever (can be minimal or absent) Focus of infection
Water, Saline and/or Plasma Loss Rapid body weight loss Poor tissue turgor Inadequate input or abnormally increased output via skin, stomach, rectum or kidneys Demonstration of "Third Space"		

53 — 5. DETERMINATION OF SEVERITY AND CAUSES OF SHOCK

HISTORY

Details of events leading to development of shock and a detailed history of prior health are usually of greater assistance in determination of the cause, type and prognosis of shock than in determination of the patient's immediate status. However, a history of trauma, operative procedures, exposure to poisonous substances (including drugs and medications), infection, fever and focal pain may be significant. In addition, estimates of prior blood loss, duration of vomiting and diarrhea and comparison with normal body weight can be of great importance in planning an effective therapeutic regimen. Inability of the patient to give a coherent history is an indication of impaired brain cell function and may represent inadequate perfusion.

53 — 6.   EXAMINATION FOR SHOCK

Examinations preceded by an asterisk (*) should be done at once.

SKIN

*Gross bleeding seen at or beneath the skin surface.
Burns — surface area, degree, depth (**25**).
Turgor.
*Color.
*Temperature.
Rash, petechiae or purpura.
Capillary filling.
Infections or wounds.
Otoscopic inspection.

CENTRAL NERVOUS SYSTEM

*Sensorium.
*Pupils — size and reactivity.
Papilledema.
Gross focal pathologic neurologic signs (motor or sensory loss, reflexes, rectal sphincter tone, pathologic toe signs).
Meningeal irritation (**30 — 16.** *Meningitis;* **48 — 41.** *Meningitis in Children*).

CARDIOPULMONARY VASCULAR SYSTEM

*Pulse rate and rhythm.
*Respiratory rate.
*Approximate tidal volume (See also **15 — 7.** *Ventilation Test.*)
*Blood pressure.
Jugular vein size.
Lungs — breath sounds, dullness, tympany.
Heart — gross size, thrills, quality of heart tones, murmurs.

ENTERIC SYSTEM AND ABDOMEN

Odor of breath.
Presence of oral blood, blood in the stool (**42 — 22.** *Rectal Bleeding*)

TABLE 3. IDENTIFICATION OF DEGREE OF SEVERITY OF SHOCK

TEST OR SIGN		NORMAL OR AVERAGE	DEGREE OF SHOCK		
			Preshock State to Mild Shock	*Moderate*	*Moderately Severe to Severe*
Sensorium	Orientation	Time Place Person Well-oriented	Oriented	Fairly well-oriented	May be confused and disoriented
	Enunciation	Distinct	Normal—slurred words	Somewhat slowed and few slurred words	Slow and slurred to monosyllabic utterances and groans
	Content	Appropriate; structured sentences	Sentences normal	Slow sentences or phrases and words	Often incoherent
Pupils	Size	Equal (2 to 4 mm.)	Normal	Normal	Normal to dilating or dilated
	Constriction with light	Rapid	Rapid	Rapid	Slow or nonreactive
Pulse	Rate	60 to 100/min.	110 to 120/min.	120 to 150/min.	Maximal
	Amplitude	Full	Full amplitude to slight decrease	Variable: mild decrease	Thready
Blood pressure (mm. of Hg.)	Systolic	120 to 145	Normal or slightly low	Decreased—often 40 to 50 mm. of Hg. below usual B.P.	Less than 80 to unobtainable
	Diastolic	60 to 90	Normal or slightly low	Decreased, but less so than systolic	40 to 50 to unobtainable
	Pulse pressure	40 to 70	30 to 40	20 to 30	Less than 20

	Patient flat	Fills to anterior border of sternocleidomastoid muscle	Normal to trace of filling	Trace to no filling	No filling
Jugular vein filling			May be full in septic shock or grossly distended in cardiogenic shock		
Urinary output via catheter — ml./min.	0.6 to 15		0.6 to 0.3	0.4 to 0.6	0.3 or less
ml./10 min.	6 to 15		6 to 8	4 to 6	3 or less
Tilt test — Rapid lying to sitting position — Pulse	Transient increase		Increased	Rapid	Already maximal
Blood pressure	Less than 10 mm. decrease		10 to 25 mm. decrease	25 to 50 mm. decrease	Marked decrease to unobtainable
Symptoms	No "lightheadedness"		No lightheadedness	Lightheadedness	Unable to sit up
Therapeutic, if whole blood loss	– – –		Probably do not transfuse	Transfuse!	Transfuse!
Est. blood loss	– – –		To 750 ml.	1000 to 1250 ml.	1500 to 1750 ml. or more
Est. % blood volume loss	– – –		15%	20 to 25%	More than 30 to 35%
Capillary blanching test — Blanching of forehead skin with thumb pressure	Return of circulation in 1.25 to 1.5 sec.		1.25 to 1.5 sec.	More than 1.5 sec.	Pallor before and after test
			Note: With hypercapnea, there may be almost instantaneous return		
Central venous pressure	Normal (3 to 8 cm. of saline)		Normal	Low	Extremely low
			May be elevated in cardiogenic shock		

or foreign substances (**36 — 5.** *Foreign Bodies in Gastrointestinal Tract*).
    Abdominal distention, tenderness, guarding or masses.
    Organomegaly, including area of splenic dullness.
    Widening of the aorta.

GENITOURINARY SYSTEM

    See **38.** *Genitourinary Tract Emergencies.* A bimanual pelvic examination should be done in women, followed later by a speculum examination, with rectal examination if posterior cul-de-sac pathology is suspected.

MUSCULOSKELETAL SYSTEM (See also 44. Musculoskeletal Conditions)

    A thorough visual inspection should be made followed by rapid but careful checking for evidence of injury to the neck, thorax, back, pelvis and extremities. Massive soft tissue trauma should be evaluated carefully.
    Various tests (Table 3) act as rough guides in determination of the magnitude of shock. No single test should be used as the sole determining factor regarding the degree or cause of shock. See **53 — 7.** *Treatment of Shock* regarding further evaluation of causative factors after obtaining the preliminary data outlined above.

53 — 7.   TREATMENT OF SHOCK

    No protocol, regardless of its length or structure, can take the place of frequent close observation of the patient and appropriate individual adjustments in treatment. The following recommendations represent a broad outline of a satisfactory approach to management of a person who presents in deep shock, with no history of onset or past history available and no evidence of acute pulmonary congestion. If pulmonary congestion is present, the therapeutic approach recommended under pulmonary edema (**51**) should be utilized.
    Evaluation of a person who is in shock begins the moment that the physician first sees the patient. During this initial survey, the physician should expedite management by initiating various tests, monitoring procedures and treatment. Therapy must take into consideration not only correction of immediate deficits and replacement of current losses but also normal physiologic requirements.

Moderate and severe shock must be treated energetically and corrected as soon as possible using periodic monitoring to evaluate progress. On the other hand, persons in mild shock who are making satisfactory progress toward normalcy should be treated conservatively and cautiously – especially the very young, the very old and persons with underlying chronic organic diseases.

CHRONOLOGIC STEPS IN TREATMENT OF SHOCK

1. Check vital signs rapidly (pupils, pulse, respirations, blood pressure).

2. Clear the airway and institute resuscitation (**11**) if necessary, continuing until the condition has stabilized.

3. Control gross bleeding.

4. Insert an intravenous catheter (preferably) or a No. 15 needle. Use a blood pressure cuff first to take a blood pressure reading and then as a precision tourniquet. Do a saphenous or other vein cutdown if necessary.

5. Draw blood specimens for:

    (a) Hemoglobin, hematocrit, white blood count and differential (1 tube of citrated blood).

    (b) Serum sugar, CO_2, sodium amylase, BUN and potassium (1 tube of clotted blood).

    (c) Type and cross-match for blood transfusions (1 tube).

    (d) Obtain 1 extra tube of clotted blood for special tests as needed (e.g., serum acetone, barbiturates, bromide, bilirubin, enzymes).

    (e) If gross hemorrhage is present which does not seem to be related to proportionate trauma, take a blood specimen for prothrombin time, fibrinogen content and platelet count.

    (f) Note the gross clotting time and put aside a sample for evaluation of clot retraction. If a patient with hemorrhage has been taking anticoagulation drugs (**49 – 79**), start indicated intravenous therapy at once after drawing blood for prothrombin time.

6. Start an infusion of 5% dextrose in normal saline (or of 5% dextrose in half normal saline in children), unless an unusual situation such as hypernatremia is suspected. If shock is associated with coma (**29**), give 25 ml. of 50% dextrose in water intravenously at once. If obvious hypovolemic shock from blood loss is present, start dextran and then blood intravenously as soon as available.

7. Resume and complete the rapid physical examination (**53 – 5**).

8. Obtain any available information concerning onset and past history.

9. Insert a urinary bladder catheter (**14 – 3.** *Catheterization*) and start initial minute-by-minute recording until the output becomes adequate. Obtain an immediate urinary specific gravity, sugar, acetone and pH and send a specimen to the laboratory for culture and microscopic examination.

10. Test responses to sitting (tilt test) if not in severe shock and to the capillary blanching test (Table 3).

11. Obtain a standard 12 lead electrocardiogram – evaluate particularly for myocardial infarction (**26 – 12**), cardiac arrhythmias and electrolyte imbalance.

12. Recheck vital signs and urine output (Table 3).

13. Insert a nasogastric tube and observe the aspirate for volume, color and blood. Save specimen for possible later examination if poisoning suspected.

14. Gavage with 500 ml. of 1/6 molar sodium lactate. Maintain suction if gastric distention or blood is present.

15. Insert a venous pressure catheter if the patient is in severe shock or is very old or young.

16. If the patient is febrile and toxic, obtain 3 to 6 blood cultures in rapid succession. Culture any wounds or drainage. Perform a lumbar puncture (**14 – 11**) if meningeal irritation, coma or focal central nervous system deficit is present. Culture throat, any petechiae, and – in females – the cervix. Make Gram stains of any probable sources of infection and start immediate appropriate massive antibiotic therapy (**30 – 41.** *Antimicrobial Drugs of Choice*).

17. If urinary output is scanty (4 to 6 ml. in 10 minutes) or absent, inject 100 ml. of a 25% solution of mannitol intravenously. If the urine volume doubles in the next 10 minutes, continue to force appropriate fluids (blood or saline); if there is no increase, fluids must be given very cautiously.

18. Obtain additional laboratory tests as required, based on current condition and response to therapy (arterial pH, pCO_2, pO_2, blood volume) and proceed with therapy for the type and degree of shock (Tables 3 and 4) and with treatment of underlying causes.

MAINTENANCE OR RESTORATION OF BLOOD AND TISSUE FLUID VOLUME

Before Whole Blood Is Available

1. Saline solution intravenously at once. If superficial veins are

collapsed or unsatisfactory, it is simple and safe to use a femoral vein until a cutdown can be done.

2. Plasma volume expanders. These solutions, given intravenously without blood-typing, are satisfactory and safe temporary

TABLE 4. TREATMENT OF SHOCK BY TYPES

KEY:	++	Prime factor
	+	Generally indicated
	±	Variable — based on clinical state
	0	Not indicated or not necessary

TREATMENT	HYPOVOLEMIC SHOCK	CARDIOGENIC SHOCK	SEPTIC SHOCK
Insurance of an adequate airway and ventilation	++	++	++
Control of hemorrhage	++	0	0
Control of pain and apprehension	++	++	++
Correction of acidosis	++	++	++
Oxygen under positive pressure	+	++	+
Conservation of body heat	++	++	++
Saline and electrolytes	++	±	+
Plasma volume expanders	++	± (LMW Dextran)	±
Whole blood	++	0	±
Vasopressors; cardiotonic drugs	±	++	±
Vasodilators	±	±	+
Antibiotics	±	±	++
Steroids	±	±	++

substitutes for whole blood. If a plasma volume expander is to be used, 10 ml. of venous blood should be collected before infusion is started. This blood specimen should be sent to the laboratory, or with the patient if he is being transferred, so that cross-matching for later blood transfusions will be facilitated.

When Whole Blood Is Available

Transfusion of adequate amounts of whole blood (**14 — 13. Transfusions**) takes a precedence over all other measures in the treatment of hypovolemic shock. The blood volume of an average adult male is about 5000 ml.; as much as 700 to 800 ml. can be lost in some instances without clinical signs of shock (**53 — 4** and Table 3). Hematocrit and hemoglobin determinations are of limited value in the initial management of shock, although they may be significant after 6 to 8 hours.

When large amounts of blood bank (storage) blood (properly cross-matched) are used, calcium gluconate (2 ml. of 10% solution after each 300 to 400 ml. of blood infusion) may be added to combat excess citrate from the blood preservative. If Type O Rh negative blood (universal donor) is used for the first emergency transfusion, it must be used for subsequent transfusions (unless 2 weeks have elapsed) because of possible acquired sensitivity to minor antigens. In severe hypovolemic shock, the total blood transfusion volume may equal approximately ½ of the patient's estimated blood volume. In severe shock from blood loss, massive replacement may be required using as many sites of transfusion as are necessary (**14 — 13. Transfusions**). Unless conditions such as central nervous system damage, heart disease or severe anemia (hematocrit less than 20%) are present, undertransfusion is more likely to occur than overtransfusion.

Control of metabolic acidosis by intravenous injection of sodium bicarbonate solution (3.75 gm. in 50 ml. of saline solution), repeated every 30 minutes as required or according to specific schedules as in cardiac arrest (**11 — 2**) or diabetic coma (**43 — 10**).

VASOPRESSOR AND CARDIOTONIC MEDICATIONS

The vasopressor drugs can be valuable adjuncts in treatment of shock, particularly cardiogenic shock and shock in which the skin is warm (rather than cold and clammy); however, because they may decrease visceral perfusion — especially of the kidneys — their use should be deferred in hypovolemic shock at least until normal blood volume has been or is nearly restored. As a rule, they should bc given slowly in 500 to 1000 ml. of intravenous fluids. The most effective of the vasoconstrictors are:

1. Phenylephrine hydrochloride (Neo-Synephrine), 3 to 5 mg., added to 500 to 1000 ml. of intravenous solution. This drug is a powerful alpha mimetic and raises blood pressure, slows the heart and increases venous pooling.

2. Ephedrine sulfate, 10 to 25 mg. intravenously, directly or in 500 to 1000 ml. of solution.

3. Levarterenol bitartrate (Levophed, norepinephrine), 4 mg., given slowly intravenously in 1000 ml. of 5% dextrose in water or saline and continued for as long as necessary. The speed of intravenous injection should be controlled by blood pressure readings every 2 minutes until a plateau with the systolic pressure slightly below normal has been reached. A plastic catheter inserted into a vein – by cutdown if necessary – is preferable to a needle because ex travasation of levarterenol bitartrate into soft tissues will cause sloughing. If long-continued use is necessary and blanching along the course of the vein develops, the site of injection should be changed at once. If extravasation into the soft tissues does occur, infiltration of the area through multiple punctures, using a fine (No. 26) needle, with 5 to 10 mg. of phentolamine methanesulfonate (Regitine) and 150 turbidity reducing units (TRU) of hyaluronidase dissolved in 15 ml. of normal salt solution may prevent extensive necrosis.

4. Metaraminol bitartrate (Aramine) subcutaneously, intramuscularly or intravenously. This drug in small doses has a beta-adrenergic effect and decreases blood pressure, increases the heart rate and decreases venous pooling. In large doses it acts as an alpha-mimetic, with a rise in blood pressure, a decrease in pulse rate and an increase in venous pooling. It has the advantage of ease of administration – it can be injected subcutaneously, intramuscularly or intravenously. Intravenously, a plastic catheter is not necessary since sloughing of the soft tissues (see levarterenol bitartrate, above) does not follow extravenous infiltration.

METHOD	DOSE	RAPIDITY OF ACTION
Subcutaneously	2 to 10 mg.	10 to 20 min.
Intramuscularly	2 to 10 mg.	7 to 10 min.
Intravenously (directly)	0.5 to 5 mg.	1 to 2 min.

By infusion, 15 to 100 mg. in 500 ml. of normal salt solution or 5% dextrose in saline or water can be given. The rate of administration should be controlled by frequent blood pressure readings.

VASODILATORS

Use of vasodilators for control of vasoconstriction occurring during shock is not as important as avoidance of aggravation of the underlying condition with vasoconstrictive drugs — particularly in hypovolemic and septic shock — and judicious correction of blood, plasma, water and saline loss (**6**). In some complex cases of shock, the test triad of monitoring urine volume, central venous pressure (CVP) and blood volume (by a rapid bedside method such as radioactive albumin) can be valuable. If blood volume, CVP and urine volume are low, give blood, plasma or saline as required. If blood volume and CVP approach or exceed normal before the urine volume rises, give isoproterenol (Isuprel) in dextrose and water solution, 2 to 3 mcgm./min.

In some patients — particularly those in cardiogenic or septic shock, utilization of the inotropic and vasodilatory effects of isoproterenol (Isuprel) given by drip infusion of 2 to 3 mg. in 1000 ml. of 5% dextrose in water may be helpful. Cautious administration of a vasodilator may help to control pulmonary venous congestion occurring during the course of treatment of shock.

CORTICOSTEROID THERAPY

In cases of severe hypersensitivity (**21 — 1**. *Anaphylactic Shock*) or endocrine failure shock (**33 — 1**. *Acute Adrenal Cortical Insufficiency;* **33 — 3**. *Acute Parathyroid Intoxication;* **33 — 5**. *Hyperthyroid Emergencies;* **43 — 15**. *Hyperthyroid Crises*) which do not respond satisfactorily to general measures, corticosteroids may be indicated. In severe septic shock, methylprednisolone sodium succinate (Solu-Medrol), 80 mg. intravenously, repeated every 4 hours, may be life-saving. In children the intravenous dose should be not less than 0.5 mg. per kilogram of body weight per 24 hours. Provided corticosteroid therapy has not been in use for more than 3 days, administration can be discontinued abruptly without ill-effects; if it has been used for longer periods, it should be gradually decreased.

Control of pain. Morphine sulfate intravenously may be used in small doses if the patient is acutely apprehensive and in severe pain, provided chest injuries (**28**) or head injuries (**41**) are not present. Pentazocine lactate (Talwin), 30 mg. intravenously does not cause significant respiratory depression and is an effective anodyne.

Transportation for hospitalization and definitive treatment should be arranged as a considered risk as soon as the patient's condition has stabilized. Speed of transportation is not as important as care in transportation in full compliance with speed and traffic regulations. Intravenous fluids, respiratory assistance and supportive therapy should be continued during transportation if necessary, preferably under supervision of a physician or registered nurse.

53 — 8. RESPONSIBILITIES OF THE ATTENDING PHYSICIAN IN CASES OF SHOCK

1. To recognize the signs and symptoms (**53 — 4**) promptly and to begin adequate corrective and maintenance treatment (**53 — 7**) based on present-day concepts of the pathophysiology of shock as soon as possible.

2. To guard against aggravation of the patient's condition by unnecessary moving for examination, x-rays or diagnostic procedures.

3. To avoid superimposing additional insult by premature wound repair, manipulation of fractures or dislocations or administration of prophylactic injections.

4. To minimize excitement caused by solicitous family or friends, or by any overenthusiastic law enforcement officers, newspaper reporters, cameramen, insurance representatives or unauthorized curious persons.

5. To record in detail all findings and treatment (and reasons therefor).

6. To make the decision regarding transfer for definitive care and to make a permanent record of reasons for such transfer.

7. To contact the hospital to which the patient is being sent (if being transferred) so that proper equipment and personnel will be standing by and delay in definitive treatment minimized.

54. SKIN AND MUCOUS MEMBRANE CONDITIONS

The skin surface area of an averaged-sized adult (70 kg., 154 lb.) is about 1.73 square meters (18½ square feet) — most of it under the frequent narcissistic inspection and palpation stressed by present-day advertising, radio commercials and television. The same applies to a lesser degree to inspectable and palpable areas of mucous membrane. This self-inspection probably is a definite contributory factor in the increasing number of persons requesting immediate treatment for alleged dermatologic and mucous membrane emergencies—supposed variations from the usual in color, temperature, texture, shape or sensation of the surface of some part of the body.

Although the majority of dermatologic conditions do not require urgent therapy as a means of saving life or function, many of them do cause acute discomfort which can be relieved by prompt and appropriate therapy.

54—1. ALLERGIC REACTIONS See 21

54—2. ANGIOEDEMA See **21—2; 48—4.** *Angioedema in Children*

54—3. BITES See **24; 61.** *Venoms*

54—4. BURNS See **25; 48—14.** *Burns in Children;* **63—4.** *Thermal Effects of a Nuclear Blast*

54—5. CONTAGIOUS DISEASES See **30—40.** *Common Exanthems*

54—6. DERMATITIS

Contact. Many of these cases are caused by exposure to irritating substances at work. *(See* **75.** *Workmen's Compensation Cases.)* Removal from exposure is the most important part of treatment. (See also **54—11.** *Poison Oak, Ivy and Sumach;* **54—16.** *Urushiol Contact Dermatitis.)*

Exfoliative. This serious condition is most frequently the result of drug therapy and may involve not only the skin but also mucous membranes. Arsenic preparations (**49—96.** *Arsphenamine*) are notorious offenders; severe cases have been reported following prolonged phenylbutazone (Butazolidin) therapy (**49—593**).

TREATMENT
1. Discontinuance of the offending drug.
2. Sedation as required.

3. Control of intense pruritis by cold compresses. Trimeprazine tartrate (Temaril), 2.5 mg. orally every 4 to 6 hours, may give subjective relief, although it has no effect on the underlying cause.

4. Oral and/or topical steroids, preferably under the direction of a dermatologist.

54−7. DRUG REACTIONS

Practically every drug in therapeutic use can cause acute edema, angioedema, pruritus and urticaria in sensitive individuals, sometimes severe enough to require emergency care. See **21.** *Allergic Reactions* and **49.** *Poisoning, Acute.*

54−8. ECZEMA

Acute itching, weeping areas occasionally bring sufferers for emergency care; more commonly, however, acute secondary infection superimposed on chronic eczematous areas due to circulatory stasis requires bed rest, elevation and antibiotic therapy.

54−9. HIVES See **54−17.** *Urticaria*

54−10. PARESTHESIAS

Variations in normal sensation of the skin are disturbing and, fortunately, often result in an emergency visit early enough in a cerebrovascular or other potentially serious condition so that neurologic and medical evaluation can be done and preventive therapy begun.

54−11. POISON OAK, IVY AND SUMACH (See also **54−16.** *Urushiols*)

The skin lesions caused by these plants are caused by a fixed non-volatile oil, toxicodendrol, and, contrary to general belief, are not contagious and do not spread.

TREATMENT

1. Washing of exposed parts with nonmedicated soap and hot water as soon as possible after exposure. Sponging with a fat solvent such as equal parts of ether and acetone may be helpful.

2. Local application of soothing lotions or of sodium bicarbonate

paste. Preparations containing phenol (carbolic acid) should not be used.

3. Administration of sedatives and analgesics to control itching and burning.

4. Hospitalization if there is generalized skin involvement, especially of the face or genitals, if secondary infection is present, or if the pain, itching and burning are severe and intractable.

5. Administration of cortisone by mouth in full doses for 2 days, then gradually decreasing doses for 5 days. Poison oak or ivy antigens should not be administered during the acute state. Their use may result in serious aggravation or complications.

54—12. PRURITUS ANI

Itching in and around the anus and rectum may be so persistent and severe that it is practically unbearable. Persons suffering from this condition may scratch so forcibly that they tear off strips of skin, subcutaneous tissue and mucous membrane with their fingernails. Antipruritic medications may give some relief; those most commonly used are as follows:

1. Ergotamine tartrate, 0.5 mg. subcutaneously.

2. Thiamine chloride, 50 to 100 mg. subcutaneously.

3. Epinephrine hydrochloride (Adrenalin), 0.5 to 1 ml. of 1:1000 solution subcutaneously.

4. Tripelennamine hydrochloride (Pyribenzamine), 50 to 100 mg. by mouth 3 times a day.

5. Trimeprazine tartrate (Temaril), 2.5 mg. by mouth every 4 to 6 hours.

COMMON CAUSES OF PRURITUS ANI ARE:

Fissure-in-Ano. See **37—6.**

Food Allergy
TREATMENT

1. Give sedatives and antihistaminics by mouth.

2. Treat secondary infection from scratching by sitz baths and application of bacitracin (Parentracin) ointment.

3. For local application prescribe 1 of the following:

Dibucaine hydrochloride (Nupercaine) ointment (1%).
Fluorohydrocortisone acetate (Florinef) cream (0.25).
Pramoxine hydrochloride (Tronothane) cream (1%).
Tripelennamine hydrochloride (Pyribenzamine) cream (1%).

4. Arrange for further medical care, preferably by an allergist.

Fungous Infection

TREATMENT

1. Prescribe sedatives by mouth.

2. Treat secondary infection from scratching by hot sitz baths and bacitracin (Parentracin) ointment.

3. Give symptomatic relief, if possible, by local application of:

Dibucaine hydrochloride (Nupercaine) ointment (1%).
Fluorohydrocortisone acetate (Florinef) ointment (0.2%).
Pramoxine hydrochloride (Tronothane) cream (1%).
Resorcinol lotion.
Whitfield's ointment.

Hemorrhoids. See 37—6.

Medications

The wide use of antibiotics, especially the tetracyclines, has resulted in a very stubborn type of pruritus ani resulting from suppression of the normal intestinal organisms.

TREATMENT

1. Discontinuance of the offending medication.

2. Local application of dibucaine hydrochloride (Nupercaine) ointment (1%).

3. Prescription of vitamin B complex in large doses, orally or parenterally.

4. Inclusion of buttermilk and/or cottage cheese in the daily diet.

5. Assurance of the patient that the condition will clear completely with time.

Pinworms (Oxyuriasis) (37—20) are frequently the cause of anal itching in children; occasionally in adults.

TREATMENT

1. Pyrivinium pamoate (Povan) orally, 5 mg. per kilogram of body weight, should be given to the patient and all members of the family or other close contacts. Tablets should be swallowed whole to avoid staining the teeth.

2. Personal care to prevent contamination and reinfection through hands, fingernails, etc.

3. Sanitary measures.

Boil all bed linen, underclothes, washcloths and towels daily.

Scrub toilet seats daily.

Sterilize metallic objects used by the patient by baking in a hot oven for at least 10 minutes.

54−13. PRURITUS VULVAE See 39−11

The causes and treatment are the same as outlined in **54−12.**
Pruritus Ani.

54−14. STINGS See 56

54−15. SUNBURN See 25−28

For systemic effects, see **57−8.** *Sunstroke.*

54−16. URUSHIOL CONTACT DERMATITIS (See also 54−11.
   Poison Oak, Ivy and Sumach)

Many plants of the urushiol category (anacardiaceae family) may
cause acute contact dermatitis.

COMMON NAMES	DISTRIBUTION	MODES OF CONTACT
Cashew Nut Shell Oil (**49−176**) (Cashew oil).	Africa, Central America, East Indies, India.	Electrical insulation, glues, printer's ink, resins, swizzle sticks.
Ginkgo Tree (Maidenhair Tree). Indian Marking Nut (Washerman Itch).	China, Europe, Japan, U.S.A. (southeast), India, Malaya.	Cosmetics, lacquerware, soaps. Laundry marking ink.
Lacquer Tree (Japanese Lacquer Tree).	China, India, Japan.	Bar rails, bracelets, ornamental wooden novelties.
Mango ("Apple of the Tropics," "King of Fruits").	California, Central America, Florida, Hawaii, Mediterranean.	Direct−plant or fruit to skin; in-direct−particles in air, contaminated insects or animals.
Oakleaf Poison Ivy (**54−11**) (Eastern Oakleaf, Poison Ivy).	U.S.A. (southeast).	Same as Mango (above).
Poison Ivy (**54−11**) (Poison Creeper, Markweed).	Canada, China, Mexico, Taiwan, U.S.A. (except southwest).	Same as Mango (above).

COMMON NAMES	DISTRIBUTION	MODES OF CONTACT
Poison Oak (**54—11**) (Western Poison Oak, Yeara).	U.S.A. (Pacific coast).	Same as Mango (above).
Poison Sumach (**54—11**) (Poison Dogwood, Poison Elder, Swamp Sumach).	U.S.A. (southeast).	Same as Mango (above).
Rengas Tree (Black Varnish Tree).	Malaya.	Furniture, wood carvings.

For treatment, see **54—11**. *Poison Oak, Ivy and Sumach.* Antihistaminics are of no value in treatment.

54—17. URTICARIA (See also 21. *Allergic Reactions*)

Characterized by the appearance on the skin and mucous membranes of pruritic reddened or whitish swellings of various sizes and shapes called wheals, acute urticaria may be either exogenous or endogeneous, usually the former.

EXOGENOUS CAUSES

Animal dander.
Animal serums used in injections.
Commercial chemicals such as DDT (**49—243**).
Drugs.

Feathers.
Food—especially berries, chocolate, fish, nuts and spices.
Perfumes and cosmetics.
Physical factors—heat, cold, light.

ENDOGENOUS CAUSES

Microorganisms.
Parasites.
Products of altered metabolism.

Psychogenic stimuli.
Secretion from endocrine glands.

TREATMENT

1. Epinephrine hydrochloride (Adrenalin), 0.5 to 1.0 ml. of 1:1000 solution intramuscularly, or, in severe cases, intravenously.

2. Immediate tracheostomy (**14—12**) if the wheals involve the mucous membrane of the throat (see **21—2; 48—4**. *Angioedema in Children*).

3. Antihistamines by mouth.

4. Vasoconstrictors such as ephedrine by mouth.

5. Corticosteroid therapy.

6. Hospitalization if response to the measures given above is not satisfactory of if a tracheostomy has been done.

54—18. VARICOSE ECZEMA AND ULCERS See 54—8

54—19. VINCENT'S ANGINA (Ulcerative Stomatitis, Trench Mouth)

This acutely contagious ulcer-forming inflammation of mucous membranes is caused by a fusiform bacillus and a coarsely coiled spirochete, both of which can usually be identified in smears. The gums and mucous membranes of the mouth and throat are commonly involved but the external ear, internal nares, female genitalia and glans penis are occasionally the sites of infection.

SIGNS AND SYMPTOMS. Reddened painful mucosa, later covered with a grayish white adherent membrane which on removal leaves punctate bleeding areas. Laboratory studies may be necessary to differentiate it from diphtheria (**30—4**) and from infectious mononucleosis. General malaise, chills and fever may be present, especially in children. Some adults show no systemic reaction, even in the presence of extensive mucous membrane involvement. There may be pain on swallowing if the oral cavity is involved, and blood-stained oral or mucous membrane secretion if the membrane is disturbed. A leukopenia is usually present.

TREATMENT

1. Isolation and sterilization of all dishes, eating utensils, washcloths, towels.

2. Close attention to oral and other personal hygiene.

3. Removal of crusts and cleansing of sloughs with hydrogen peroxide.

4. Application of sodium perborate paste to the gums or other affected areas.

5. Administration of penicillin, 1.2 million units intramuscularly daily for 4 days. Tetracycline in large doses by mouth should be substituted if the patient gives a history of sensitivity to penicillin.

6. Referral for specialist care if the systemic reaction is severe, or if the condition is extensive or extending. Permanent damage to the gums and mucous membranes may occur without proper and prolonged treatment.

54—20. X-RAY (RADIATION) BURNS See 25—33

55. SOFT TISSUE INJURIES

Soft tissue injuries of varying degrees of severity make up the bulk of cases treated on any emergency service.

55—1. ABDOMINAL INJURIES (See also **19.** *Abdominal Pain*)

Nonpenetrating injuries caused by direct blunt trauma to the abdominal wall are far more common than penetrating or perforating injuries and may be so severe that hemorrhage and shock (**53**) cause death before any treatment can be given, or so slight that no treatment is required. Between these two extremes lies the intermediate field in which accurate diagnosis and prompt and proper treatment can influence the chance of recovery.

The severity of the trauma inflicted on an underlying viscus by a blunt object depends upon the force exerted, the size and shape of the striking object, the location of impact, the ability of the person struck to give way with the blow or to tighten his muscles in preparation for it, and the strength of the abdominal musculature.

NONPENETRATING ABDOMINAL INJURIES IN ORDER OF FREQUENCY

STRUCTURE INVOLVED	PER CENT (*Approximate*)
Spleen	26.0
Kidneys	24.0
Intestines	16.5
Liver	15.5
Abdominal wall	4.5
Retroperitoneal hemorrhage	3.5
Mesentery	3.0
Pancreas	1.5
Diaphragm	1.0
Other	4.5

More than 80% of abdominal injuries from blunt trauma are the result of automobile accidents; industrial accidents (**75**) account for another 10%. The mortality from nonpenetrating abdominal injuries is about three and one-half times that for penetrating injuries, probably owing in great part to the difficulty in making an accurate diagnosis.

For treatment, see under the organ involved.

Absolute indications for laparotomy, no matter what viscus is suspected, are:

1. Pneumoperitoneum demonstrable by x-rays.

2. Abdominal paracentesis which yields blood [must be associated with clinical signs of active bleeding or evidence of contamination from contents of a hollow viscus (stomach contents, bile, feces, urine)].

3. Secondary collapse following recovery from primary posttraumatic shock, with localized evidence of abdominal injury.

Penetrating abdominal injuries

TREATMENT

1. Treatment of shock (**53 – 7**).

2. Application of a sterile dressing to the external wound.

3. Immediate hospitalization for close observation and probable laparotomy.

Perforating abdominal injuries are usually bullet wounds (**55 – 6**) or stab wounds (**55 – 33**).

TREATMENT

1. Treatment of shock (**53 – 7**).

2. Application of sterile dressings to entrance and exit wounds.

3. Hospitalization for definitive care. Any observations which might be of value to law enforcement agencies (powder marks on clothing, powder burns on skin, course of wound tract) should be recorded on the emergency chart.

55 – 2. ABRASIONS (For corneal abrasions, see 35 – 32)

TREATMENT

1. Thorough scrubbing with soap and water for removal of embedded foreign material is essential. If necessary, a narcotic can be given, topical anesthetic applied or procaine or lidocaine (Xylocane) block anesthesia used to control pain during the cleansing process. If removal of all embedded foreign bodies and devitalized tissue from the skin or subcutaneous structures cannot be accomplished under topical or local anesthetic, hospitalization for administration of general anesthesia may be necessary to prevent permanent and disfiguring tattooing.

2. Extensive abrasions should be dressed with petrolatum gauze. As a rule nitrofurazone (Furacin) or bismuth tribromophenate

(Xeroform) gauze should not be used unless definite evidence of infection is present. Collodion dressings should not be used routinely because they are difficult to remove and because they may promote anaerobic growth. Application of compound tincture of benzoin to the surrounding skin followed by sterile gauze and Elastoplast under slight tension makes a satisfactory dressing.

3. All patients who have sustained extensive pavement or gravel burns should receive tetanus immune-globulin (TIG) or tetanus toxoid (**16**).

55 – 3. BITES See **24**

55 – 4. BLADDER INJURIES See **38 – 1**

55 – 5. BRAIN INJURIES See **41.** *Head Injuries;* **48 – 9.** *Brain Injuries in Children*

55 – 6. BULLET WOUNDS

Whenever possible, the exact site of entry, the course of the bullet and the point of exit should be described in detail in the patient's record. The presence or absence of powder burns or marks on the skin and clothing should be noted. If the bullet is recovered, it should be turned over to the proper law enforcement officers. For treatment, see **55 – 1.** *Abdominal Injuries,* and the discussion of the body area involved. All cases require protection against tetanus (**16**).

55 – 7. BURNS See **25; 48 – 14.** *Burns in Children*

55 – 8. CARDIAC INJURIES See **26 – 22.** *Hemopericardium with Tamponade*

55 – 9. CHEST INJURIES See **28**

55 – 10. CONTUSIONS (See also **55 – 1.** *Abdominal Injuries*)

Mild contusions. Ordinary contusions (provided fracture has been ruled out) need only symptomatic treatment to reduce pain and swelling. The patient should be instructed to limit use of an extremity, given crutches or a splint if indicated and instructed regarding application of hot or cold compresses at home. As a general rule, cold is more effective for the first day; after 24 hours, hot compresses or contrast baths may be used. Marked relief, especially of throbbing fingers and toes, may be obtained by gentle inunction of the injured part for 10 to 15 minutes every 3 or 4 hours with a 2.5% ointment of hydrocortisone acetate in neomycin sulfate (Neo-Cortef).

Severe contusions, especially of the extremities, may require elevation and snug elastic bandages to prevent and control intramuscular bleeding. Hyaluronidase, 300 TRU in 1 ml. of normal saline solution, injected directly into a hematoma may be of benefit.

55 – 11. CRUSH INJURIES

Crushing injuries to the chest may cause serious damage without external evidence of trauma.

1. Alveolar rupture and hemorrhage, especially in children (**28 – 3**).

2. Cardiac contusion with or without severe symptoms such as myocardial infarction (**26 – 12**), hemopericardium (**26 – 22**) and cardiac arrest (**26 – 7**). Milder contusions may result in ECG changes (ST segment variations and T-wave flattening) which persist for lengthy periods.

3. Diaphragmatic damage (**28 – 6**).

4. Fractured ribs and sternum (**28 – 2**).

5. Mediastinal hemorrhage (**28 – 1**).

6. Tension pneumothorax (**28 – 5**).

Crushing injuries to the extremities may cause severe damage not apparent on initial examination. X-rays are indicated in all cases. See also **48 – 65.** *Wringer Injuries.*

Crushing injuries to the low back or flanks may cause severe kidney damage (**38 – 2**). Hematuria, gross or microscopic, is present in 75 to 80% of cases.

55 – 12. DIAPHRAGMATIC INJURIES See 28 – 6

55 – 13. DUODENAL RUPTURE

Severe blunt nonpenetrating trauma to the upper abdomen or back may cause retroperitoneal rupture of the duodenum. X-ray studies are the only preoperative method of diagnosis. Suspicion of duodenal rupture requires immediate exploratory laparotomy.

55–14. EAR INJURIES See 32–4

55–15. EYE INJURIES See 35–29 to 35–37

55–16. FOREIGN BODIES See 38–6

For removal of fishhooks in soft tissue, see Figure 30 (page 612).

55–17. GALLBLADDER AND BILE DUCT INJURIES

Because of its sheltered location, the gallbladder and its duct system are rarely injured by blunt trauma unless there is also extensive liver damage (**55–21**). It may, however, be injured by penetration or perforation. Suspicion or evidence (usually by abdominal paracentesis) of gallbladder or duct damage calls for immediate exploratory laparotomy.

55–18. GREASE GUN INJURIES

Severe injuries, usually to the hand, may result from injection through a small puncture wound in the skin of lubricating grease under as much as 600 lbs. per square inch pressure. Following the tracts of least resistance (fascial compartments, intermuscular septa, tendon and nerve sheaths), the grease may dissect for considerable distance in the brief moment of contact. Even with extensive damage, immediate pain is unusual but becomes agonizing within a few hours due to tissue ischemia. Since the grease is not radiopaque, x-rays are of little, if any, value in determining the extent of damage.

TREATMENT
1. Anodynes or narcotics for control of pain.
2. Release of tension and removal of the contaminant as an urgent emergency procedure. Wide surgical exposure with painstaking debridement, usually under regional nerve block, must be done to minimize permanent disability.
3. Intensive and prolonged antibiotic therapy.

55–19. INTESTINAL INJURIES

Rupture or perforation of any portion of the bowel calls for immediate surgical exploration and repair. A history of possible

OFF THE HOOK . . . with thread

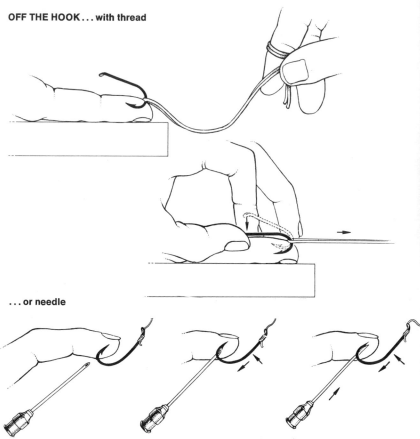

. . . or needle

Figure 30. A, B, To fish for fishhooks, you'll need about four feet of line. Loop the line around the curve of the hook and wrap the ends several times around your forefinger. Then take the hook's eye and shank in the thumb and forefinger of your free hand and push down, disengaging the barb. Finally, align the string with the shank's long axis — and yank. C. To remove a hook without using a string, all you need is an 18-gauge disposable needle. Introduce the needle along the barbed side of the hook, with the bevel toward the inside of the hook curve. D, Apply slight pressure upward on the hook shank, so that the barb is disengaged from the flesh. Then push the needle gently upward and rotate until the lumen locks firmly over the barb. E, Keeping the needle locked over the barb with gentle upward pressure, rotate the hook shank slightly upward and the hook curve downward until needle and hook are removed through the original wound. (From Longmire, W. T., Jr., Emergency Medicine, Vol. 3, No. 7, p. 98, July, 1971.)

trauma, with some immediate severe abdominal pain followed by a brief pain-free period, is typical. Demonstration by x-ray of free air under the diaphragm is conclusive, but absence of air does not rule out perforation.

55 – 20. LACERATIONS

Before treatment of any laceration the presence or absence of damage to nerves, tendons and other deep structures should be determined by tests of function and recorded in the emergency record.

PREPARATION FOR REPAIR

1. Cleanse the area around the wound for at least 2 inches, clipping any hair which may protrude into the wound.

2. Give preliminary sedatives, anodynes or narcotics as needed to control pain, apprehension and restlessness except in infants and small children (**4**).

3. Cover the wound with sterile gauze; cleanse the surrounding skin with a mild detergent such as pHisoHex and with soap and water. Irrigate thoroughly with saline.

4. Remove the gauze and scrub the laceration with bland non-medicated soap and water, loosening and removing foreign bodies; follow with copious irrigations with sterile saline, using a bulb syringe or gravity apparatus. Remove any excess saline with sterile gauze; then paint with tincture of quaternary ammonium chloride (QAC), tincture of thimerosal (Merthiolate) or tincture of iodine (1/4 strength).

5. If tetanus-immune globulin (TIG) or toxoid is indicated (**16**), it may be given before the patient is taken to surgery. In apprehensive, excited or undisciplined children, all injections except local anesthesia should be postponed until after surgical repair.

6. If cleansing the wound is extremely painful, it should be performed under 1 or 2% procaine or lidocaine (Xylocaine) infiltration or block anesthesia.

PRINCIPLES OF TREATMENT

1. **Repair** (control of hemorrhage, debridement, primary closure) is safe within 6 hours of injury. This time may be extended at the discretion of the physician if the wound is not grossly contaminated or obviously infected. In certain instances delay in repair may be necessary while a valid operative permit is being obtained (**69 – 15**).

2. **Small lacerations** may be closed by adhesive butterflies or Steri-Strips and pressure dressings applied after irrigation and ruling out of the presence of foreign bodies. X-rays (**18**) should be taken if the history suggests the possibility of radiopaque foreign material.

3. **Sterile operating room technique** is essential in all cases. All persons in the operating room, *including the patient* (unless a face screen is in use or the laceration involves the face or head), should be capped and masked. The surgeon must wear a cap, mask and sterile gloves, and the surgery nurse's hair should be confined. A sterile operating gown should be worn if a lengthy or extensive repair is necessary.

4. **A tourniquet** should be used to insure a bloodless field whenever the location of the laceration will allow. Strips of rubber dam or heavy rubber bands clamped with a hemostat make excellent finger tourniquets. A blood pressure cuff inflated to 20 mm. of mercury above systolic pressure works very well on the arm or leg. In lengthy procedures the tourniquet should be relaxed for a few seconds every hour. At the conclusion of the procedure, the patient should be examined carefully for loss of temperature and light touch perception indicative of blocking of conduction through the peripheral nerves by the localized pressure of the tourniquet ("tourniquet paralysis").

5. **Anesthesia**

Infiltration or local block with 1 or 2% procaine or lidocaine (Xylocaine) is the method of choice for emergency use.

If another physician or an anesthetist is present, short light inhalation anesthesia [nitrous oxide, ether, vinyl ether (Vinethene) or ethyl chloride] or intravenous Pentothal Sodium may be given (not in children). Because of the danger of aspiration of stomach contents and subsequent development of pneumonia, general anesthesia should never be started until at least 6 hours after the last meal. If a general anesthetic is used, *the patient must be watched at all times until fully conscious.*

Brachial plexus blocks, sciatic blocks and spinal anesthesia should not be attempted as emergency procedures unless under the direction of an anesthesiologist or physician experienced in their use.

Nerve blocks at the wrist or above the ankle are satisfactory if the physician is familiar with the technique.

Anesthesia (preferably local regional block) should be used while repairing lacerations requiring suturing unless:

The patient is comatose or in such condition that he does not feel pain.

Closure of the laceration can be obtained with 1 or 2 sutures.

Acute sensitivity to local anesthetic agents (**49 — 72**) is present.

The patient requests repair without anesthesia on religious or other grounds.

Cooperation of the patient cannot be obtained.

6. **Examination of the wound under anesthesia for:**

Extent and severity.

Foreign bodies, superficial or embedded.

Severence of, or damage to, muscles, tendons, blood vessels or nerves.

Fractures and dislocations.

Hematomas.

Any openings into joints, tendon sheaths or fascial spaces through which contamination might be introduced. If examination under anesthesia shows such severe or extensive damage that emergency repair would be difficult or lengthy, a sterile bandage should be applied, the patient given a sedative and hospitalization for repair arranged. The physician to whom the patient is being sent should whenever possible be contacted by telephone and full details given. A summary of findings and treatment should be sent with the patient.

7. **Debridement.** The object of debridement is to convert a wound lined with damaged and potentially infected tissue into a surgically clean wound. Therefore, starting with the skin and working toward the depths of the wound, all damaged tissues should be removed by sharp dissection, sparing nerves, tendons, blood vessels, joint capsules and articular surfaces. Hematomas should be evacuated and bleeding vessels clamped and tied, using No. 000 plain catgut, fine silk or No. 40 or 50 cotton. Buried sutures should be kept to a minimum. No disinfectants, antiseptics or medications of any type should be painted, sprinkled, sprayed or insufflated into the wound.

Debridement should be limited in certain areas. The most important of these are:

The eyelids. Lacerations in this region should be thoroughly cleansed and closed with fine Dermalin (Figure 19) to prevent ectropion (**35 — 8**) or entropion (**35 — 11**).

The hand and fingers (**40 — 5**).

The face. Adequate closure should be obtained with the expectation of possible revision by a plastic surgeon at a later date.

The lips, especially in the region of the vermilion line.

The penis (38 — 4).

In these areas little if any tissue should be removed unless gross contamination or maceration is present. Skin edges should be approximated without tension and sutured loosely without inverting or overlapping (Figure 31).

8. **Closure**

Obliteration of dead spaces by mattress sutures of No. 000 plain catgut, fine silk or No. 40 or 50 cotton. Buried sutures should be kept to a minimum.

Careful approximation of skin edges without undue tension, using interrupted sutures of No. 40 or 50 cotton or fine Dermalin (Figure 31). All external knots should be placed away from the approximated skin edges.

Essential structures (tendons, nerves, blood vessels, joints and bone) *must* be covered. In some instances a pedicle graft (with the base proximally) can be swung from the immediate neighborhood and the resultant defect covered with a split graft.

Completely severed soft tissue, if small and not macerated (fingertips, portions of the nose and ear) may be cleansed and sutured in place as full thickness grafts.

9. **Dressings**

A petrolatum gauze or a Telfa nonadherent dressing should be applied over the sutures, covered with sterile gauze and the surrounding area painted with compound tincture of benzoin. When this has dried enough to be "tacky," an elastic pressure bandage should be applied. On any portion of an extremity, care should be taken to allow for postoperative edema. Tight nonelastic circular bandages completely around an extremity should never be applied.

Nitrofurazone (Furacin) and bismuth tribromophenate (Xeroform) gauze should not be used for the original dressing unless evidence of gross infection has been noted.

Collodion dressings should not be applied directly over the wound, but collodion is useful for anchoring the edges of dressings, especially on the face.

10. **Immobilization.** In some areas of the body, motion may interfere with healing. Limited activity, splinting, use of a sling or Velpeau bandage, plaster of Paris immobilization or crutches may be indicated. Elevation of an injured extremity will help to control swelling, throbbing and pain.

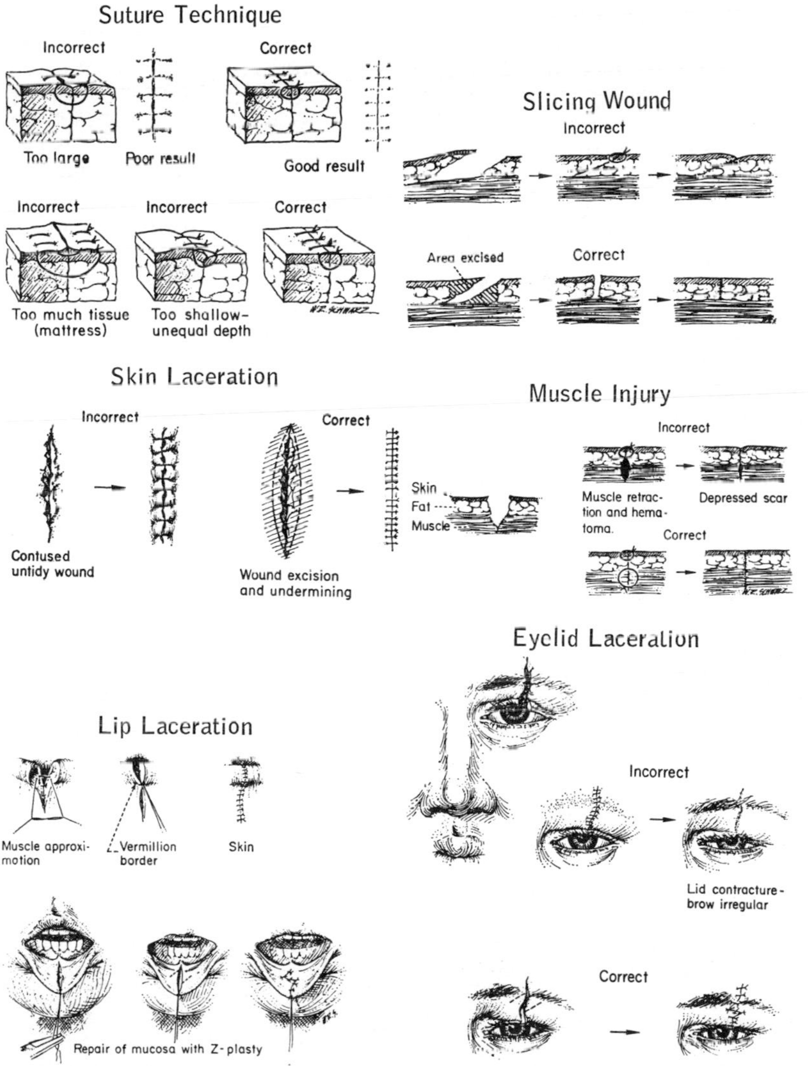

Figure 31. Repair of lacerations. (Modified from Curtin, J. W.: Illinois Med. J., Vol. 129, No. 6, 1966.)

11. Postoperative care

Specific instructions must be given to the patient regarding recheck examination (see **64 – 2** for suggested recheck examination form). All grossly contaminated or severely crushed or contused injuries must be rechecked in 24 hours; so should injuries in which debridement only, without closure, has been done. All finger, hand, wrist or elbow injuries should be seen by a physician on the day following surgical repair. Minor lacerations should be inspected in not more than 3 days. Tetanus immune globulin (TIG) or tetanus toxoid should be given routinely (**16**) unless the condition is minimal or of a type which, in the opinion of the attending physician, does not require this protection. Penicillin or broad spectrum antibiotics may be indicated if gross contamination or infection has been noted or if repair has been delayed more than 6 hours after injury. Sedatives and anodynes to last only until the next scheduled recheck visit should be prescribed or furnished.

55 – 21.   LIVER INJURIES

If severe blunt trauma to the right lower ribs or abdomen (usually the result of vehicular or industrial injury) without external evidence of injury has occurred and severe shock (**53**) not explainable by other injuries is present, damage to the liver should always be suspected. Usually, however, hepatic damage is associated with other injuries (fractured ribs, fractured pelvis, ruptured diaphragm, mediastinal hemorrhage) and is signaled by upper abdominal pain, tenderness and spasm. Right shoulder pain may be present, often only on deep inspiration.

TREATMENT

Treatment of shock (**53 – 7**) before and during transfer for laparotomy.

55 – 22.   NASAL INJURIES See **45 – 5**; **55 – 20**. *Lacerations*

55 – 23.   NERVE INJURIES See **40 – 6**. *Nerve Injuries in the Hand;* **46 – 8**

55 – 24.   PAINT SPRAY GUN INJURIES

High pressure compressed air paint spray guns used in industry may cause extensive damage which often is overlooked because of the lack of initial pain and the minute wound of entrance. Fortunately, the extent of damage usually can be accurately determined by x-ray examination after removal of all paint from the surface of the injured part.

For treatment, see **55 — 18.** *Grease Gun Injuries.*

55 — 25. PANCREATIC INJURIES

Blunt trauma to the abdomen, usually from automobile accidents, and usually associated with other serious injuries, is a common cause of traumatic pancreatitis. Injury limited to the gland is usually the result of bullet or stab wounds. Serum amylase levels are of value in diagnosis.

TREATMENT

Wide exposure at laparotomy, with opening of the lesser omental sac to allow inspection of the complete gland for ecchymoses, edema, fat necrosis, tears of the capsule and parenchyma and retroperitoneal hematomas, and for surgical procedures as indicated.

55 — 26. PENETRATING WOUNDS (See also **26 — 22.** *Hemopericardium;* **28 — 9** to **28 — 12.** *Penetrating Chest Wounds;* **35 — 29** to **35 — 37.** *Eye Injuries;* **55 — 28.** *Puncture Wounds*)

This general category covers all types of injuries, usually but not necessarily caused by small pointed objects, in which there is a wound of entrance but none of exit. Diagnosis is usually apparent and treatment [exploration, debridement, closure, protection against tetanus (**16**)] well-standardized; therefore, the mortality is less than in injuries resulting from blunt force without external evidence of injury.

55 — 27. PERFORATING WOUNDS

Through-and-through wounds with unmistakable skin defects at the points of entrance and exit are usually caused by bullets. The mortality is less than for contusions caused by blunt force or for penetrating wounds because surgical exploration without delay is more frequently and promptly carried out.

55−28. PUNCTURE WOUNDS (See also 55−26; 27)

Conservative Treatment.

Superficial cleansing, bandaging, protection against tetanus by administration of tetanus-immune globulin (TIG) or toxoid (**16**) and prophylactic antibiotics if indicated are all that is required in the majority of cases. Large, deep or grossly contaminated puncture wounds should be handled in the same manner as lacerations (**55−20**).

Puncture wounds requiring special treatment.

1. *Bites.* See **24.**
2. *Chest injuries involving the pericardium* (**26−22**) *or pleura* (**28−9**).
3. *Eye injuries.* See **35−29** through **35−37.**
4. *Foreign bodies.* See **36.**
5. *Grease gun injuries.* See **55−18.**
6. *Gunshot wounds.* Treatment varies with the caliber and type of bullet (hard- or soft-nosed), and the tract of the projectile into or through the body. Protection against tetanus (**16**) is always indicated. Removal of the bullet is often contraindicated.
7. *Hemorrhaging puncture wounds* usually can be controlled by pressure or, if on an extremity, by a properly applied tourniquet. Extension of the wound under local or general anesthesia with evacuation of hematomas and identification and ligation of the bleeding vessels may be necessary.
8. *Paint spray gun injuries.* See **55−24.**
9. *Peritoneal or visceral puncture.* If perforation or penetration of the peritoneum or of solid or hollow abdominal viscus is known or suspected, immediate hospitalization is mandatory. Pretransportation treatment of shock (**53−7**) is essential.
10. *Stab wounds.* See **55−33.**
11. *Stings.* See **56.**
12. *Stud and staple gun injuries.* See **55−36.**
13. *Tear gas gun injuries.* See **55−37.**

55−29. SCALP WOUNDS See 41−21

55−30. SPINAL CORD INJURIES See 44−11; 46−11

55−31. SPLENIC INJURIES

Injuries to the spleen represent the largest group (approximately 26%) in most statistical series concerned with the effects of blunt trauma. Automobile injuries represent the largest part of this group. Rupture of the spleen is often associated with rib fractures and other chest and abdominal traumatic pathology.

SIGNS AND SYMPTOMS. Upper abdominal pain which may vary markedly in intensity and tenderness and muscle spasm or guarding in the left upper quadrant, sometimes extending below the umbilicus. Left shoulder pain, elicited by pressure over the left upper quadrant and by deep inspiration, is present in about 50% of cases. Bleeding may be temporarily tamponaded by perisplenic hematomas, with irreversible circulatory collapse (**53.** *Shock*) when capsular rupture occurs – sometimes several weeks after injury.

TREATMENT
Splenectomy as soon as the condition is recognized. If the diagnosis is in doubt, or conservative measures are used for any reason, cross-matched blood should be available for immediate use.

55 – 32. SPRAINS AND STRAINS See **44 – 60.** *Sprains;* **63 – 12.** *Sprains and Strains in Wartime*

55 – 33. STAB WOUNDS (See also **55 – 26.** *Penetrating Wounds*)

The treatment of stab wounds depends upon the injury tract, the structures involved and the length of time since injury. Close observation for several hours, followed by surgical exploration, may be required to determine the true extent of injury, particularly if the weapon used has produced a very small entrance wound (hatpins, ice picks, thin knife blades).

55 – 34. STINGS See **56**

55 – 35. STOMACH INJURIES

Penetrating wounds of the stomach are usually associated with other abdominal damage and require immediate surgical repair. Blunt trauma may cause rupture of the stomach wall, particularly if scarring from old ulceration is present.

55 – 36. STUD AND STAPLE GUN INJURIES

A modern stud driving device used in the construction industry utilizes small explosive powder charges for propulsion of rivets and studs. As a result, it offers 2 sets of hazards:

55−37. TEAR GAS PEN AND GUN INJURIES

1. The bullet-like effect of the stud or rivet. For treatment, see **55−6.** *Bullet Wounds;* **55−26.** *Penetrating Wounds.*

2. The gunpowder danger from the charge. Any break in the skin is an indication for protection against tetanus (**16**).

Large industrial staple guns, spring propelled, may cause severe soft tissue and bone injuries. For treatment, see **55−20.** *Lacerations;* **55−26.** *Penetrating Wounds.*

55−37. TEAR GAS PEN AND GUN INJURIES

The increasing use of small tear gas pistols for self-defense has resulted in permanent impairment of sensation and mobility when the gun has exploded in the user's hand−apparently from imbedding of particles of the lacrimating agent, alpha-chloroacetophenone, in nerve and muscle tissue. Serious eye injuries have been reported.

TREATMENT (except for eye injuries)

1. Thorough debridement with removal of imbedded foreign bodies, followed by thorough irrigation.

2. Application of a sterile dressing, leaving the wound open.

3. Reference for follow-up care in 1 or 2 days. Reexploration of the wound in 3 to 4 weeks may be necessary.

TREATMENT OF EYE INJURIES

See **49−192.** *Chloroacetophenone (Mace).*

55−38. TRACHEOBRONCHIAL INJURIES

Rupture of the trachea or of the bronchi can be caused by direct trauma, such as steering wheel impact, by heavy glancing blows to the chest, and by falls. Increased intraluminal pressure with a closed glottis may be a factor. Tremendous cervical and facial emphysema ("puffball like") may be rapidly fatal. Tension pneumothorax (**28−5**) may require treatment. In some cases, immediate tracheostomy (**14−12**) followed by thoracotomy may have a successful outcome; in all cases, immediate hospitalization for close observation and possible emergency surgical intervention is indicated.

55−39. WHIPLASH INJURIES See **44−58.** *Neck Injuries;* **46−11**

55−40. WINDSHIELD GLASS INJURIES

Prior to 1966 plate glass was used for windshields and side windows of automobiles. Impact caused shattering into large

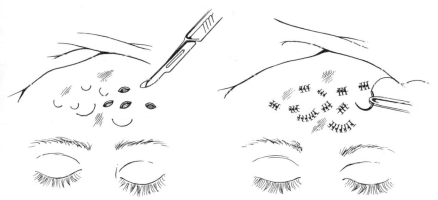

Figure 32. Striking the head against a shatterproof windshield causes many small lacerations and avulsion flaps and injuries. Whenever possible, the smaller injuries should be excised elliptically to convert irregular scars to linear ones and minimize scarring. (From Emergency Medicine, Vol. 4, No. 5, p. 160, May, 1972.)

knife-like fragments with sharp cutting edges which could—and did—inflict severe injuries, especially lacerations of the face and neck.

In 1966, safety regulations made the use of shatter-proof glass mandatory. Since on impact this type of glass breaks into many small shards, facial injuries it causes usually consist of small puncture wounds and elliptical lacerations (Figure 32).

TREATMENT

1. Thorough irrigation and inspection and palpation for possible foreign bodies.

2. Debridement with conversion of elliptical lacerations into straight lines, corresponding whenever possible to the normal skin lines of the face.

3. Careful approximation of subcutaneous tissues with 4–0 plain catgut followed by closure of skin edges with 6–0 nylon (Figure 32), with removal of the stiches in about 5 days. Antibiotic therapy based on cultures should be begun at once if there is any evidence of infection.

4. Protection against tetanus (**16**).

Revision of disfiguring scars should be postponed until at least 6 months after injury to allow the scars to mature.

55 — 41. WRINGER INJURIES See **48 — 65**

55 — 42. ZIPPER INJURIES See **48 — 66**

56. STINGS

See also **24.** *Bites;* **61.** *Venoms.*

Approximately 50% of deaths from venomous stings are due to Hymenoptera (bees, fire ants, hornets, wasps, yellow jackets); 80% of these deaths occur within 2 hours of the sting.

56 — 1. BEE STINGS

These are common and may be dangerous. Extremely great sensitivity (natural or acquired) to hymenoptera venom may be encountered and constitutes an acute emergency. These patients present the clinical picture of severe anaphylactic shock and require immediate energetic handling as a lifesaving measure (**21**). Epinephrine hydrochloride (Adrenalin), 0.5 to 1 ml. of 1:1000 solution, should be given subcutaneously or slowly intravenously followed by therapy for shock (**53 — 7**) and hospitalization.

Persons known to be sensitive to Hymenoptera venom, especially those over 40 years of age with known heart disease, should have available an emergency kit for immediate treatment of insect bites and stings. This kit should contain the following:

1. Tweezers for removal of the stinger. These should be used, however, only if removal of the stinger cannot be accomplished by gentle teasing with a fingernail — compression with tweezers may cause additional injection of venom.

2. A tourniquet.

3. A disposable hypodermic syringe (with needle) containing 1 ml. of 1:1000 epinephrine hydrochloride (Adrenalin).

4. An aerosol inhalator containing epinephrine hydrochloride (Adrenalin) or isoproterenol solution.

5. Antihistamine tablets (oral).

SYMPTOMATIC LOCAL TREATMENT

Cold compresses, application of tincture of iodine, ammonia or baking soda, or magnesium sulfate (Epsom salts) soaks will usually give relief. The "stinger" (from the honeybee only) should be identified and removed if present.

Desensitization to Hymenoptera venom sometimes is practical but should always be supervised by an allergist. A polyvalent extract against the bumblebee, fire ant, honeybee, hornet, wasp and yellow jacket is available commercially.

56 — 2. CADDIS FLY STINGS

Acute allergic reactions have been reported, especially in the Great Lakes area of the United States, from stings from this fly. For treatment, see **21.** *Allergic Reactions;* **56 — 1.** *Bee Stings.*

56 — 3. CATERPILLAR STINGS

Among the larvae which can cause severe reactions from venom carried in the hair are the brown-tail moth, buck moth, flannel moth, Io moth, range caterpillar, saddleback caterpillar, tussock moth and white moth. The venom is a polypeptide which causes local edema, swelling and acute pain. Vomiting, convulsions and shock may occur in children.

TREATMENT

1. Thorough washing of the site of the sting, followed by application of ammonia, baking soda or tincture of iodine.

2. Control of pain by aspirin, codeine or morphine. Intravenous injection of 10 ml. of 10% calcium gluconate may be effective.

3. Supportive and symptomatic care (**49 — 4**).

56 — 4. CORAL STINGS

The toxicity of venom from coral varies with the variety but may cause acute allergic reactions (**21**).

56 — 5. FIRE ANT STINGS (See also **61.** *Venoms*)

Although these ants also bite, toxic effects are caused by venom injected through a spine on the ant's abdomen. Since the ants move and sting quickly (each ant 3 or 4 times), 3000 to 5000 stings have been reported on one person following disturbance of an ant mound.

SIGNS AND SYMPTOMS. Immediate development of an umbilicated pustule surrounded by a reddened acutely painful halo, with severe, burning, stinging pain at and for some distance around the site of the sting. The temperature is usually elevated. Dyspnea, cyanosis and acute respiratory depression may develop rapidly.

TREATMENT

1. Artificial respiration (**11 — 1**) in severe cases.
2. Treatment of allergic reactions (**21 — 1**).
3. Protective sterile dressing over pustular areas.
4. Control of pain. Narcotics may be necessary for 12 to 24 hours.

PROGNOSIS. Although fatalities from respiratory collapse have been reported from multiple stings, complete recovery in 3 to 5 days usually occurs.

56 — 6. HYMENOPTERA STINGS See **56 — 1**. *Bee Stings;* **61**. *Venoms*

56 — 7. LARVAL STINGS See **56 — 3**. *Caterpillar Stings*

56 — 8. MARINE ANIMAL STINGS See **56 — 4**. *Coral Stings;* **56 — 9**. *Portuguese Man-of-War Stings;* **56 — 12**. *Sea Anemone Stings;* **56 — 13**. *Stingray;* **56 — 14**. *Tropical Jellyfish Stings;* **61**. *Venoms*

56 — 9. PORTUGESE MAN-OF-WAR STINGS

Stings from these marine creatures are relatively common in persons participating in water sports. Severe pain, local swelling and anaphylactic shock (**21**) may occur. Aggravation of preexistent heart disease in elderly persons may be fatal.

TREATMENT

1. Remove any adherent tentacles at once, with the hands wrapped in cloth or protected by gloves.
2. Treat shock (**53 — 7**).
3. Wash with water followed by dilute ammonia; coat with sodium bicarbonate paste.
4. Give tripelennamine hydrochloride (Pyribenzamine), 50 mg. orally every 4 hours.
5. Inject 10 ml. of 10% calcium gluconate intravenously.

56 — 10. PUSS CATERPILLAR STINGS (See also **56 — 3**. *Caterpillar Stings*)

Of the more than 50 species of larvae which may produce toxic effects from venoms contained in the hair, the larval stage of the flannel moth is the most common. It is known in different localities by various names – el perrito ("little dog"), Italian asp, possum bug, puss caterpillar, wooly slug and wooly worm. In appearance it is a blob of neatly combed brown fur, shaped like a Brazil nut and 20 to 30 mm. long. The venom is contained in hidden clusters of specialized hair on the back; it is not found in all hairs.

For treatment, see **56 – 3.** *Caterpillar Stings.*

56 – 11. SCORPION STINGS (See also 61. *Venoms*)

The seriousness of toxic reactions to scorpion stings varies with the species, with the site of the sting and with the age of the victim. Infants and small children account for most of reported fatalities.

European scorpion – relatively nontoxic.

North American scorpion – moderately toxic, especially to infants and small children.

South American scorpion – extremely toxic.

In all age groups, the victim develops precordial pain, vertigo, vomiting, cephalgia, visual disturbances, impairment of speech, exquisite local pain, circulatory and respiratory depression, fibrillary twitching, glucosuria and hyperglycemia. Blindness, occasionally permanent, may occur. Fatal toxic myocarditis has been reported.

TREATMENT

1. Compress the sting site with ice and with ammonium hydroxide solution.

2. Control pain by rapid acting barbiturates, intramuscularly or intravenously, and calcium gluconate (10 ml. of 10% solution) intravenously. Morphine and synthetic narcotics are not, as a rule, effective in control of the exquisite pain at the sting site.

3. Administration of anti-scorpion serum after testing for sensitivity. (See **12.** *Serum Sensitivity and Desensitization.*

4. Hospitalization for close observation and symptomatic and supportive care (**49 – 4**).

56 – 12. SEA ANEMONE ("Sea Nettle") STINGS

Many varieties and sizes of sea anemone contain toxic venoms. Tiny anemones recently discovered off the Australian coast are rated among the world's most poisonous organisms. The Australian and Philippine sea wasp has been responsible for a considerable number of fatalities. It is possible that some of the cases of "drown-

ing" in proficient swimmers are in fact due to overwhelming reaction to these venoms.

For treatment, see **56 – 9**. *Portuguese Man-of-War Stings.*

56 – 13.   STINGRAY (Stingaree) STINGS

Wounds caused by the stingray are common in the South Pacific
and have been reported from Gulf of Mexico and California resorts
where water sports are popular. Both the fresh water and salt water
varieties are dangerous. They are characterized by large, jagged,
irregular wounds which may in themselves be fatal and by severe localized pain or, in some instances, numbness of the whole affected extremity, caused by venom carried in the integumentary
sheath of the ray's serrated stinger. Nausea, vomiting, headache,
dizziness and painful, shallow respiration, with pallor and cyanosis,
usually is present. After 1 or 2 hours, severe intractable generalized
myalgia, often associated with muscle spasm, develops. Severe
shock (**53**) may be irreversible and terminal if the chest or abdomen
has been penetrated.

TREATMENT

1. Thorough irrigation of the wound (provided the pleura or peritoneum has not been perforated).

2. Sedation by intramuscular or intravenous barbiturates.

3. Control of severe pain by local heat and morphine sulfate subcutaneously or intravenously.

4. Surgical removal of the serrated stinger or sheath, followed
by thorough debridement.

5. Hospitalization for care in all cases after treatment of shock
(**53 – 7**). Unless extensive debridement is done, large, slow-healing
ulcers may develop at the site of the sting.

56 – 14.   TROPICAL JELLYFISH STINGS See also **56 – 9**. *Portuguese Man-of-War Stings;* **56 – 12**. *Sea Anemone Stings*)

These cause local pain and generalized myalgia. Severe systemic
reactions are rare. The muscle pain usually yields readily to intravenous administration of 5 to 10 ml. of 10% calcium gluconate
solution, but in some cases codeine or morphine sulfate may be
necessary. Local treatment as given under *Portuguese Man-of-War
Stings* (**56 – 9**) should be used.

56—15. WASP (Hornet, Yellow Jacket) **STINGS**

Wasp stings may cause reactions similar to but more severe than bee stings (**56—1**). Acute anaphylactic reactions (**21**) may be terminal. The treatment is the same as for bee stings except that there is no buried stinger to be removed. For emergency kit and desensitization, see **56—1.** *Bee Stings.*

57. TEMPERATURE VARIATION EMERGENCIES

57—1. COLD INJURIES (Cold Allergy or Sensitivity, Chilblain, Frostbite, Immersion Foot, Trench Foot) (See also **57—5.** *Hypothermia*)

The exact mechanism of injury from exposure to low temperatures is unknown, but vascular changes with sludging of the blood undoubtedly are important factors. There is a wide variation in the ability of different individuals to tolerate cold. The chances of injury by exposure to low temperature are increased by a darkly pigmented skin, advanced age, poor general physical condition, anoxia (as in high altitude climbing or flying) and previous trauma, especially cold injury. For the effects of wind velocity, see Figure 33.

Accurate determination of the extent of tissue damage at the time of the original examination is impossible.

TREATMENT

1. Rest in a recumbent position.

2. Rapid rewarming by moist heat after the injured person has reached a safe place where there will be no chance of refreezing. It is better to postpone rapid rewarming for a few hours than to be forced to repeat the process. The solution should be kept between 36.7°C. (98°F.) and 40°C. (104°F.).

3. After rewarming, exposure to air at room temperature—at about 21°C. (69.4°F.)—is most satisfactory.

4. Administration of analgesics for severe pain. Morphine sulfate, 8 to 15 mg. subcutaneously or intravenously, may be necessary in severe cases; codeine sulfate, 0.06 gm., meperidine hydrochloride (Demerol), 50 to 100 mg., or pentazocine lactate (Talwin), 15 to 30 mg., may give relief if the pain is moderate.

Wind chill factor chart

Estimated wind speed (in mph)	Actual Thermometer Reading (° F)											
	50	40	30	20	10	0	-10	-20	-30	-40	-50	-60
	EQUIVALENT TEMPERATURE (° F.)											
calm	50	40	30	20	10	0	-10	-20	-30	-40	-50	-60
5	48	37	27	16	6	-5	-15	-26	-36	-47	-57	-68
10	40	28	16	4	-9	-24	-33	-46	-58	-70	-83	-95
15	36	22	9	-5	-18	-32	-45	-58	-72	-85	-99	-112
20	32	18	4	-10	-25	-39	-53	-67	-82	-96	-110	-124
25	30	16	0	-15	-29	-44	-59	-74	-88	-104	-118	-133
30	28	13	-2	-18	-33	-48	-63	-79	-94	-109	-125	-140
35	27	11	-4	-20	-35	-51	-67	-82	-98	-113	-129	-145
40	26	10	-6	-21	-37	-53	-69	-85	-100	-116	-132	-148
(Wind speeds greater than 40 mph have little additional effect.)	LITTLE DANGER (for properly clothed person). Maximum danger of false sense of security.			INCREASING DANGER Danger from freezing of exposed flesh.			GREAT DANGER					

Trenchfoot and immersion foot may occur at any point on this chart.

Figure 33. Wind chill factor chart. (From Earle, A. S., et al.: Patient Care, December, 1972. Copyright © Miller & Fink Corporation, Darien, CT. All rights reserved.)

5. Administration of human tetanus immune globulin (TIG) or toxoid (**16**).

6. Adequate prophylactic antibiotic therapy.

7. Observation until the extent of damage can be determined.

Do Not

1. Rub or compress the affected part with ice, snow or cold water. Massage or friction of any type is harmful.

2. Attempt to evacuate blebs or blisters.

3. Allow use, especially weight bearing, unless absolutely necessary (evacuation from disaster areas, etc.).

4. Apply pressure dressings or ointments of any type.

5. Allow excessive use of tobacco or snuff.

6. Administer anticoagulants, corticosteroids or vasodilators; they are of no value and may do harm.

7. Debride sloughing areas or perform any type of amputation except in the presence of a spreading virulent infection; unnecessary loss of tissue may result.

57−2. HEAT CRAMPS

Depletion of body fluid sodium chloride by prolonged excessive sweating may result in a pale skin, extreme thirst, nausea, dizziness, rapid strong pulse and normal or slightly elevated temperature. Muscular twitching (sometimes generalized as in epilepsy) and severe painful muscle cramps may be present if the salt depletion is extreme.

TREATMENT
1. Complete rest in a cool place.
2. In severe cases, normal salt solution, 1000 ml. intravenously to correct dehydration and salt depletion; milder cases will respond rapidly to oral intake of hypotonic salt solution (1 level teaspoonful of table salt and 1/2 teaspoonful of baking soda in 1000 ml. of water) or salt tablets.
3. Complete and rapid recovery practically always occurs. Hospitalization generally is not required.

57−3. HEAT EXHAUSTION (Heat Prostration)

This relatively common condition is caused by prolonged exposure to heat, often with high humidity. Fatalities are rare; when they do occur there is generally underlying cardiac or other pathology. The clinical picture is the result of peripheral vasomotor collapse and is characterized by a pale clammy skin; subnormal, normal or slightly elevated temperature; a fast, weak pulse; hypotension; dilated pupils; nausea; vomiting; generalized weakness and stupor deepening into coma.

TREATMENT
1. Move to cooler and less humid surroundings.
2. Allow fluids as desired if able to swallow; if not, give normal saline intravenously.
3. Give stimulants if the pulse is very weak or hypotension is severe:
Strong black coffee by mouth, or caffeine sodiobenzoate, 0.5 gm. intramuscularly.

Atropine sulfate, 1.0 to 1.5 mg. subcutaneously or slowly intravenously.

Amphetamine sulfate, 15 mg., slowly intravenously.

4. If recovery is slow, identify and treat underlying pathology.

57 — 4. HEAT HYPERPYREXIA (Heatstroke) (See also 57 — 6. *Iatrogenic Heatstroke*)

Failure of adequate elimination of body heat from breakdown of the sweating apparatus is invariably fatal unless recognized early and treated energetically. All untreated patients will die. Even with rapid and energetic treatment, the mortality is above 50%. The clinical picture is startling, with a hot *dry* skin, at first ruddy, but later becoming gray; a rapid full pulse, later becoming weak and thready and slow deep respirations later becoming of Cheyne-Stokes type. The pupils are dilated, and an offensive body odor is usually present. Muscular twitching and epileptiform convulsions with early loss of consciousness may occur. There is always a rapidly increasing body temperature, which may reach 44°C. (111.2°F.).

TREATMENT

1. Immediate reduction of body temperature by cold water baths, ice compresses, chilled saline enemas, sponging with alcohol, evaporation of water sprayed on the body or application of hypothermia blankets. *The rectal temperature must be reduced to 39°C. (102.2°F.) as rapidly as possible* by whatever means are available.

2. Constant vigorous massage of the extremities to promote circulation of the cooled blood to all parts of the body.

3. Intravenous cardiac and respiratory stimulants. Large amounts of intravenous fluids should be avoided because of the danger of pulmonary edema (**51**).

4. Oxygen inhalations under positive pressure by face mask if cyanosis is present.

5. Control of convulsions by sedation with rapidly acting barbiturates, chloral hydrate or paraldehyde. During convulsions protection from injury (especially tongue biting) and insurance of an adequate airway are essential.

6. Hospitalization as soon as possible. Cooling measures should be continued during transportation to a hospital.

DIFFERENTIAL DIAGNOSIS

	HEAT CRAMPS (SEE 57-2)	HEAT EXHAUSTION (HEAT PROSTRATION) (SEE 57-3)	HEAT HYPERPYREXIA (HEATSTROKE) (SEE 57-4)
Skin	Pale—excessive perspiration	Pale, cool and clammy	Hot, dry—at first ruddy, later gray
Body temperature	Normal or slightly elevated	Usually normal, but may be sub-normal or slightly elevated	Rapidly increasing rise—up to 39° C.
Pulse	Rapid, strong	Rapid, weak	Rapid and full early; later weak and thready
Respiration	Normal	Normal	Slow and deep early; later Cheyne-Stokes
Blood pressure	Normal	Decreased	Increased early; later decreased
Pupils	Normal	Dilated	Dilated
Body odor	Normal perspiration	Normal	Offensive
Muscle cramps	Severe	None	None
Convulsions	Generalized twitching	Rare	Epileptiform type early in course
Nausea and vomiting	Mild nausea—rarely vomiting	May be prolonged	Usually does not occur
State of consciousness	Normal	Stupor—coma in severe cases	Early loss of consciousness
Pain	Severe (from muscle cramping)	Headaches in mild cases	Only at onset
Treatment	Rest in a cool place. Correction of dehydration	Removal from excessive heat and humidity. Correction of dehydration. Supportive and symptomatic care	*Immediate* reduction of body temperature. Control of convulsions. Cardiac and respiratory support

DIFFERENTIAL DIAGNOSIS

	HEAT CRAMPS (SEE 57 — 2)	HEAT EXHAUSTION (HEAT PROSTRATION) (SEE 57 — 3)	HEAT HYPERPYREXIA (HEATSTROKE) (SEE 57 — 4)
Hospitalization	Not necessary	Rarely necessary unless underlying cardiac or other pathology is present	Essential, with cooling measures during transportation
Prognosis	Complete recovery without residual ill effects	Good in absence of severe preexistent underlying pathology	Hopeless in untreated cases; poor (50% mortality) in treated cases. Surviving cases may have permanent mental damage

57 — 5. HYPOTHERMIA (For localized effects, see 57 — 1)

Chilling of the whole body from exposure to natural elements or during therapeutic procedures (cardiac and vascular surgery, treatment of certain poisonings) results in progressive decrease of physiologic processes which eventually becomes irreversible. The ability to survive hypothermia depends on the length of exposure, inherent constitutional factors (some persons tolerate low temperatures better than others), environmental factors (altitude, barometric pressure, humidity) and physical condition (age, nutritional status, preexistent disease). Survivals from rectal temperatures as low as 23.3°C. (74°F.) have been reported.

TREATMENT

Slow rewarming

1. Application of blankets.

2. Determination of urinary output by retention catheter. Intravenous fluids must be limited until kidney function is reestablished, usually 12 to 18 hours after institution of treatment.

3. Careful search for and treatment of underlying disease processes. Hypothermia may completely mask the usual signs and symptoms of infection and other diseases and make the effects of

commonly used drugs such as digitalis, steroids, insulin and anti-coagulants completely unpredictable until the body temperature approaches normal.

Rapid rewarming. This is necessary if the rectal temperature is close to the lethal limit.

1. Application of heat under close supervision by any and all means available, including hot fluids by mouth, electric blankets, electric heaters, gastric lavage with warm solutions, warm water enemas and hot water bottles. The rate of body temperature increase is not related to the methods used and rarely exceeds 0.6°C. (1.2°F.) per hour.

2. Insertion of a retention catheter for observation of kidney function.

3. Recognition and symptomatic treatment of the 2 frequent complications of rapid rewarming—cardiac arrhythmias, which may progress to cardiac arrest (**26 – 7**), and hypertension.

4. Recognition and treatment of underlying pathologic conditions (**57 – 5**).

5. Avoidance of the detrimental measures outlined in **57 – 1**.

57 – 6. IATROGENIC HEATSTROKE (See also 57 – 4)

During periods of excessively hot weather with high humidity, hospitalized persons with impaired sweat secretion are especially susceptible to heatstroke. The significance of the clinical picture of impending heatstroke may be overlooked or misinterpreted in persons under anesthesia if drapes and covering prevent adequate heat loss; in quadriplegics, hemiplegics and paraplegics in whom the perspiration-control mechanism has been short-circuited; in persons on medications which inhibit sweating, especially atropine and phenothiazines; and in psychiatric patients whose mental symptoms are dramatic enough to divert attention from the signs and symptoms of impending heatstroke (**57 – 4**).

TREATMENT
See *Heat Hyperpyrexia* (**57 – 4**).

57 – 7. LOW SALT SYNDROME

Hot humid temperatures increase the body's need for salt; hence, the widespread use of salt tablets in industries where high temperatures are the usual environment (steel and aluminum furnaces, engine rooms of ships).

57—8. SUNSTROKE

Infants and small children are peculiarly susceptible to the effects of hot weather salt depletion, which may be confused with other serious conditions, such as brain concussion (**48—9**) or contusion (**48—11**).

SIGNS AND SYMPTOMS. Lethargy, loss of appetite, nausea, vomiting, opisthotonus, convulsive seizures and stupor deepening into coma. Low spinal fluid chlorides are usually present.

TREATMENT

1. Oxygen by face mask or tent as required.

2. Intravenous administration of normal saline solution for correction of salt deficiency and fluid imbalance (**6**).

3. Control of convulsions by sedative suppositories [dosage according to age or weight (**4**)].

4. Prophylactic measures for hospitalized infants consist of daily oral administration of Darrow's solution and glucose water. In older children, addition of 0.5 to 1.5 gm. of salt to the daily diet is usually effective.

57—8. SUNSTROKE

Although "sunstroke" properly applies only to heat hyperpyrexia (**57—4**) developing following direct exposure to hot sun, the term is often used loosely for cases of heat exhaustion (**57—3**) in which there has been disturbance in the state of consciousness, provided there is a history of exposure to sunlight. In many instances, a mixed picture may be present; however, a rapidly rising body temperature associated with a hot dry skin makes immediate energetic treatment as outlined under *Heat Hyperpyrexia* (**57—4**) mandatory.

58. TOOTHACHE

58—1. PAIN

Pain from injuries, disease or extraction of the teeth may be severe. Temporary relief of acute discomfort can often be given.

TREATMENT

1. Codeine sulfate, 0.03 to 0.06 gm., and acetylsalicylic acid (aspirin), 0.6 gm. by mouth, every 2 to 4 hours.

2. Application of oil of cloves. A local anesthetic ointment such as 4% butacaine (Butyn) with 1:1500 nitromersol (Metaphen) rubbed into the painful area and surrounding gum tissues will usually give relief for 4 to 6 hours.

3. Packing of cavities with a thick paste prepared by mixing oil of cloves and powdered zinc oxide. A few cotton fibers may be added for body.

4. The need for dental care at the earliest possible opportunity should be stressed.

58-2. AERODONTALGIA

A minute pocket of air beneath a filling or cap may cause excruciating pain in divers on ascent to the surface. Treatment consists of replacement of the dental repair even if ordinary methods of detection fail to show any defect.

58-3. ALVEOLAR ABSCESSES See 20-1

58-4. POSTEXTRACTION BLEEDING See 42-42

59. VASCULAR DISORDERS

Various types of severe catastrophes can occur from acute pathology involving the vascular system (arteries, veins and lymphatics).

59-1. ARTERIAL INJURIES

Immediate recognition of severe injuries to major arteries, followed by prompt and proper surgical treatment, may be lifesaving or may eliminate the necessity for amputation. Surgical techniques are available for repair of defects in major arteries by direct suturing, venous grafts or prosthetic grafts; even extremely small arteries can at times be repaired successfully using a microscopic lens device for better visualization.

TYPES OF ARTERIAL INJURY

1. *Contusion.* Vasospasm resulting from damage to the intima may give a clinical picture suggestive of complete vessel transection.

2. *Compression* against a bony prominence, usually near the elbow, wrist, knee or ankle.

3. *Laceration* may result in fatal external or internal hemorrhage. Small lacerations may cause more prolonged bleeding than complete severance because the injured vessel cannot retract into the surrounding soft tissues.

4. *Severance*—complete.

Severe arterial damage results in the appearance of bright red blood, often spurting, if a channel to the surface is available, in the development of a rapidly increasing hematoma which becomes hard and tense when anatomic limits are reached or by bleeding into actual or potential body cavities. Exsanguination may occur unless control is accomplished (**42–1**). Pulsations in the arteries distal to the injury may be decreased or absent. Shock (**53**) usually is present. There may be intense pain from ischemia or pressure on surrounding structures, or increased, disturbed or decreased sensation.

TREATMENT

1. Control of major hemorrhage (**42–1**). This is a lifesaving measure and takes precedence over all other therapeutic measures.

Methods:

(a) Application of external pressure by a tight-fitting bandage.

(b) Application of a tourniquet to an extremity proximal to the injury. The pressure of the tourniquet must be above systolic pressure. Every effort should be made to preserve collateral circulation. An improperly applied tourniquet may increase or prolong, not control, hemorrhage.

(c) Clamping with a hemostat proximal to the injury. To prevent additional damage to the artery, the hemostat should be placed as close as possible to the site of injury.

(d) Packing of natural or traumatic cavities with sterile gauze, or application of internal pressure by use of a balloon or other expanding device.

2. Treatment of shock (**53–7**).

3. Release of compression by reduction of displaced fractures or dislocations as soon as evidence of arterial compression is recognized, or whenever the possibility of compression of a major artery

is suspected from the position of displaced bone fragments or joint surfaces.

4. Hospitalization for definitive surgical care *as soon as possible* in all cases of known or suspected major arterial damage. The time lag between injury and repair must be kept to a minimum for a successful result.

59-2. INTRACRANIAL HEMORRHAGE

Bleeding within the cranium is one of the common causes of catastrophic incidents known as cerebrovascular accidents (CVAs) or "strokes" which we define as *the rapid onset of focal neurologic signs and symptoms or coma due to disruption of blood supply to or from the brain.* See also **59-4.** *Cerebral Embolism;* **59-7.** *Cerebral Thrombosis;* **59-8.** *Transient Focal Cerebral Ischemia.* Table 5 (page 640) indicates features in the differential diagnosis of common causes of strokes; the need for accurate diagnosis to assure appropriate treatment is evident (see Table 6, pages 644-645).

Epidural hemorrhage. See **41-19; 48-26.** *Extradural Hemorrhage in Children.*

Intracerebral hemorrhage

COMMON CAUSES

Degeneration of cerebral arteries and arterioles secondary to arteriosclerosis and atherosclerosis.

Congenital weakness of blood vessel walls (saccular aneurysms, berry aneurysms).

Hypertension.

Blood dyscrasias; primary or secondary, due to the effects of medications such as anticoagulants (**42-34**).

Trauma.

Damage of arterial walls secondary to arteritis, congenital malformations, infections and toxins.

SIGNS AND SYMPTOMS are highlighted by the sudden onset, usually with activity, of intense headache, nausea, vomiting and (frequently) coma. Neurologic signs of paralysis and paresis depend upon the location and extent of the hemorrhage. Blood in the spinal fluid and evidence of secondary meningeal irritation may be present.

TREATMENT

1. *General supportive measures.* The measures outlined in Table 5 are applicable to patients with strokes resulting in similar disabil-

(*Text continues on page 648*)   **page 639**

TABLE 5. DIFFERENTIAL DIAGNOSIS OF COMMON CAUSES OF STROKES

	FOCAL CEREBRAL ISCHEMIA	CEREBRAL THROMBOSIS	CEREBRAL EMBOLISM	INTRACEREBRAL HEMORRHAGE
Onset	Sec. to min.	Min. to hours	Sudden	Rapid; min. to 1 or 2 hours
Duration of signs and symptoms	Sec. to min.	Permanent if related to infarction; potentially reversible if related to edema and ischemia	Rapid improvement may occur depending on collateral flow	Permanent if related to infarction; potentially reversible if related to edema and ischemia
Activity	Positive if related to decreased cardiac output	Usually occurs at rest	Probably not related to activity	Usually occurs during activity
Contributing or associated diseases	Peripheral and coronary atherosclerosis, hypertension	Peripheral and coronary atherosclerosis, hypertension	Atrial fibrillation, aortic and mitral valvular disease, myocardial infarction, atherosclerotic plaques	Hypertensive cardiovascular disease, coagulation defects
Sensorium	Usually conscious	Usually conscious	Usually conscious	Coma common
Nuchal rigidity	Absent	Absent	Absent	Frequently present

Location of cerebral deficit	Focal or "arterial syndrome"	Focal or "arterial syndrome"	Focal or "arterial syndrome"	Focal; "arterial syndrome" not common
Convulsions	Rare	Rare	Rare	Common
Cerebrospinal fluid	Usually normal	Usually normal	Usually normal	Bloody; normal if hemorrhage entirely intracerebral
Skull x-rays	May show calcification of intracranial arteries	Possible arterial calcification and pineal shift from edema	Usually normal	May show pineal shift from hemorrhage, edema, or hematoma
Angiography	Single or multiple narrowed areas of aortic arch or of neck or cerebral arteries	Same as focal cerebral ischemia plus arterial obstruction	Site of arterial obstruction; may be normal after a few hours	Avascular area; displacement and stretching of surrounding arteries and veins
Recurrence in survivors	Common	Common	Common	Common

(Modified from Cain, H. D., and Smith, E.: "Principles in Management of Cerebrovascular Accidents," *Hospital Medicine*, October 1965.)

(Table continues)

TABLE 5. DIFFERENTIAL DIAGNOSIS OF COMMON CAUSES OF STROKES (*Continued*)

	SUBARACHNOID HEMORRHAGE	SUBDURAL HEMORRHAGE	EXTRADURAL HEMORRHAGE	BRAIN TUMOR
Onset	Sudden; variable progression	Insidious, occasionally acute	Rapid; usually minutes to hours	Usually very slow; rapid with hemorrhage
Duration of signs and symptoms	Variable; complete clearing may occur in days or weeks	Hours to months	Initial fluctuating course common, then steadily progressive	Gradually progressive; permanent
Activity	More frequent during activity	Usually but not always related to head trauma	Almost always related to trauma	Unrelated to activity
Contributing or associated diseases	Intracerebral arterial aneurysms, trauma, tumor	Chronic alcoholism	Any condition that predisposes to trauma	If metastatic, primary focus
Sensorium	Coma common	Generally clouded	Rapidly advancing coma	Slow progressive loss
Nuchal rigidity	Present except immediately	Absent	Absent	Absent

	Diffuse; aneurysm may give focal sign before and after hemorrhage	Frontal-lobe signs common, ipsilateral pupil may dilate	Temporal-lobe signs, dilatation of ipsilateral pupil and high intracranial pressure	Focal – area of tumor
Location of cerebral deficit				
Convulsions	Common	Infrequent	Common	Variable; Jacksonian type most common
Cerebrospinal fluid	Grossly bloody; increased pressure	Normal to slight elevation of protein	Increased pressure, usually normal color and cells	Increased protein and pressure
Skull x-rays	Usually normal; may show calcified aneurysm	Frequently contralateral shift of pineal	Frequently fracture across middle meningeal artery groove	May show pineal shift, calcification
Angiography	Outline of one or more aneurysms (unless filled with blood)	Avascular subdural mass	May demonstrate site of bleeding, avascular mass	Identification of mass, vascularity
Recurrence in survivors	Common	Can recur after surgery	None with adequate initial surgery	Varies with type of tumor

(Modified from Cain, H. D., and Smith, E.: "Principles in Management of Cerebrovascular Accidents," *Hospital Medicine*, October 1965.)

TABLE 6. GOALS AND METHODS OF SUPPORTIVE TREATMENT IN ACUTE PHASE OF CVAs AND COMPARABLE DISABILITIES

ORGAN SYSTEM	GOALS	METHODS OF TREATMENT
Skin	Prevention of pressure ulcers	Changing position every two hours Keeping all pressure off reddened or blanched skin Keeping skin dry and clean
Respiratory tract	Maintenance of a clear airway	Suctioning; tracheostomy if necessary Draining of secretions by postural positioning Encouragement of periodic deep breathing and coughing; use of ancillary chemical and mechanical agents as necessary Liquefaction of secretions by adequate hydration and use of aerosols, and by instillation of saline drops if a tracheostomy tube is in place Administration of antibiotics if clinical or x-ray evidence of pulmonary infection is present
Cardiovascular system	Maintenance of adequate blood pressure for perfusion of vital organs	Judicious use of vasopressors and blood transfusions Preservation of vasomotor tone by early mobilization, including sitting and use of standing table or bed
	Reduction of peripheral thrombophlebitis	Wrapping of lower extremities from toes to upper thighs with elastic bandages Early mobilization

TABLE 6. GOALS AND METHODS OF SUPPORTIVE TREATMENT IN ACUTE PHASE OF CVAs AND COMPARABLE DISABILITIES *(Continued)*

ORGAN SYSTEM	GOALS	METHODS OF TREATMENT
Gastrointestinal system	Maintenance of hydration, electrolyte balance, and anabolism	Administration of adequate fluids, minerals, calories, and vitamins, orally, through gastric tube or parenterally
	Promotion of normal bowel function	Proper bowel-training program
Genitourinary system	Assurance of complete urinary elimination	Catheter drainage if necessary
	Reduction of infection, protection and preservation of the upper urinary tract	Adequate hydration and removal of catheter as soon as possible. Antibacterial medications
Central nervous system	Avoidance of further depression of CNS	Restriction of sedatives. Avoidance of narcotics
	Control of convulsive seizures	Diphenylhydantoin as needed
	Counteracting usual depression	Proper attitude and counseling; use of centrally acting antidepressant drugs
Musculoskeletal system	Maintenance of normal range of joint-motion	Daily exercise, passive and then active as indicated. Proper positioning with footboards, pillows, and removable splints. Avoidance of excessive passive stretching against spastic muscles
	Maintenance of tone of uninvolved as well as affected muscles	Early mobilization. Supervised resistive exercises. Use of a standing table or bed

(Modified from Cain, H. D., and Smith, E.: "Principles in Management of Cerebrovascular Accidents," *Hospital Medicine,* October 1965.)

TABLE 7. GOALS IN PREVENTION AND TREATMENT OF CEREBROVASCULAR ACCIDENTS

TYPE OF STROKE	GOALS	METHODS USED TO ACHIEVE GOALS
Arterial occlusion	Removal of occlusion	Thrombectomy or embolectomy
	Reduction of thrombus propagation	Anticoagulant therapy Endarterectomy
	Prevention of formation of new thrombi	Anticoagulant therapy Endarterectomy
	Prevention of formation of new emboli	Conversion of atrial fibrillation to sinus mechanism Antibiotic treatment of bacterial endocarditis Mitral commissurotomy, ablation of left atrial appendage in mitral stenosis Endarterectomy Anticoagulant therapy
	Improvement of blood flow to cerebrum	Enlargement toward normal of arterial channels arising from aortic arch and carotid vessels Endarterectomy Arterial bypass Vasodilatation
	Correction of pathologic conditions decreasing cardiac output and oxygen-carrying capacity of the blood	Treatment of congestive heart failure and serious arrhythmias Blood transfusions for severe anemia
	Reduction of cerebral edema	Corticosteroids Hypertonic agents intravenously (e.g., urea, hypertonic glucose)

Intracranial hemorrhage	Establishment of normal blood coagulability	Correction of congenital or acquired coagulation defects Avoidance of anticoagulants if hemorrhage may occur or has occurred
	Reduction of cerebral intra-arterial pressure	Hypotensive drugs Postural position (tilt table) Ligation of, or Salibi clamp on, common carotid artery Ligation of intracranial artery
	Control of ruptured aneurysm	Surgical reinforcement or isolation (depending on anatomic location and accessibility)
	Elimination of hematoma	Surgical evacuation and control of bleeding
	Reduction of oxygen need of brain	Hypothermia

(Modified from Cain, H. D., and Smith, E.: "Principles in Management of Cerebrovascular Accidents," *Hospital Medicine*, October 1965.)

ities, no matter what the cause. Early active exercise is restricted in patients with extensive intracranial bleeding, particularly subarachnoid hemorrhage (below).

2. *Specific measures.* Treat any contributing blood-coagulation disorders such as hemophilia, thrombocytopenia or conditions resulting from medication with heparin or warfarin-like drugs (**42 — 34.** *Anticoagulant Therapy*).

Reduce moderate to severe hypertension cautiously. Rapid reduction of the blood pressure to "normal" may cause the clinical condition to deteriorate because of inadequate perfusion levels. See also *Hypertensive Crisis* (**26 — 11**).

Subarachnoid hemorrhage of severe degree occurs most frequently from a ruptured saccular aneurysm. Signs, symptoms and precipitating causes are similar to those outlined under intracerebral hemorrhage (above); however, in general, the onset is more catastrophic, the coma is more severe and the cerebrospinal fluid shows more red blood cells.

TREATMENT AND PROGNOSIS

Treatment is similar to that outlined for intracerebral hemorrhage (above) except that immediate surgery may be definitive and lifesaving. If the only signs are meningeal irritation from blood or mild neurologic deficits, *immediate* arteriograms, followed by surgery if indicated, give the best statistical chance of survival. Hypothermia may be of value in some cases. Dexamethasone (Decadron), 15 to 25 mg. intravenously, and/or mannitol (Osmitrol) intravenously may help to relieve cerebral edema.

Subdural hemorrhage. (See also **41 — 20; 48 — 32.** *Head Injuries in Children.*)

This condition usually arises from a tear in one of the cerebral veins entering the dural sinuses, caused by direct trauma to the frontal or occipital region. Since the hemorrhage is venous and its pressure less than in extradural hemorrhage (**41 — 19; 48 — 32.** *Head Injuries in Children*) signs are slower in developing, sometimes requiring weeks. However, an acute subdural hematoma, suspected on the basis of alteration of conscious state, unilateral pupillary dilation and focal sensory and motor changes will usually require emergency care.

TREATMENT

Hospitalization for diagnostic localizing examinations and probable craniotomy. For supportive treatment, see Table 6 on pages 644–645.

59 — 3.   DISSECTING AORTIC ANEURYSM

The defect which leads to weakening of the aortic wall is usually cystic central necrosis. Increased stress on the aortic wall from increased intracranial pressure, hypertension or trauma may precipitate acute signs and symptoms consisting of abdominal or thoracic pain (which may be minimal or excruciating, sudden or progressive), pallor, sweating and shock (53). There may be pathologic discrepancies in the blood pressure and pulses between the two arms or between the arms and legs and signs of ischemia or infarction of the brain, kidney, myocardium or spinal cord. Widening of the aorta may be demonstrable by palpation or radiologic studies.

TREATMENT

1. Immediate hospitalization.
2. Absolute rest.
3. Barbiturates and opiates as necessary for control of restlessness, pain and apprehension.
4. Treatment of shock (**53 — 7**). The blood pressure should be kept at the minimal level to maintain adequate perfusion of vital organs. Cautious reduction of moderate or severe hypertension is indicated.
5. Evaluation for surgical treatment.

PROGNOSIS.   The mortality from dissecting aortic aneurysms is in the 75 to 80% range; a much better prognosis is offered if the aneurysm can be repaired prior to dissection.

59 — 4.   EMBOLISM

An embolus of either cardiac or noncardiac origin may cause infarction of any organ of the body. The diagnosis is usually made by evidence of sudden infarction and/or malfunction of the involved organ plus determination of the presence of a probable source of the embolus. In general, emergency therapy is designed to be supportive, to reduce the source of likelihood of other emboli and to allow performance of a surgical embolectomy if indicated and possible.

CEREBRAL EMBOLI

Cerebral emboli usually arise from a cardiac source and may be due to myocardial infarction (**26 — 12**), chronic atrial fibrillation (**26 — 3**) or endocarditis (**26 — 6**). Another source may be atherosclerotic plaques from major arteries of the neck. Signs and symptoms, which generally correspond to the neurologic areas supplied by the occluded artery, have a sudden onset.

TREATMENT

1. Supportive. (See under **59−2** for general supportive treatment.)

2. Surgical attack of thromboembolic occlusions in completed strokes generally has not given favorable results. Surgical approach to remove the source of past and future emboli may be considered (e.g., prosthetic replacement of diseased and defective cardiac valves; endartectomy of grossly atherosclerotic major neck vessels).

3. Anticoagulation may be considered for reduction of thrombotic emboli if evidences of infection and secondary hemorrhage are *not* present.

PULMONARY ARTERY EMBOLISM

Lodging of a clot large enough to completely occlude the bifurcation of the common pulmonary artery ("saddle embolus") results in sudden collapse and death within minutes. Resuscitative measures are ineffective.

Embolization of medium-sized and small branches of the pulmonary artery:

SIGNS AND SYMPTOMS vary with size and number of occluded arteries; most frequently recognized are those cases with sudden onset of severe chest pain, dyspnea, cyanosis, extreme anxiety and apprehension. Hemoptysis may occur. Tachycardia (sinus or atrial) and signs of shock (**53**) may appear. Physical findings vary; there may be none or those previously mentioned−a pleuritic friction rub, increased pulmonary second sound and pleural effusion.

Further diagnostic measures may include enzyme studies (LDH, SGOT and bilirubin), roentgenographic studies (PA and lateral of chest, pulmonary arteriography), radioisotope lung scan, end-tidal and arterial pCO_2 and electrocardiograms taken immediately and at 6 and 12 hours (Transient atrial arrhythmias, prominent P waves, S_1Q_3 pattern, right bundle branch block, nonspecific ST-T changes or no electrocardiographic abnormality may be present.) Differential diagnosis from other cardiac and pulmonary diseases [myocardial infarction (**26−12**), pneumonia (**52−14**), pericarditis (**26−16**) and septic shock (**53**)] may be difficult.

TREATMENT

(See also **51**. *Pulmonary Edema.*)

Therapy varies with the severity of the clinical condition and with available medicosurgical resources.

1. Position of comfort.

2. Oxygen by intranasal catheter or face mask.

3. Heparin, 10,000 units intravenously, followed by maintenance anticoagulation.

4. Morphine sulfate, 10 mg. subcutaneously for pain. Segmental pain may be relieved by intercostal nerve blocks.

5. Treatment of shock (**53**) by intravenous drip infusion of isoproterenol (Isuprel), 0.05 to 0.10 mg., diluted to 125 ml. in 5% dextrose in water, administered over a 30 minute period and/or levarterenol bitartrate (Levophed), 4 ml. of 0.2 ml., per cent solution in 1000 ml. of 5% dextrose in water by intravenous catheter drip infusion with frequent blood pressure monitoring.

6. Application of elastic wraps evenly to both legs from toes to groin. Elevate the foot of the bed slightly; have the patient lie with knees straight.

7. Indications regarding referral for and institution of pulmonary embolectomy are still variable and under evaluation but include:

Availability of an experienced surgical team and cardiopulmonary bypass unit.

Clinical and preliminary supportive evidence of a major embolism.

Evidence by x-rays, electrocardiograms or direct measurement of rapidly increasing pulmonary artery pressure.

Pulmonary arteriographic or radioactive isotope evidence of gross vascular bed involvement.

PROPHYLACTIC MEASURES FOR PREVENTION OF RECURRENCE OF PULMONARY ARTERY EMBOLI

Persons who have had previous emboli, thrombophlebitis, pelvic inflammatory disease or tumor, endocardial disease, patients who are bedfast for long periods, those with chronic disability and victims of accidents are especially prone to develop pulmonary emboli. Although prophylactic treatment is not properly a part of emergency care, the essential features are outlined here because of their importance and applicability to many patients seen with major emergencies.

1. Maintenance of proper fluid balance and prevention of dehydration (**6**).

2. Insistence on early activity and frequent changes in position in postoperative or debilitated patients.

3. Encouragement of active and passive leg exercises.

4. Positioning with no pillows under the knees; foot of the bed or leg supports of wheel chair slightly elevated.

5. Firm, even application of compression bandages or elastic stockings from toes to upper thighs in patients with lower extremity thrombophlebitis and subsequent necessary prolonged bed rest.

6. Administration of anticoagulant therapy under careful control and observation for those with a high likelihood of thromboembolism. Heparin is the drug of choice initially.

7. Reduction of weight to a normal range.

EMBOLUS IN PERIPHERAL ARTERIES

Whether the blocking of a peripheral artery is due to embolism or arteriosclerotic thrombus, the emergency treatment for the artery is similar. Recognition of the condition and proper handling may be the deciding factors in saving a limb or a life.

SIGNS AND SYMPTOMS. Acute pain, usually severe, pallor, coldness and numbness of the affected extremity, absence or gross diminution of pulsation in the arteries distal to the lesion and puffiness and pitting edema if there is concomitant venous involvement.

TREATMENT

1. Protect the extremity from mechanical injury and place in a level or slightly dependent position.

2. Relieve pain and vasospasm by morphine sulfate, 10 to 15 mg. subcutaneously or intravenously; papaverine hydrochloride, 0.2 gm. by mouth, or 30 to 60 mg. intraarterially proximal to the occlusion (if the embolism is in a small distal artery), and atropine sulfate, 0.6 mg. subcutaneously or intravenously.

3. Transfer to a hospital as soon as possible. Immediate embolectomy (frequently removal with a Fogarty catheter) or paravertebral sympathetic nerve blocks may be indicated.

4. After obtaining control specimens, begin anticoagulation therapy, preferably with heparin, 10,000 units intravenously, initially if indicated.

AIR EMBOLISM (Arterial Embolism) (See also **23 — 5.** *Diving Hazards;* **59 — 9.** *Venous Air Embolism*)

In an adult of average weight, 60 to 80 ml. of air in the vascular tree may be a lethal amount, although the speed of entry, pressure and position of the patient may cause marked variations in the amount which can be tolerated.

CAUSES

Intrinsic air in the alveoli, pulmonary cavity or pleural cavity (pneumothorax).

Extrinsic air accidentally injected during diagnostic procedures, open operations and traumatic incidents.

SIGNS AND SYMPTOMS. Dizziness, cold clammy skin, thready pulse, extreme hypotension, dyspnea and cyanosis often followed by Cheyne-Stokes respiration. Convulsions, coma and localized neurologic signs (hemiplegia, blindness) may be present. Confirmatory findings are detection of air in the retinal vessels by ophthalmoscopic examination, appearance of sharply defined areas of pallor in the tongue (Liebermeister's sign), "marbling" of the skin and bubbling of air mixed with blood from a skin incision. X-ray demonstration of air in the cerebral vessels is sometimes possible. Coronary artery involvement can give the characteristic electrocardiographic changes of myocardial injury or infarction (**26 – 12**).

TREATMENT

1. Keep the patient's head down.
2. Give symptomatic supportive therapy (artificial respiration, oxygen under positive pressure, support of circulation, etc.).
3. Hospitalize immediately for further treatment.

59 – 5. SYNCOPE (Fainting, Vasodepressor Syncope)

Transient loss of consciousness is not a serious condition unless the patient is injured in falling. Various mechanisms may lead to collapse of arterial vasomotor tone and temporary insufficiency of cerebral circulation; thorough investigation should be made to determine the underlying cause. See **26 – 20**. *Stokes-Adams Attacks* and **50 – 11** for differential diagnosis.

TREATMENT

1. Recumbent position until recovered.
2. Inhalations of aromatic spirits of ammonia.
3. Treatment of any injuries sustained in falling.
4. Ephedrine, 25 mg. to 50 mg. orally.
5. Prevention of repeated falling; instructions for mild preliminary exercises and gradual arising when orthostatic hypotension is present.
6. Prohibit operation of motor vehicles or exposure to potentially hazardous situations (height, moving machinery) if recurrence is likely until effective preventative treatment is established.

59 – 6. THROMBOANGIITIS OBLITERANS (Buerger's Disease)

The extremely severe pain caused by this progressive condition may bring the patient for emergency relief.

59 – 7. THROMBOSIS

TREATMENT OF ACUTE EPISODES

1. Bed rest with positioning of the involved extremity for most comfort and least blanching.

2. Papaverine hydrochloride, 30 to 60 mg. intravenously. Larger doses, up to 100 mg. intravenously, may be given in severe cases.

3. Tetraethylammonium chloride (Etamon), 200 mg. dissolved in 20 ml. of physiologic salt solution, intravenously. This solution should be given very slowly with close observation for the onset of acute and delayed hypotension, nausea and abdominal distention Check the blood pressure after injection of each 5 ml. of solution.

4. For severe pain, codeine sulfate or morphine sulfate may be required. Check for possible addiction to narcotics (**2 – 4**).

5. Hospitalization may be indicated if the acute pain cannot be controlled by the measures given above, or if the patient shows signs of possible addiction to narcotics.

59 – 7. THROMBOSIS

Cerebral and major arteries of neck. Signs, symptoms and treatment are similar to emboli (**59 – 4**) occurring in the same arteries, except that the onset is frequently slower. Thrombolysins have not proved their value in treatment. For treatment of completed stroke due to cerebral thrombosis, statistics favor non-use of anticoagulants except possibly in vertebral-basilar artery thrombosis. Acute surgery for thrombectomy is usually too late for preservation or restoration of cerebral function, and restoration of blood flow in the acute postinfarction period may be further injurious to the softened, swollen brain tissue.

Peripheral artery thrombosis. See **59 – 4.** *Embolism of Peripheral Arteries.*

59 – 8. TRANSIENT FOCAL CEREBRAL ISCHEMIA

Recurrent episodes of cerebral ischemia lasting from seconds to a few minutes may give any of the signs and symptoms of a "stroke," but the patient reverts spontaneously to his prior normal or near normal state.

TREATMENT

1. Obtain and record an accurate history of events.

2. Auscultate for bruit over major neck arteries, palpate carotid and temporal arteries and record blood pressure in both arms.

3. Refer the patient to a vascular or neurosurgeon for diagnostic evaluation which may include lumbar subarachnoid puncture, arteriography and electroencephalography. Surgical removal of large atherosclerotic lesions in major branches of the aortic arch and arteries of neck may prevent recurrence of ischemia and development of completed strokes.

4. Anticoagulation is effective in reducing the number of recurrences.

5. Evaluate for any associated hypertensive or cardiac problems.

59 – 9. VENOUS AIR EMBOLISM

This condition may follow diagnostic injection of air (peritoneum, pleura, subarachnoid space); retroperitoneal trauma; operation on the head, neck and genitourinary tract; administration of fluids into, or removal of blood from, any vein or extreme changes in atmospheric pressure (**23.** *Barotrauma*).

SIGNS AND SYMPTOMS. Deep inspiration followed by coughing exhalation, then a few attempts at breathing followed by apnea. The blood pressure drops and the pulse becomes weak or imperceptible.

TREATMENT

1. Immediate left lateral position.

2. Artificial respiration followed by administration of oxygen under positive pressure by endotracheal catheter and rebreathing bag.

3. Immediate hospitalization for aspiration of air from the right atrium, preferably by open operation.

59 – 10. PHLEBOTHROMBOSIS (See also **59 – 4.** *Pulmonary Artery Embolism*)

Few clinical signs may be produced even in the presence of extensive thrombotic involvement of the deep veins of the lower extremities and the pelvic veins. These thrombi may dislodge and migrate; phlebothrombosis is the most common cause of pulmonary embolism (**59 – 4**).

SIGNS AND SYMPTOMS. Moderate elevation of temperature, unilateral leg edema with enlargement of thigh and calf and positive Homan's sign (pain in the calf of the involved leg on forced dorsiflexion of the foot).

TREATMENT

1. Complete rest; 10° to 15° elevation of the extended extremity.

2. Application of moist heat.
3. Treatment of pain and vasospasm.
4. Anticoagulation with sodium heparin, 10,000 units intravenously, after obtaining a preliminary coagulation time.
5. Referral to a hospital for observation and care.
6. Surgical consultation regarding thrombectomy or removal of thrombus with a Fogarty catheter is indicated if there is gross edema and evidence of extensive femoral/iliac vein involvement. Recurrent emboli may require inferior vena cava ligation.

59—11. THROMBOPHLEBITIS

Thrombophlebitis is usually an inflammation of a superficial vein, with infection and varicosities contributing factors. The commonest sites are the veins of the lower extremities, although veins in any portion of the body may be involved.

SIGNS AND SYMPTOMS. Severe pain with redness and induration over the course of the vein, fever (sometimes chills) and swelling of the extremity. Embolization may occur and cause pulmonary artery occlusion, but it is much less common than with phlebothrombosis (**59—10**).

TREATMENT
1. Bed rest.
2. Heat (hot, moist compresses are best) at about body temperature.
3. Elevation of the extremity about 6 inches above the heart level to allow lymphatic-venous drainage.
4. Avoidance of dehydration by oral and intravenous administration of fluids (**6**).
5. Compressive wrapping or elastic stockings from toes to above knee when upright or ambulatory.
6. Hospitalization if the condition persists, if deep vein involvement occurs or if any signs of emboli appear [treat as for phlebothrombosis (**59—10**)].

59—12. VARICOSE VEINS

Esophageal varices. See **37—4**. *Hemorrhage from the Gastrointestinal Tract.*
Hemorrhoids. See **37—6**. *Anorectal Conditions.*

Postinjection thrombophlebitis. Inflammation of a vein wall of varying degrees of severity may follow local injection of varicose veins with sclerosing solutions. For treatment, see **59 – 11** (*above*).

Postligation hemorrhage. Bleeding may occur several days after surgical procedures for ligation of varicose veins of the lower extremities.

TREATMENT

1. Sedation by barbiturates subcutaneously or intravenously.

2. Application of local pressure.

3. Hospitalization if bleeding is persistent or if blood loss has been extreme.

Pruritus due to varicose eczema. The itching caused by chronic eczema, especially that secondary to degenerative changes in the vessels of the lower legs, may be severe enough to bring the patient for emergency care.

TREATMENT

1. Sedation by barbiturates.

2. Application of local anesthetic preparations such as calamine lotion with 1% phenol (*do not bandage or compress*) or dibucaine (Nupercaine) ointment.

3. Referral to a dermatologist for definitive care.

Rupture of a varicose vein of an extremity. Rupture of a varicosity may be spontaneous or traumatic and may cause stubborn and persistent bleeding severe enough to result in secondary anemia. The bleeding is usually not enough to cause symptoms of shock.

TREATMENT

1. Elevate the extremity; restrict activity.

2. Apply direct pressure by an elastic bandage or gauze fluffs held in place by a roller elastic bandage.

3. Administer sedation as needed, preferably by rapid-acting barbiturates.

4. Place mattress sutures of No. 40 or No. 50 cotton, under local anesthesia if necessary.

5. Refer for further surgical care, preferably within 24 hours.

Varicose ulcers with secondary infection and cellulitis

TREATMENT

1. Limit activity.

2. Elevate the extremity.

3. Give oral tetracyclines, 250 to 500 mg. 4 times a day the 1st day; then 250 mg. 4 times a day.

4. Wash twice daily with pHisoHex solution. Apply petrolatum or bacitracin (Parentracin) gauze dressings covered with fluffs and an elastic bandage for gentle pressure.

5. Hospitalize if the cellulitis is extensive or spreading in spite of conservative treatment or if the cooperation of the patient in regard to limitation of activity cannot be obtained.

59 – 13. LYMPHATIC SYSTEM EMERGENCIES

Lymphangitis. Uncontrolled infection in an extremity, frequently of streptococcal origin, will cause involvement of the lymphatics and adjacent blood vessels. The condition is identified by pain, tenderness, swelling and characteristic superficial red streaks in the involved extremity.

TREATMENT

1. Antibiotics, broad spectrum or penicillin.

2. Moist heat and hypertonic solutions such as magnesium sulfate locally.

3. Rest and elevation of the extremity.

4. Analgesics.

Obstruction. Enlargement of lymph nodes secondary to various types of pathology may cause acute obstruction of the superior vena cava or extrahepatic bile ducts. Treatment is primarily surgical. Lymph fluid may clot if stagnant for long periods.

59 – 14. RAYNAUD'S PHENOMENA AND REFLEX NEUROVASCULAR SYNDROME

In this condition, severe vascular spasm – usually in the distal upper extremities – is associated with uncomfortable paresthesias, pain, pallor of the fingers during the arteriospasm phase, cyanosis during the venospasm phase and then rubor and residual edema of digits (probably due to venospasm, diapedesis of proteins through capillary walls during the ischemic phase and clotting of lymph fluids in lymphatic channels). Trophic ulcers in edematous fingers and small areas of gangrene – usually at the tips of the fingers – may occur.

Precipitation of events by exposure to cold is characteristic. The idiopathic type (Raynaud's disease) occurs almost entirely in women. Numerous other causes of the reflex neurovascular syndrome (shoulder-hand syndrome) are associated with Raynaud's

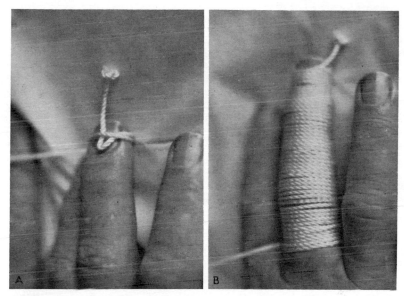

Figure 34. Technique of compressive centripetal wrapping. A, A small loop of string is placed over the fingernail before the first coil of the helix is turned. B, Firm, contiguous, centripetal wrapping is rapidly performed. Immediately upon completion of helix of desired length, the protruding distal lip of string is pulled and the total wrapping is removed centripetally. (From Cain, H. D., and Liebgold, H. B.: Arch. Phys. Med., Vol. 48, 1967.)

phenomenon (e.g., occlusive arterial disease, neurogenic lesions, trauma, collagen diseases).

Patients with these conditions may present themselves for emergency evaluation and treatment because of acute discomfort in hand and/or shoulder or because of presence of tender pregangrenous or gangrenous lesions.

TREATMENT

1. Mild sedation with phenobarbital, 15 to 30 mg. 4 times a day orally, or diazepan (Valium), 5 mg. orally 3 or 4 times a day.

2. Mild analgesics. Avoid narcotics.

3. Evaluate and treat any underlying contributing cause.

4. Avoid exposure to cold and improve body and extremity warmth with clothing.

5. Mild vasodilatation with tolazoline hydrochloride (Priscoline), 25 to 50 mg. orally 4 times a day.

6. Encourage full use of extremity – dystrophic changes and disability will ensue otherwise.

7. Reduction of discomfort, improved range of motion, healing of trophic ulcers and improved circulation occur with rapid reduction of edema in the digits by use of centripetal concentric compression. Ordinary string is wrapped *firmly* and rapidly from the distal to proximal portion of each edematous digit (Figure 34) and then removed *immediately,* in the same manner as removing a ring from a swollen finger. Place thin sterile gauze over any ulceration. Rewrap periodically until the edema is completely gone.

8. Stellate ganglion blocks may be of value.

9. Severe recurrent vasospastic events warrant referral for surgical consultation regarding sympathectomy.

60. VENEREAL DISEASES

60 – 1. CHANCRE (Hard Chancre)

This primary lesion of syphilis appears from 10 to 60 days (usually about 3 weeks) after exposure. No medication or treatment which might block the diagnosis should be prescribed, or be allowed to be applied, until a darkfield examination has been done. When the diagnosis of syphilis has been established treatment is as outlined in **60 – 5.** *Syphilis.*

60 – 2. CHANCROID (Soft Chancre)

No emergency treatment is indicated. The patient should be referred to his private physician or to a venereal disease clinic for care and should be warned against the local application of medications of any type, since this may block diagnosis by darkfield examination.

60 – 3. GONORRHEA For prophylaxis, see **60 – 6** and **60 – 7**

No matter what history is given by the patient, if a urethral discharge is present in a male, a smear should be taken by the attending

physician and stained and examined for the presence of gram negative intracellular diplococci. Additional smears and cultures should
be sent to a laboratory for examination. The same applies to females
with profuse whitish vaginal discharge, or who are suspected of
being asymptomatic carriers of infection. Cultures from the anus
and pharynx may be necessary in certain cases. If the clinical
picture and gram stain indicates gonorrhea, treatment should be
started without waiting for further confirmatory laboratory findings.

TREATMENT

1. Aqueous procaine penicillin G, 4.8 million units intramuscularly, plus probenicid (Benemid), 1 gm. orally. Patients who
are allergic to penicillin should be given oxytetracycline, 1.5 gm.
intramuscularly, followed by 0.5 gm. 4 times a day orally for 7 days.

2. General measures:

Support of the scrotum and contents by a suspensory or athletic
supporter.

Limitation of activity.

Intake of large amounts of fluids, avoiding alcoholic drinks of
all types.

3. Instruction to male patients to obtain further medical attention after 7 days even if the urethral discharge clears completely.
Female patients should be impressed with the need for gynecologic
care as soon as possible. The possibility of homosexual transmission
should always be kept in mind.

For prophylactic measures, see **60 — 6** and **60 — 7**.

Gonorrhea is a reportable disease (**10**).

60 — 4. LYMPHOPATHIA VENEREUM (Venereal Lymphogranuloma)

Formerly believed to be caused by a virus, this condition is now
known to be caused by obligate intracellular parasites called Chla-
mydiae which are spread by sexual contact.

SIGNS AND SYMPTOMS. Minute (often undemonstrable) lesions
at site of entry, development of enlarged lymphatic nodes ("bu-
boes") which may suppurate and become fistulous. Scarring and
stricture of the rectum may develop. Lymphopathia venereum is
a reportable disease (**10**).

TREATMENT

1. Instruction regarding sterilization of bedding, clothing, towels,
and dressings.

2. Tetracycline orally, 1 gm. initially, then 0.5 gm. every 6 hours.

3. Sulfadiazine, 1 gm. orally every 4 hours.

4. Arrangement for further medical care or reference to a public health clinic.

60 – 5. SYPHILIS

The reverse side of the standard Confidential Morbidity Form (**10**) *must* be completed on all cases.

PRIMARY LESIONS (Chancres) (See also **60 – 1**. Chancres)

These should not receive emergency treatment. The patient should be told not to apply any medication of any type but to report to his physician or to a venereal disease clinic as soon as possible for diagnosis and treatment. Primary cases are reportable (**10**). For treatment of established cases, see below (secondary lesions).

SECONDARY LESIONS

Secondary syphilitic lesions are reportable (**10**) and require energetic and prolonged treatment. As soon as the diagnosis has been established, one of the following intramuscular therapy regimens should be begun:

1. Benzathine penicillin G, 1.2 million units intramuscularly into each buttock (total 2.4 million units) immediately.

Or

2. Procaine penicillin G with 2% aluminum monostearate (PAM), 2.4 million units at once, followed by 1.2 million units every 3 days for 2 doses (total 4.8 million units).

Or

3. Aqueous procaine penicillin G, 600,000 units daily for 8 days (total 4.8 million units).

Oral administration of penicillin is not effective.

If the patient is allergic to the penicillins, a broad spectrum antibiotic such as erythromycin or tetracycline orally should be substituted, with a total dosage of 40 gm. given in divided doses every 6 hours over a period of 10 days (1 gm. every 6 hours for 10 days). If late syphilis or cardiovascular or neurosyphilis is present, the dose of broad spectrum antibiotic should be doubled, with careful follow-up, including spinal fluid examinations.

TERTIARY (LATE) SYPHILIS

Gastric Crisis in Tabes Dorsalis

This condition may simulate an acute surgical abdomen (**19**). Since the vomiting is of central origin, the usual antispasmodics and antinauseants are of little value.

Treatment

1. Put the patient to bed and give a retention enema prepared as follows:

> Chloral hydrate, 2 to 4 gm.
> Sodium bromide, 2 to 4 gm.
> Water to make 15 ml.

2. If step 1 does not give relief after 2 or 3 hours of observation, the patient should be hospitalized.

3. The use of opium derivatives or synthetic narcotics should be avoided in gastric crises because of their lack of efficacy and of the strong possibility of addiction. Pentazocine lactate (Talwin) intramuscularly in 30 mg. doses every 3 hours may give relief.

Lightning Pain in Tabes

Treatment

All types of therapy are symptomatic, empirical and often unsuccessful.

1. Penicillin, 1.2 million units, or tetracyclines intramuscularly, as outlined above.

2. Thiamine hydrochloride, 20 mg. intravenously.

3. Narcotics may be necessary but should be used with caution because of possible addiction. Codeine sulfate is the narcotic of choice. Pentazocine lactate (Talwin), 30 mg. slowly intravenously or intramuscularly is effective in some cases.

Paretic Mental Disturbances

These conditions may require hospitalization after temporary control of the patient by large doses of barbiturates and/or chloral hydrate. Physical restraint is often necessary until adequate sedation can be accomplished. Chlorpromazine hydrochloride (Thorazine), 50 to 100 mg. intramuscularly may assist in sedation.

Cardiovascular Syphilis

This late development is usually characterized by signs of aortic insufficiency or of ascending aortic aneurysm. Treatment consists of penicillin or broad spectrum antibiotics as outlined above, plus symptomatic and supportive care.

60–6.   PROPHYLAXIS AGAINST POSSIBLE EXPOSURE TO VENEREAL DISEASE

If facilities are available, the following immediate venereal prophylactic routine may be used for male patients.

1. Have the patient urinate.
2. Instruct the patient to wash the external genitalia thoroughly with soap and water.
3. Give penicillin, 2.4 million units intramuscularly, unless there is a history of sensitivity to penicillin, in which case a tetracycline or erythromycin should be substituted (**60–5**).
4. Instruct the patient to report to his physician or to a public venereal disease clinic for further care.

If facilities and time are not available for the procedure outlined above, the patient should be:

1. Referred to his physician for care.
2. Given the address of the closest public health prophylactic station.
3. Given tetracycline, 1 gm. orally.

Female patients should be instructed to obtain medical care at once. Penicillin, 2.4 million units (or tetracycline, 1 gm. orally if the patient is penicillin-sensitive), should be given intramuscularly, together with routine instructions for cleansing and douching.

60–7.   PROPHYLAXIS AFTER EXPOSURE TO KNOWN CASES

GONORRHEA

Patients known to have been exposed to gonorrhea in the ten days previous to examination should be given 2.4 million units of aqueous penicillin G intramuscularly or 1.5 gm. of oxytetracycline hydrochloride in a single oral dose.

SYPHILIS

A history of exposure to infectious syphilis in the 90 days previous to examination requires intramuscular administration of 2.4 million units of penicillin G benzathine. Large doses of tetracycline or erythromycin orally should be substituted if the patient is sensitive to penicillin.

61. VENOMS

SOURCE	LOCAL REACTION	TYPE OF SYSTEMIC TOXIC REACTION	SEVERITY OF SYSTEMIC REACTION	DANGEROUS TO LIFE?
Adder (**24–19.** *Snake Bites*)	Moderate	Hemolytic Neurotoxic	+++	Yes
Ants (except fire ants) (**24–1**)	Severe	Endothelial	+	Only to hypersensitive persons
Bee (**56–1**)	Moderate	Endothelial, histaminic,	+++ (Acute sensitivity common)	Yes – about ½ of fatalities from venoms are due to Hymenoptera
Black widow spider (**24–4**)	Severe pain for 10 to 15 minutes	Neurotoxic	++ to +++	Rarely fatal in adults unless an especially vascular part of body has been bitten; high mortality in children
Boomslang (**24–19.** *Snake Bites*)	Moderate	Hemotoxic	+++	Yes
Brown spider (**24–5**)	Blebs followed by sloughing	Necrotizing	++	Yes – a few fatalities have been reported
Bushmaster (**24–19.** *Snake Bites*)	Marked swelling	Hemolytic and neurotoxic	+++	Yes

SOURCE	LOCAL REACTION	TYPE OF SYSTEMIC TOXIC REACTION	SEVERITY OF SYSTEMIC REACTION	DANGEROUS TO LIFE?
Cantril (**24 — 19.** *Snake Bites*)	Swelling and discoloration	Hemolytic, neurotoxic and hemotonic	+++	Yes
Centipede	Moderate pain, swelling	Local irritant only	+	No
Cobra (**24 — 19.** *Snake Bites*)	Minimal	Hemolytic and neurotoxic	+++	Yes
Coelenterates	Nettle-like	Necrotizing, allergic	++	Yes — a few fatalities have been reported
Cone shells	Minimal	Not identified	+++	Yes — Stings of large varieties have been lethal
Copperhead (Highland moccasin) (**24 — 19.** *Snake Bites*)	Severe pain and swelling	Mixed hematoxic and neurotoxic	+++	Yes — death is caused by a curare-like paralysis (see **49 — 234**)
Coral	Moderate, lacerations heal slowly, prone to secondary infection	Not identified	+	No
Coral snake (harlequin snake) (**24 — 19.** *Snake Bites*)	Minimal	Neurotoxic	+++	Yes

Fer-de-lance (24–19. Snake Bites)	Severe local pain	Neurotoxic	+++	Yes
Fire ants (56–5)	Severe burning pain	Mixed—hemotoxic, cardiorespiratory depressant	++	Usually not. A few fatalities have been reported following massive stinging
Flea (24–10)	Varies in individuals	Anticoagulant—allergic reactions common	+	No
Frog [Kokoi frog (Colombia)]	Slight	Neurotoxic	+++	Yes—the deadliest venom known
Gila monster (24–11)	Severe	Hemotoxic	++	Yes—mortality rate is 1% in adults, 5% in small children
Hornets (56–6. Hymenoptera)	See Hymenoptera (below)		++	See Hymenoptera (below)
Hymenoptera (56–6)	Moderate to severe allergic reactions common	Histaminic, hemolytic, neurotoxic	++	Yes—about 1/2 of fatalities from venoms are due to Hymenoptera
Krait (24–19. Snake Bites)	Severe	Neurotoxic	+++	Yes
Marine snails	See Coneshells	(above)	++	Yes
Mosquito (24–16)	Varies, may be severe	Allergic, disease carrier (certain varieties)	+ to ++	No
Octopus	Slight	Neurovascular, respiratory depressant	++	Yes—A few fatalities have been reported

SOURCE	LOCAL REACTION	TYPE OF SYSTEMIC TOXIC REACTION	SEVERITY OF SYSTEMIC REACTION	DANGEROUS TO LIFE?
Rattlesnake (**24—19.** *Snake Bites*)	Marked swelling and discoloration	Mixed hematoxic, neurotoxic, and histaminic	+++	Yes – about 11% of reported rattlesnake bites are fatal
Sandflies (**62—18**)	Very slight	Febrile, acute arthralgic	++	No
Scorpion (**56—11**)	Usually numbness, rarely severe pain	Hemolytic neurotoxic	+++	Yes – high mortality rate in children under 1 year; adults generally survive
Sea snakes (**24—19.** *Snake Bites*)	Usually mild	Hematoxic, neurotoxic	+++	Yes – a few varieties are deadly
Sea urchins	Slight, nettle-like	Not identified	+	No
Sea wasps	Slight	Anaphylactic shock	+++	Yes
Stingray (**56—13**)	Severe, from penetration of spines	Neurotoxic, cardiotoxic	+++	Yes – particularly if the thoracic or abdominal wall has been penetrated
Stonefish	Severe; pain often almost unbearable	Anaphylactic, neurotoxic, respiratory depressant	+++	Yes – antivenin for some varieties is available

Tarantula (**24–21**)	Moderate to very severe, especially in children	None	++	No
Ticks (**24–22**)	Usually mild	Usually mild local reaction only, but ticks may transmit disease or cause paralysis	+ to +++	No – unless serious disease transmitted
Vipers (**24–19.** *Snake Bites*)	Severe	Hemotoxic	+++	Yes
Wasp (**56–6.** *Hymenoptera*)	See Hymenoptera (above)	See Hymenoptera (above)	+++	See Hymenoptera (above)
Water moccasin (cottonmouth, gapper, trapjaw) (**24–19.** *Snake Bites*)	Moderate pain and swelling	Mostly neurotoxic but some hemotoxic	+++	Yes
Water snakes (common type)	Moderate due to tooth marks	None	+	No
Wood ticks (certain varieties) (**24–22**)	None	Neurotoxic	+ to ++	Yes – progressive paralysis may cause death if tick is not completely removed. Serious disease may be transmitted
Yellow jackets (**56–6.** *Hymenoptera*)	See Hymenoptera (above)	See Hymenoptera (above)	+++	See Hymenoptera (above)

62.   VIRAL INFECTIONS

62—1.   ARBOVIRAL INFECTIONS (Arthropod-borne Viruses)

SYNDROMES

1. *Encephalitis* or meningoencephalitis caused by numerous viral strains:
Eastern equine.
Western equine.
St. Louis.
California.
Hong Kong.
Japanese B.
Russian spring-summer and diphasic meningoencephalitis.
Murray Valley (Australia).
2. *Dengue-like fevers* (**62—4**)—3 to 7 days' duration.
Colorado tick fever.
Sandfly fever (**24—18**).
Chikungunya and o'nyong nyong fevers (Africa).
3. *Hemorrhagic fevers*
Hemorrhagic fevers of South Asia, Crimea and Argentina.
Kyasanur Forest disease (India).
Yellow fever (**30—39**).
TREATMENT
No specific therapy is available. Antibiotics are of no value and should be used only in the presence of bacteriologic complications. Efficient symptomatic and supportive care is often effective.

62—2.   CHICKENPOX (Varicella) See **30—3.**

62—3.   COMMON COLD (See also **52—3.** *Coryza*)

SIGNS AND SYMPTOMS.   General malaise, coryza, sore throat and cough.
TREATMENT
Symptomatic only. The following measures may be advised, although the most effective measures (1 and 2) will rarely be carried out by the patient.
1. Bed rest.
2. Large amounts of fluids by mouth.

3. Acetylsalicylic acid (aspirin), 0.6 gm. orally every 4 hours

4 Mild sedation by small doses of barbiturates by mouth.

5. Phenylephrine hydrochloride (Neo-Synephrine) nose drops (0.25% buffered solution). Amphetamine (Benzedrine) inhalers may give temporary relief; however, excessive or prolonged use may result in rebound edema of the mucous membranes.

6. Any thick, syrupy cough mixture to allay throat tickling. Brown mixture and elixir terpin hydrate, with or without codeine sulfate or dihydrocodeinone bitartrate (Hycodan), are satisfactory. Vaporizers or aerosols may give subjective relief.

62 — 4. DENGUE (Dandy Fever, Breakbone Fever)

This acute but rarely fatal viral infection is transmitted by the Aedes mosquito. Although it is more common in tropical climates, it has been reported in temperate zones. The incubation period is 5 to 10 days.

SIGNS AND SYMPTOMS. Sudden rise in temperature — 39.4 to 40.6° C. (103 to 105° F.) associated with a slow pulse. There is usually an intense headache with general malaise and prostration, often associated with severe myalgia and arthralgia, especially of the muscles of the back. A cyanotic, blotchy appearance of the face and soreness behind the eyeballs with severe pain on eye movements are characteristic. There is usually generalized adenopathy with splenic enlargement and deferred appearance of a generalized morbilliform rash, usually starting on the back of the hands and feet. Leukopenia is usually present.

TREATMENT

1. Bed rest, preferably in a darkened room to minimize movements of the eyes.

2. Large doses of salicylates, with or without codeine, by mouth for headache and hyperpyrexia.

3. Calcium gluconate, 10 ml. of 10% solution intravenously for acute muscle and joint pain.

PROGNOSIS. Complete recovery in from 10 to 14 days. Hospitalization for careful nursing care may be necessary.

62 — 5. ENCEPHALITIS, ACUTE

Many conditions which have been reported as being due to infectious organisms are grouped together under this general heading (see **62 — 1.**) In addition, the following clinical entities are among those which may manifest themselves as encephalitis:

Chickenpox (**30 – 3**).
Measles (**30 – 15**).
Mumps (**30 – 17**).
Herpes simplex (**35 – 14; 62 – 9**).
Lymphopathia venereum (**60 – 4**).
Poliomyelitis (**30 – 21**).

Laboratory investigation is necessary to determine the etiology since, in general, all are characterized by high fever [often to 41° C. (106°F.)], general malaise, acute restlessness, severe headache, severe generalized myalgia and sometimes palsies.Delirium, convulsions (especially in children) and coma may be present.

Blood specimens for identification of viral strains must be refrigerated, packed in special containers and sent at once to a properly qualified laboratory.

TREATMENT

1. Tepid sponging to reduce fever.

2. Codeine sulfate, 0.03 gm., and acetylsalicylate acid (aspirin), 0.6 gm. by mouth for headaches.

3. Chloral hydrate, 0.5 to 1.0 gm. by mouth, repeated as necessary for adequate sedation.

4. Barbiturates, preferably sodium pentobarbital (Nembutal), 120 to 200 mg. intravenously for extreme restlessness or convulsions.

5. Immediate transfer to a hospital equipped for isolation and treatment.

62 – 6. FOOT AND MOUTH DISEASE (Aphthous Fever)

This is characterized by a moderate temperature elevation and the formation of vesicles on the buccal membrane of the mouth and between the fingers and toes. The acutely contagious virus may be transmitted from infected animals by milk and butter.

TREATMENT

Symptomatic only. Mouthwashes may be prescribed. Complete recovery within 2 weeks is to be expected.

62 – 7. GERMAN MEASLES (Rubella) See **30 – 24**

62 – 8. HEPATITIS

Two types are recognized:

Infective hepatitis. IH is characterized by an abrupt acute onset,

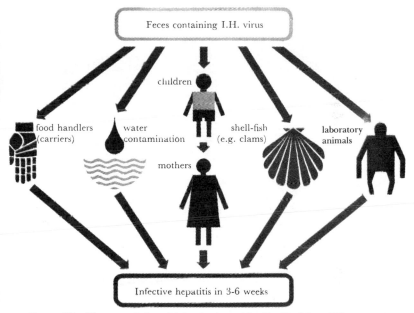

Figure 35. The transmission of infective hepatitis. (Modified from Abbottempo.)

usually with a high fever. It is transmitted by feces (Figure 35) and has an incubation period of 3 to 6 weeks.

TREATMENT

Immediate hospitalization. Hemorrhagic complications may be serious.

Homologous serum hepatitis. SH is transmitted by infected blood or plasma or by the use of inadequately sterilized instruments (Figure 36). This type is rarely encountered as an emergency because its onset is usually insidious, with an incubation period of 3 to 6 months.

TREATMENT

Hospitalization on a nonemergency basis for determination of the amount of liver damage, and appropriate symptomatic and supportive therapy.

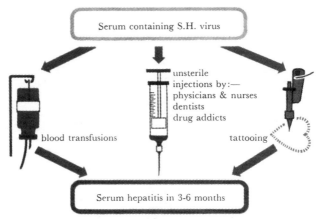

Figure 36. The transmission of serum hepatitis. (Modified from Abbottempo.)

62—9. HERPES SIMPLEX (See also 35—14. *Ophthalmic Herpes*)

All adults probably have latent infection. Vesicles may form when the body resistance is low for any reason, or after direct stimuli such as bright sunlight. Encephalitis (**62—5**) may be a serious complication, especially in children.

TREATMENT

Local application of zinc oxide ointment to prevent cracking and secondary infection, followed by referral to an internist or dermatologist for further care, is all that is required in most cases, unless the eyes are involved (**35—14**). Acute encephalitis (**62—5**) requires immediate hospitalization.

62—10. INFLUENZA (See also 30—11)

Incubation period. 1 to 5 days.

SIGNS AND SYMPTOMS. Sudden onset, usually with acute catarrhal symptoms and fever of 38.9 to 40.6°C. (102 to 105°F.) followed by severe, generalized myalgia, chest pain, marked pharyngitis and purulent bronchitis, often associated with sinusitis. In children, otitis media (**32—13**) may develop. Pneumonia, usually involving both lower lobes, may occur. Acute gastrointestinal symptoms may be present and the blood may show a leukopenia.

TREATMENT

1. Home care is usually possible except when a severe pneumonic process is indicated by clinical or x-ray examination.

2. Bed rest.

3. Large amounts of fluids, especially fruit juices, by mouth.

4. Soft diet.

5. Phenylephrine hydrochloride (Neo-Synephrine) nose drops (0.25% buffered solution).

6. Control of high fever by repeated sponging or application of cold compresses. These measures, with sedation by sodium pentobarbital (Nembutal) suppositories, are essential to prevent the development of convulsions or coma in children.

7. Antibiotics and sulfonamides have no effect on influenzal conditions and should be used only for associated bacterial infections.

62 – 11. INTERSTITIAL PNEUMONIA (Viral Pneumonia)
(See also 48 – 45. Pneumonia in Children)

The causative organism for acute interstitial pneumonia may be a filterable virus or an obligate intracellular parasite (30 – 41).

Incubation period. 10 to 14 days.

SIGNS AND SYMPTOMS. Insidious onset with systemic symptoms more marked than respiratory symptoms. Severe headaches and general malaise are usually present, with a slight intermittent temperature rise, usually not over 38.8°C. (102°F.). The pulse is relatively slow. Physical signs in the lungs are usually minimal but striking x-ray changes (increase in size of hilar shadow; soft, patchy infiltration, most marked near the hilum) are usually present. The white blood count is normal or decreased.

TREATMENT

1. Acetylsalicylic acid (aspirin), 0.6 gm., with or without codeine sulfate; or sodium salicylate, 1 gm., with sodium bicarbonate, orally every 4 hours for joint and muscle pain. If the myalgia is severe, 10 ml. of 10% calcium gluconate intravenously may give relief.

2. Large amounts of fluids by mouth or intravenously if the patient shows evidence of dehydration.

3. Tetracyclines or chloramphenicol if due to mycoplasma.

4. Oxygen therapy if dyspnea or cyanosis is present.

5. Ammonium chloride or dihydrocodeinone bitartrate (Hycodan) cough mixtures.

6. Bed rest at home is generally adequate. Hospitalization is rarely necessary.

PROGNOSIS. Complete recovery almost invaribly occurs. Complications are rare, although extreme weakness and lassitude may persist for several weeks.

62-12. MEASLES (Rubeola) See 30-15.

62-13. MUMPS (Epidemic Parotitis) See 30-17

62-14. MYOSITIS (Myofibrositis) See 44-57

62-15. PLEURODYNIA

Supposedly caused by a virus, pleurodynia may be encountered as an emergency because of the sudden onset of high fever associated with rapid breathing and acute chest pain. In children, acute abdominal pain may simulate a surgical emergency.

TREATMENT
1. Bed rest.
2. Codeine sulfate, 0.06 gm., and acetylsalicylic acid (aspirin), 0.6 gm. by mouth. Morphine sulfate in small doses subcutaneously may be necessary for relief of acute pain in older children and adults. Pentazocine lactate (Talwin), 15 to 30 mg. intramuscularly, often is effective for control of pain.
3. Because acute symptoms usually subside in 24 hours with recurrence within a few days, medical check-up during the quiescent period should be recommended.

62-16. POLIOMYELITIS (Infantile Paralysis, Heine-Medin Disease) See 30-21; 46-9. *Paralysis;* 48-49. *Respiratory Paralysis*

62-17. RABIES (Hydrophobia)

This acute infectious disease has been reported in badgers, bats (insectivorous and vampire types), cats, coons, coyotes, dogs, domestic farm animals, foxes, jackals, mongooses, skunks, squirrels, weasles, wildcats and wolves. It may be transmitted to human beings by:
1. A bite of a rabid animal.
2. Licking of any superficial abrasion of the skin by a rabid animal.

3. Contact of oral secretion from a patient suffering from rabies with any break in the attendant's skin.

4. Exposure to (possibly inhalation of) dust in caves infested with rabid or rabies-carrying bats.

Incubation period. Two weeks to 12 months, usually 15 days to 5 months.

SIGNS AND SYMPTOMS

1. Redness, swelling and pain around the healed scar at the point of entry.

2. Severe encephalitic symptoms – headache, insomnia, restlessness, irritability and increased sensitivity to stimuli.

3. Development in 2 or 3 days after the initial symptoms of an acute excitement stage characterized by extreme restlessness with intermittent maniacal outbursts, spasm of the muscles of deglutition and respiration, frothing of the mouth, bloody saliva and vomitus and slow rise in temperature to 41.7°C. (107°F.).

4. Terminal paralytic stage characterized by total exhaustion, coma and death from cardiac collapse.

TREATMENT

If there is no suspicion or proof that the animal is rabid, the treatment should consist of:

1. Local cleansing. Lacerations should be thoroughly washed with green soap and water, debrided, irrigated and sutured.

2. Administration of human tetanus immune globulin (TIG), 250 units intramuscularly. A booster injection of tetanus toxoid may be substituted or added if the patient gives a history of adequate active immunization (**16**).

3. Penicillin, 1.2 million units, intramuscularly followed by chlortetracycline (Aureomycin) or oxytetracycline (Terramycin), 250 mg., every 4 hours by mouth.

4. Immediate reporting of the incident to the proper local authorities for impounding, observation and possible postmortem examination of the animal. As a rule, impounded animals are kept under observation for 10 days; if they show no evidence of illness during this period, the danger of rabies is negligible. *The animal should never be destroyed* by the victim, his family or friends; if it has been killed, the body must be saved and turned over as soon as possible to the proper public health authorities.

If the animal is known to have, or suspected of having, rabies, treatment should consist of:

1. Thorough local cleansing of the wound with green soap and

water. Lacerations should be spread and the depths of the wound washed thoroughly. Puncture wounds should *not* be probed or extended surgically because of the danger of spreading the virus.

2. Administration of human tetanus immune globulin (TIG), 250 units. If the patient has been actively immunized in the past, a booster of tetanus toxoid should be given in addition to the human tetanus immune globulin (**16**).

3. Administration of hyperimmune serum (HIS), 55 units per kilogram (2.2 lb.) of body weight, and/or rabies vaccine (RV) as outlined below. Hyperimmune serum must be given as soon as possible; it has no effect after 72 hours.

TREATMENT OF ESTABLISHED RABIES

1. Transfer to a properly equipped hospital as soon as possible.

2. Give morphine sulfate, 15 to 30 mg., subcutaneously or intravenously *as often as necessary to control pain*. Respiratory assistance should be given as required.

3. Control convulsions and spasm by:

Ether, chloroform or ethyl chloride inhalations—to the point of coma if necessary.

Chloral hydrate, 1 to 3 gm. rectally.

Tribromoethanol (Avertin), 60 to 100 mg. rectally.

4. *All persons who come in contact with the patient must wear rubber gloves and observe extreme precautions*. The saliva, even if dry, is very infectious for 12 to 38 hours.

TREATMENT OUTLINE (See table on page 679).

PROGNOSIS. Rabies has a very high mortality rate if the disease has become established. Fortunately, the lag in the development of symptoms after exposure allows time for observation of the animal and laboratory proof of rabies by examination of the brain for Negri bodies. Recent development of a fluorescent-dye method by which rabies can be detected in animals in 15 minutes may allow more prompt and efficient management of suspected cases of rabies in the near future.

62−18. SANDFLY FEVER

This fever is caused by a virus transmitted to humans by sandfly bites. Its course is brief and never fatal.

SIGNS AND SYMPTOMS. Fever—usually not over 39.4°C. (103°F.) —lasting 3 to 4 days, and painful joints and muscles. The usual course is slow recovery of normal strength; weakness and lassitude often persist for several weeks.

TREATMENT OF RABIES

| TYPE OF EXPOSURE | CONDITION OF ANIMAL | | TREATMENT* |
	At Time of Exposure	After 10 Days' Observation	
Licking — skin intact	Rabid	Dead	RV daily × 14
Licking — abrasions present	Rabid	Dead	HIS daily × 2; RV daily × 14
	Healthy	Signs of rabies	Start RV at first sign
Bites other than of face and head	Healthy	Healthy	None
	Healthy	Signs or proof of rabies	Start RV at first signs
	Signs suggestive of rabies	Healthy	Start daily RV at once; discontinue on 5th day if animal is healthy
	Rabid, escaped, not identified, any wild animal	—	HIS daily × 2; RV daily × 14 to 21
Bites of face or Head	Healthy	Healthy	HIS daily × 2
	Signs suggestive of rabies	Healthy	HIS daily × 2; RV daily-discontinue on 5th day
	Rabid, escaped, not identified; any wild animal	—	HIS daily × 2; RV daily × 14 to 21

*HIS, Hyperimmune Serum; RV, Rabies Vaccine (Duck Embryo).
*A new rabies vaccine prepared in human diploid cells is still being tested and should be commercially available in the near future. It has the advantages of requiring only 2 to 3 daily injections instead of the 14 to 21 injections required by duck embryo rabies vaccine.

TREATMENT
1. Limited activity, preferably bed rest.
2. Copious fluids.
3. Local heat and codeine sulfate, 0.03 gm., and acetylsalicylic acid (aspirin), 0.6 gm., for myalgia. Severe cases may require intravenous injections of 10 ml. of 10% calcium gluconate solution.

62 — 19. SMALLPOX (Variola (See **30 — 30; 30 — 40.** *Common Exanthems*

62 — 30. YELLOW FEVER See **30 — 39**

63. WARTIME EMERGENCIES

In addition to combatant casualties, injuries and illnesses of varied types and severity may result among the civilian population during wartime. The results of food and water contamination, bombing of various types, blast injuries, bullet wounds, shrapnel injuries, effects of gases, bacterial and viral infections, burns, concussions, contusions, dislocations, fractures, infectious and contagious diseases, lacerations, effects of radioactivity, stress-induced psychiatric symptoms and aggravation of preexistent conditions could conceivably require the best possible treatment in the shortest possible time. When tremendous numbers of casualties occur, as in area saturation bombing or nuclear blasts, on-site treatment must of necessity be restricted to the simplest possible effective procedures with removal of the victims to a safe area for definitive care as soon as possible.

In wartime, emergency treatment and management of many conditions will vary in important details from that outlined in previous sections in this book. The most important points are summarized in the following paragraphs.

63 — 1. BACTERIAL OR VIRAL INFECTIONS (Biological Warfare)

In spite of highly publicized and supposedly sacred covenants between nations, inoculation of the population in a given area through bombing or sabotage is always a possibility during war-time. It is impossible to outline in advance any emergency procedures to cope with such a situation. However, the well-known public health principles applicable to any epidemic should be put into effect as soon as possible. These principles are segregation of cases, decontamination and symptomatic treatment, followed by specific therapy and preventive inoculations as soon as the causative organisms have been identified and their sensitivities determined.

Decrease in resistance of the body to infection may also be expected to occur following mass or nuclear bombing or other wartime emergencies. Interference with normal sleep, poor food, extreme fatigue and mental strain may also contribute to this morbid picture.

63 – 2.   BLAST INJURIES

Direct blast effects usually consist of multiple massive contusions of the lungs and are characterized by dyspnea, cyanosis and unconsciousness. External signs of trauma may be completely absent. Cardiac contusion cases may be in shock (**53**) or show marked bradycardia and irregularities.

TREATMENT

1. Insurance of an adequate airway.

2. Administration of oxygen under positive pressure by face mask or endotracheal catheter and rebreathing bag. Mouth-to-mouth methods of artificial respiration (**11 – 1**) may be necessary while awaiting mechanical facilities or when such facilities are not available in sufficient quantity.

3. Strong coffee or tea by mouth or injection of caffeine sodiobenzoate, 0.5 gm. intramuscularly.

4. Treatment of shock (**53 – 7**). Administration of excessive amounts of fluids should be avoided because of the danger of development of pulmonary edema (**51**).

5. Transfer from the disaster site for definitive care as soon as possible.

Indirect blast effects are caused by striking, or being struck by, objects and are similar to those encountered in industry, automobile accidents, explosions or in the home. Although therapy may of necessity have to be modified by lack of supplies and properly trained personnel, the best emergency treatment possible under the circumstances should be administered, with arrangements for evacuation as soon as possible to an area where more thorough care can be given.

63 – 3. EXPLOSIVE AND FIRE BOMBS

These may cause many casualties if employed in saturation or area bombing. The types of injuries to be expected are the same as given under blast injuries (**63 – 2**) and nuclear bombs (**63 – 4**), except that the effects of radioactivity (**63 – 4**) would not be present.

63 – 4. NUCLEAR (Atomic, Hydrogen) BOMBS

Although nuclear bombs have been characterized as "just bigger and better bombs," certain effects resulting from ionizing radiation are peculiar to them. If an atomic or hydrogen bomb is exploded at a considerable distance above the earth's surface, gamma rays and, under certain circumstances, neutrons may cause serious and fatal injury. Extreme thermal radiation also may cause flash burns (**25 – 14**) as well as secondary burns. If the fireball comes in contact with the earth's surface, the blast and thermal effects are decreased, but the ground or water is contaminated with fission products. Radioactive fallout, although it may have serious delayed effects, is not an urgent emergency problem in the ordinary sense; however, determination of the intensity of radioactive contamination is essential for estimating prognosis.

Blast injuries, if direct (**63 – 2**), need no practical consideration following nuclear bombing, since any person close enough to be injured by blast pressure would undoubtedly be killed by other effects. For indirect blast injuries, see **63 – 2.**

Ionizing radiation effects may be caused by:

Alpha rays, emitted by unfissioned bomb residue containing plutonium or uranium. If even small amounts of an alpha-emitting substance are deposited in the bones, under certain circumstances serious damage may occur from long-term bombardment of tissues.

Beta rays, emitted from fission products. Although they are relatively nonpenetrating as compared with gamma rays, the products by which they are emitted may enter the body through inhalation, ingestion or through a break in the skin. Many of these products have the same tendency as alpha rays to localize in the bones and cause severe signs and symptoms, often delayed, through constant bombardment.

Gamma rays, liberated for only a few seconds after a high air burst and similar in effect to a high energy x-ray machine. Their range in air varies directly with the size of the bomb, and they may be lethal for several miles from the point of explosion. These rays have a tremendous penetrating power and are the most important causative factor in radiation injuries.

Neutrons, formed by the combination of a positively charged proton and an electron. These particles have a relatively short range as compared with gamma rays; their chief importance is that, on striking the surface of the earth, they may cause fission products which emit beta or gamma rays. Persons relatively close to a nuclear blast may be shielded by a barrier from gamma rays but may develop acute symptoms from neutron exposure.

63 – 5. EVALUATION AND TREATMENT OF RADIATION INJURIES

The distance from the exploding bomb and the measurement of the amount of radiation exposure have been considered as possible criteria for determining the need for, and extent of, treatment. Too many variables are involved to make either method alone practical, but a combination of this information with the tempo of the effects and the clinical picture is a feasible method by which radiation injuries can be divided into 3 groups:

Supralethal doses of radiation. In these cases survival is improbable.

SIGNS AND SYMPTOMS

1. Development of persistent severe vomiting not more than 2 hours after exposure, followed by high fever, diarrhea, tenesmus and dehydration.

2. Rapid development of extreme prostration, with death in a few hours or days.

TREATMENT

Treatment of this group of cases, based on the hope that temporary support of life might conceivably result in regeneration of damaged tissues, would be prolonged and expensive and require large amounts of supplies and drugs which could be better utilized in treatment of persons with greater chances of survival. Therefore, refusal of treatment to persons receiving supralethal doses of radiation might be necessary. If treatment of this category of patients were decided upon, transfer from the disaster site to an adequately equipped hospital would be necessary. If by use of sedatives and antispasmodics and by maintenance of fluid balance (6) the patient could be kept alive for 10 to 12 days, it would be possible (although not probable) that recovery might take place. A relatively small percentage of cases would fall into this group because of the more rapid lethal blast and thermal effects.

Sedation. Any available barbiturates can be used, preferably those with a relatively prolonged effect, such as phenobarbital. Paraldehyde, chloral hydrate and bromides also may be of value, as may any of the numerous tranquilizer drugs.

Control of nausea and vomiting

1. Chlorpromazine hydrochloride (Thorazine), 25 to 50 mg. by mouth or intramuscularly.

2. Prochlorperazine dimaleate (Compazine), 5 to 10 mg. by mouth.

3. Meclizine hydrochloride (Bonine), 25 mg., in tablets or chewing gum.

4. Atropine sulfate, 0.5 to 1.0 mg. subcutaneously or intravenously 3 times a day.

5. Adiphenine hydrochloride (Trasentine), 30 mg. with or without phenobarbital; 20 mg. by mouth 3 to 4 times a day.

6. Amphetamine sulfate (Benzedrine) or dextroamphetamine sulfate (Dexedrine), 5 mg. 3 to 4 times daily by mouth.

7. Pyridoxine hydrochloride (Vitamin B_6), 50 to 100 mg. orally 3 to 4 times daily, or 25 to 50 mg. intravenously.

Cardiovascular support

1. Ephedrine sulfate, 50 mg., by mouth 3 times a day, or 25 to 30 mg. in 500 to 1000 ml. of 5% dextrose in saline or water intravenously.

2. Levarterenol bitartrate (Levophed) intravenously or metaraminol bitartrate (Aramine) intramuscularly or intravenously.

Fluid and electrolyte replacement (6)

1. Saline and other fluids – by mouth if possible. One level teaspoonful of table salt and ½ teaspoonful of baking soda dissolved in 1000 ml. of water makes a satisfactory hypotonic solution for oral use.

2. Sodium bicarbonate, 1000 ml. of 2% solution by rectum per day.

3. Saline or Ringer's solution intravenously if supplies and equipment are available.

Potentially lethal doses of radiation. Survival of members of this group of patients will depend to a great extent upon adequate medical care. The clinical picture of potentially lethal dosage is as follows:

1. Nausea and vomiting coming on within a short time (usually within 2 hours) of exposure.

2. Spontaneous cessation of vomiting within 24 hours.

3. An asymptomatic period of 1 to 3 weeks.

4. Late (after 1 to 3 weeks) development of severe infections, purpura, epilation, oral and cutaneous lesions and bloody diarrhea.

TREATMENT

The only emergency treatment indicated is that aimed at the acute symptoms of the first few hours – sedatives, antispasmodics and fluid replacement (**6**).

Sublethal doses of radiation. Symptoms and signs of this group will, in general, be the same as for potentially lethal doses of radiation (above), except that:

1. There will usually be no vomiting on the day of exposure.

2. Late symptoms will be much milder or may not appear at all.

3. The late development of a leukopenia may be the only clinical evidence of radiation damage.

TREATMENT

No emergency treatment is known which will influence the development or severity of late symptoms in any way.

Do Not

1. Waste whole blood, plasma, plasma volume expanders or intravenous fluids as emergency supportive measures in this group of patients, unless other associated conditions make their use imperative. Replacement fluids (**6**) should not be given intravenously if oral or rectal administration is practical. Increased bleeding tendencies and decreased resistance to infection may make any type of hypodermic administration hazardous.

2. Administer antibiotics. They will be far more beneficial in treatment of other conditions.

3. Prescribe corticosteroids; they do no good and possibly may do harm.

63 – 6. THERMAL EFFECTS

Burns of all degrees and extent, often associated with other severe injuries, may follow a nuclear blast. Except for napalm burns (**25 – 20**) and phosphorus burns (**25 – 22**), these burns differ in no way from those encountered in civilian emergency practice (**25; 48 – 14.** *Burns in Children*).

TREATMENT

Through instruction of Civilian Defense units and stockpiling of supplies, the following method of management would seem to be practical:

1. Treat shock (**53 – 7**). Whenever possible, hypotonic solution should be given by mouth, supplemented if necessary by plasma volume expanders intravenously (**6**). As much as 10 liters (quarts) of hypotonic solution, prepared by dissolving 1 level teaspoonful of table salt (sodium chloride) and ½ teaspoonful of baking soda (sodium bicarbonate) in 1000 ml. (1 quart) of water, can be given orally to severe burn cases during a 24 hour period.

2. Cut off or remove soiled or charred clothing.

3. Cleanse gently with soap and water and a weak detergent solution after administration of anodynes or narcotics if pain is severe. No debridement should be attempted and no antiseptic or disinfectant solutions should be used.

4. Apply a securely anchored sterile dressing. This may consist of petrolatum gauze or a similar material if available, or of a simple type of dry dressing stockpiled in many localities. This dressing consists of a large cellulose pad faced with fine mesh gauze which is applied directly to the burned surface and held in place with bandage or adhesive. With this method, elastic pressure bandages are not necessary.

5. Fasten burn dressings so that slipping will not take place. Although the original dressing may become discolored from serous drainage, it should not be disturbed for at least 1 week unless evidence of gross infection is present.

6. *Do not* apply any of the following substances to burns of any degree or extent:

Alcoholic preparations of any type.

Aluminum powder.

Antibiotic solutions, salves, ointments or creams.

Boric, picric or tannic acid.

Butter, grease, lard, paraffin or wax.

Gentian violet or other dyes.

Proprietary burn salves, creams or lotions.

Silver nitrate solutions.

7. Limit motion of the burned areas by splinting or slings whenever possible.

8. Arrange for disposition of cases:

Hospitalize if:

More than 25% of the body surface of an adult is involved (**25 – 1**). For children, see **48 – 14**.

Less than 25% of the body area is involved (**25 – 1**), but the eyes, eyelids, nose, mouth, respiratory tract, genitalia or feet are severely damaged.

Other severe injuries are present.

Arrange for ambulatory care for all other burn cases (**25**).

63 – 7.   BULLET WOUNDS

On-site treatment should be limited to insurance of an adequate airway, respiratory assistance (**11 – 1**) and control of hemorrhage (**42 – 1**) and shock (**53 – 7**), with transfer as soon as possible to a hospital equipped for definitive care.

63 – 8.   BURNS See **25; 48 – 14.** *Burns in Children;* **63 – 6.** *Nuclear Bomb Thermal Effects*

63 – 9.   FRACTURES AND DISLOCATIONS (See also **44.** *Musculoskeletal Disorders*)

Under wartime conditions reduction of fractures or dislocations should not be attempted unless evidence of acute circulatory embarassment or nerve pressure is conclusive. The injured part should if possible be splinted in a position of minimal discomfort, pain controlled and evacuation arranged. Open fractures should be protected by a sterile dressing and given prophylaxis against tetanus (**16**) if necessary. No sulfonamide powder, antibiotic powder or ointment of any kind should be applied to any open fracture. Oral or parenteral antibiotics should be given only if a delay of more than 6 hours before definitive treatment can be obtained is anticipated.

63 – 10.   MEDICAL EMERGENCIES

In wartime many chronic medical conditions can be aggravated by physical and mental stress and require emergency care. Poor food, nervous strain, exposure, prolonged excitement and overexertion can trigger disabling, sometimes fatal, increases in symptoms primarily caused by preexistent metabolic disorders, infections and other chronic conditions. Even small doses of ionizing radiation will cause decreased general body resistance with the usual complications.

It has been estimated that about 2% of all casualties following a major wartime catastrophe would involve known or latent diabetics. Persons requiring insulin would be furnished enough to control their condition so that they could be evacuated from the disaster area. The dosage of insulin can be calculated accurately enough by the Benedict urine test:

Benedict Test	Units of Regular Insulin
Blue (negative)	None
Green (1 plus)	5
Yellow (2 plus)	10
Orange (3 plus)	15
Red (4 plus)	20

Clinitest and Acetest strips also can be used to determine the severity of diabetes and the amount of insulin necessary.

63 – 11. POISON GASES (Chemical Warfare)

If in violation of world-wide international covenants chemical warfare is ever used again, it is probable that phosphate ester "nerve gases" will almost completely supplant lacrimators, pulmonary irritants, irritant smokes and vesicants (**49 – 832.** *War Gases*). All of the "nerve gases" are strongly cholinesterase-inhibiting and result in profound stimulation of the parasympathetic nervous system. For treatment, see **49 – 546.** *Organic Phosphates.*

63 – 12. SPRAINS AND STRAINS (See also **44 – 60.** *Sprains*)

Mass casualties represent the only valid indication for treatment of damaged ligaments and adjacent structures by immediate infiltration with a local anesthetic. Control of pain by this procedure will often allow ambulatory evacuation, even in severe sprains of the lower extremities or back, but may result in serious permanent disabilitiy from laxity of ligamentous structures.

For routine treatment of sprains and strains, see **44 – 60.** *Sprains* and topics treating of the part of the body involved.

ADMINISTRATIVE, CLERICAL AND MEDICOLEGAL PRINCIPLES AND PROCEDURES

64. ABANDONMENT

64—1. ACCEPTANCE OF PATIENTS

Legally, no physician is compelled to respond to any emergency call or undertake emergency examination or treatment in any situation whatever, just as he is not compelled legally to respond to any other request for services. Theoretically, he need give no explanation for his refusal to render aid or to accept responsibility. However, once he has given advice (even by telephone) or has examined or treated the patient, the physician-patient relationship has been established. From then on he is responsible for the patient's care until his responsibility has been shifted to another physician either by the original attendant or by the patient or his agents.

Ethically, certain situations may arise in which refusal to establish the physician-patient relationship might result in social and professional criticism in spite of the generally accepted precept incorporated in the Principles of Medical Ethics — "A physician may choose who he will serve." The three situations most commonly encountered in which it is unethical to refuse treatment are:

1. **If no other medical help is available.** This situation occurs most often in traffic accident cases and has been clarified in many localities by "Good Samaritan" laws which specify that a physician giving on-site emergency treatment (which must conform with accepted methods) need not continue with the care of the patient unless he so desires. The physician does have the responsibility, however, of seeing that the injured person is turned over to a law enforcement officer, ambulance attendant or other responsible person.

2. **If assistance in an emergency is requested.** Unfortunately, no absolute precise definition of what constitutes an "emergency" has ever been established. The previous concept (that an emergency consists of an unforeseen condition requiring immediate medical care to save life or preserve function) has been modified and expanded by judicial interpretation in different areas in different and conflicting ways. In addition, there is often a considerable discrepancy between the view of lay persons (including patients) and physicians as to what constitutes an "emergency" case.

Refusal of a request for medical care must be based on a definite reason, which can be substantiated later if necessary — for instance, physical (or mental) impairment of the physician — or previous professional commitments. Referral of the patient to another physician may not be adequate justification; neither may specialization be claimed on the part of the physician — in the patient's mind a doctor is a doctor and he expects help.

No person who reports to an emergency department should be refused advice or treatment — the act of coming to the emergency department constitutes a request for treatment.

Requests for emergency care may be made by the injured or ill individual in person or by telephone or by someone else in his behalf. If any questions regarding the patient's complaints or condition are asked by the physician (or by his nurse or other representative) and any recommendations given, or treatment prescribed, a physician-patient relationship has been established which can be terminated only by specific notification (**64−2**).

3. **If refusal of treatment constitutes abandonment.** Social censure, criticism and condemnation and civil lawsuit can follow refusal of a physician to give further advice or treatment to a person with whom a physician-patient relationship is in effect, provided the patient has a genuine need for the attention he requests.

64−2. PREVENTION OF POSSIBLE LEGAL ACTION

Failure of the attending physician to take reasonable steps to complete specific arrangements for follow-up care after emergency treatment and to stress the possible ill-effects of lack of such care may constitute a basis for legal action by the patient (or his natural or legal guardians) on the grounds of abandonment. A practical method of prevention of this type of claim consists of sending the patient (or his legal guardian) a brief letter explaining the need for further medical care and outlining the possible consequences of lack of care. This letter should be sent by registered mail, with return receipt requested. A copy of this letter and the return receipt (or the undelivered original letter) should be made a part of the patient's permanent record. As an added protection the following form (Instructions for Follow-Up Care) has been found to be of value, especially in clinics, offices and stations where large numbers of emergency cases are treated. This form should be completed in duplicate. The original should be given to the patient when emergency care is completed and the copy placed in the patient's record.

INSTRUCTIONS FOR FOLLOW-UP CARE

The examination and treatment which you have received has been on an emergency basis only and has not been intended to be a substitute or replacement for complete medical care. For your protection, I hereby suggest that in order to prevent possible complications you follow the recommendations checked below:

☐ Telephone your private physician for an appointment

on_____
(Date)

☐ Report at once to your private physician.

☐ Report at once to_____Hospital.

☐ Telephone for an appointment in the_____

Clinic at_____on_____
(location)   (date)

☐ Report back to this Emergency Department on_____

_____at   A.M.
(date)   P.M.

☐ Other (specify)_____

Date_____   Signed_____M.D.

---

65.   CERTIFICATES

65-1. BIRTH CERTIFICATES

The signature of the attending physician (or licensed midwife in some localities) in black permanent ink is required on all certificates covering live births and stillbirths.

For uniformity in reporting to public agencies, the following criteria are in general use:

65 – 2. LIVE BIRTH

Any infant born at any age, which after birth shows any sign of life, even momentarily (heart beat, impulse in cord or respiratory activity).

65 – 3. PREMATURE BIRTH

Any infant under 2500 gm. (5½ lbs.) in weight, regardless of length or age.

65 – 4. STILLBIRTH

Any infant born dead (no heart beat, impulse in cord or respiratory activity) and weighing 1000 gm. (2 lb. 3 oz.) or more regardless of length or age.

65 – 5. ABORTION

Any infant born dead and weighing under 1000 gm. (2 lbs. 3 oz.), regardless of length or age.

65 – 6. DEATH CERTIFICATES

Whenever an infant weighing 2500 gm. or more shows signs of life (**65 – 2**), even momentarily, both a birth certificate (**65 – 1**) and a death certificate must be completed and signed by the attending physician or coroner. Abortions (**65 – 5**) do not require completion of any certificate; however, a notation must be made in the emergency record and signed by the attending physician.

A death certificate must be completed within a given time (usually 15 or 24 hours) on every death case, no matter what the cause. For detailed information regarding coroner's (medical examiner's) responsibility, see **3 – 5**.

66. EMERGENCY CASE RECORDS

In many instances, legal actions against physicians and hospitals are based upon incidents alleged to have occurred at the time of initial emergency treatment (**68.** *Malpractice*). Therefore, to protect the physician and hospital as well as the patient, meticulous care should be used in completion, filing and safekeeping of detailed accurate, legible records on all emergency cases.

66 – 1. EMERGENCY CHARTS, CARDS OR SHEETS

A detailed record of each emergency case interviewed, examined and/or treated should be written and signed (not initialed) by the attending physician as soon as possible after the patient is seen.

The record on each case should be written legibly in ink and should contain the following information:

Chief complaints. What brings the patient in?

History of onset

1. Illness – duration, type of onset, chronological development of symptoms, previous attacks.

2. Injuries – When? Where? How? Previous injuries, including possible aggravation by present incident.

Physical findings. Temperature, respiration, pulse and blood pressure should be recorded in severe cases or when shock or evidence of infection is present. Neurologic examination should be done whenever the history or findings suggest possible head, spinal cord or peripheral nerve injury; other special examinations (orthopedic or urologic) may be indicated. Negative as well as positive findings should be recorded.

X-rays. The attending physician's interpretation of any films should be recorded (**18**). Careful examination of the wet films generally will disclose any pathology present. A confirmatory reading by a roentgenologist should be obtained as soon as possible.

Laboratory results. The results of any laboratory tests performed by, under the direction of, or by order of the attending physician should be recorded.

Diagnosis or impression. Whenever possible, a specific diagnosis should be given. If this is not possible, the impression or working diagnosis can be used. "Deferred" *should never be used.*

TREATMENT

1. Medications administered or prescribed.

2. Therapy for shock – time, type and amount.

3. Splints – type, time applied.

4. Supportive measures – artificial respiration, analeptics, oxygen.

5. Gastric lavage – with what? Results?

6. Tourniquet—time applied and removed.
7. Surgical repair—anesthesia, number and type of sutures.
8. Immunizing or prophylactic procedures.
9. Antibiotics.
10. Instructions regarding home treatment, with number of doses of medication prescribed.

Disposition

1. Sent home? How? With whom? At what time?
2. Referred? To whom? (Specify name and address of physician.) A follow-up care form (**64-2**) should be completed in duplicate and the original given to the patient. The duplicate copy should be made a part of the patient's record.
3. Hospitalized? Where? At what time? By private car or ambulance?

If the patient and/or his family or legal guardian refuses to follow the advice of the attending physician regarding disposition or treatment, it should be explained in the presence of witnesses that the attending physician will not be responsible for further developments. The patient (or the parents or guardian) should be given a "Release from Responsibility" form (**66-3**) to sign. This should be witnessed by 2 persons over 18 years of age (*not* by the attending physician) and should be made a part of the patient's record. Refusal to sign the "Release from Responsibility" form should be indicated by a witnessed note to that effect in the record.

As further protection for the physician whose advice has been refused, a letter specifying that the patient-physician relationship has been severed and that further medical care should be obtained elsewhere should be sent as soon as possible to the last known address of the patient (or his guardian). This letter should be sent by registered mail, with return receipt requested. A copy, together with the returned receipt (or the undelivered original letter), should be incorporated in the patient's record.

Estimated temporary disability. This information is often necessary for completion of insurance forms. Whenever the patient is told by the physician to discontinue work (housework or in industry), it should be indicated as:

Estimated Temporary Disability (ETD) .... (days, weeks, months).

All emergency records *must* be signed by the attending physician with his full name. Initials only should never be used.

66 – 2. EMERGENCY CASE LOG

In those offices, admitting departments, stations or wards which handle emergency cases, a current and chronologic emergency log should be kept by clerical or nursing personnel in addition to the records or charts completed by the attending physician. This log should be a permanent record, typed or written in ink, and should contain the following information:

Classification code (private, industrial, insurance coverage).
Date and time registered.
Name in full, including middle initial (if no middle initial, indicate as N.M.I.). If the patient is a minor, the legal guardian's name, address and telephone number should be given.
Address and telephone number.
Date of birth (if not known, indicate apparent age).
Sex.
Brought for emergency care by (self, family, guardian, friends, police, ambulance).
Brought from (home, address, site of accident, name of hospital).
Type of case (pediatric, surgical, medical, obstetric, undetermined).
Diagnosis. If a specific diagnosis has not been given on the medical record by the examining physician, the working or symptom diagnosis should be entered. "Deferred" *should never be used.*
Treatment, in brief.
Disposition – home, to work, hospitalized, referred (to whom?).
Condition – good, fair, poor, critical, deceased.
Time discharged from emergency care.
Out by (self, friends, ambulance).
Follow-up care – specific instructions.
Name (not initials), of the attending physician.

66 – 3. RELEASE FROM RESPONSIBILITY

Occasionally a patient, or his guardian, will refuse to follow the recommendations for treatment or disposition made by the examining physician. In cases of this type a "Release from Responsibility" form (page 697) should be signed by the patient (or his natural or legal guardian) in the presence of 2 witnesses. This signed and witnessed release should be made a permanent part of the emergency record.

66 – 4. UNUSUAL OCCURRENCE REPORTS

Emergency practice is prone to unusual occurrences because of the types of cases which are handled. Any incidents which fall into any of the following categories should be covered by a detailed note

---

RELEASE FROM RESPONSIBILITY
(*Cross out portions which do not apply*)

Date_____Time_____ m.

I hereby certify that of my own free will I am removing my

_____ _____ _____from the
(self, son, daughter, husband, wife, ward)

_____
(Office, Clinic, Hospital)

against the recommendation and advice of_____ _____M.D.,
and that I am hereby refusing further examination, tests, and
treatment. I hereby acknowledge that I have been informed of, and
understand, the possible consequences of such removal and/or refusal. Having full knowledge of the risks involved, and realization of
the dangers that may result from removal of the patient and/or refusal of recommended examination, tests, and treatment, I hereby

agree to hold the_____ _____ _____
(Office, Clinic, Hospital)

and____ _____ _____, M.D.

and all others concerned blameless and free from any and all liability
for any direct or indirect injuries or ill-effects which may result by
reason of removal of the patient, and/or refusal of examination,
tests, and treatment.

Witness_____ ____Signed_____ _____

Witness_____ ____   Relationship to Patient___ _____
                                    (self, mother, father, husband,
                                    wife, guardian)

---

made in the patient's record and by an entry in the emergency log
(**66 – 2**).

Omission, incorrect administration or improper dosage of any
drug or medication ordered or prescribed by the attending physician.

Incidents which cause, or which might be construed as causing,
bodily injury to a patient or other persons.

Serious reactions caused by drugs or other substances administered or prescribed in the treatment of emergency conditions.

Accidents, breaks in technique or unusual incidences during examination and/or treatment.

Incidents occurring in the entrance to or on the property or grounds of the emergency station, office, clinic, ward or hospital, which might be construed as causing or contributing to mental or physical suffering or injury−direct or indirect−to a patient or visitor. (Injuries to emergency personnel or police officers are covered under the compensation acts and require the usual industrial form [75−2].)

Loss or alleged loss of clothing, money, jewelry or other personal effects.

Complaints of any nature made by a patient or visitor−no matter if trivial or apparently unsubstantiated.

66−5. PERMITS AND AUTHORIZATIONS See **69**

66−6. DEATH CASES See **3**

66−7. SUBROGATION (Liability) **Cases** See **67**

66−8. WORKMEN'S COMPENSATION (Industrial) **Cases** See **75**

67. LIABILITY AND SUBROGATION CASES

Many of the cases treated as emergencies result from direct or indirect trauma (assault, auto accidents, railroad wrecks, industrial accidents) which may be the basis for future litigation of considerable complexity; therefore, it is the responsibility of the attending physician to see that *on first examination* all evidences of injury are noted in detail on the patient's chart. These include superficial contusions, abrasions and lacerations, as well as more serious injuries. The exact location and severity (slight, moderate, severe) should be noted in detail on the emergency record.

X-rays should be taken whenever necessary to establish, confirm or rule out traumatic, preexistent or other relevant conditions (18−1).

Any evidence of or tests for any degree of intoxication from alcohol, narcotics or other drugs should be entered on the clinical record with enough detail to refresh the physician's memory in case he should be required to testify in court at a later date.

68. MALPRACTICE

68−1. NEGLIGENCE

Malpractice actions against physicians are usually based on allegations of negligence. In order to prove negligence, the complainant must, as a rule, present evidence concerning the following points (sometimes referred to as the *Four D's*):

Duty. The existence of a physician-patient relationship (**64−1**) assumes a duty of the physician toward the patient.

Dereliction of duty. See **68−3**.

Direct causation. An unbroken chain of causation from the derelict act, or acts, to the condition of which the patient complains must be proved.

Damage. Proof of general damages (pain, suffering, physical dysfunction or disfigurement) and/or special damages (loss of earnings, medical and hospital expenses, necessary travel and other indirect costs) must be presented.

Negligence may consist of:

Omission of proper and recognized methods of examination and treatment.

Commission of improper, unauthorized, experimental or non-recognized methods of examination or treatment. Application of the legal doctrine of *res ipsa loquitur* may result in inference of actionable negligence from the fact of injury itself, without corroborating medical evidence. Malpractice action for assault may be based on alleged lack of informed consent (**69−15**) on the part of the patient.

68−2. STATUTES OF LIMITATION

This rule varies in different jurisdictions, but generally statutes of limitation run from the time that the patient becomes aware of the damaging incident, not from the date of the procedure.

68 – 3. STANDARDS OF CARE IN EMERGENCY CASES

The criteria by which proper and recognized methods of examination and treatment are determined have changed markedly during the last few years. Formerly the general ("Locality") rule was usually stated as follows: "A physician is required to exercise or use such reasonable and ordinary care, skill and diligence as a physician in good standing in the same area in the same general line of practice, ordinarily used in like cases." At the present time the same standards of knowledge, skill and experience are applied to a general practitioner in a remote rural area as to a specialist in a sophisticated urban medical center.

It is sometimes assumed that a lower standard of care is required in the management and treatment of emergency cases than in nonurgent situations and that the ordinary criteria for determining negligence do not apply in these circumstances. No reliable legal support can be found for these assumptions.

The available time or degree of urgency (**17.** *Urgency Evaluation — Triage*) does not in any way modify a physician's duty to use reasonable care; this duty remains the same at all times. However, the degree of skill required of the physician may vary according to the skill that good physicians exercise in like cases and circumstances. A correct test is whether or not the physician took such action as a skillful and experienced physician would have taken under similar circumstances.

68 – 4. MALPRACTICE INSURANCE

All physicians, especially those who handle a large volume of emergency cases, should be covered adequately by malpractice insurance with a reliable company. The insurance policy should contain the specific provision that no claim can be paid or settled by the company without the approval of the insured physician.

68 – 5. ROUTINE SAFEGUARDS AGAINST MALPRACTICE ACTIONS

Completion and careful preservation of accurate, detailed and legible records on every patient. The length of time that these records are required by law to be preserved varies in different localities, but records on children must be kept until they reach their majority.

Utilization of maximum skill, knowledge and judgment in examination, treatment and disposition.

Insistence on competent consultation in problem cases.

Avoidance of quasi-experimental, controversial or nonaccepted procedures.

Explanation to the patient (or his legal guardian) *in advance* of the purpose, extent, expected results, possible complications and estimated expense of any procedure (see **69–15**. *Informed Consent*). Under no circumstances should any express, specific or implied guarantee or warranty be suggested, given or endorsed.

Notation in the patient's record, in detail and in a noncritical fashion, of any complications or unusual situations related directly or indirectly to the management of the case.

Avoidance of direct, indirect or implied criticism of the work of or the results obtained by other physicians, even under extreme provocation.

Use of courtesy, kindness, sympathy and tact in all relationships with the patient, family, relatives, friends or other interested parties.

69. PERMITS AND AUTHORIZATIONS IN RELATION TO EMERGENCY CASES

(Some of the forms in this section are modified from "Medicolegal Forms with Legal Analysis" published by the Law Department of the American Medical Association and from "Reference Manual of Permits, Consents and/or Releases; Hospital Administrative Procedure No. 1–10" prepared by the office of the Area Administrator, Kaiser Foundation Hospitals, Oakland, California. The "Consent to Medical Examination Following Sexual Assault" (**69–14**) is modified from a form in use at the Michael Reese Hospital, Chicago.)

Some of the following permits and authorizations have been referred to in the preceding text. All have been found useful in the management of emergency cases.

69—1. ACCESS TO EMERGENCY RECORDS (See also 69—8)

To_____, Administrator, _____Hospital.
    I hereby authorize you to furnish a copy of the medical records of

_____, covering the period from
    (Name of patient or "myself")

_____19_____to_____19_____to, or to allow

those records to be inspected or copied by,_____

I hereby release_____Hospital, all members of its
staff, and you personally from all legal responsibility or liability that
may arise from the act I have authorized above.

                                Signed_____

                                Date_____

Witness_____

Approved_____M.D., Attending Physician.

69—2. ADMISSION OF OBSERVERS

                        Date_____19_____

Patient_____ Age_____

Room or Ward_____

    I hereby authorize my attending physician_____M.D.

and the_____Hospital
to permit the presence of such observers as they may deem fit to
admit, in addition to physicians and hospital personnel, while I
am undergoing operative surgery, childbirth, examination, treatment.

(Cross out portions   Signed_____
  which do not apply)
                          Spouse_____

                  Witness_____

69–3. **AUTOPSY PERMIT** See 3–6.

NAME OF DECEASED_____AGE_____SEX_____

RACE_____MARITAL STATUS_____DATE OF BIRTH_____

   1. I hereby authorize_____ M.D., and such persons as he may designate, to perform and attend a complete autopsy, including brain and spinal cord, on the remains of my

_____ _____for the purpose of determining the cause of death. Authority is also granted for the preservation and study of any and all tissues or parts which may be removed. This authority shall be limited only by the following express conditions:

_____

   2. It is understood that due care will be taken to avoid mutilation or disfigurement of the body.

         Signature of spouse,
         legal guardian or
         next of kin*_____

         Address_____

         Relationship to
         the deceased____ _____

Signature of Witness_____

Address_____

City and State_____ Date_____

*For explanation of "Next of Kin," see **3–6**.

69 — 4. **BLOOD ALCOHOL TEST** See 15 — 1

Witnesses should be disinterested adults, not the attending physician, his nurse, or a law enforcement officer.

I hereby request a blood specimen for determination of alcohol content from _____
(Patient's name)

_____
(Address)

by authorization of my supervisor, _____
(Capt., Sgt., or Chief)

Witness _____ Signed _____

Witness _____

Badge No. _____

Police Dept. _____

Date _____ Time _____.

_____

Date _____ Time _____

I, the undersigned, hereby authorize withdrawal of blood for the purpose of determination of the alcohol content.

Witness _____ Signed _____

Witness _____

---

69 – 5.   BLOOD TRANSFUSION (See also 69 – 32. Refusal of Blood or Blood Derivatives)

To:_____M.D.
(Attending physician)

and_____Hospital. Date_____19___

    1. I hereby request and authorize administration of a blood

transfusion to_____   _____and
(Insert "myself" or name of patient)
such additional transfusions as may be deemed necessary and advis-

able by_____M.D. or physicians specifically
designated by him.

    2. It is understood and agreed that_____M.D., or the
physicians designated by him, will be responsible only for the performance of their own individual professional acts, and that blood
typing and selection of compatible blood are the responsibilities of
those who actually perform the necessary laboratory tests.

    3. It has been fully explained, and it is understood, that blood
transfusions do not always produce a desirable result and that there
is a possibility of ill-effects, including hepatitis and/or other diseases, from such transfusion or transfusions.

    4. It has been clearly explained, and it is understood, that cir-
cumstances may make detailed cross-matching tests impractical or
impossible and that immediate need may make necessary the use
of existing stocks of blood which may not include the most compatible blood types.

    5. It is understood, and hereby expressly agreed, that blood sup-
plied in accordance with this agreement is incidental to the rendition
of services and that no requirement, guarantee or warranty of fitness
or quality shall apply.

Signature of patient_____

        *When patient is a minor or
incompetent to give consent:*

        Signature of person authorized to sign consent for

        patient_____

        Address_____

        Relationship to
        patient_____

Witness_____

Address_____

69 – 6. **BLOOD PLASMA TRANSFUSION** (See also **69 – 32.** *Refusal of Blood or Blood Derivatives*)

To_____M.D. and
(Attending physician)

_____Hospital. Date_____19___

   1. I hereby request and authorize administration of blood plasma

to_____in such amounts and at such
(Insert "myself" or name of patient)

times as may be deemed necessary and advisable by_____M.D.
or physicians specifically designated by him.
   2. It has been fully explained, and it is understood, that blood plasma does not always produce a desirable result and that it is a product made from mixed blood obtained from many persons and that sometimes it may cause hepatitis and/or other diseases.
   3. It is understood, and hereby expressly agreed, that the blood plasma supplied in accordance with this agreement is incidental to the rendition of services and that no requirement, guarantee or warranty of fitness or quality shall apply.

Signature of patient_____

       When patient is a minor or
       incompetent to give consent:

       Signature of person authorized to sign consent for patient

_____

       Address_____

       Relationship to patient_____
Witness:

   Signature_____

   Address_____

69 — 7. DIAGNOSTIC PROCEDURES (Arteriograms, Arthrograms, Bronchograms, Cisternal Puncture, Myelograms, Paracentesis, Spinal Puncture, Sternal Puncture, Other Procedures Requiring Injection of a Radiopaque Material)

PATIENT_____AGE_____

DATE_____TIME_____A.M.

    I hereby request and authorize_____M.D.

to perform upon_____the following
               ("myself" or name of patient)

diagnostic procedure:_____.
I have been fully informed of the risks and possible consequences involved and understand that unforeseen results may occur.

               Signed_____

               Relationship to patient_____
The foregoing consent was read, discussed and signed in my presence, and in my opinion the person so signing did so freely and with full knowledge and understanding.

               Witness_____

---

69 – 8. DISCLOSURE OF INFORMATION BY PATIENT'S PHYSICIAN (See also **69 – 1.** *Access to Emergency Records*)

1. I hereby authorize_____M.D.

to disclose complete information to_____

concerning medical findings and treatment of_____
(name or "myself")

from _____ 19____ until the date of conclusion of such treatment.

2. Furthermore, I authorize the physician specified above to testify without limitation as to all medical findings and to all treatment administered to the undersigned, in any legal action, suit or proceedings to which I am, or may become, a party, and I hereby waive on behalf of myself and any persons who may have an interest in the matter, all provisions of law relating to the disclosure of confidential medical information.

Signed_____

Place_____

Date_____

Witness_____

69 – 9. **DISPOSAL OF BODY** (Antemortem Bequest) (See also **69 – 33.** *Universal Donor Card*)

I hereby instruct that my body be delivered immediately after death

to the_____Hospital, _____,

(address)

through the local coroner, to be preserved and/or used in such manner as may seem desirable for purposes of medical teaching and research.

Signature_____

Address_____

Date_____

Witnesses: Addresses:

_____   _____

_____   _____

69 – 10. **DISPOSAL OF DEAD FETUS***

Date_____

We hereby authorize and request that_____
Hospital preserve for scientific purposes, or dispose of, the dead fetus

or body of the baby born to_____on_____, 19___
in accordance with customary medical practice. All claims to the body are hereby relinquished.

Signed_____(mother)

Signed_____(father)

Witness_____

*This consent should be executed by both parents if possible. An unmarried mother's consent is sufficient.

69–11. DISPOSAL OF A SEVERED OR AMPUTATED PART OR ORGAN

Date_____

I hereby authorize the_____Hospital to preserve for scientific purposes, or to use in grafts upon living persons, or to otherwise dispose of in a proper and suitable manner,

the tissues, parts, or organs of_____
(Name of patient or "myself")
specified below.

_____
(Parts or organs)

Signed_____

Relationship to patient
(Self, parent, legal guardian)_____

Witness_____

Witness_____

69 – 12. EMERGENCY CARE WITHOUT A SURGERY PERMIT

The degree of emergency as evaluated by the examining physician is the deciding factor in the handling of patients who are unable to sign their own treatment permits because of minority or mental condition, and whose natural or legal guardians are not available. These cases can be divided into three main groups by means of the time element:

Immediate treatment required [Gross Hemorrhage, Acute Poisoning, Cardiac Emergencies, Respiratory Embarrassment (**17.** *Urgency Evaluation – Triage)*]. In these cases there is a definite *positive* obligation for treatment without delay. While the patient is being prepared for and undergoing treatment, every effort should be made to locate the natural or legal guardian by telephone, telegraph or other means. The cooperation of law enforcement and social service agencies of the community can often be obtained.

Before emergency surgery or procedures of any type are undertaken, the Immediate Treatment Form (p. 712) must be signed by 2 licensed physicians and made a part of the patient's permanent record.

In addition, a standard informed consent treatment permit (**69 – 15**) signed by the natural or legal guardian, or telegraphic or telephonic permission (**69 – 31,** *below*), should be obtained at the earliest opportunity.

TREATMENT WITHIN 6 TO 12 HOURS REQUIRED (Lacerations, Open Fractures, etc.).

In these cases, further attempts should be made by the means previously outlined to obtain permission from the natural or legal guardian. If the *safe period of delay* has passed without obtaining permission, an Immediate Treatment Permit (p. 712) should be completed and treatment given.

TREATMENT POSTPONABLE FOR OVER 12 HOURS WITHOUT DANGER TO THE LIFE OR HEALTH OF THE PATIENT (Simple Fractures, Dislocations Without Nerve or Vascular Pressure Symptoms)

In these cases, every attempt should be made within the set time limit to obtain proper authorization before proceeding with surgical or other care. Copies of telegrams, letters, etc., should be attached to the patient's record. In order to retain control of the patient, hospitalization while attempting to locate the natural or legal guardian may be indicated. If proper written, telephonic or telegraphic authority has not been obtained at the end of the *safe waiting period*, the treatment necessary to prevent injury to health or serious permanent disability may be performed, provided full information regarding the need for the procedure has been made a part of the record, and an Immediate Treatment Permit (below) has been signed by 2 licensed physicians in the presence of 2 witnesses.

IMMEDIATE TREATMENT PERMIT

(Patient a minor, mentally incompetent or unable to sign because of condition; natural or legal guardian not available.)

Date ＿＿＿＿ Time ＿＿＿＿ m.

We, the undersigned physicians, licensed to practice in the State of

＿＿＿＿＿＿＿＿, hereby certify that it is our considered opinion that

＿＿＿＿＿＿＿＿＿, ＿＿＿＿＿, is in need of immediate treat-
(Name of patient)   (Age)
ment to save life and/or to prevent serious disability and/or deformity.

We further certify that unsuccessful attempts have been made for a reasonable time to communicate with the parents, spouse, or legal guardian of the patient named above, and that in our professional judgment further delay in rendering treatment will seriously increase the danger to the patient's life and health.

Witness ＿＿＿＿＿＿＿＿＿ Signed ＿＿＿＿＿＿＿＿, M.D.

Witness ＿＿＿＿＿＿＿＿＿ Signed ＿＿＿＿＿＿＿＿, M.D.

Miscellaneous provisions concerning emergency permits

1. The signer must be clearly aware of the nature of his consent.

2. Persons witnessing signatures must be mentally competent and 18 years of age or older.

3. When emergency procedures are performed without the signature of the patient or his natural or legal guardian, a properly signed and witnessed permit should be obtained at the earliest possible opportunity and incorporated in the emergency record.

4. Permits signed with an "X" should be witnessed by 2 adult persons able to write their names.

5. Surgery or other treatment necessary to prevent a cosmetic or functional defect requires a validly signed operative or treat-

ment permit based on informed consent (**69 – 15**). This requirement also applies to elective surgery of any type. These procedures cannot be performed under an Immediate Treatment Permit.

6. No person who has temporary custody only of a minor has any legal right to authorize treatment of any kind.

7. The authority of a duly appointed legal guardian supersedes that of a parent or spouse.

8. Grandparents, adult brothers, sisters, close relatives, etc. *cannot sign a permit for a minor* [except *in loco parentis* (**69 – 21.** *below*)].

9. Permits should be signed *before any preoperative medication is given to the patient.*

10. If a patient qualified to give permission specifically prohibits any procedure verbally or in writing before becoming incompetent or irresponsible, the procedure cannot be performed under any circumstances, even as a lifesaving measure, in many localities (see **69 – 32.** *below*).

11. Because the father and mother are charged equally with the control and custody of a child, express prohibition by 1 parent prevents any treatment even though the other has given permission. This applies even if the parents are separated and can be overruled only if the laws in the particular locality provide for the issuance of treatment orders by juvenile or other courts.

12. When marriage of a minor, divorce, annulment, legal guardianship, or *in loco parentis* relationship is claimed as a basis for exceptions to the usual rules regarding treatment permits, adequate proof to substantiate the claim should be required.

69 – 13. ENTRUSTMENT OF CARE OF MINORS*

Parents or legal guardians who wish to leave their children or wards under the care of another adult during working hours, overnight, while on vacation trips, etc., can ensure prompt emergency care by completing and signing a document of the type shown on page 714. The signed and witnessed document should be kept in the possession of the adult designated to authorize care during the parents' or guardian's absence, to be presented to the attending physician in the case of an emergency involving the persons specified thereon.

---

*Any person under 18 years of age.

69 – 13. ENTRUSTMENT OF CARE OF MINORS

TO WHOM IT MAY CONCERN:

(Cross out words which do not apply)

This is to certify that I/we,_____

_____the_____
(names in full)   (mother, father, legal guardian)

of the persons listed below, do hereby constitute and appoint

_____
(name in full)   (address)

my/our true and lawful attorney, solely, and with the power to authorize and consent to the administration of any anesthetic or medical treatment to, and the performance of whatever operations or removal of tissue decided to be necessary by the attending physician,

on the below named minor(s) for the period from_____to
(date)

_____, inclusive.
(date)

NAME	AGE OR DATE OF BIRTH

WITNESSED BY:

_____   _____
Name   Name   Relationship

_____   _____
Address   Name   Relationship

_____   _____
Name   Address

_____
Address
                    Date of signing_____

69 — 14. EXAMINATION FOR CRIMINAL SEXUAL ASSAULT
(For detailed outline of required history and examination, see **9.** *Rape*)

CONSENT TO MEDICAL EXAMINATION FOLLOWING SEXUAL ASSAULT

I, _____ _____, voluntarily request

_____ _____M.D., his medical and
nursing assistants and associates, to conduct an examination to determine
the medical implications of an alleged sexual assault made upon me. I fully
understand this examination will include tests for presence of sperm and
venereal disease, as well as clinical observations for physical evidence of
penetration of and/or injury to my reproductive organs.

I fully understand the nature of the examination and the fact that medical
information gathered by this means may be used as evidence in a court of
law or in connection with the enforcement of public health rules and laws.

I hereby grant permission to_____ _____
Hospital and its agents for the release of this and related information to
authorized officials when deemed necessary or advisable and I herewith

save and hold harmless said_____ _____
Hospital and its agents from any and all claims of injury, whatsoever, which
may in any manner result from the release of such information.
This will certify that I am of legal age and capacity to consent to this examination and that I fully understand all of its implications.

_____   _____
              Witness   Signature of Patient

TO BE SIGNED BY PARENTS OR GUARDIANS
OF MINOR PATIENT

This will certify that while I am not of legal age to consent to this examination, I fully understand all of its implications.

                                          _____
                                                    Signature of Patient

(Form continued on page 716.)

69—15. INFORMED CONSENT

(Continued)

I, _____ , in my capacity as

_____ of the patient,
      (father, mother, guardian, etc.)

_____ , do hereby grant permission to

_____ Hospital and its agents,

as specified above, to conduct this examination on my _____ .
                                                       (son, daughter, ward)

_____   _____
          Witness   Signed

                  Date of signing _____

69—15. INFORMED CONSENT

No longer is a blanket authorization covering any and all medical, surgical and laboratory procedures considered adequate for emergency or other medical care. It is becoming more and more generally accepted that before he gives his consent, the patient is entitled to accurate and detailed information not only regarding the projected operation, diagnostic procedure or therapy but also concerning recognized risks, possible complications and their effects and available alternative methods of treatment.

To protect the attending physician and his assistants, the anesthesiologist and the clinic or hospital and its personnel against subsequent allegations by the patient, his legal guardian or heirs (usually triggered by a result below the expectations of the patient or his family or by a dispute concerning charges) that the patient (or his legal guardian) was not informed of or did not have full understanding of possible risks and/or complications at the time that permission was given, the authorization should whenever possible incorporate the following points:

1. Date. If more than a few hours elapse between signature of the authorization and the time that the procedure is begun, the claim may be made that the patient had changed his mind during

page 716

the interim and that, therefore, the procedure was done without legal authorization.

2. Time of consent. The exact time at which permission is given should be indicated and should always be before administration of any drug or medication which might be construed as interfering in any way with the patient's complete comprehension and sound judgment.

3. The scheduled procedure – in lay terms if possible – with the name of the physician who will personally perform it (unless otherwise specified).

4. A general statement in nontechnical language of recognized risks and complications of the procedure and possible adverse consequences.

5. A specific statement that no guarantee of the results of the procedure has been made or implied and that alternative methods of treatment have been discussed.

6. A properly executed and witnessed signature of the patient or of his legal guardian. If the patient is physically unable to sign his name he should make a mark with a pen held by or against any portion of his body. His full name should then be written or printed after the mark, with the notation "_____, his mark" and properly witnessed.

7. Witnesses to the patient's signature must be disinterested adults – not the attending physician.

The following General Information About Surgery form covers all the points outlined above and should be used to supplement the Routine Operative and Treatment Permit (**69 – 19**).

GENERAL INFORMATION ABOUT SURGERY

You and your doctor have decided that for the further diagnosis or treatment of your illness or condition, an operation is necessary. Surgical procedures of any type involve the taking of risks, ranging from minor to serious (including the risk of death) but today are generally safe, helpful and often lifesaving. It is important to be aware of the following possible risks before you give your consent to the operation that you and your physician are planning.

A surgical procedure, whether minor or serious, involves cutting skin, tissue or organs. The following may be the reactions of your body to an operation.

1. Infection – invasion of tissue by bacteria or other germs occurs to some degree whenever a cut or incision is made. In most instances, the natural defense mechanisms of the body heal the affected area without difficulty. In some instances antibiotic medicines are prescribed and at times additional surgical measures may be necessary.

2. Hemorrhage – cutting of blood vessels and accompanying bleeding occurs in every incision. This is usually easily controlled. At times blood transfusions are

required to replace excessive blood loss. If blood transfusions are given there is a small additional risk of liver inflammation. There is no way to completely predict this undesired reaction. In simple operations there is usually less blood loss than in major ones, but not always. There are instances when excessive bleeding occurs after the original operation (major or minor) is completed, and additional action must be taken to control delayed bleeding.

3. Drug reactions—unexpected allergies, lack of proper response or illness caused by the drugs can occur. It is important for you to inform your physician of any problems you have had with drugs and to let him know which medications you now take regularly.

4. Anesthesia reactions—there may be unusual or expected responses to the gases, drugs or methods used which can lead to difficulties with lung, heart or nerve function. Except in unusual situations or emergencies you are not allowed to eat or drink for several hours prior to surgery in order to prevent the effects of vomiting. Your reactions to surgery continue to be observed in the recovery room during the period immediately after the operation.

5. Blood vessel inflammation and clotting—when they happen together, thrombophlebitis results; blood clots may separate and move into other organs and cause more damage.

6. Injury to other organs—because of closeness of other organs to the area being operated on, it may be unavoidable that other organ functions are affected. The stress of surgery may also harm other organ systems. Required adjustments in the treatment will be made by your physician in response to these conditions.

7. Other concerns—it is not possible to list here all the possible risks and complications and their variations, which may arise in any surgical operation or procedure. Each situation depends upon the condition of health and the purpose and nature of the operation. Your physician is willing to discuss any further details with you.

ALTERNATIVES TO TREATMENT

Other ways of managing your illness, which may range from doing nothing to taking different measures, should be considered. Since you and your doctor have decided upon surgery as the treatment indicated, do not hesitate to discuss the reasons and the alternatives. Because there are risks involved in any operation, with no guarantee or assurance of a successful result, it is important that you clearly understand and agree to it as the decision of your choice.

I have read the above information and am satisfied that I understand it. I have discussed with my physician any particular doubts, problems, or concerns I may have regarding the intended surgery or procedure. I have no further questions regarding possible risks, complications, and alternatives to the intended treatment.

Date   Name

Witness

If the patient does not wish to be informed he should sign the following form in lieu of the General Information about Surgery form (above).

Following the discussion I have had with my doctor regarding my condition, I prefer not to know in any detail the common risks of any surgical procedure.

Date _____ Name _____

Witness _____

69–16. IN LOCO PARENTIS See **69–21**

19–17. MATURE MINORS See **69–20**

69–18. NALORPHINE HYDROCHLORIDE (Nalline)
TEST AUTHORIZATION See **15–3**

69–19. OPERATIVE AND TREATMENT PERMIT (General)
(See also **69–15.** *Informed Consent*)

General considerations. Whenever possible, an informed consent treatment permit, including permission for operative procedures (**69–15**) should be signed by the patient (or his natural or legal guardian), properly witnessed and made a permanent part of the medical record before any treatment is given. Legally, treatment against the explicit or implied wish of the patient or of his natural or legal guardian may constitute actionable assault. Practically, it is generally considered that the following types of treatment can be given without authorization and that omission may be considered as evidence of improper care and negligence (**68–1; 68–3**).

1. Cleansing and irrigation of a wound (not debridement) with coaptation of the edges by adhesive straps or "butterflies" and application of protective sterile bandages.

2. Application of temporary splints (not casts) to prevent aggravation of an injury by motion.

3. Oral or rectal administration of medications.

4. Artificial respiration, or assistance to respiration, by any expired air, manual or mechanical means, including inhalation by tent, catheter or mask, of air, oxygen or other nonanesthetic gases.

In contrast, the following procedures should not be done without a properly signed permit unless an immediate threat to life or health is present:

1. Surgical procedures, major or minor, emergency or elective.
2. Administration of local or general anesthesia.
3. Insertion of a needle for any reason whatsoever. This includes intracutaneous, subcutaneous, intramuscular, intravenous or intraspinal injections of all types, as well as the withdrawal of blood, spinal fluid, etc., for diagnosis or treatment.
4. Gastric lavage or gavage.
5. Catheterization.
6. Application or changing of corrective splints or casts.

The best definition of a danger or threat to life or health which would warrant proceeding without proper authorization is as follows:

It must involve a threat which carries danger of major incapacities, permanent or irreversible, through impairment or loss of a function, organ or structural unit of the body.

A satisfactory form of general operative and treatment permit is shown on page 721.

69 – 20.   PERSONS WHO MAY SIGN THEIR OWN EMERGENCY TREATMENT PERMITS

Any mentally competent person over 18 years of age. The decision regarding mental competency must be made by the attending physician, provided it has not been established by court action.

Any mentally competent male over 16, or female over 15, who is married or divorced or whose marriage has been annulled. Such persons are considered as being emancipated from parental control; hence, they can sign their own permits in many states.

"Mature" minors. In some states, unmarried minors between 16 and 18 may, under certain circumstances, sign emergency permits. These circumstances are as follows:

1. When the consent of the natural or legal guardian cannot be obtained within the time limit available to save life or prevent suffering or permanent disability.

CONSENT TO OPERATION, ADMINISTRATION OF ANESTHETICS, AND THE RENDERING OF OTHER MEDICAL SERVICES

1. I authorize _____ M.D., and/or his associates, assistants of his choice, and personnel assigned by the Hospital, to perform the following operation or procedure upon me _____

   _____

   and/or to do any other procedures that in (his) (their) judgment may be advisable for the patient's well-being, including such procedures as are considered medically advisable to remedy conditions discovered during the procedure or operation. I am satisfied with my understanding of the nature of the operation or procedure, the more common risks associated with it, including the potential for serious harm, and alternative methods of treatment, which have been explained to me by _____.
   No warranty or guarantee has been made as to the result or cure.

2. I hereby authorize and direct the above named Hospital, Medical Group, physician and/or his associates and assistants, to provide such additional services for me as he or they may deem medically advisable, including, but not limited to, the selection and administration of anesthesia and the performance of pathology and radiology services.

3. I hereby authorize the Hospital to dispose of any severed tissue or member in accordance with accustomed hospital practice.

4. (Other) _____

   _____

Date _____ Signed: _____

Hour: _____ Witness: _____
(If patient is a minor or is unable to sign, complete the following:)
Patient is a minor _____, or is unable to sign because _____

Signed: _____

Witness; _____ Relationship: _____

2. When the natural or legal guardians are not available, but the minor has presented himself for treatment accompanied by older relatives and with a parent's knowledge, provided there is no reason to suspect that 1 or both of the parents' consent would not have been given had they been available.

69–21. PERSONS WHO MAY SIGN PERMITS FOR MINORS*

A natural parent. If the parents have been legally divorced, the parent to whom the court has awarded custody of the child must sign the permit. The signatures of both parents are desirable, although not essential, in cases of this type.

In the rare instances where there is a difference of opinion between undivorced parents, emergency treatment of any type *cannot be given* if specifically prohibited by 1 of the parents, unless there is a provision in the law of the specific locality for the issuance of a treatment order by juvenile or other courts.

A legal guardian, duly appointed by court order.

The husband of a married female over 15, or the wife of a married male over 16, if the patient is mentally incompetent, and provided the patient has not expressly prohibited the procedure verbally or in writing before the onset of mental incompetence.

In loco parentis. Any person who, in the *permanent* absence of the parents, has assumed parental obligations without the formalities of legal adoption is *in loco parentis*. For example, if an uncle or grandparent receives a niece, nephew or grandchild into his household as a member of his family, he assumes the rights and duties of the lawful parent. Since permanent, not temporary, custody is required, the important factor to determine in each case is whether the child has actually been deserted or abandoned by the parents. To constitute abandonment there must be actual desertion, accompanied by the intention to sever complete, or as completely as possible, the parental relationship.

69–22. PERSONS WHO MAY SIGN PERMITS FOR LEGALLY ADJUDGED MENTALLY INCOMPETENT ADULTS

A legally appointed guardian, usually a parent, spouse or close relative, but in some instances a nonrelated person. In this case,

---

*A minor is any person under 18 years of age.

the legal guardian alone can sign permits, and his decision takes precedence over that of a parent or spouse.

69 – 23. PERSONS WHO MAY SIGN PERMITS FOR ADULTS WHO ARE TEMPORARILY MENTALLY INCOMPETENT FROM SERIOUS DISEASE OR INJURY

A spouse, provided that the patient has not expressly prohibited the procedure verbally or in writing before becoming mentally irresponsible.

A legal guardian. If a mentally irresponsible patient is brought for emergency care without accompanying identification (transients, auto accident cases, alcoholics, attempted suicides, etc.), handling must be in accordance with the rules outlined under **69 – 12.** *Emergency Care without a Surgery Permit.*

69 – 24. PHOTOGRAPHING OF PATIENTS

Photographing by newspaper cameramen of injured or ill persons undergoing emergency care should never be allowed without written permission of the patient or, if a minor, of a parent or legal guardian. Under no circumstances should photographs of unconscious, dazed or mentally irresponsible adult patients be allowed, even if permission has been given by the spouse, unless such photographs are needed by law enforcement agencies.

For medical articles, teaching, etc., the permit on page 724 is acceptable.

69 – 25. STERILIZATION PERMIT

If a surgical procedure which might cause sterility must be performed on an emergency – not elective – basis, an authorization such as the one on page 725 *must* be signed by both husband and wife and properly witnessed *before the operation is begun.*

69 – 26. TACIT CONSENT See **15 – 1.** *Blood Analysis*

69 – 27. TELEGRAPHIC CONSENT See **69 – 31**

69 – 28. TELEPHONIC CONSENT See **69 – 31**

CONSENT TO TAKING AND PUBLICATION OF PHOTOGRAPHS

Patient_____

Place_____

Date_____

In connection with the medical services which I am receiving

from my physician, _____M.D., I consent that photographs may be taken of me, or of parts of my body, under the following conditions:

1. The photographs may be taken only with the consent of the physician designated above and under such conditions and at such times as he may approve.

2. The photographs shall be taken by my physician or by a photographer approved and designated by him.

3. Any and all photographs taken as specified above shall be used for medical purposes only.

4. If, in the judgment of my physician, medical research, education, or science will be benefited by their use, such photographs, and information relating to my case, may be published and republished, either separately or in connection with each other, in professional journals or medical books, or used for any other purpose which my physician may deem proper in the interest of medical education, knowledge, or research; provided, however, that it is specifically understood that in any such publication or use I shall not be identified by name.

5. The aforementioned photographs may be modified or retouched in any way that my physician, in his discretion, may consider desirable.

Signed_____

(patient)

Witness_____

I hereby authorize and direct_____M.D.,

or the attending physicians of the_____Hospital, to

perform the following operation upon_____,

(name of patient or "myself")

and to perform any other procedures which they may, in their absolute discretion, deem advisable or desirable during this operation.

_____

(name or description of operation)

_____

It has been explained to me, and I understand, that as a result of the operation or operations specified above I may (or will probably) be sterile. I understand that the word "sterility" means that I will be unable to reproduce, and, in giving my consent to the operation specified above and/or other procedures deemed desirable, I have in mind the possibility or probability of such a result. I hereby release

_____M.D., the attending physicians of the

_____Hospital, and the hospital, its agents and employees from any liability or responsibility for my present condition or for any condition that may result from said operation or procedures.

Date_____Hour_____Signed_____

(Patient)

Witness_____

Witness_____

I join in authorizing the performance upon my wife (husband) of the operation and procedures specified and consented to above. It has been explained to me, and I understand, that as a result of the operation, and/or procedures, my wife (husband) may be sterile.

Date_____Hour_____Signed_____

(Husband) (Wife)

Witness_____

69 – 29. TELEVISING OF OPERATION

PATIENT_____PLACE_____DATE_____

In the interest of medical education and knowledge, I hereby consent to the televising of the operation which is scheduled to be

performed upon me on or about_____19_____

I hereby authorize_____M.D. and the_____
Hospital to admit to the operating room the cameramen and technicians and other persons who are to participate in the televising of this operation.

Witness_____   Signed_____

---

69 – 30. TERMINATION OF PREGNANCY PERMIT

(Not to be used for therapeutic abortion – this is not an emergency procedure.)

TERMINATION OF PREGNANCY RELEASE: (Other than therapeutic abortion)

I, the undersigned, am advised by the attending physicians of the

_____Hospital that I may be in a condition of abortion. I hereby declare that neither the physicians nor any persons employed by or connected with said hospital have performed any act which may have contributed directly or indirectly to the interruption of my pregnancy and do hereby release said hospital and the attending physicians from any liability or responsibility for my condition. I hereby consent and direct the attending physicians to terminate my pregnancy as an urgent medical necessity and for my physical welfare. I further release the attending physicians and the hospital and its employees from all liability for any results and consequences that may occur from the termination of my pregnancy.

Date_____Hour_____Signed_____
                                              (Patient)

Witness_____Approved_____
                                      (Husband)

Witness_____Approved_____

                                      _____
                                      (Parents, if a Minor)

69–31. TYPES OF VALID EMERGENCY TREATMENT PERMITS

WRITTEN

Authorizations should always be signed if possible. If the patient is illiterate or physically unable to write, but is mentally competent, he should make an X, with assistance if necessary. The certification by 2 witnesses should be as follows:

"John Doe (his mark)"   Witness _____
                            Witness _____

TELEGRAPHIC. A copy of the telegraphic authorization must be made a permanent part of the record.

TELEPHONIC. This is valid provided 2 persons listen in on the line and both record the time and circumstances in the patient's record. A substantiating written authorization should be obtained as soon as possible.

VERBAL. Verbal permission or silent (tacit) acquiescence of a mentally competent adult is a valid consent, but often difficult or impossible to prove at a later date. Therefore, a properly witnessed written consent (**69–15**) should be obtained at the earliest possible opportunity.

69–32. REFUSAL OF BLOOD OR BLOOD DERIVATIVES

At least one religious group (Jehovah's Witnesses) will not allow administration of blood or blood derivaties, even as a lifesaving measure. In circumstances of this type, to protect the attending physician and the hospital, the following form should be signed by the patient and spouse, by parents of a minor or by the legal guardian of a mentally incompetent person.

Because of religious beliefs, I hereby expressly forbid the administration of human blood or any of its derivatives to _____
during this hospitalization. I hereby release the hospital, its personnel and the attending physician from any responsibility whatsoever for any unfavorable reactions or untoward results due to my refusal to permit the use of blood or its derivatives. It has been clearly explained and I fully understand the possible consequences of such refusal.

Date _____   Signed _____

Witness _____   Spouse _____

                               Parents _____

                               Legal Guardian _____

69—33. UNIFORM DONOR CARDS (to be signed and carried with you).

(Face)

UNIFORM DONOR CARD

OF _____

Print or type name of donor

In the hope that I may help others, I hereby make this anatomical gift, if medically acceptable, to take effect upon my death. The words and marks below indicate my desires.

I give: (a) _____ any needed organs or parts

(b) _____ only the following organs or parts

_____

Specify the organ(s) or part(s)

for the purposes of transplantation, therapy, medical research or education;

(c) _____ my body for anatomical study if needed.

Limitations or special wishes, if any: _____

(Reverse)

Signed by the donor and the following two witnesses in the presence of each other:

_____	_____
Signature of Donor	Date of Birth of Donor
_____	_____
Date signed	City & State
_____	_____
Witness	Witness

This is a legal document under the Uniform Anatomical Gift Act or similar laws.

---

70. RELEASE OF INFORMATION

The physician who treats an emergency case, and all emergency personnel working under his supervision, direction or control, should always keep in mind that medical information obtained during the physician-patient relationship is confidential and privileged, and cannot be divulged without proper authorization (**69−8**) from the patient (or his legal guardian) except by due process of law. Therefore, only factual nonmedical information (name, address, age, how brought in, attending physician, disposition, etc.) can be given to members of the family, friends, attorneys, claim adjustors, investigators, reporters or other interested persons, unless a proper authorization has been signed by the patient or his legal guardian. If an accident requires investigation and report by a law enforcement agency, is covered by the provisions of city, county or state emergency contracts or concerns a member of the merchant marine or armed services, a brief report, preferably in lay terms, covering the diagnosis, prognosis and disposition may be given to the investigating officer or to the proper law enforcement authorities subject to the following restrictions:

FOR POLICE CASES

The following items of public information may be given *without* the patient's consent:

1. **Identity:** (a) Name, (b) marital status, (c) sex, (d) age, (e) occupation, (f) firm or company employing patient and (g) address.

2. **Nature of the accident:** (a) Injured by automobile, explosion, shooting; (b) if there is a fracture, it is not to be described in any way except to state the member involved; and (c) more than a statement that it is simple or open may not be made.

3. **Injuries of the head:** (a) A simple statement that the injuries involve the head may be made; (b) it may not be stated that the skull is fractured; (c) no opinion as to the severity of the injury or prognosis should be given.

4. **Internal injuries:** (a) It may be stated that there are internal injuries, but nothing more specific as to the location of the injuries, and (b) a statement that the condition is serious may be made.

5. **Unconsciousness:** (a) If the patient is unconscious when he is brought to the hospital, a statement of this fact may be made; (b) the cause of unconsciousness, however, should not be given.

6. **Cases of poisoning:** (a) A statement may be made that the patient is being treated for suspected poisoning; (b) information as to the trade name of poisoning substances must not be given; (c) no statement concerning the possibility of accident or suicide may be made; (d) make no prognosis; (e) if patient has ingested a poisonous compound, do not identify it by trade name but only by a general name, i.e., caustic, cleaning compound, etc.

7. **Shooting:** (a) A statement may be made that there is a penetrating wound and the general location; (b) no statement may be made as to how the accident occurred, i.e., accidental, suicidal, homicidal or in a brawl, nor may the environment under which the accident occurred be mentioned.

8. **Stabbing:** The same general statements may be made for stabbing as for shooting accidents (above).

9. **Intoxication:** No statement may be made as to whether or not the patient is intoxicated.

10. **Burns:** (a) A statement may be made that the patient is burned, also of the general location on the body; (b) a statement as to how the accident occurred may be made only when the absolute facts are known; and (c) no prognosis may be given.

11. **Attending physician:** Hospitals may state to the representatives of newspapers, radio stations, or television stations the name of the attending physician of private patients and refer such representatives to the physician for information about the case. The name is given with the understanding, however, that it is not to be used without the physician's consent.

FOR OTHER THAN POLICE CASES

If the patient is conscious and can communicate with the doctor or nurse in charge, or relatives, he should be asked whether he will permit any information to be given. His decision is final. If the patient agrees to permit information to be given, the conditions are identical with those outlined above.

Conditions requiring an immediate report to the proper law enforcement authorities are:

1. Wounds or injuries of any degree, extent or results, self-inflicted with known or suspected suicidal intent.

2. Wounds or injuries inflicted by another person, or persons, by means of a club, knife, gun, pistol or any other potentially deadly weapon. This includes fists or hands if the assailant is, or

has been, a professional pugilist, or has been trained in judo or karate.

3. Injuries or illnesses resulting from conditions which might be dangerous to the general populace.

4. Criminal abortions, proved or suspected.

5. Injuries resulting from violation of any law. This includes minor trafic accidents, with or without property damage or injuries to others.

6. Bites—animal, bat or human.

7. Industrial conditions, i.e., injuries or illnesses covered by state or federal compensation laws (**75**).

8. Conditions or injuries in which objective findings on examination are not in accordance with the history.

Since the reports completed by law enforcement officers become public documents, medical information thereon is not privileged and can be divulged without specific authorization from the patient or his legal guardian.

Written reports concerning diagnosis, treatment and prognosis may be drawn up at the request of insurance adjustors, attorneys or other interested parties, provided a properly witnessed written authorization (**69—8**) signed by the patient (or the parent or legal guardian if the patient is a minor or has been legally declared incompetent) has been completed and made a part of the file, and provided the permission of the emergency physician who treated the case (or his superior in a hospital or plant emergency department) has been obtained.

Specific authorization is not a requirement for release of information concerning an industrial case (**75**). By requesting medical care under the provisions of any of the several workmen's compensation acts, the patient waives the physician-patient relationship.

The oral or written request or permission of a patient's spouse to release medical information is not adequate if the patient is mentally competent to make the decision regarding release of information.

71. RESPONSIBILITIES OF PHYSICIANS EXAMINING AND TREATING EMERGENCY CASES

1. To be available at all times if assigned to an emergency department, room, station or ward.

2. To examine, evaluate and give prompt and proper treatment to all persons requiring emergency care in accordance with accepted medical standards.

3. To decide whether or not persons requesting examination and treatment do, in fact, require emergency care. This very important decision is the responsibility solely of the emergency physician. Under no circumstances should it be made by a nurse, orderly, aide or clerk.

4. To treat patients in order of urgency (**17.** *Urgency Evaluation — Triage*).

5. To supervise, instruct, direct and assume responsibility for professional assistants, nurses, orderlies, clerks, attendants and other emergency department personnel.

6. To be familiar with the location of, indications for and adjustment and application of the various types of mechanical diagnostic and therapeutic equipment available in the emergency and critical care units.

7. To be familiar with the application to emergency situations of rites of various religious denominations and sects (**3—8**).

8. To be aware of the laws and ordinances relating to emergency situations of the political subdivision in which he is practicing.

9. To be familiar with and abide by staff association constitution and by-laws, and the hospital's rules, regulations and standing orders, including details of any formally outlined disaster plan, if on duty in an emergency department, room or ward.

10. To be familiar with accepted actions, doses, side effects and toxicity of commonly used drugs.

11. To arrange for future medical management of all persons with whom he has established a physician-patient relationship through examination, treatment or advice, with full knowledge of

his responsibility until another physician takes over active supervision (**64.** *Abandonment*).

12. To evaluate the condition of each patient before transfer or referral to be certain that such transportation or referral will not decrease the patient's chances of recovery or survival. In borderline cases, if, in the considered judgment of the emergency physician, transportation is indicated and feasible, supportive measures (oxygen, plasma volume expanders, vasopressor drugs, etc.) should be continued in the ambulance, preferably under the supervision of a physician, registered nurse or trained ambulance attendant. The résumé sent with the patient should indicate the attending physician's reasons for transfer (see No. 13, below).

13. To complete and send with any referred or transferred patient a medical résumé giving diagnosis and treatment. This résumé should be enclosed in a sealed envelope and a copy made a permanent part of the emergency record.

14. To determine and certify the cause and time of death in terminal cases and to certify to dead on arrival (DOA) cases (**3 – 4**).

15. To cooperate with family members, clergy, members of law enforcement agencies, press, photographers and other interested persons within the limits established by the physician-patient relationship, applicable legal restrictions and staff and hospital regulations.

16. To use courtesy, consideration, tact and kindness in his relations not only with his patients but also with accompanying members of the family, relatives, neighbors or other interested persons.

17. To complete a detailed, concise, accurate *and legible* record on each patient, specifying not only *what* was done but also *why* it was done.

72. SERVICE PERSONNEL AND DEPENDENTS

Only supportive emergency care and measures to prevent aggravation of a condition should be given to members of any of the branches of the Armed Services and their dependents – enough to insure arrival at the closest Armed Services or Government hospital or clinic in satisfactory condition. Obvious or suspected fractures and dislocations should not be x-rayed unless, in the opinion of the attending emergency physician, films are necessary for adequate interim care. The injured parts should be splinted (with an inexpensive type of splint if possible), and pain, shock, etc. controlled by the usual measures. Transportation, by government ambulance if necessary, usually can be arranged by telephonic communication with the proper government facility in the vicinity.

73. SUBPOENAS

73—1. APPEARANCE IN RESPONSE TO SUBPOENA

Any physician can be subpoenaed to appear in person at any time before any court, any administrative agency or any investigative board by any party to any legal action. Attendance at the specified time and place is mandatory provided a legal subpoena (**73—4**) has been properly served and accepted (**73—5**). Noncompliance constitutes contempt of court and can be punished accordingly.

73—2. RELIEF FROM UNREASONABLY SHORT NOTICE

If a physician is served with a subpoena which specifies appearance before an administrative agency, investigative board or court on unreasonably or unusually short notice (for example, service at 5 P.M. to appear the next day at 9:30 A.M.), he or his attorney usually can obtain relief by informing the clerk of the agency, board or court of other pressing medical duties, with the request that attendance be continued to a later time so that arrangements can be made in advance for attendance.

73—3. DUCES TECUM

A subpoena duces tecum is a court, administrative board or law enforcement investigative agency order which requires production of certain specified documents at a specified place at a given time. This material may include original x-rays and business office records in addition to the medical chart.

73−4. REQUIREMENTS FOR A LEGAL SUBPOENA

1. Specification of the date, time and place of appearance.
2. Signature of the proper official of the issuing court, board or administrative agency.
3. Impress of the official seal of the issuing agency, board or court on the original document.

73−5. PROPER SERVICE

This, as a rule, is considered to mean presentation of the original subpoena (with its impressed official seal) to the subpoenee for inspection, and payment in advance of the appropriate witness fee plus mileage at the established rate per mile from the place at which the subpoena is served to the location of the court or agency at which the subpoenee is ordered to appear.

74. TESTIMONY IN COURT

Any physician is required by law to appear before an investigative agency, administrative agency or in court in response to a properly completed and served subpoena (**73−4; 75−5**). He may be required to appear as a factual (nonmedical) witness (**74−1**), as a medical witness (**74−2**) or as an expert medical witness (**74−3**).

74−1. NONMEDICAL TESTIMONY

In some instances a physician may be called upon to testify regarding an incident concerning which he has firsthand (not hearsay) knowledge. As a witness he has the same rights, privileges and obligations as any other witness and is entitled to the nominal witness fee (plus mileage). This fee and mileage allowance must be paid in advance by the server at the time that the subpoena is served.

74−2. MEDICAL TESTIMONY

Any physician may be required to testify regarding findings on medical examination or treatment of any patient under his care, subject to the privileged communication rule. This means that confidential information obtained during examination or treatment, or at any other time when the patient-physician relationship is in effect, cannot be divulged except under certain circumstances. These circumstances vary in details in different localities but in general are:

1. With the permission of the patient (or his legal guardian).
2. In criminal cases.
3. In civil cases where there is a question of the mental competency of a deceased person.
4. In personal injury or wrongful death cases.
5. In certain will contests.

The usual medical witness fees apply unless prior arrangements have been made with the attorney. However, if the line between medical testimony and testimony as an expert witness (**74–3**) is crossed by the request of legal counsel for either side for interpretation of the factual medical testimony or for a medical opinion of any type, the physician may request that the presiding officer of the agency, board or court classify him as an expert witness (**74–3**).

74–3. EXPERT WITNESS

Any person who possesses more knowledge than the court about the subject involved may be classified as an "expert witness." Therefore, in medical matters any physician may be qualified as an expert witness even if he is not particularly trained or experienced in a given specialty, and even if he has not actually examined or treated the patient.

An expert medical witness may be required to answer hypothetical questions under oath and to give his opinion concerning diagnosis, disability, further treatment and prognosis. Whenever possible, questions should be answered by "Yes" or "No," but if qualifications are required, they will usually be allowed by the presiding judge or hearing officer. If sufficient facts to permit an accurate and fair answer have not been incorporated in the hypothetical question, the physician may so state and defer his answer until the presiding officer has given a ruling regarding the need for further information.

74−4. PREPARATION OF A COURT CASE

1. Careful review of the written records made at the time of prior examinations.

2. Pretrial conferences with the attorney.

3. Arrangements regarding expert witness fees should be made with the attorney in advance of court appearance. These fees vary in different localities, but they are usually based on the time spent in preparation, pretrail conferences and anticipated time in court. *Under no circumstances* should this fee be on a contingent basis. It should always apply in full, regardless of the outcome of the case−won, lost, dismissed or settled out of court.

74−5. OBLIGATIONS OF A PHYSICIAN AS A WITNESS

To dress and act in a respectful, conservative and dignified manner. To give testimony distinctly with candor, sincerity and accuracy, avoiding medical terminology as much as possible and explaining those medical terms which are used. Above all, "talking down" to the jury in a condescending manner should be avoided. The original medical record can often be used for reference but if so used is admissible as evidence.

To avoid taking sides, especially by coloring testimony or acting as a medical advocate in other ways.

To remain calm, even-tempered and alert under cross-examination; and to avoid trying to appear clever in debate.

To keep differences of opinion with other physicians on an impersonal professional level.

To abide scrupulously by any and all rulings made by the trial judge or presiding officer. Questions concerning privileged information or other similar matters can be asked directly of, and decided by, the judge or hearing officer.

75. WORKMEN'S COMPENSATION (INDUSTRIAL) CASES

75−1. MANAGEMENT ON INITIAL VISIT

Special forms for reporting industrial cases (injuries or illnesses caused by or arising out of employment) are used almost universally. *All medical information on these forms must be filled out in full by the emergency physician at the first examination.* written permission of the patient is not necessary; by requesting treatment as an industrial case, all rights to a confidental patient-physician relationship are waived. If, after examination, the physician concludes that the injury or illness of which the patient complained was not caused by or did not arise out of employment, he should so inform the patient and write "Nonindustrial" across the face of the industrial form. From this point, any advice or treatment is on a nonindustrial basis.

75−2. COMPLETION OF FIRST REPORT OF INJURY

Reports to employers, insurance carriers and governmental agencies must be completed and submitted as soon as possible after the first examination. Therefore, for adequate reporting, it is essential that all spaces on the industrial form be filled in. The following is an explanation of the subheadings found on many industrial injury and illness forms.

Diagnosis. This must be specific and descriptive and must indicate the severity of the condition. "Bruised finger" is worthless for industrial reporting purposes; "mild contusion volar surface distal phalanx left index finger" gives a clear picture of the location, type and severity of the injury. If a definite diagnosis cannot be established, a symptom diagnosis should be given. "Diagnosis deferred" is worthless and should never be used.

Descriptive names for the digits of the hand should always be given, i.e., thumb, index finger, middle (or long) finger, ring finger and little finger. "First," "second," etc., should never be used. Finger joints should be specified, i.e., "metacarpophalangeal," "proximal interphalangeal" and "distal interphalangeal," not "first," "second" and "third."

Negative findings are of value in diagnosis and prognosis. Examples: "Concussion of the brain—mild. Neurologic examination negative." "Laceration volar surface middle phalanx left ring finger—tendons and nerve supply not injured." "Severe contusion right supra-orbital ridge. No evidence of damage to eye."

P. D. (Permanent disability). On the initial visit, only an estimate regarding ultimate permanent disability can be made. Answer "Yes" or "No." If "Yes," specify:

Amputation—exact level.

Expected loss of function from limited motion, weakness or deformity – slight, moderate or marked.

Cosmetic disfigurement sometimes constitutes a ratable permanent disability. For instance, an extensive disfiguring scar on the face might be a handicap in the labor market, while a scar on any portion of the body which is usually covered would not be.

Accident sole cause? In the majority of cases the answer is "Yes." Certain unusual circumstances, such as syncope (**59 – 5**) causing a fall with resultant injury or symptoms developing in a previously asymptomatic hernia (**37 – 5**), do occur. These should be specified under "Contributing Causes."

Previous impairment. Under this heading preexistent conditions such as arthritis, limited function from old trauma or disease, previous operative procedures etc., should be listed. Aggravation of a preexistent condition by an industrial injury is a frequent and legitimate cause of compensable temporary or permanent disability.

TREATMENT

Include under this heading surgical procedures, splinting, casting, medications, elastic bandages, immunizing injections, administration of anesthetics and antibiotics, and instructions regarding home care. If suturing has been done, the number and type of sutures should be specified.

X-rays. "Yes" or "No." If taken, give impression or working diagnosis, subject to later confirmation by a roentgenologist (**18**).

Hospitalized. Give date of hospitalization, name and location of hospital and method of transportation (private car, ambulance, etc.).

FURTHER TREATMENT (LENGTH). This is important information for insurance companies or employers, because a reserve to meet all expenses of the case usually is set up as soon as the First Report of Injury is received. It is better to overestimate than to underestimate the treatment period.

Disability (how long). If no time loss from work is anticipated, indicate as "N. T. L." (No Time Lost). If in the opinion of the examining physician the patient is unable to work, the expected duration of disability should be given in days, weeks or months. As in the case of length of treatment, it is better to overestimate than to underestimate.

To return. The patient should be told to return at a specified time on a specified date, and this date entered on the form. Vague instructions such as "Return if doesn't feel better" or "P. R. N." should never be used. If discharged from care, so state.

Referred to. If "To Return" has been filled out, this space can be left blank. Otherwise, specify the physician to whom the patient is being referred or the hospital to which he has been instructed to report.

APPENDIX

TABLE OF APPROXIMATE METRIC AND APOTHECARY EQUIVALENTS
(1 ml. is approximately equal to 1 cc.)

LIQUID

0.03 ml. – ½ minim	4 ml. – 1 fluidrachm
0.05 ml. – ¾ minim	5 ml. – 1¼ fluidrachms
0.06 ml. – 1 minim	8 ml. – 2 fluidrachms
0.10 ml. – 1½ minims	10 ml. – 2½ fluidrachms
0.20 ml. – 3 minims	15 ml. – 4 fluidrachms
0.25 ml. – 4 minims	30 ml. – 1 fluidounce
0.30 ml. – 5 minims	50 ml. – 1¾ fluidounces
0.50 ml. – 8 minims	100 ml. – 3½ fluidounces
0.60 ml. – 10 minims	200 ml. – 7 fluidounces
0.75 ml. – 12 minims	250 ml. – 8 fluidounces
1.00 ml. – 15 minims	500 ml. – 1 pint
2.00 ml. – 30 minims	1000 ml. – 1 quart
3.00 ml. – 45 minims	4000 ml. – 1 gallon

WEIGHT

0.10 mg. – 1/600 grain	40.00 mg. – ⅔ grain
0.12 mg. – 1/500 grain	50.00 mg. – ¾ grain
0.15 mg. – 1/400 grain	60.00 mg. – 1 grain
0.20 mg. – 1/300 grain	75.00 mg. – 1¼ grains
0.25 mg. – 1/250 grain	100.00 mg. – 1½ grains
0.30 mg. – 1/200 grain	0.12 gm. – 2 grains
0.40 mg. – 1/150 grain	0.15 gm. – 2½ grains
0.50 mg. – 1/120 grain	0.20 gm. – 3 grains
0.60 mg. – 1/100 grain	0.25 gm. – 4 grains
0.80 mg. – 1/80 grain	0.30 gm. – 5 grains
1.00 mg. – 1/60 grain	0.40 gm. – 6 grains
1.20 mg. – 1/50 grain	0.50 gm. – 7½ grains
1.50 mg. – 1/40 grain	0.60 gm. – 10 grains
2.00 mg. – 1/30 grain	0.75 gm. – 12 grains
3.00 mg. – 1/20 grain	1.00 gm. – 15 grains
4.00 mg. – 1/15 grain	1.50 gm. – 22 grains
5.00 mg. – 1/12 grain	2.00 gm. – 30 grains (½ drachm)
6.00 mg. – 1/10 grain	3.00 gm. – 45 grains
8.00 mg. – ⅛ grain	4.00 gm. – 60 grains (1 drachm)
10.00 mg. – ⅙ grain	5.00 gm. – 75 grains
12.00 mg. – ⅕ grain	6.00 gm. – 90 grains
15.00 mg. – ¼ grain	8.00 gm. – 2 drachms
20.00 mg. – ⅓ grain	10.00 gm. – 2½ drachms
25.00 mg. – ⅜ grain	15.00 gm. – 4 drachms
30.00 mg. – ½ grain	30.00 gm. – 1 ounce

APPROXIMATE LIQUID MEASURES
(1 ml. is approximately equal to 1 cc.)

HOUSEHOLD MEASURE	METRIC	APOTHECARY
1 to 2 drops equal (varies with viscosity, specific gravity, type and fullness of container, etc.)	0.06 ml. or	1 minim
1 teaspoonful equals about	4.00 ml. or	1 fluidrachm
1 dessertspoonful equals about	8.00 ml. or	2 fluidrachms
1 tablespoonful equals about	15.00 ml. or	4 fluidrachms
1 teacupful equals about	120.00 ml. or	4 fluidounces
1 glassful equals about	250.00 ml. or	8 fluidounces
1 pint equals about	500.00 ml. or	16 fluidounces
1 quart equals about	1000.00 ml. or	32 fluidounces
1 gallon equals about	4000.00 ml. or	128 fluidounces

LENGTH

INCHES	CENTIMETERS	CENTIMETERS	INCHES
1	2.5	1	.4
2	5.1	2	.8
4	10.2	3	1.2
6	15.2	4	1.6
8	20.3	5	2.0
12	30.5	6	2.4
18	46	8	3.1
24	61	10	3.9
30	76	20	7.9
36	91	30	11.8
42	107	40	15.7
48	122	50	19.7
54	137	60	23.6
60	152	70	27.6
66	168	80	31.5
72	183	90	35.4
78	198	100	39.4

1 in. = 2.54 cm.	1 cm. = 0.3937 in.

APPROXIMATE CONVERSION TABLES—POUNDS AND KILOGRAMS

KILOGRAMS TO POUNDS		POUNDS TO KILOGRAMS	
kg.	lb.	lb.	kg.
1 —	2.204	1 —	0.454
2 —	4.4	2 —	0.9
3 —	6.6	3 —	1.4
4 —	8.8	4 —	1.8
5 —	11.0	5 —	2.3
6 —	13.2	6 —	2.7
7 —	15.4	7 —	3.2
8 —	17.6	8 —	3.6
9 —	19.8	9 —	4.1
10 —	22.0	10 —	4.5
15 —	33.0	15 —	6.8
20 —	44.0	20 —	9.1
25 —	55.0	25 —	11.4
30 —	66.0	30 —	13.6
35 —	77.0	35 —	15.9
40 —	88.0	40 —	18.2
45 —	99.0	45 —	20.5
50 —	110.0	50 —	22.7
55 —	121.0	55 —	25.0
60 —	132.0	60 —	27.3
65 —	143.0	65 —	29.6
70 —	154.0	70 —	31.8
75 —	165.0	75 —	34.1
80 —	176.0	80 —	36.4
85 —	187.0	85 —	38.7
90 —	198.0	90 —	40.9
95 —	209.0	95 —	43.2
100 —	220.0	100 —	45.4
		125 —	56.8
		150 —	68.2
		175 —	79.5
		200 —	90.8

APPENDIX

To convert:

Milliliters into grams

Sp. gr. × ml. = gm.

Grams into milliliters

$$\frac{gm.}{sp.\ gr.} = ml.$$

Grains into grams

$$\frac{gr.}{15} = gm.$$

Milliliters into ounces

$$\frac{ml.\ \times\ sp.\ gr.}{28.35} = oz.$$

Ounces into milliliters

$$\frac{oz.\ \times\ 28.35}{sp.\ gr.} = ml.$$

TABLE OF COMMON DOSE CONVERSIONS
(GRAINS TO GRAMS, APPROXIMATE)

$1/200$ gr. =	0.3 mg.
$1/150$ gr. =	0.4 mg.
$1/120$ gr. =	0.5 mg.
$1/100$ gr. =	0.6 mg.
$1/60$ gr. =	1 mg.
$1/30$ gr. =	2 mg.
$1/4$ gr. =	15 mg.
$1/2$ gr. =	30 mg.
1 gr. =	60 mg.
$1\frac{1}{2}$ gr. =	100 mg. (0.1 gm.)
5 gr. =	300 mg. (.3 gm.)
$7\frac{1}{2}$ gr. =	500 mg. (.5 gm.)
10 gr. =	600 mg. (.6 gm.)
15 gr. =	1000 mg. (1 gm.)

COMPARATIVE THERMOMETER READINGS

FAHRENHEIT	CENTIGRADE		FAHRENHEIT	CENTIGRADE
96.0	35.5		101.4	38.5
96.2	35.6		101.6	38.6
96.4	35.7		101.8	38.7
96.6	35.8		102.0	38.9
96.8	35.9		102.2	39.0
97.0	36.1		102.4	39.1
97.2	36.2		102.6	39.2
97.4	36.3		102.8	39.3
97.6	36.4		103.0	39.4
97.8	36.6		103.2	39.6
98.0	36.7		103.4	39.7
98.2	36.8		103.6	39.8
98.4	36.9		103.8	39.9
98.6	37.0		104.0	40.0
98.8	37.1		104.2	40.1
99.0	37.2		104.4	40.2
99.2	37.3		104.6	40.3
99.4	37.4		104.8	40.4
99.6	37.6		105.0	40.6
99.8	37.7		105.2	40.7
100.0	37.8		105.4	40.8
100.2	37.9		105.6	40.9
100.4	38.0		105.8	41.0
100.6	38.1		106.0	41.1
100.8	38.2		108.0	42.2
101.0	38.3		110.0	43.3
101.2	38.4			

To convert Centigrade into Fahrenheit:

Multiply by 9, divide by 5, and add 32 $\left(°F = \frac{°C \times 9}{5} + 32 \right)$

To convert Fahrenheit into Centigrade:

Subtract 32, multiply by 5, divide by 9 $\left(°C = \frac{°F - 32 \times 5}{9} \right)$

Clinical ranges, °F and °C

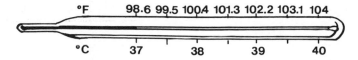

BLOCK CHEMISTRY FINDINGS IN HEALTH AND DISEASE

	MINIMAL QUANTITY NECESSARY FOR DETERMINATION	NORMAL RANGE, VALUES/100 ML.	CONDITIONS IN WHICH VARIATIONS FROM NORMAL MAY OCCUR	
			Increase	Decrease
Glucose	5 ml. of serum, oxalated whole blood or plasma, 0.1 ml. (Micromethod)	80 to 120 mg.	Diabetes mellitus; hyperthyroidism; acromegaly; hemochromatosis; adrenal tumors, cortical or medullary	Hyperinsulinism, Addison's disease, adenoma or carcinoma of islands of Langerhans
Total serum protein	5 ml. of serum	6.0 to 7.5 gm.	Dehydration (see Globulin, below)	Cachectic illnesses, renal disease, severe burns, malnutrition, liver disease
Albumin	5 ml. of serum	3.5 to 5.5 gm.	Dehydration	Renal disease, malnutrition, liver disease
Globulin	5 ml. of serum	2.5 to 3.0 gm.	Chronic infectious diseases such as tuberculosis, syphilis malaria, rheumatoid arthritis, kala-azar, lymphogranuloma venereum. sarcoidosis. cirrhosis, myeloma, carcinomatosis, lupus erythematosus, polyarteritis	

Albumin-Globulin (A/G) Ratio		1.3:1 to 3:1	See Albumin and Globulin, above
Fibrinogen	5 ml. of oxalated plasma	0.25 to 0.5 gm.	Liver disease, cachexias, afibrinogenemia, post partum
Nonprotein nitrogen (NPN)	5 ml. of serum, oxalated whole blood or plasma	25 to 38 mg.	Most infectious diseases, conditions producing inflammation or destruction, traumatic injuries
Urea nitrogen (BUN)	5 ml. of serum, oxalated whole blood or plasma	8 to 20 mg.	Renal disease, urinary obstruction; cardiac failure; intestinal obstruction, gastrointestinal hemorrhage; metallic poisoning; dehydration and shock
Creatinine	5 ml. of serum, oxalated whole blood or plasma	1 to 2 mg.	Same as Nonprotein Nitrogen
Uric acid	5 ml. of serum, oxalated whole blood or plasma	2 to 5 mg. (women), 3 to 7 mg. (men)	Renal disease, urinary obstruction, metallic poisoning
Calcium	5 ml. of serum	9 to 11 mg., 4.5 to 6.0 mEq./L.	Gout, nephritis, eclampsia, leukemia
			Hyperparathyroidism, parathyroid administration, vitamin D overdosage, sarcoidosis
			Severe liver damage
			Hypoparathyroidism, severe nephritis, uremia, rickets, steatorrhea

(Table continues)

BLOOD CHEMISTRY FINDINGS IN HEALTH AND DISEASE (Continued)

| | MINIMAL QUANTITY NECESSARY FOR DETERMINATIONS | NORMAL RANGE, VALUES/100 ML. | CONDITIONS IN WHICH VARIATIONS FROM NORMAL MAY OCCUR | |
			Increase	Decrease
Phosphorus (inorganic)	5 ml. of serum	2.5 to 3.5 mg. (adults), 3 to 5 mg. (children)	Nephritis, uremia, rickets, hypoparathyroidism	Hyperparathyroidism
Sodium	5 ml. of serum or plasma	315 to 340 mg., 136 to 145 mEq./L.	Cerebral lesions (occas.), primary water deficit	Addison's disease, severe diarrhea, high fevers, diabetic acidosis, renal insufficiency
Potassium	5 ml. of serum or plasma	14 to 20 mg., 3.6 to 5.0 mEq./L.	Addison's disease; renal insufficiency	Diabetic acidosis, hyperadrenocorticism, severe diarrhea, familial periodic paralysis
Chlorides	5 ml. of serum or plasma	355 to 376 mg., 98 to 106 mEq./L.	Nephritis, eclampsia, cardiac failure	Gastrointestinal disturbances, febrile conditions, acidosis, vomiting, shock
Cholesterol	5 ml. of serum	150 to 250 mg.	Lipoid nephrosis, amyloidosis, biliary cirrhosis, myxedema, obstructive jaundice, diabetes	Advanced liver disease

Determination	Amount required	Normal values	Increased in	Decreased in
Cholesterol esters	5 ml. of serum	60 to 80% of total cholesterol	Obstructive jaundice, biliary cirrhosis	Severe liver disease
Total lipids	5 ml. of serum	570 to 820 mg.	Nephrosis, diabetes, arthritis, hypothyroidism	
Serum acid phosphatase	5 ml. of serum	1 to 3 King-Armstrong units, 0 to 1 Bodansky units	Metastasizing prostatic carcinoma	
Serum alkaline phosphatase	5 ml. of serum	8 to 13 King-Armstrong units, 1 to 4 Bodansky units	Increased osteoblastic activity (Paget's disease, osteogenic sarcoma, osteoplastic bone metastases, rickets, hyperparathyroidism); obstructive jaundice	
CO_2 combining power	5 ml. of serum taken under mineral oil	45 to 70 vol./100 ml, 21 to 30 mEq./L.	Emphysema, chronic vomiting, alkalosis	Acidosis, ketosis; bowel obstruction, diarrhea; traumatic shock

INDEX

Page numbers in *italics* indicate illustrations.

INDEX

Anthrax, 170
Antibiotics, poisoning from, 378. See also specific drugs.
Anticoagulant therapy, hemorrhage in, 269
Anticoagulants, poisoning from, 379
Antidepressants, tricyclic, poisoning from, 528
Antidote(s), neutralization of poison by, 360
universal, in poisoning, 362
Antifebrin, poisoning from, 364
Antifreeze, poisoning from, 429
Antihistaminics, poisoning from, 379
Antimicrobial drugs, 182, 183
Antimony, poisoning from, 379
Antiperspirants, poisoning from, 415
Antipyrine, poisoning from. See *Aminopyrine.*
Antu, poisoning from, 380
Anuria, in children, 338
Anus, abscess of, 85
Aortic aneurysm, dissecting, 649
Aphthous fever, 672
Apical abscess, 85
Apiol, poisoning from. See *Triorthocresyl phosphate.*
Apomorphine hydrochloride, poisoning from, 380
Apothecary and metric equivalents, 741
Appendicitis, acute, 226
Apple(s) bitter, poisoning from, 410
devil's, poisoning from, 414
thorn, poisoning from, 414, 524
Apricot pits, toxicity of, 373
Arabic, gum, poisoning from, 363, 547
Aralen diphosphate, poisoning from, 405
Arbor vitae, poisoning from, 547
Arboviral infections, 670
Arecoline, poisoning from, 380
Argemone oil, poisoning from, 381
Arm-weight traction method, for reduction of shoulder dislocations, 57
Arnica, poisoning from, 381, 548
Arrest, cardiac. See *Cardiac arrest.*
Arrhythmias, agonal, 145
Arsacetin, poisoning from, 381
Arsenic, poisoning from, 381
precipitation of, 361
Arsenic color pigments, poisoning from, 382

Arsenic trioxide, poisoning from, 382
Arsenic trisulfide, poisoning from, 382
Arseniuretted hydrogen, poisoning from, 382
Arsine, poisoning from, 382
Arsinima triloba, poisoning from, 382
Arsphenamine, poisoning from, 383
Artane, poisoning from, 383
Arterial embolism, 652
pulmonary, 650
Arterial injuries, 637
types of, 638
Artery(ies), compression of, 638
contusion of, 638
intracranial, rupture of, headaches from, 153
laceration of, 638
mesenteric, occlusion of, 229
peripheral, embolus of, 652
pulmonary, embolism of, 650
severance of, 638
Arthritis, 279
of cervical spine, headaches from, 147
Arthropod-borne viruses, 670
Artificial respiration, manual methods of, 40
mechanical methods of, 41, *41*
mouth-to-airway, 40
mouth-to-mask, 40
mouth-to-mouth, 38, *38, 39*
mouth-to-nose, 39
Asari, poisoning from, 436
Asarum europaeum, poisoning from, 383
Asbestos, poisoning from, 383
Asphalt burns, 119
of eye, 121
Asphyxia neonatorum, 319
Asphyxiation, 95-97
Aspidium, poisoning from, 383
Aspiration, catheter, in tracheostomy, 64
pericardial sac, 53
peritoneal, 54
Aspirin, poisoning from, 383
peak salicylate levels in, *506*
Asterol dihydrochloride, poisoning from, 384
Asthma, 577
in children, 320
moderate attacks of, treatment of, 579

Asthma (*Continued*)
  treatment of acute severe broncho-
    spasm in, 578
  remedies for, poisoning from, 384
ATA, poisoning from, 371
Atabrine, poisoning from, 500
Atomic bombs, injuries from, 682
Atrial fibrillation, 128, *130*
Atrial flutter, 128, *130*
Atropine sulfate, poisoning from, 384
Auramine, poisoning from, 384
Aureomycin, poisoning from, 379
Auripigment, poisoning from, 382
Aurothioglucose, poisoning from, 440
Aurothioglycolanilide, poisoning from,
  440
Autopsy(ies), in coroner's cases, 9
  in noncoroner's cases, 9
  permits for, 9, 703
  religious restrictions on, 11
Autumn crocus, poisoning from, 548
Avantine, poisoning from, 453
Avertin, poisoning from, 527
Azalea, poisoning from, 548
Azo dyes, poisoning from, 424

Baby powders, poisoning from, 384
Bacillary dysentery, 171
Bacilli, antimicrobial drugs of choice
  for, 183
Bacitracin, poisoning from, 378, 385
Back injuries, 279
  crushing, 610
Bacterial endocarditis, acute, 128
Bacterial food poisoning, 433
Bacterial infections, wartime, 680
BAL, poisoning from, 385
Balloon fish, poisoning from, 434
Balsam, of Peru, poisoning from, 489
Banana oil, poisoning from, 373
Banana peel scrapings, as hallucinogen,
  441
Banthine, poisoning from, 464
Barbenyl, poisoning from, 490
Barbiturates, addiction to, 4
  poisoning from, 385
  prescription restrictions on, 30
  short-term effects of, 443
Barium, precipitation of, 361

Barium compounds, poisoning from, 386
Barotrauma, 97
Barracuda, food poisoning from, 387,
  434
  bites, 105
Bartholin gland abscesses, 240
Baseball finger, 246, 247, 291
Bass, sea, poisoning from, 434
Bat bites, 105
Battered child syndrome, 321
Bead tree, poisoning from, 460
Bean(s), broad, poisoning from, 431
  calabar, poisoning from. See
    Physostigmine.
  castor, poisoning from, 400, 550
  djenkol, poisoning from, 423
  fava, poisoning from, 431
  jequirity, poisoning from, 453
  Mexican jumping, poisoning from, 469
  stinging, poisoning from, 472
  Windsor, poisoning from, 431
Bee stings, 624
Bee venom, 665
Beech creosote, poisoning from, 411
Beechnut, poisoning from, 387
Belladonna, poisoning from, 387
Belladonna alkaloids, poisoning from,
  387
Bell's palsy, 306
Benadryl, poisoning from. See *Anti
  histaminics.*
Bends, 98
Benedict urine test, 688
Benne oil, poisoning from, 509
Bennett's fracture, 246
Benzahex, poisoning from, 388
Benzalkonium chloride, poisoning from,
  536
Benzanthrone, poisoning from, 387
Benzedrine, poisoning from, 373
Benzene, poisoning from, 388
Benzene hexachloride, poisoning from,
  388
Benzethonium chloride, poisoning from,
  389
Benzidine, poisoning from, 389
Benzidine dyes, poisoning from, 424
Benzol, poisoning from, 388
Benzpyrene, poisoning from, 389
Benzylchloride, poisoning from, 389
Beryllium, poisoning from, 389

Coma (*Continued*)
  cerebral hypoxia and, 169
  cerebrovascular disorders and, 169
  fat embolism and, 169
  hepatic, 164
  in acute infections, 159
  in diabetes mellitus, 160
    differential diagnosis, 161
    in children, 332
    treatment of, 162
  in emphysema, 163
  in epilepsy, 164
  in poisoning, 165, 362
  in uremia, 165
  myxedema, 195
  of unknown etiology, 166
  postoperative, and cerebral hypoxia, 169
    and cerebral thrombosis, 169
    and hypothermia, 170
    from anesthetics, 168
    prolonged, 168
  rare causes of, 166
Communicable diseases, 170–186. See also specific diseases.
Compound 42, poisoning from, 534
Compound 497, poisoning from, 419
Compound 1068, poisoning from, 402
Compound 3956, poisoning from, 526
Compressed air sickness, 98
Compression, cardiac. See *Cardiac compression.*
Compressive centripetal wrapping, technique of, 659
Concussion, brain, 255
  headaches from, 148
Cone shell venom, 666
Coniine, poisoning from, 410
Conjunctiva, adhesions of, 205
  burns of, 206
  foreign bodies in, 206
  intense light and, 206
  lacerations of, 207
Conjunctivitis, 201
  differential diagnosis of, 214
Consciousness, state of, in head injuries in children, 340
Consent(s), for emergency treatment. 701–728
  informed, definition of, 716
  tacit, definition of, 68

Constipation, headache from, 148
Contact dermatitis, 600
Contact lenses, removal of, 212
  methods of, 213
  suction cup for, 214
Contagious diseases, 170–186
Contusions, 609. See also specific organ or part of body.
  severe, 610
Convulsions. See also *Convulsive seizures.*
  in children, 328
    treatment of, 329
  in poisoning, 362
Convulsive seizures, 186–188
  in adults, 186
  in children and adolescents, 186
  neonatal and infantile, 186
Copper, poisoning from, 410
Copper acetoarsenite, poisoning from. See *Arsenic.*
Copper arsenite, poisoning from. See *Arsenic* and *Arsenic color pigments.*
Copperhead snake venom, 666
Coprinus afromentarius, poisoning from, 434
Coral snake venom, 666
Coral stings, 625
Coral venom, 666
Cord compression. See *Spinal cord, compression of.*
Cordifolia, poisoning from, 548
Corn campion, poisoning from, 368
Corn cockle, poisoning from, 368
Corn rose, poisoning from, 368
Cornea, burns of, 208
  contusions of, 208
  foreign bodies in, 208
  ulcers of, 201
  wounds of, penetrating, 209
    superficial, 208
Coroner's death cases, 8
  autopsies in, 9
Corozate, poisoning from, 423
Corrosive sublimate, poisoning from, 390
Corticosteroid therapy, hemorrhage from, 269
  in shock, 598
Corticotropin, poisoning from, 411
Cortisone, poisoning from, 411
Coryza, 580

Fainting, 572, 653
Falls, in children, 336
False grape, poisoning from, 488
False morel, poisoning from, 445, 473
Familial periodic paralysis, 309
Fat embolism, and coma, 169
Fava beans, poisoning from, 431
Febrile headaches, 148
Fecal impaction, 219
Felons, 87
Femur, test for injury to, 72
Fenfluramine hydrochloride, poisoning from, 431
Ferbam, poisoning from, 423
Fer-de-lance venom, 667
Fern, male, poisoning from, 383
Ferric salts, poisoning from. See *Iron salts.*
Ferrous salts, poisoning from. See *Iron salts.*
Fetus, dead, permit for disposal of, 709
Fever, aphthous, 672
  breakbone, 671
  dandy, 671
  dengue-like, causes of, 670
  headaches from, 148
  hemorrhagic, 670
  parrot, 175
  polymer fume, 495
  Rocky Mountain spotted, 114
  sandfly, 678
  scarlet, 176
    differential diagnosis of, 180
  typhoid, 178
  typhus, 178
  undulant, 178
  yellow, 179
Fibrillation, atrial, 128, *130*
  cardiac, in cardiac arrest, 44
  ventricular, *131,* 144
Fibrinogen, value range of, 747
Fibromyositis, 151
Finger, baseball, 246, *247,* 291
Finger cherry, poisoning from, 553
Finger joints, contusions of, 245
Fire ant stings, 625
Fire ant venom, 667
Fire bombs, injuries from, 682
Fire bush, poisoning from, 559
Fire extinguishers, poisoning from, 431
Fire thorn, poisoning from, 559
Fireworks, poisoning from, 431

Fish poisoning, 434
Fishhooks, removal of, *612*
Fissures, anorectal, 225
Flanks, crush injuries to, 610
Flash burns, 122
Flavins, poisoning from, 424
Flea bites, 108
Flea venom, 667
Fluid(s), basic daily requirements for, 24
  cerebrospinal, normal values of, 60
  emergency replacement of, 22–27
    basic requirements in, 24
    in adult burns, 26
    in radiation injuries, 684
    management of, 22
    output estimation in, 25
    solutions for, 26
    oral, for mass casualty use, 27
  spinal, normal values, in children, 330
Flukes, parasitic, 230
Fluorescein sodium, poisoning from, 425
Fluorides, poisoning from, 432
Fluoroacetates, poisoning from, 432
Fluoroscopic examination, 78
Fluorosilicates, poisoning from, 432
Flutter, atrial, 128, *130*
"Fly agaric," poisoning from, 472
Food allergy, and pruritus ani, 602
  headaches from, 148
Food poisoning, bacterial, 433
  chemical, 433
Foot, immersion, 629
Foot and mouth disease, 672
Foreign bodies, 215–219. See also specific organ involved.
Formaldehyde, poisoning from, 437
Formalin, poisoning from, 437
Formic acid, poisoning from, 437
Four-o'clock, poisoning from, 553
Fowler's solution. See *Arsenic.*
Foxglove, poisoning from. See *Digitalis.*
Foxtails, in ear, 215
Fracture(s), 287. See also specific part of body involved.
  Bennett's, 246
  boxer's, 246, 290
  Colles', 289
  greenstick, 288
  requiring hospitalization, 293
  Smith's, 289
  wartime, 687
French chalk, poisoning from, 517

INDEX

Infection(s), acute, coma in, 159
  arboviral, 670
  as cause of respiratory obstruction
    in children, 345
  bacterial, wartime, 680
  excitement in, 198
  fungous, and pruritus ani, 603
  of ear or tooth, headaches from, 154
  parasitic, 228, 230
  respiratory, in children, 348
  shigella. See *Dysentery, bacillary.*
  streptococcal, hemolytic, 172
  viral, 670–680
  wartime, 680
Infectious mononucleosis, 180
Influenza, 172, 674
Information, medical, release of, 729–732
  permit for, 702, 708
Informed consent, definition of, 716
Inhalation, smoke, 97. See also
    Asphyxiation.
  in children, 352
Inhalation anesthetics, poisoning from, 374
Injections, intraglossal, 52
  prophylactic, in head injuries, 254
Injuries. See also specific parts of body
    involved.
  requiring tetanus immunization, 73–76
Ink, indelible, poisoning from, 450.
    See also *Aniline dyes* and *Hand,
    puncture wounds of.*
  poisoning from. See *Aniline dyes* and
    Silver salts.
Ink eradicators, poisoning from. See *Hy-
    pochloric acid* and *Oxalic Acid.*
Inkberry, poisoning from, 558
Inky caps, poisoning from, 554
Insect(s), bites, 109. See also name of
    specific insect.
  on eyelids, 209
  in ears, 215
Insect powder, Persian, poisoning from, 498
Insomnia, 569
Insulin, poisoning from. See *Diabetes
    mellitus.*
Insulin shock, 160
  differential diagnosis, 161
  treatment of, 162

Interstitial pneumonia, 675
Intestinal injuries, 611
Intestinal obstruction, in children, 342
Intestinal tract, foreign bodies in, in
    children, 337, 339
Intocostrin, poisoning from, 412
Intoxication, alcohol, clinical examina-
    tion for, 68
    tests for, 67
      blood analysis, 67
      breath analysis, 67
      interpretation of, 69
  citrate, in blood transfusions, 66
  paint thinner, 522
  parathyroid, acute, 193
Intracerebral hemorrhage, 639
  differential diagnosis of, 640
Intracranial artery, rupture of, and
    headache, 153
Intracranial hemorrhage, 639
Intraglossal injections, 52
Intraperitoneal perforation, 221
Intravenous anesthetics, poisoning from.
    See *Pentothal sodium.*
Intravenous emergency equipment, 19
Inversine, poisoning from, 460
Iodates, poisoning from, 451
Iodides, poisoning from, 451
Iodine, poisoning from, 451
Iodoform, poisoning from, 451
Iodopyracet, poisoning from, 423
Ipecac, poisoning from, 451
  fluidextract of, poisoning from, 360
Iproniazid, poisoning from, 452
Iridocyclitis, 204
  differential diagnosis of, 214
Iris, of eye, injuries to, 210
  poisoning from, 554
Iritis, 204
  differential diagnosis of, 214
Iron oxide, poisoning from. See *Iron
    salts* and *Metal fumes.*
Iron salts, poisoning from, 452
Irritant poisons, 359
Ischemia, cerebral, transient focal, 654
  as cause of stroke, 640
Ischioanal abscesses, 88
Ischiorectal abscess, 228
I-sedrine, poisoning from, 425
Islet cell tumor, hypoglycemia in, 193
Isodrin, poisoning from, 452

INDEX

Lead acetate, poisoning from. See *Lead salts*.
Lead arsenate, poisoning from, 455
Lead arsenite, poisoning from, 455
Lead chromate, poisoning from, 455
Lead oxide, poisoning from, 455
Lead salts, poisoning from, 435, 455
Legal responsibilities of physician, in accepting patients, 690
  in follow-up care, 691
Lemon grass oil, poisoning from, 456
Lenses, contact, removal of, 212
  suction cup for, *214*
Leprosy, 172
Lethane, poisoning from, 456
Levopropoxyphene, poisoning from, 456
Lewisite, poisoning from, 534
Liability cases, 698
Librium, poisoning from, 402
Ligustrum vulgare, poisoning from. See *Privet*.
Lilacin, poisoning from, 519
Lily, of the valley, poisoning from, 555
  spider, poisoning from, 560
Lime, poisoning from, 456
Lindane, poisoning from, 388
Linseed oil, contamination of. See *Lolium temulentum*.
Lipids, in blood, value range of, 749
Lipsticks, poisoning from, 456. See also *Cosmetics*.
Liquid measures, 742
Lithium chloride, poisoning from, 456
Liver, injuries to, 618
  yellow atrophy of, in pregnancy, 313
Lixivium, poisoning from, 458
Llama bites, 110
Lobelia, poisoning from, 457, 555
Lockjaw, 176. See also *Tetanus*.
Locust, poisoning from, 555
Lolium temulentum, poisoning from, 457
Lomotil, poisoning from, 457
Lorchel, poisoning from, 445
Low salt syndrome, 635
LSD, poisoning from. See *Hallucinogens*.
  short-term effects of, 443
Lubricating oil, poisoning from, 480
Luminal, poisoning from, 490
Lunate dislocations, 282

Lungs, hemorrhage from, 265
  removal of poisons from, 359
Lupine, poisoning from, 556
Lye, poisoning from, 458
Lymphangitis, 658
Lymphatic system, obstruction of, 658
Lymphatic system emergencies, 658
Lymphogranuloma, venereal, 661
Lymphopathia venereum, 661
Lysergic acid diethylamide (LSD), poisoning from. See *Hallucinogens*.
  short-term effects of, 443

Macassar oil, poisoning from. See *Safrole*.
Mace, poisoning from, 403, 533
Magnesium, burns from, 122
  deficiency of, myalgia from, 296
  poisoning from, 458
Magnesium oxide. See *Metal fumes*.
Magnesium sulfate, poisoning from, 459
Magnolia, poisoning from, 556
Maki-maki, poisoning from, 521
Malaria, 172
Malathion, poisoning from, 459
Male fern, poisoning from, 383
Malleolar fractures, 292
Malpractice, 699–701
  insurance for, 700
  safeguards against, 700
Mancellier, poisoning from, 447
Manchineel poisoning from. See *Hippomane mancilla*.
Mandrake, poisoning from, 556
Maneb, poisoning from, 423
Manganese, poisoning from, 459
Manganese oxide, poisoning from. See *Metal fumes*.
Mango, poisoning from, 556, 604
Manic-depressive psychoses, 567. See also *Psychiatric emergencies*.
  excitement in, 198
Manzinello, poisoning from, 447
Maphrasen, poisoning from. See *Arsphenamine*.
Marcozole, poisoning from, 465
Marigold, marsh, poisoning from, 396
Marihuana, poisoning from, 459, 556
  short-term effects of, 443
Marine animal stings, 626

Marine snail venom, 667

Marsalid, poisoning from, 452

Marsh marigold, poisoning from, 396

Masterwort, poisoning from, 446

Mastoiditis, 189

Matches, poisoning from, 460

Mayapple, poisoning from, 556

Meadow saffron, poisoning from. See *Colchicine.*

Measles, 173, 180

  German, 175, 180

Mecamylamine, poisoning from, 460

Mecholyl, poisoning from, 460

Medical bag, emergency, contents of, 14–21

Medical examiner's death cases, 8

  autopsy in, 9

Medications. See also *Drugs.*

  and pruritus ani, 603

  for emergency medical bag, 16

Melia azedarach, poisoning from, 460

Melitoxin, poisoning from, 418

Meniere's disease, 304

Meningeal irritation, headaches from, 150

Meningitis, 173

  in children, 343

Meningococcemia, in children, 344

Menorrhagia, 240

Menses, absence of, 240

Menstruation, painful, 240

  profuse, 240

Mental disturbances. See also *Psychiatric emergencies.*

  paretic, in syphilis, 663

Menthol, poisoning from, 460

Meperidine, poisoning from, 415

Meperidine hydrochloride, poisoning from, 461. See also *Demerol.*

Mephobarbital, poisoning from. See *Barbiturates.*

Meprobamate, poisoning from, 461

Merbromin, poisoning from, 462

Mercaptans, poisoning from, 461

Mercuric salts, precipitation of, 361

Mercurochrome, poisoning from, 462

Mercurous chloride, poisoning from, 396

Mercury, ammoniated, poisoning from, 372

  poisoning from, 462

Mercury antiseptics, poisoning from, 462

Mercury diuretics, poisoning from, 462

Mercury oxycyanide, poisoning from, 463

Merthiolate, poisoning from. See *Mercury antiseptics.*

Mescal, poisoning from, 463

Mescaline, short-term effects of, 443

Mesenteric artery occlusion, 229

Metabolism, cellular, methods for rapid monitoring of, 587

  disorders of, 272–279

  in children, 319

Metacarpals, fractures of, 245, 290

Metafuel, poisoning from, 464

Metal(s), burns from, of eye, 121

  poisoning from, 435

  precipitation of, 361

Metal fumes, poisoning from, 463

Metaldehyde, poisoning from, 464

Metaphen, poisoning from. See *Mercury antiseptics.*

Metatarsals, fractures of, 292

Methacholine, poisoning from, 460

Methadone, poisoning from, 464

  short-term effects of, 444

Methamphetamine hydrochloride, poisoning from. See *Amphetamines* and "*Speed-balls.*"

Methanol, poisoning from, 466

Methantheline bromide, poisoning from, 464

Methapyrilene hydrochloride, poisoning from, 465

Methedrine, poisoning from, 513

Methenamine, poisoning from, 447, 465

Methimazole, poisoning from, 465

Methophenobarbital, poisoning from. See *Barbiturates.*

Methophinan hydrobromide, poisoning from, 465

Methoxychlor, poisoning from, 466

Methyl acetate, poisoning from, 466

Methyl alcohol, poisoning from, 466

Methyl bromide, poisoning from, 467

Methyl cellosolve, poisoning from, 467

Methyl chloride, poisoning from, 467

Methyl formate, poisoning from, 468

Methyl hydrate, poisoning from, 466

Methyl iodide, poisoning from, 468

Methyl parafynol, poisoning from, 468

Mycifradin, poisoning from, 378
Myelograms, permit for, 707
Myfradin, poisoning from. See *Antibiotics.*
Myocardial infarction, acute, *132, 133,* 138
Myochrysine, poisoning from, 440
Myofascitis, 151
Myofibrositis, 296
  headaches from, 151
Myringotomy, incision for, *191*
Myristicin, poisoning from, 474
Mysoline, poisoning from, 497
Mytilotoxism, 435
Myxedema, compounded by narcotics, 195
Myxedema coma, 195

Nabam, poisoning from, 423
Nail polish, poisoning from, 474
Nail polish removers, poisoning from See *Acetone.*
Nalline test, in narcotic addiction, 71
Nalophrine hydrochloride test, in narcotic addiction, 71
Napalm, burns from, 124
Naphazoline hydrochloride, poisoning from, 497
Naphtha, poisoning from. See *Benzene.*
Naphthalene, poisoning from, 474
Naphthol, poisoning from, 475
Naphthylamine, poisoning from, 475
α-Napthylthiourea, poisoning from, 380
Narcissus, poisoning from, 475, 557
Narcotics, addiction to, 4
    restrictions on treatment, 5
    tests for, 71
  antidote for, 361
  in emergency cases, 27–30
  prescription restrictions on, 30–34
Narcylene, poisoning from, 366
Nasal conditions, 300–303
Nasal packing, anterior, 52
Nasal septum, abscesses of, 88
  injuries to, 303
Naso-orbital fractures, *213*
Nasopharyngeal packing, 53
Nasopharyngitis, in children, 350

Nausea, control of, in radiation injuries, 684
Neck, dislocations of, 296
  fractures of, 296
  hemorrhage from, 266
  severe strains of, 297
  "whiplash" injuries of, 297, 308
Negligence, definition of, 699
Neoarsphenamine, poisoning from. See *Arsphenamine.*
Neocinchophen, poisoning from. See *Cinchophen.*
Neomercazole, poisoning from, 397
Neomycin, poisoning from, 378
Neosalvarsan, poisoning from. See *Arsphenamine.*
Neostigmine bromide, poisoning from, 475
Nephritis, 237
Nerve gases, poisoning from. See *Organic phosphates* and *War gases.*
Nerve injuries, in hand, 250
  peripheral, 309
Nerve poisons, 359
Neuralgia, 305
  trigeminal, 308
Neuritis, 305
  alcoholic, 306
  peripheral, 306
    in pregnancy, 307
  retrobulbar, 307
Neurologic disorders, 303–312
Neuropathy, peripheral, paralysis due to, 309
Neurotoxins, 359
Neurovascular syndrome, reflex, 658
Neutrons, radiation effects of, 683
Niacin, poisoning from, 476
Nickel, poisoning from, 476
Nickel carbonyl, poisoning from, 476
Nicotine, poisoning from, 476
Nicotinic acid, poisoning from, 476
Nifos, poisoning from. See *Organic phosphates.*
Night blooming cereus, poisoning from, 557
Nightshade, poisoning from, 513
  woody, poisoning from, 424
Niran, poisoning from. See *Organic phosphates.*
Nitrates, poisoning from, 477

INDEX

Pyridine HCl, poisoning from, 465
Pyrocantha, poisoning from, 559
Pyrocatechol, poisoning from, 499
Pyrogallic acid, poisoning from, 499
Pyrogallol, poisoning from, 499
Pyrogenic reactions, in blood trans-
    fusions, 66
Pyrolan, poisoning from, 499

Q-137, poisoning from, 489
QAC, poisoning from, 499
Quaternary ammonium salts, poisoning
    from, 499
Quicklime, poisoning from, 500
Quicksilver, poisoning from. See
    Mercury.
Quinacrine, poisoning from, 500
Quinidine, poisoning from, 500
Quinine, poisoning from, 500
Quinophen, poisoning from. See *Cincho-
    phen.*
Quinsy, 89

Rabies, 676
    treatment outline for, 679
Racephedrine, poisoning from, 425
Radial head subluxations, 284
Radiation, burns from x-rays, 79
    injuries from, cardiovascular support
        in, 684
        control of nausea in, 684
        evaluation and treatment of, 683
        fluid and electrolyte replacement in,
            684
        sedation in, 684
    lethal doses of, 684
    sublethal doses of, 685
Ragwort, poisoning from, 559
Ranunculus scleratus, poisoning from,
    501
Rape, 34–35
    seminal fluid test for, 73
    suspected, permit for examination for,
        715
Rat bites, 110
Rat killers, poisoning from, 501
Rat's bane, poisoning from, 417

Rattlesnake venom, 668
Rauwolfia alkaloids, poisoning from, 501
Rayless goldenrod, poisoning from, 430
Raynaud's phenomena, 658
Rectum, abscess of, 85
    bleeding from, 266, 267
    prolapse of, 224
    stricture of, 226
Red cedar, poisoning from, 547
Red sage, poisoning from, 555
Red snapper, poisoning from, 434
Red squill, poisoning from, 502
Reflex changes, in head injuries in
    children, 340
Reflex neurovascular syndrome, 658
Refrigerating agents, poisoning from,
    372, 502
Refusal of blood or derivatives, 727
Relaxation headaches, 152
Release, for refusal of blood, 727
    from responsibility, 696, 719
    of medical information, 729–731
        by physician, permit for, 702, 708
Religious rites, after death, 11, 12
    for premature infants, 11
    in abortion, 11
    in critical cases, 11
Rengas tree, dermatitis from, 605
Reserpine, poisoning from, 501
Resorcinol, poisoning from, 502
Respiration, artificial, 38. See also
    Artificial respiration.
Respiratory distress, 574
Respiratory failure, in poisoning, 361
Respiratory infections, in children, 348
Respiratory obstruction, in children,
    causes of, 345
    localization of, 346
Respiratory paralysis, in anterior polio-
    myelitis, 351
Respiratory tract, mucous membrane
    burns of, 123
Respiratory tract conditions, 577–585
Resuscitation, 37–47. See also *Artificial
    respiration.*
    after cardiac arrest, 45
    expired air methods, 38, *38,* 39
    heart-lung, 46, 47, *48*
    manual methods, 40
    mechanical methods, 41, *41*
    mouth-to-mouth, 38, *38,* 39

page 784

INDEX

Wheezing, in children, 355
"Whiplash" injuries, of neck, 297, 308
White cedar, poisoning from, 460
White flag, poisoning from, 483
White hellebore, poisoning from, 532
White sanicle, poisoning from, 430
White snakeroot, poisoning from, 430
White vitriol, poisoning from, 537
Whitlows, 87
Whooping cough, 179
Whortleberry, poisoning from, 530
Wild animal bites, 114
Wild cherry, poisoning from, 550
Wild pepper, poisoning from, 552
Wild sage, poisoning from, 555
Wild tobacco, poisoning from, 561
Wild tomato, poisoning from, 561
Wild wood vine, poisoning from, 488
Wind chill factor chart, 630
Windshield glass, injuries from, 622
    repair of, 623
Windsor bean, poisoning from, 431
Wisteria, poisoning from, 562
Withdrawal symptoms, with chronic
    morphinism, 471
Wood, poisoning from, 535
Wood alcohol, poisoning from, 466
Wood creosote, poisoning from, 411
Wood naphtha, poisoning from, 466
Wood spirit, poisoning from, 466
Wood tick venom, 669
Woodbine, American, poisoning from,
    488
Woody nightshade, poisoning from, 424,
    548
Wool sorters' disease, 170
Workmen's compensation cases, 737–
    740
Wormseed, poisoning from, 400
Wormwood, poisoning from, 363
Wounds, bullet, of chest, 158
    gunshot, 620
    penetrating, 619
    perforating, 619
    puncture, 620
    removal of poisons from, 359
    stab, 621
        of chest, 158
    tetanus-prone, 74
Wringer injuries, in children, 356
Wrist joint, fractures of, 289

X-rays, 77–79
    burns from, 79, 126
    indications for, 77
    interpretation of, 78
    ownership of, 78
    protection of gonads during, 79
    transferral of, 78
Xylene, poisoning from. See *Benzene.*
Xylol, poisoning from. See *Benzene.*

Yage, poisoning from, 442
Yatren, poisoning from. See *Oxyquino-
    lone derivatives.*
Yellow atrophy of liver, in preg-
    nancy, 313
Yellow cedar, poisoning from, 547
Yellow fever, 179
Yellow jacket stings, 629
Yellow jacket venom, 669
Yellow jasmine, poisoning from, 439
Yew, English, poisoning from, 518
    poisoning from, 562
Yucca, poisoning from, 560

Zeneb, poisoning from, 423
Zephiran, poisoning from, 536
Zerlate, poisoning from, 423, 536
Zinc, food poisoning from, 436
Zinc arsenate, poisoning from, 536
Zinc arsenite, poisoning from, 536
Zinc chloride, poisoning from, 536
Zinc cyanide, poisoning from, 536
Zinc dimethyldithiocarbamate, poison-
    ing from, 536
Zinc oxide, poisoning from, 537
Zinc phosphide, poisoning from, 537
Zinc stearate, poisoning from, 537
Zinc sulfate, poisoning from, 537
Zinc vitriol, poisoning from, 537
Zipper injuries, in children, 357
Ziram, poisoning from. See *Zerlate.*
Zygadenus venenosus, poisoning from,
    537
Zygoma, fracture of, *212*